FIRST AID FOR THE® USMLE STEP 1 2008

TAO LE, MD, MHS
Assistant Clinical Professor of Medicine and Pediatrics
Chief, Section of Allergy and Immunology
Department of Medicine
University of Louisville

VIKAS BHUSHAN, MD
Diagnostic Radiologist

DEEPAK A. RAO, MS, MPhil
Medical Scientist Training Program
Yale University

LARS GRIMM
Yale University
Class of 2008

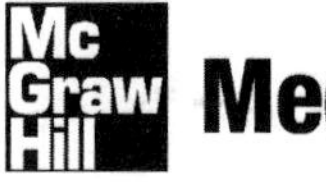

Medical

New York / Chicago / San Francisco / Lisbon / London / Madrid / Mexico City
Milan / New Delhi / San Juan / Seoul / Singapore / Sydney / Toronto

The ***McGraw·Hill*** *Companies*

First Aid for the® USMLE Step 1 2008: A Student to Student Guide

1 2 3 4 5 6 7 8 9 0 QPD/QPD 0 9 8 7

ISBN 978-0-07-149868-5
MHID 0-07-149868-0
ISSN 1532-6020

Notice

Medicine is an ever-changing science. As new research and clinical experience broaden our knowledge, changes in treatment and drug therapy are required. The authors and the publisher of this work have checked with sources believed to be reliable in their efforts to provide information that is complete and generally in accord with the standards accepted at the time of publication. However, in view of the possibility of human error or changes in medical sciences, neither the authors nor the publisher nor any other party who has been involved in the preparation or publication of this work warrants that the information contained herein is in every respect accurate or complete, and they disclaim all responsibility for any errors or omissions or for the results obtained from use of the information contained in this work. Readers are encouraged to confirm the information contained herein with other sources. For example and in particular, readers are advised to check the product information sheet included in the package of each drug they plan to administer to be certain that the information contained in this work is accurate and that changes have not been made in the recommended dose or in the contraindications for administration. This recommendation is of particular importance in connection with new or infrequently used drugs.

This book was set in Electra LH by Rainbow Graphics.
The editor was Catherine A. Johnson.
Project management was provided by Rainbow Graphics.
The production supervisor was Phil Galea.
The designer was Marsha Cohen/Parallelogram.
Quebecor World Dubuque was printer and binder.

This book is printed on acid-free paper.

DEDICATION

To the contributors to this and future editions, who took time to share their knowledge, insight, and humor for the benefit of students.

and

To our families, friends, and loved ones, who supported us in the task of assembling this guide.

CONTENTS

CONTRIBUTING AUTHORS

RAVISH AMIN
University of Medicine and Dentistry of New Jersey
Class of 2010

JESSE BIBLE
Yale University
Class of 2008

WENDY A. CIOVACCO
Yale University
Class of 2009

CHRISTOPHER KINSELLA, JR.
Drexel University
Class of 2009

YASHA MODI
Yale University
Class of 2008

MINA SAFAIN
Yale University
Class of 2009

MARK SCHLANGEL
Yale University
Class of 2009

NADIYA BABAR SHAFI, MD
Resident, Department of Pathology and Laboratory Medicine
University of Louisville

CHRISTINA L. SHENVI, PhD
Yale University
Class of 2009

AMANDA SILVERIO
Yale University
Class of 2009

VINITA TAKIAR, MPhil
Medical Scientist Training Program
Yale University

NEIL VASAN
Medical Scientist Training Program
Yale University

MATTHEW VESTAL
Yale University
Class of 2009

FACULTY REVIEWERS

DIANA M. ANTONIUCCI, MD, MAS
Assistant Professor of Medicine, Division of Endocrinology
University of California, San Francisco

SUSAN BASERGA, MD, PhD
Professor of Molecular Biophysics and Biochemistry, Genetics, and Therapeutic Radiology
Yale University

LINDA S. COSTANZO, PhD
Professor of Physiology
Virginia Commonwealth University

JOSEPH E. CRAFT, MD
Professor of Medicine and Immunobiology
Yale University

STUART D. FLYNN, MD
Associate Dean, Academic Affairs
Professor, Departments of Pathology and Basic Medical Sciences
The University of Arizona

WILLIAM GANONG, MD
Lange Professor of Physiology Emeritus
University of California, San Francisco

FRED GORELICK, MD
Professor of Medicine and Cell Biology
Yale University and VAMC West Haven

RAJESH JARI, MD, MSC
Resident in Physical Medicine and Rehabilitation
Johns Hopkins University

BERTRAM KATZUNG, MD, PhD
Professor of Pharmacology
University of California, San Francisco

SHANTA KAPADIA, MD
Lecturer, Surgical Anatomy and Experimental Surgery
Yale University

WARREN LEVINSON, MD, PhD
Professor of Microbiology and Immunology
University of California, San Francisco

ETHAN P. MARIN, MD, PhD
Fellow, Section of Nephrology
Yale University

PETER MARKS, MD, PhD
Associate Professor, Hematology
Yale University

CHRISTIAN MERLO, MD, MPH
Instructor, Medicine
Division of Pulmonary and Critical Care Medicine
Johns Hopkins University

DANIEL MUNDY, MD
General Psychiatry Attending
Yale University

DHASAKUMAR S. NAVARATNAM, MD
Assistant Professor, Neurology and Neurobiology
Yale University

ALAN PAO, MD
Assistant Professor of Medicine
Division of Nephrology
Department of Medicine
Stanford University

SANJIV J. SHAH, MD
Assistant Professor of Medicine
Division of Cardiology, Department of Medicine
Northwestern University

STEPHEN F. THUNG, MD
Assistant Professor, Department of Ob/Gyn
Yale University

FOREWORD

The purpose of *First Aid for the® USMLE Step 1: A Student-to-Student Guide* is to help medical students and international medical graduates review the basic medical sciences and prepare for the United States Medical Licensing Examination Step 1 (USMLE Step 1). Preparing for this examination can be a stressful, difficult, and costly task. This book helps students make the most of their limited time, money, and energy. As is often the case in medical school, we found that the best advice a student can receive is from other medical students. We also recognized that certain basic science topics and details are "popular" and appear frequently on examinations. With this in mind, *First Aid for the® USMLE Step 1* was started in 1989.

As we studied for the USMLE, we examined and evaluated scores of review books and thousands of sample questions. We kept track of useful study strategies, frequently tested facts, and helpful mnemonics through a simple computer database. The printed database was first distributed to the medical school class of 1992 at the University of California, San Francisco (UCSF). The next year, a revised edition was self-published under the name *High-Yield Basic Science Boards Review: A Student-to-Student Guide.* This guide was distributed to the UCSF class of 1993 and to numerous faculty and medical students at various institutions.

Two years ago, *First Aid for the USMLE Step 1* was reorganized into a partial organ system–based format. We feel that this change has substantially improved the book in several ways. First, this format reflects the evolving curriculum in U.S. medical schools. Second, by keeping a general principles section, we have not had to disperse this important information into what can sometimes be awkward organ system headings. *First Aid for the USMLE Step 1* has four major sections:

Section I: Guide to Efficient Exam Preparation is a compilation of general student advice and study strategies for taking the computerized USMLE Step 1.

Sections II: High-Yield General Principles and **Section III: High-Yield Organ Systems** contain short descriptions of frequently tested facts and concepts as well as mnemonics, diagrams, and high-quality photo illustrations to facilitate learning.

Section IV: Top-Rated Review Resources is designed to save students time and money by identifying high-quality, reasonably priced review and sample examination books and software. The comments and ratings are based on our analyses and on an annual nationwide random sampling of third-year medical students.

First Aid for the® USMLE Step 1 is not designed to be a comprehensive text or the sole study source for the USMLE Step 1; it is meant as a guide to one's preparation for the USMLE Step 1. The material in this book has been written to strengthen one's familiarity with a large number of topics in a short, fact-based review. The authors do not advocate blindly memorizing the lists of facts, and we hope medical students realize that memorization cannot replace an understanding of the concepts that underlie these key points.

Entries in *First Aid for the® USMLE Step 1* originated from hundreds of students, international medical graduates, and faculty members, who synthesized the facts, notes, and mnemonics from a variety of textbooks, review books, lecture notes, and personal notes. We regret the inability to reference each individual fact or mnemonic owing to the diverse and often anecdotal sources. Although the material has been reviewed by faculty members and medical students, errors and omissions are inevitable. We urge readers to identify errors and suggest improvements. We regret that some students may find certain mnemonics trivializing or offensive. The mnemonics are meant solely as optional devices for learning.

The authors and McGraw-Hill intend to continue updating *First Aid for the® USMLE Step 1* so that the book grows in quality and scope and continues to reflect the material covered on the USMLE Step 1. If you have any study strategies, high-yield facts with mnemonics, or book reviews for the next edition, please e-mail us. (See How to Contribute, p. xv.) Any student or faculty member who submits material subsequently used in the next edition of *First Aid for the® USMLE Step 1* will receive personal acknowledgment in the next edition and a $10 gift certificate per complete entry. Good luck in your studies!

PREFACE

With the 2008 edition of *First Aid for the® USMLE Step 1*, we continue our commitment to providing students with the most useful and up-to-date preparation guide for the USMLE Step 1. This edition represents a major revision in many ways and includes:

- A revised and updated exam preparation guide for the USMLE Step 1. Includes detailed analysis as well as study and test-taking strategies for the FRED format.
- Revisions and new material based on student experience with the 2007 administrations of the computerized USMLE Step 1.
- Expanded USMLE advice for international medical graduates, osteopathic medical students, podiatry students, and students with disabilities.
- Over a thousand frequently tested facts and useful mnemonics, including hundreds of new or revised entries.
- A high-yield collection of over 175 glossy photos similar to those appearing on the USMLE Step 1 exam.
- An in-depth guide to hundreds of recommended basic science review and sample examination books, based on a nationwide survey of randomly selected third-year medical students.

The 2008 edition would not have been possible without the help of the hundreds of students and faculty members who contributed their feedback and suggestions. We invite students and faculty to continue sharing their thoughts and ideas to help us improve *First Aid for the® USMLE Step 1*. (See How to Contribute, p. xv.)

Louisville	Tao Le
Los Angeles	Vikas Bhushan
New Haven	Deepak A. Rao
New Haven	Lars Grimm

ACKNOWLEDGMENTS

This has been a collaborative project from the start. We gratefully acknowledge the thoughtful comments, corrections, and advice of the many hundreds of medical students, international medical graduates, and faculty who have supported the authors in the continuing development of *First Aid for the USMLE Step 1*.

Thanks to Noam Maitless for the original book design, as well as Evenson Design Group, Ashley Pound, and Elizabeth Sanders for design revisions. For support and encouragement throughout the process, we are grateful to Thao Pham and Jonathan Kirsch, Esq.

Thanks to Selina Franklin and Louise Petersen for organizing and supporting the project. For editorial support, an enormous thanks to Andrea Fellows. A special thanks to Rainbow Graphics, especially David Hommel and Susan Cooper, for remarkable editorial and production work.

For submitting contributions and corrections, thanks to Blake Alkire, Rebecca Altschul, Fernando Bobis, Justin Chan, Nelson Conley, Daisy Cortes, Brad Fuller, Vivek Gupta, Betty Huo, Christopher Kinsella, Kevin Lee, Victor Marmolejos, Matthew McRae, Mark McRae, Christopher P. Miller, Sneha Patel, Chaithra Prasad, Marion Protano, Gabriel Sarah, Jonathan Schwartz, Rehan Shamim, R.M. Singa, Saranya Srinivasan, Gurmeet Sran, Kelly J. Tenbrink, and Jonathan Trager.

For completing book surveys, thanks to Daniel M. Halperin, Ellen Vollmers, Lauren Abern, Michelle Lynn Diaz, Samreen Hasan, Seth Goldstein, Yasha S. Modi, Daniel Rosenbaum, Eric Matthew Karlin, Aaron Aday, Ankit Patel, Brynn Utley, Crystal Hung, Jennifer Austin, Jimmy Carlucci, Jonathan Seccombe, Kevin Perry, Megan Herceg, Theresa Marsh, Rakesh, Josh M. Heck, Nupur Adam Prater, Christopher da Fonseca, Crystal Wang, David Shield, Geoffrey Kannan, Helena A. Hart, Jaimin G. Shah, Jeffrey Fiorenza, Jerry Chao, Jessica Woan, Justin Chen, Lindsey Shultz, Michelle Marie Walther, Rebecca Dezube, Ryan Childers, Sarah Stechschulte, Susanna Thomas Valley, Tina Kao, Alena Klimava, Catherine Dale, Feng-Yen Li, Liat Corcia, Lisa Hofler, Evelyn Osemeikhian, Simon Conti, and Christina L. Shenvi.

Thanks to Kristopher Jones, Kristina Panizzi, and Peter Anderson of the Department of Pathology, University of Alabama at Birmingham, for use of images from the Pathology Education Instructional Resource Digital Library (http://peir.net). Special thanks to Dr. Raoul Fresco for his generous contributions to the glossy photo section.

Finally, thanks to Ted Hon, one of the founding authors of this book, for his vision in developing this guide on the computer, and to Chirag Amin for his enormous contributions as an editor and author over many editions.

Louisville Tao Le
Los Angeles Vikas Bhushan
New Haven Deepak A. Rao
New Haven Lars Grimm

HOW TO CONTRIBUTE

This version of *First Aid for the® USMLE Step 1* incorporates hundreds of contributions and changes suggested by faculty and student reviewers. We invite you to participate in this process. We also offer **paid internships** in medical education and publishing ranging from three months to one year. Please send us your suggestions for:

- Study and test-taking strategies for the new computerized USMLE Step 1
- New facts, mnemonics, diagrams, and illustrations
- High-yield topics that may reappear on future Step 1 exams
- Personal ratings and comments on review books that you have examined

For each entry incorporated into the next edition, you will receive a **$10 gift certificate** per entry from the author group, as well as personal acknowledgment in the next edition. Diagrams, tables, partial entries, updates, corrections, and study hints are also appreciated, and significant contributions will be compensated at the discretion of the authors. Also let us know about material in this edition that you feel is low yield and should be deleted.

The preferred way to submit entries, suggestions, or corrections is via our blog:

www.firstaidteam.com

Otherwise, please send entries, neatly written or typed or on disk (Microsoft Word), to:

First Aid Team
914 N. Dixie Avenue, Suite 100
Elizabethtown, KY 42701

Contributions received by June 30, 2008, receive priority consideration for the 2009 edition of *First Aid for the® USMLE Step 1.*

NOTE TO CONTRIBUTORS

All contributions become property of the authors and are subject to editing and reviewing. Please verify all data and spellings carefully. In the event that similar or duplicate entries are received, only the first entry received will be used. Include a reference to a standard textbook to facilitate verification of the fact. Please follow the style, punctuation, and format of this edition if possible.

INTERNSHIP OPPORTUNITIES

The author team of Le and Bhushan is pleased to offer part-time and full-time paid internships in medical education and publishing to motivated medical students and physicians. Internships may range from three months (e.g., a summer) up to a full year. Participants will have an opportunity to author, edit, and earn academic credit on a wide variety of projects, including the popular *First Aid* series. English writing/editing experience, familiarity with Microsoft Word, and Internet access are required. Go to our blog **www.firstaidteam.com** to apply for an internship. A sample of your work or a proposal of a specific project is helpful.

HOW TO USE THIS BOOK

Medical students who have used previous editions of this guide have given us feedback on how best to make use of the book.

It is recommended that you begin using this book as early as possible when learning the basic medical sciences. You can use Section IV to select first-year course review books and Internet resources and then use those books for review while taking your medical school classes.

Use different parts of the book at different stages in your preparation for the USMLE Step 1. Before you begin to study for the USMLE Step 1, we suggest that you read Section I: Guide to Efficient Exam Preparation and Section IV: Top-Rated Review Resources. **If you are an international medical graduate student, an osteopathic medical student, a podiatry student, or a student with a disability,** refer to the appropriate Section I supplement for additional advice. Devise a study plan and decide what resources to buy. We strongly recommend that you invest in at least one or two top-rated review books in each subject. *First Aid* is not a comprehensive review book, and it is not a panacea that can compensate for not studying during the first two years of medical school. Scanning Sections II and III will give you an initial idea of the diverse range of topics covered on the USMLE Step 1.

As you study each discipline, **use the corresponding high-yield-fact section in *First Aid for the® USMLE Step 1* as a means of consolidating the material and testing yourself** to see if you have covered some of the frequently tested items. Work with the book to integrate important facts into your fund of knowledge. Using *First Aid for the® USMLE Step 1* as a review can serve as both a self-test of your knowledge and a repetition of important facts to learn. High-yield topics and vignettes are abstracted from recent exams to help guide your preparation.

Return to Sections II and III frequently during your preparation and fill your short-term memory with remaining high-yield facts a few days before the USMLE Step 1. The book can serve as a useful way of retaining key associations and keeping high-yield facts fresh in your memory just prior to the examination.

Reviewing the book immediately after the exam is probably the best way to **help us improve the book in the next edition.** Decide what was truly high and low yield and **send in your comments or your entire annotated book.**

First Aid Checklist for the USMLE Step 1

This is an example of how you might use the information in Section I to prepare for the USMLE Step 1. Refer to corresponding topics in Section I for more details.

Years Prior

- ☐ Select top-rated review books as study guides for first-year medical school courses.

Months Prior

- ☐ Review computer test format and registration information.
- ☐ Register six months in advance. Carefully verify name and address printed on scheduling permit. Call Prometric for test date ASAP.
- ☐ Define goals for the USMLE Step 1 (e.g., comfortably pass, beat the mean, ace the test).
- ☐ Set up a realistic timeline for study. Cover less crammable subjects first. Review subject-by-subject emphasis and clinical vignette format.
- ☐ Simulate the USMLE Step 1 to pinpoint strengths and weaknesses in knowledge and test-taking skills.
- ☐ Evaluate and choose study methods and materials (e.g., review books, practice tests, software).
- ☐ Ask advice from those who have recently taken the USMLE Step 1.

Weeks Prior

- ☐ Simulate the USMLE Step 1 again. Assess how close you are to your goal.
- ☐ Pinpoint remaining weaknesses. Stay healthy (exercise, sleep).
- ☐ Verify information on admission ticket (e.g., location, date).

One Week Prior

- ☐ Remember comfort measures (loose clothing, earplugs, etc.).
- ☐ Work out test site logistics such as location, transportation, parking, and lunch.
- ☐ Call Prometric and confirm your exam appointment.

One Day Prior

- ☐ Relax.
- ☐ Light review of short-term material if necessary. Skim high-yield facts.
- ☐ Get a good night's sleep.
- ☐ Make sure the name printed on your photo ID appears EXACTLY the same as the name printed on your scheduling permit. You will not be allowed to take the exam unless the names match EXACTLY.

Day of Exam

- ☐ Relax. Eat breakfast. Minimize bathroom breaks during the exam by avoiding excessive morning caffeine.
- ☐ Analyze and make adjustments in test-taking technique. You are allowed to review notes/study material during breaks on exam day.

After the Exam

- ☐ Celebrate, regardless.
- ☐ Send feedback to us at **www.firstaidteam.com.**

SECTION I

Guide to Efficient Exam Preparation

▶ INTRODUCTION

Relax.

This section is intended to make your exam preparation easier, not harder. Our goal is to reduce your level of anxiety and help you make the most of your efforts by helping you understand more about the United States Medical Licensing Examination, Step 1 (USMLE Step 1)—especially what the new FRED computer-based testing (CBT) is likely to mean to you. As a medical student, you are no doubt familiar with taking standardized examinations and quickly absorbing large amounts of material. When you first confront the USMLE Step 1, however, you may find it all too easy to become sidetracked and not achieve your goal of studying with maximal effectiveness. Common mistakes that students make when studying for the boards include the following:

- "Stressing out" owing to an inadequate understanding of the computer-based format
- Not understanding how scoring is performed or what your score means
- Starting *First Aid* too late
- Starting to study too late
- Using inefficient or inappropriate study methods
- Buying the wrong books or buying more books than you can ever use
- Buying only one publisher's review series for all subjects
- Not using practice examinations to maximum benefit
- Not using review books along with your classes
- Not analyzing and improving your test-taking strategies
- Getting bogged down by reviewing difficult topics excessively
- Studying material that is rarely tested on the USMLE Step 1
- Failing to master certain high-yield subjects owing to overconfidence
- Using *First Aid* as your sole study resource

In this section, we offer advice to help you avoid these pitfalls and be more productive in your studies. To begin, it is important for you to understand what the examination involves.

▶ USMLE STEP 1—THE CBT BASICS

The USMLE assesses a physician's ability to apply knowledge, concepts, and principles that are important in health and disease and that constitute the basis of safe and effective patient care.[2]

Some degree of concern about your performance on the USMLE Step 1 examination is both expected and appropriate. All too often, however, medical students become unnecessarily anxious about the examination. It is therefore important to understand precisely what the USMLE Step 1 involves. As you become familiar with Step 1, you can translate your anxiety into more efficient preparation.

The USMLE Step 1 is the first of three examinations that you must pass in order to become a licensed physician in the United States.[1] The USMLE is a joint endeavor of the National Board of Medical Examiners (NBME) and the

Federation of State Medical Boards (FSMB). In previous years, the examination was strictly organized around seven traditional disciplines: anatomy, behavioral science, biochemistry, microbiology, pathology, pharmacology, and physiology. In June 1991, the NBME began administering the "new" NBME Part I examination, which offered a more integrated and multidisciplinary format coupled with more clinically oriented questions.

In 1992, the USMLE replaced both the Federation Licensing Examination (FLEX) and the certifying examinations of the NBME.[3] The USMLE now serves as the single examination system for U.S. medical students and international medical graduates (IMGs) seeking medical licensure in the United States.

The CBT format of Step 1 is simply a computerized version of the former paper exam.

How Is the CBT Structured?

The CBT Step 1 exam consists of seven question "blocks" of 50 questions each (see Figure 1) for a total of 350 questions, timed at 60 minutes per block. A short 11-question survey follows the last question block. The computer begins the survey with a prompt to proceed to the next block of questions. Don't be fooled! "Block 8" is the NBME survey.

Don't be fooled! After the last question block comes the NBME survey ("Block 8").

The seven question blocks on Step 1 were designed to reduce eyestrain and fatigue during the exam. Once an examinee finishes a particular block, he or she must click on a screen icon to continue to the next block. Examinees **cannot** go back and change their answers to questions from any previously completed block. However, changing answers is allowed **within** a block of questions as long as time permits.

Prometric test centers offer Step 1 on a year-round basis, except for the first two weeks in January. The exam is given every day except Sunday at most centers. Some schools administer the exam on their own campuses.

FIGURE 1. Schematic of CBT Exam.

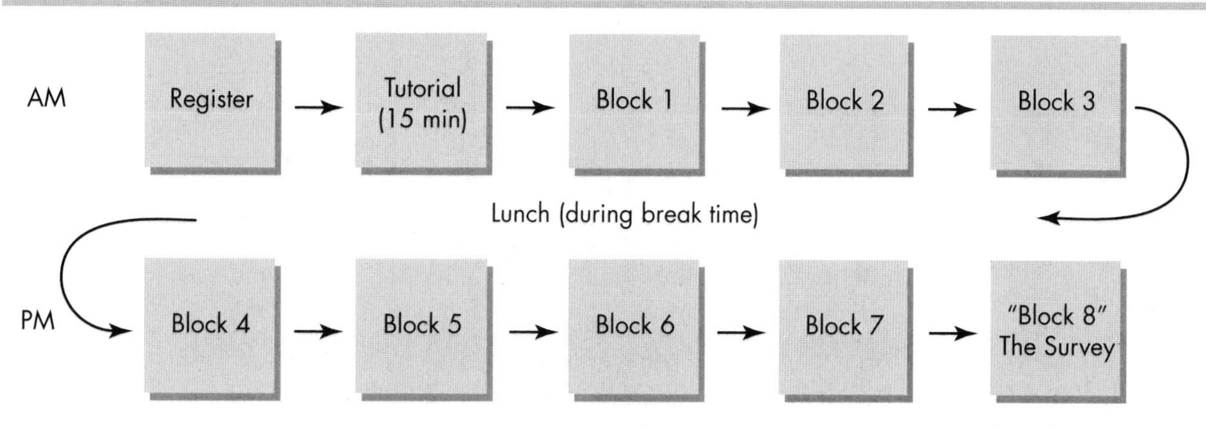

What Is the CBT Like?

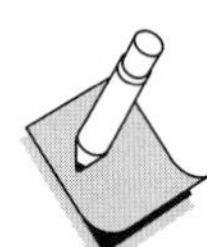

Skip the tutorial and add 15 minutes to your break time!

Because of the unique environment of the CBT, it's important that you become familiar ahead of time with what your test-day conditions will be like. Familiarizing yourself with the testing interface before the exam can add 15 minutes to your break time! This is because the 15-minute tutorial offered on exam day may be skipped if you are already familiar with the exam procedures and the testing interface (see description of CD-ROM below). The 15 minutes is then added to your allotted break time (should you choose to skip the tutorial).

For security reasons, examinees are not allowed to bring any personal electronic equipment into the testing area. This includes digital watches, watches with computer communication and/or memory capability, cellular telephones, and electronic paging devices. Food and beverages are also prohibited. The testing centers are monitored by audio and video surveillance equipment.

In 2006, the USMLE completed its transition to FRED. FRED is a computer-based format that is similar to the old forms of CBT, with minor differences.

Test illustrations include:

- *Gross photos*
- *Histology slides*
- *Radiographs*
- *EMs*
- *Line drawings*

The typical question screen in FRED consists of a question followed by a number of choices on which an examinee can click, together with a number of navigational buttons on the top of the screen. There is a countdown timer on the upper left-hand corner of the screen as well. There is also a button that allows the examinee to mark the question for review. If questions happen to be longer than the screen (which occurs very rarely), a scroll bar appears on the right, allowing the examinee to see the rest of the question. Regardless of whether the examinee clicks on the answer or leaves it blank, he or she must click the "Next" button to advance to the next question.

Some questions contain figures or color illustrations. These are typically situated to the right of the question. Although the contrast and brightness of the screen can be adjusted, there are no other ways to manipulate the picture (e.g., there is no zooming or panning).

The examinee can call up a window displaying normal lab values. In order to do so, he or she must hit the "Lab" icon on the top part of the screen. Afterward, the examinee will have the option to choose between "Blood," "Cerebrospinal," "Hematologic," or "Sweat and Urine." The normal-values screen may obscure the question if it is expanded. The examinee may have to scroll down to search for the needed laboratory values.

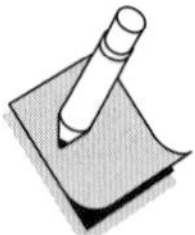

Ctrl-Alt-Delete are the keys of death during the exam. Don't touch them!

FRED allows the examinee to see a running list of questions on the left part of the screen at all times. The new software also allows examinees to highlight or cross out information by using their mouse. Finally, there is an "Annotate" icon on the top part of the screen that allows students to write notes to themselves for review at a later time. Examinees need to be careful with all of these new features, because failure to do so can cost valuable time!

What Does the CBT Format Mean to Me?

The significance of the CBT to you depends on the requirements of your school and your level of computer knowledge. If you hate computers and freak out whenever you see one, you might want to confront your fears as soon as possible. Spend some time playing with a Windows-based system and pointing and clicking icons or buttons with a mouse. These are the absolute basics, and you won't want to waste valuable exam time figuring them out on test day. Your test taking will proceed by pointing and clicking, essentially without the use of the keyboard. The free CD is an excellent way to become familiar with the test interface.

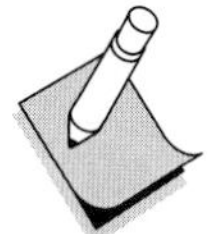

Keyboard shortcuts:

A–E—Letter choices.

Enter or spacebar—Move to next question.

Esc—Exit pop-up Lab and Exhibit windows.

Alt-T—Countdown timers for current session and overall test.

For those who feel they would benefit, the USMLE offers an opportunity to take a simulated test, or "CBT Practice Session at a Prometric center." Students are eligible to take the three-and-one-half-hour practice session after they have received their fluorescent orange scheduling permit (see below).

The same USMLE Step 1 sample test items (150 questions) available on the CD or USMLE Web site, www.usmle.org, are used at these sessions. **No new items will be presented.** The session is divided into three one-hour blocks of 50 test items each and costs about $42. Students receive a printed percent-correct score after completing the session. No explanations of questions are provided.

You may register for a practice session online at www.usmle.org.

How Do I Register to Take the Exam?

Step 1 or Step 2 applications may be printed from the USMLE Web site. The application allows applicants to select one of 12 overlapping three-month blocks in which to be tested (e.g., April–May–June, June–July–August). The application also includes a photo ID form that must be certified by an official at your medical school to verify your enrollment. After the NBME processes your application, it will send you a fluorescent orange slip of paper called a scheduling permit.

The scheduling permit you receive from the NBME will contain your USMLE identification number, the eligibility period in which you may take the exam, and two additional numbers. The first of these is known as your "scheduling number." You must have this number in order to make your exam appointment with Prometric. The second number is known as the "candidate identification number," or CIN. Examinees must enter their CINs at the Prometric workstation in order to access their exams. Prometric has no access to the codes. **Do not lose your permit!** You will not be allowed to take the boards unless you present this permit along with an unexpired, government-issued photo identification that includes your signature (such as a driver's license or passport). Make sure the name on your photo ID exactly matches the name that appears on your scheduling permit.

Test scheduling is done on a "first-come, first-served" basis. It's important to call and schedule an exam date as soon as you receive your scheduling permit.

Once you receive your scheduling permit, you may call Prometric's toll-free number to arrange a time to take the exam. Although requests for taking the

Testing centers are closed on major holidays and during the first two weeks of January.

exam may be completed more than six months before the test date, examinees will not receive their scheduling permits earlier than six months before the eligibility period. The eligibility period is the three-month period you have chosen to take the exam. Most medical students choose the April–June or June–August period. Because exams are scheduled on a "first-come, first-served" basis, it is recommended that you telephone Prometric as soon as you receive your permit. After you've scheduled your exam, it's a good idea to confirm your exam appointment with Prometric at least one week before your test date. Prometric does not provide written confirmation of exam date, time, or location. Be sure to read the *2008 USMLE Bulletin of Information* for further details.

What If I Need to Reschedule the Exam?

You can change your test date and/or center by contacting Prometric at 1-800-MED-EXAM (1-800-633-3926) or www.prometric.com. Make sure to have your CIN when rescheduling. If you are rescheduling by phone, you must speak with a Prometric representative; leaving a voice-mail message will not suffice. To avoid a rescheduling fee, you will need to request a change before noon EST at least five business days before your appointment. Please note that your rescheduled test date must fall within your assigned three-month eligibility period.

When Should I Register for the Exam?

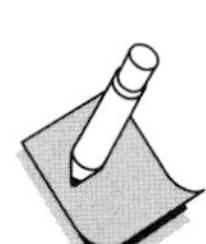

Register six months in advance for seating and scheduling preference.

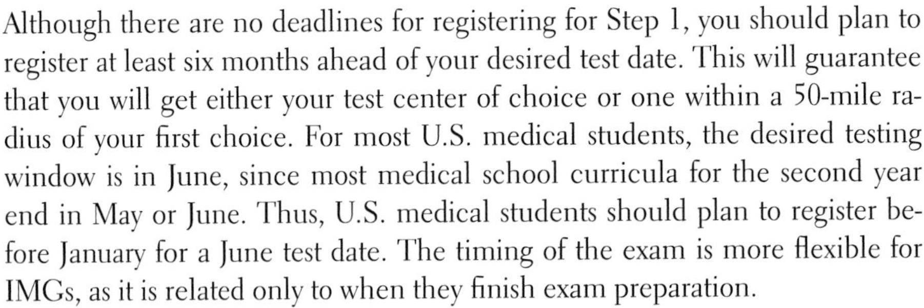

Although there are no deadlines for registering for Step 1, you should plan to register at least six months ahead of your desired test date. This will guarantee that you will get either your test center of choice or one within a 50-mile radius of your first choice. For most U.S. medical students, the desired testing window is in June, since most medical school curricula for the second year end in May or June. Thus, U.S. medical students should plan to register before January for a June test date. The timing of the exam is more flexible for IMGs, as it is related only to when they finish exam preparation.

Choose your three-month eligibility period wisely. If you need to reschedule outside your initial three-month period, you must submit a new application along with another application fee.

Where Can I Take the Exam?

Your testing location is arranged with Prometric when you call for your test date (after you receive your scheduling permit). For a list of Prometric locations nearest you, visit www.prometric.com.

How Long Will I Have to Wait Before I Get My Scores?

The USMLE reports scores three to six weeks after the examinee's test date. In August 2007, the USMLE switched from paper to electronic score reporting. Examinees will be notified via e-mail when their scores are available. Following the online instructions, examinees will be able to view, download, and print their score report. Additional information about score timetables and accessibility is available on the official USMLE Web site.

What About Time?

Time is of special interest on the CBT exam. Here's a breakdown of the exam schedule:

15 minutes	Tutorial (skip if familiar)
7 hours	60-minute question blocks
45 minutes	Break time (includes time for lunch)

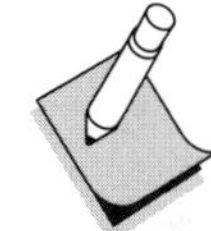

Be careful to watch the clock on your break time.

The computer will keep track of how much time has elapsed on the exam. However, the computer will show you only how much time you have remaining in a given block. Therefore, it is up to you to determine if you are pacing yourself properly (at a rate of approximately one question per 72 seconds).

The computer will **not** warn you if you are spending more than your allotted time for a break. You should therefore budget your time so that you can take a short break when you need one and have time to eat. You must be especially careful not to spend too much time in between blocks (you should keep track of how much time elapses from the time you finish a block of questions to the time you start the next block). After you finish one question block, you'll need to click the mouse to proceed to the next block of questions.

Gain extra break time by skipping the tutorial or finishing a block early.

Forty-five minutes is the minimum break time for the day. You can gain extra break time (but not time for the question blocks) by skipping the tutorial or by finishing a block ahead of the allotted time.

If I Freak Out and Leave, What Happens to My Score?

Your scheduling permit shows a CIN that you will enter onto your computer screen to start your exam. Entering the CIN is the same as breaking the seal on a test book, and you are considered to have started the exam when you do so. However, no score will be reported if you do not complete the exam. In fact, if you leave at any time from the start of the test to the last block, no score will be reported. The fact that you started but did not complete the exam, however, will appear on your USMLE score transcript.

The exam ends when all blocks have been completed or their time has expired. As you leave the testing center, you will receive a printed test-completion notice to document your completion of the exam. To receive an official score, you must finish the entire exam.

What Types of Questions Are Asked?

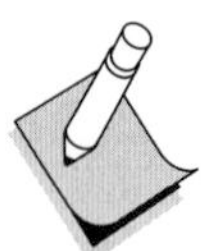

Although numerous changes had to be made to accommodate the CBT format, the question types are the same as those in previous years.

Nearly three-fourths of Step 1 questions begin with a description of a patient.

One-best-answer items are the only multiple-choice format. Most questions consist of a clinical scenario or a direct question followed by a list of five or more options. You are required to select the one best answer among the options given. There are no "except," "not," or matching questions on the exam. A number of options may be partially correct, in which case you must select the option that best answers the question or completes the statement. Additionally, keep in mind that experimental questions may appear on the exam (see Difficult Questions, p. 22).

How Is the Test Scored?

Each Step 1 examinee receives an electronic score report that includes the examinee's pass/fail status, two test scores, and a graphic depiction of the examinee's performance by discipline and organ system or subject area. The actual organ system profiles reported may depend on the statistical characteristics of a given administration of the examination.

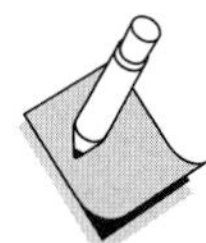

The mean Step 1 score for U.S. medical students rose from 200 in 1991 to 217 in 2005.

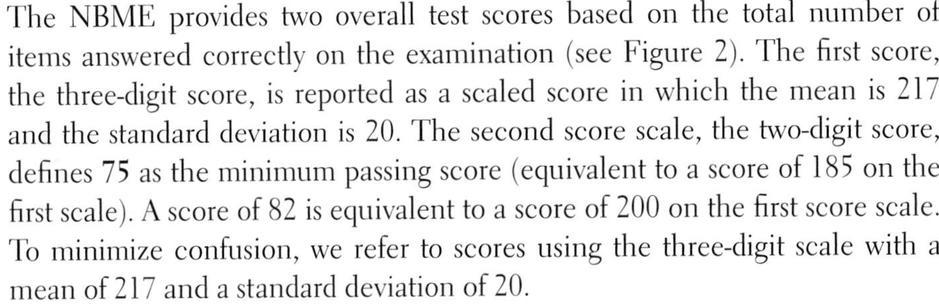

The NBME provides two overall test scores based on the total number of items answered correctly on the examination (see Figure 2). The first score, the three-digit score, is reported as a scaled score in which the mean is 217 and the standard deviation is 20. The second score scale, the two-digit score, defines 75 as the minimum passing score (equivalent to a score of 185 on the first scale). A score of 82 is equivalent to a score of 200 on the first score scale. To minimize confusion, we refer to scores using the three-digit scale with a mean of 217 and a standard deviation of 20.

A score of **185** or higher is required to pass Step 1. Passing the CBT Step 1 is estimated to correspond to answering 60–70% of questions correctly. In 2005, the pass rates for first-time test takers from accredited U.S. and Canadian medical schools was 90% (see Table 1). The NBME also reports that 99% of these test takers eventually pass. Although the NBME may adjust the minimum passing score at any time, no further adjustment is expected for several years.

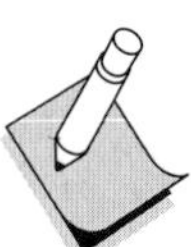

Passing the CBT Step 1 is estimated to correspond to answering 60–70% of the questions correctly.

According to the USMLE, medical schools receive a listing of total scores and pass/fail results plus group summaries by discipline and organ system. Students can withhold their scores from their medical school if they wish. Official USMLE transcripts, which can be sent on request to residency programs, include only total scores, not performance profiles.

Consult the USMLE Web site or your medical school for the most current and accurate information regarding the examination.

FIGURE 2. Scoring Scales for the USMLE Step 1.

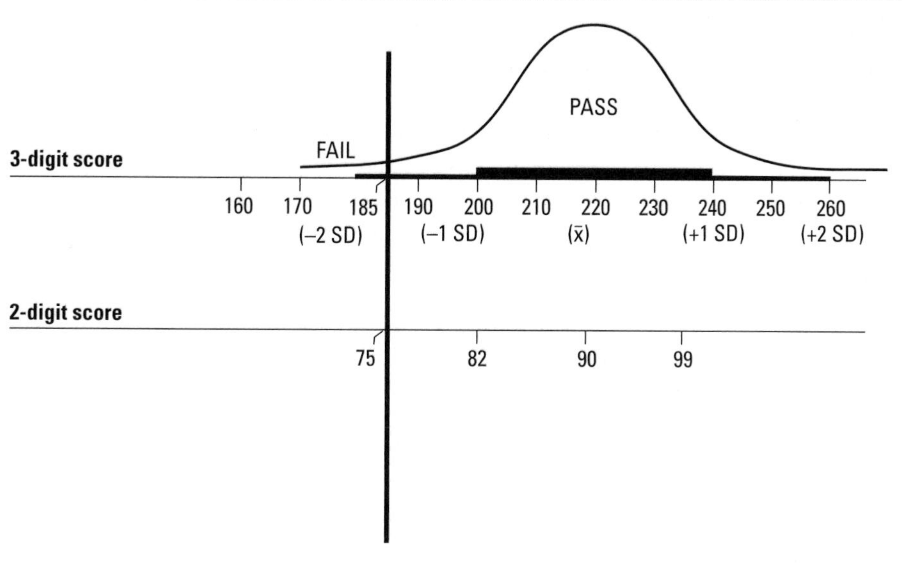

TABLE 1. Passing Rates for the 2005–2006 USMLE Step 1.[a]

	2005		2006	
	No. Tested	Passing (%)	No. Tested	Passing (%)
NBME-registered examinees (U.S./Canadian)				
Allopathic students				
First-time takers	16,799	94	16,818	95
Repeaters	1,491	65	1,349	67
Allopathic total	**18,290**	**92**	**18,167**	**92**
Osteopathic students				
First-time takers	1,265	73	1,258	77
Repeaters	66	53	67	52
Osteopathic total	**1,331**	**72**	**1,325**	**76**
Total (U.S./Canadian)	**19,621**	**90**	**19,492**	**92**
IMG examinees (ECFMG[b] registrants)				
First-time takers	13,488	68	14,585	71
Repeaters	5,911	39	6,017	39
IMG total	**19,399**	**59**	**20,602**	**61**
Total Step 1 examinees	**39,020**	**75**	**40,094**	**76**

[a]Reflects the most current data available at the time of publishing. Source: www.nbme.org.
[b]Educational Commission for Foreign Medical Graduates.

What Does My Score Mean?

For students, the most important point with the Step 1 score is passing versus failing. Passing essentially means, "Hey, you're on your way to becoming a fully licensed doc."

Beyond that, the main point of having a quantitative score is to give you a sense of how you've done aside from the fact that you've passed the exam. The two-digit or three-digit score gauges how well you have performed with respect to the content on the exam.

Since the content of the exam is what drives the score, the profile of the exam is what remains relatively constant over the years. That is to say that each exam profile includes a certain number of "very hard" questions along with "medium" and "easy" ones. The questions vary, but the profile of the exam doesn't change substantially. This ensures that someone who scored 200 on the boards yesterday has achieved a level of knowledge comparable to that of a person who scored 200 four years ago.

Official NBME/USMLE Resources

We strongly encourage students to use the free materials provided by the testing agencies (see p. 24) and to study in detail the following NBME resources, all of which are available on CD-ROM or at the USMLE Web site, www.usmle.org:

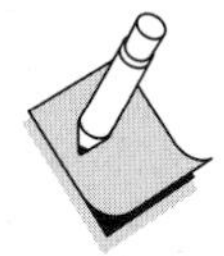

Practice questions may be easier than the actual exam.

- *USMLE Step 1 2008 Computer-based Content and Sample Test Questions* (information given free to all examinees)
- *2008 USMLE Bulletin of Information* (information given free to all examinees)
- Comprehensive Basic Science Self-Assessment (CBSSA)

The *USMLE Step 1 2008 Computer-based Content and Sample Test Questions* contains approximately 150 questions that are similar in format and content to the questions on the actual USMLE Step 1 exam. This practice test offers one of the best means of assessing your test-taking skills. However, it does not contain enough questions to simulate the full length of the examination, and its content represents a limited sampling of the basic science material that may be covered on Step 1. Moreover, most students felt that the questions on the actual 2007 exam were more challenging than those contained in that year's sample questions. Others, however, reported that they had encountered a few near-duplicates of these sample questions on the actual Step 1 exam. Presumably, these are "experimental" questions, but who knows? So the bottom line is, know these questions!

The extremely detailed *Step 1 Content Outline* provided by the USMLE has not proved useful for students studying for the exam. The USMLE even states that ". . . the content outline is not intended as a guide for curriculum development or as a study guide."[4] We concur with this assessment.

The *2008 USMLE Bulletin of Information* is found on the CD-ROM. This publication contains detailed procedural and policy information regarding the CBT, including descriptions of all three Steps, scoring of the exams, reporting of scores to medical schools and residency programs, procedures for score rechecks and other inquiries, policies for irregular behavior, and test dates.

The NBME also offers the Comprehensive Basic Science Self-Assessment (CBSSA), which tests users on topics covered during basic science courses in a format similar to that of the USMLE Step 1 examination. Students who prepared for the examination using this Web-based tool reported that they found the format and content highly indicative of questions tested on the Step 1 examination. In addition, the CBSSA is a fair predictor of USMLE performance (see Table 2).

TABLE 2. CBSSA to USMLE Score Comparison.

CBSSA Score	Approximate USMLE Step 1 Score
200	< 136
250	148
300	163
350	178
400	192
450	206
500	219
550	230
600	240
650	248
700	256
750	261
800	> 265

The CBSSA exists in two forms: a standard-paced and a self-paced format, both of which consist of four sections of 50 questions each (for a total of 200 multiple-choice items). The standard-paced format allows the user up to one hour to complete each section, reflecting the time limits of the actual exam. By contrast, the self-paced format places a four-hour time limit on answering the multiple-choice questions. Keep in mind that this bank of questions is available only on the Web. The NBME requires that users log on, register, and start within 30 days of registration. Once the assessment has begun, users are required to complete the sections within 20 days. Following completion of the questions, the CBSSA will provide a performance profile indicating each user's relative strengths and weaknesses, much like the report profile for the USMLE Step 1 exam. However, keep in mind that this self-assessment does **not** provide the user with a list of correct answers. Table 2 provides an approximate correlation of scores between the CBSSA and the USMLE. Feedback from the self-assessment takes the form of a performance profile and nothing more. The NBME charges $45 for this service, which is payable by credit card or money order. For more information regarding the CBSSA, please visit the NBME's Web site at www.nbme.org and click on the link labeled "NBME Self-Assessment Services."

▶ DEFINING YOUR GOAL

It is useful to define your own personal performance goal when approaching the USMLE Step 1. Your style and intensity of preparation can then be matched to your goal. Your goal may depend on your school's requirements, your specialty choice, your grades to date, and your personal assessment of the test's importance. Do your best to define your goals early so that you can prepare accordingly.

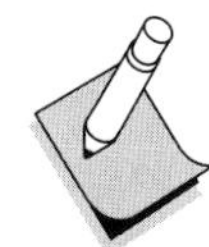

Fourth-year medical students have the best feel for how Step 1 scores factor into the residency application process.

Certain highly competitive residency programs, such as those in plastic surgery and orthopedic surgery, have acknowledged their use of Step 1 scores in the selection process. In such residency programs, greater emphasis may be placed on attaining a high score, so students who seek to enter these programs

Some competitive residency programs place more weight on Step 1 scores in their selection process.

may wish to consider aiming for a very high score on the Step 1 exam (see Figure 3). At the same time, your Step 1 score is only one of a number of factors that are assessed when you apply for residency. Indeed, many residency programs value other criteria more highly than a high score on Step 1. Fourth-year medical students who have recently completed the residency application process can be a valuable resource in this regard.

▶ TIMELINE FOR STUDY

Make a Schedule

After you have defined your goals, map out a study schedule that is consistent with your objectives, your vacation time, and the difficulty of your ongoing coursework (see Figure 4). Determine whether you want to spread out your study time or concentrate it into 14-hour study days in the final weeks. Then factor in your own history in preparing for standardized examinations (e.g., SAT, MCAT).

Time management is key. Customize your schedule to your goals and available time following any final exams.

Typically, students allot between five and seven weeks to prepare for Step 1. Some students reserve about a week at the end of their study period for final review; others save just a few days. When you have scheduled your exam date, do your best to adhere to it. Recent studies show that a later testing date does not translate into a higher score, so avoid pushing back your test date.[5] This highlights the importance of working out a realistic schedule to which you can adhere.

Another important consideration is when you will study each subject. Some subjects lend themselves to cramming, whereas others demand a substantial long-term commitment. The "crammable" subjects for Step 1 are those for which concise yet relatively complete review books are available. (See Section IV for highly rated review and sample examination materials.) Behavioral sci-

FIGURE 3. Median USMLE Step 1 Score for Matched U.S. Seniors.[a]

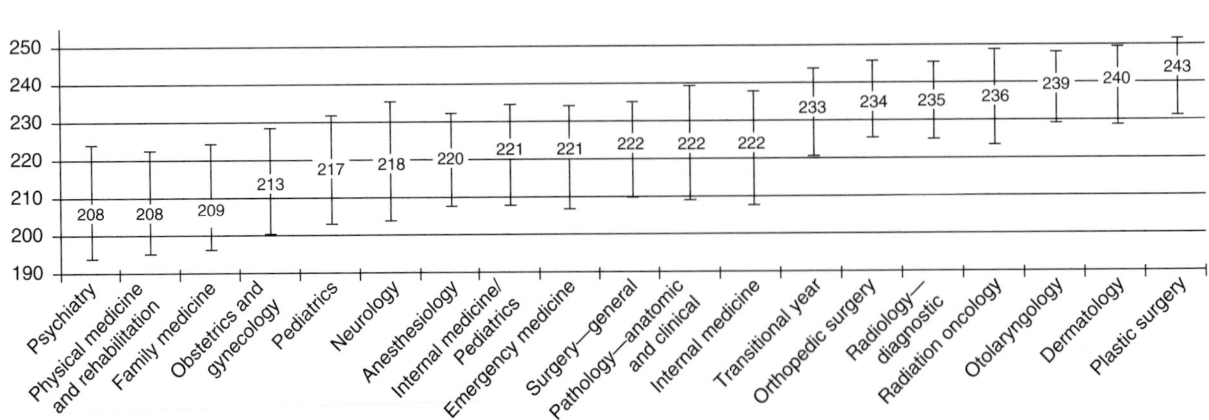

[a] Vertical lines show interquartile range. Source: www.nrmp.org.

FIGURE 4. Typical Timeline for the USMLE Step 1.

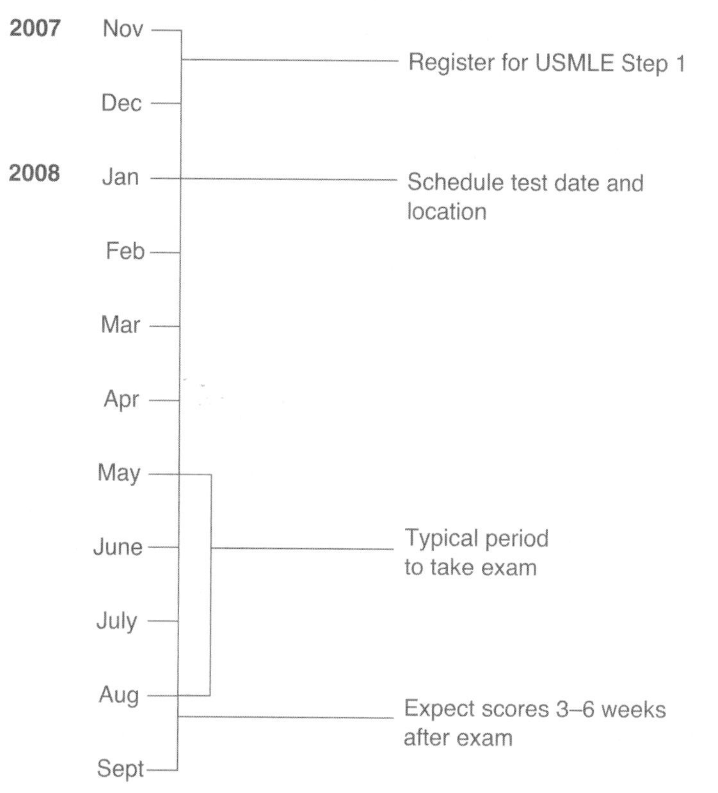

ence and physiology are two subjects with concise review books. Three subjects with longer but quite comprehensive review books are microbiology, pharmacology, and biochemistry. Thus, these subjects could be covered toward the end of your schedule, whereas other subjects (anatomy and pathology) require a longer time commitment and could be studied earlier. Many students prefer using a "systems-based" approach (e.g., GI, renal, cardiovascular) to integrate the material across basic science subjects. See Section III to study anatomy, pathology, physiology, and pharmacology facts by organ system.

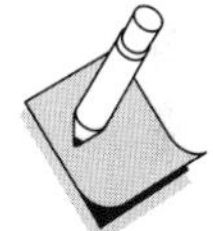

"Crammable" subjects should be covered later and less crammable subjects earlier.

Practically speaking, spending a given amount of time on a crammable or high-yield subject (particularly in the last few days before the test) generally produces more correct answers on the examination than spending the same amount of time on a low-yield subject. Student opinion indicates that knowing the crammable subjects extremely well probably results in a higher overall score than knowing all subjects moderately well.

Make your schedule realistic, and set achievable goals. Many students make the mistake of studying at a level of detail that requires too much time for a comprehensive review—reading *Gray's Anatomy* in a couple of days is not a realistic goal! Revise your schedule regularly on the basis of your actual progress. Be careful not to lose focus. Beware of feelings of inadequacy when comparing study schedules and progress with your peers. **Avoid students who stress you out.** Fo-

Avoid burnout. Maintain proper diet, exercise, and sleep habits.

cus on a few top-rated resources that suit your learning style—not on some obscure books your friends may pass down to you. Do not set yourself up for frustration. Accept the fact that you cannot learn it all. Maintain your sanity throughout the process.

You will need time for uninterrupted and focused study. Plan your personal affairs to minimize crisis situations near the date of the test. Allot an adequate number of breaks in your study schedule to avoid burnout. Maintain a healthy lifestyle with proper diet, exercise, and sleep.

Buy review books early (first year) and use while studying for courses.

Year(s) Prior

The NBME asserts that the best preparation for the USMLE Step 1 resides in "broadly based learning that establishes a strong general foundation of understanding of concepts and principles in basic sciences."[6] We agree. Although you may be tempted to rely solely on cramming in the weeks and months before the test, you should not have to do so. The knowledge you gained during your first two years of medical school and even during your undergraduate years should provide the groundwork on which to base your test preparation. Student scores on NBME subject tests (commonly known as "shelf exams") have been shown to be highly correlated with subsequent Step 1 scores.[7] Moreover, undergraduate science GPAs as well as MCAT scores are strong predictors of performance on the Step 1 exam.[8] The preponderance of your boards preparation should thus involve resurrecting dormant information that you have stored away during the basic science years.

We also recommend that you buy highly rated review books early in your first year of medical school and use them as you study throughout the two years. When Step 1 comes along, these books will be familiar and personalized to the way in which you learn. It is risky and intimidating to use unfamiliar review books in the final two or three weeks preceding the exam.

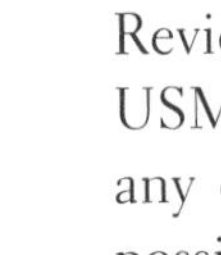

Simulate the USMLE Step 1 under "real" conditions before beginning your studies.

Months Prior

Review test dates and the application procedure. In 2008, testing for the USMLE Step 1 continues on a year-round basis (see Table 3). If you have any disabilities or "special circumstances," contact the NBME as early as possible to discuss test accommodations (see p. 56, First Aid for the Student with a Disability).

Before you begin to study earnestly, simulate the USMLE Step 1 under "real" conditions to pinpoint strengths and weaknesses in your knowledge and test-taking skills. Be sure that you are well informed about the examination and that you have planned your strategy for studying. Consider what study methods you will use, the study materials you will need, and how you will obtain your materials. Plan ahead. Get advice from third- and fourth-year medical students who have recently taken the USMLE Step 1. There might be strengths and weaknesses in your school's curriculum that you should take into account in decid-

TABLE 3. 2008 USMLE Exams.

Step	Focus	No. of Questions/ No. of Blocks	Test Schedule/ Length of CBT Exam	Passing Score
Step 1	Basic mechanisms and principles	350/7	One day (eight hours)	185
Step 2	Clinical diagnosis and disease pathogenesis	368/8	One day (nine hours)	184
Step 3	Clinical management	480/11	Two days (16 hours)	184

ing where to focus your efforts. You might also choose to share books, notes, and study hints with classmates. That is how this book began.

Three Weeks Prior

Two to four weeks before the examination is a good time to resimulate the USMLE Step 1. You may want to do this earlier depending on the progress of your review, but be sure not to do it later, when there will be little time to remedy defects in your knowledge or test-taking skills. Make use of remaining good-quality sample USMLE test questions, and try to simulate the computerized test conditions so that you can adequately assess your test performance. Recognize, too, that time pressure is increasing as more and more questions are framed as clinical vignettes. Most sample exam questions are shorter than the real thing. Focus on reviewing the high-yield facts, your own notes, picture books, and very short review books.

In the final two weeks, focus on review and endurance. Avoid unfamiliar material. Stay confident!

One Week Prior

Make sure you have your CIN (found on your scheduling permit) as well as other items necessary for the day of the examination, including a driver's license or another form of photo identification with your signature (make sure the name on your ID **exactly** matches that on your scheduling permit), an analog watch, and possibly earplugs. Confirm the Prometric testing center location and test time. Work out how you will get to the testing center and what parking and traffic problems you might encounter. If possible, visit the testing site to get a better idea of the testing conditions you will face. Determine what you will do for lunch. Make sure you have everything you need to ensure that you will be comfortable and alert at the test site.

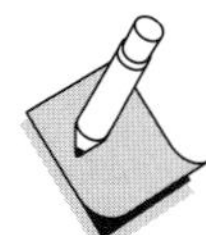

Confirm your testing date at least one week in advance.

One Day Prior

Try your best to relax and rest the night before the test. Double-check your admissions and test-taking materials as well as the comfort measures discussed earlier so that you will not have to deal with such details on the morning of

No notes, books, calculators, pagers, recording devices, or digital watches are allowed in the testing area.

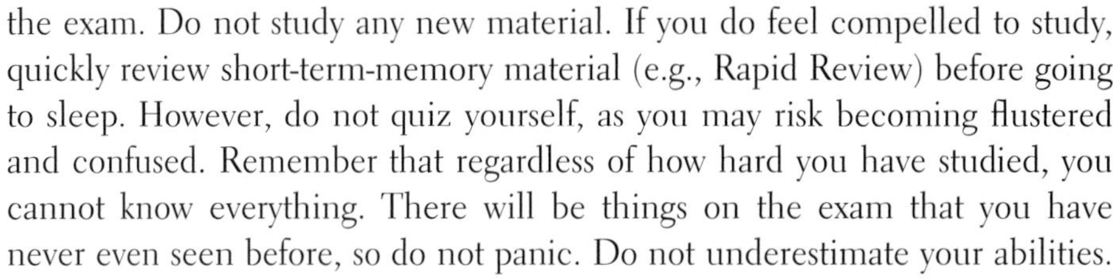

the exam. Do not study any new material. If you do feel compelled to study, quickly review short-term-memory material (e.g., Rapid Review) before going to sleep. However, do not quiz yourself, as you may risk becoming flustered and confused. Remember that regardless of how hard you have studied, you cannot know everything. There will be things on the exam that you have never even seen before, so do not panic. Do not underestimate your abilities.

Many students report difficulty sleeping the night prior to the exam. This is often exacerbated by going to bed much earlier than usual. Do whatever it takes to ensure a good night's sleep (e.g., massage, exercise, warm milk). Do not change your daily routine prior to the exam. Exam day is not the day for a caffeine-withdrawal headache.

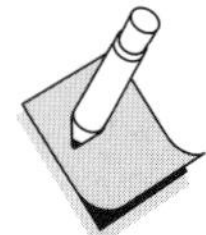

Arrive at the testing center 30 minutes before your scheduled exam time. If you arrive more than half an hour late, you will not be allowed to take the test.

Morning of the Exam

On the morning of the Step 1 exam, wake up at your regular time and eat a normal breakfast. Make sure you have your scheduling permit admission ticket, test-taking materials, and comfort measures as discussed earlier. Wear loose, comfortable clothing. Plan for a variable temperature in the testing center. Arrive at the test site 30 minutes before the time designated on the admission ticket; however, do not come too early, as this may intensify your anxiety. When you arrive at the test site, the proctor should give you a blue, laminated USMLE information sheet that will explain critical factors such as the proper use of break time. Seating may be assigned, but ask to be reseated if necessary; you need to be seated in an area that will allow you to remain comfortable and to concentrate. Get to know your testing station, especially if you have never been in a Prometric testing center before. Listen to your proctors regarding any changes in instructions or testing procedures that may apply to your test site.

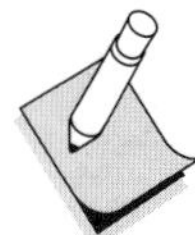

Some students recommend reviewing certain "theme" topics that tend to recur throughout the exam.

Remember that it is natural (and even beneficial) to be a little nervous. Focus on being mentally clear and alert. Avoid panic. Avoid panic. Avoid panic. When you are asked to begin the exam, take a deep breath, focus on the screen, and then begin. Keep an eye on the timer. Take advantage of breaks between blocks to stretch and relax for a moment.

After the Test

After you have completed the exam, be sure to have fun and relax regardless of how you may feel. Taking the test is an achievement in itself. Remember, you are much more likely to have passed than not. Enjoy the free time you have before your clerkships. Expect to experience some "reentry" phenomena as you try to regain a real life. Once you have recovered sufficiently from the test (or from partying), we invite you to send us your feedback, corrections, and suggestions for entries, facts, mnemonics, strategies, resource ratings, and the like (see p. xv, How to Contribute). Sharing your experience benefits fellow medical students and IMGs.

▶ IF YOU THINK YOU FAILED

After the test, many examinees feel that they have failed, and most are at the very least unsure of their pass/fail status. There are several sensible steps you can take to plan for the future in the event that you do not achieve a passing score. First, save and organize all your study materials, including review books, practice tests, and notes. Familiarize yourself with the reapplication procedures for Step 1, including application deadlines and upcoming test dates. The CBT format allows an examinee who has failed the exam to retake it no earlier than the first day of the month after 60 days have elapsed since the last test date. Examinees will, however, be allowed to take the exam no more than three times within a 12-month period should they repeatedly fail.

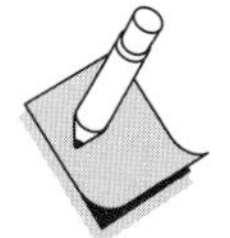

If you pass Step 1, you are not allowed to retake the exam in an attempt to raise your score.

The performance profiles on the back of the USMLE Step 1 score report provide valuable feedback concerning your relative strengths and weaknesses. Study these profiles closely. Set up a study timeline to strengthen gaps in your knowledge as well as to maintain and improve what you already know. Do not neglect high-yield subjects. It is normal to feel somewhat anxious about retaking the test—but if anxiety becomes a problem, seek appropriate counseling.

Fifty-two percent of the NBME-registered first-time takers who failed the June 1998 Step 1 repeated the exam in October 1998. The overall pass rate for that group in October was 60%. Eighty-five percent of those scoring near the old pass/fail mark of 176 (173–176) in June 1998 passed in October. However, 1999 pass rates varied widely depending on initial score (see Table 4, which reflects the most current data available at the time of publishing).

TABLE 4. Pass Rates for USMLE Step 1 Repeaters, 1999.[9]

Initial Score	% Pass
176–178	83
173–175	74
170–172	71
165–169	64
160–164	54
150–159	31
< 150	0
Overall	**67**

Although the NBME allows an unlimited number of attempts to pass Step 1, both the NBME and the FSMB recommend that licensing authorities allow a minimum of three and a maximum of six attempts for each Step examination.[9] Again, review your school's policy regarding retakes.

▶ IF YOU FAILED

Even if you came out of the exam room feeling that you failed, seeing that failing grade can be traumatic, and it is natural to feel upset. Different people react in different ways: For some it is a stimulus to buckle down and study harder; for others it may "take the wind out of their sails" for a few days; and for still others it may lead to a reassessment of individual goals and abilities. In some instances, however, failure may trigger weeks or months of sadness, feelings of hopelessness, social withdrawal, and inability to concentrate—in other words, true clinical depression. If you think you are depressed, please seek help.

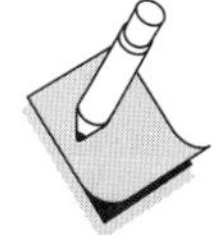

Near the failure threshold, each three-digit scale point is equivalent to about 1.5 questions answered correctly.[10]

▶ STUDY METHODS

It is important to have a set of study methods for preparing for the USMLE Step 1. There is too much material to justify a studying plan that is built on random reading and memorization. Experiment with different ways of studying, as you will not know how effective something might be until you try it. This is best done months before the test so that you can determine what works and what you enjoy. Possible study options include the following:

- Studying review material in groups
- Creating personal mnemonics, diagrams, and tables
- Using *First Aid* as a framework on which to add notes
- Taking practice computer as well as pencil-and-paper tests (see Section IV for resources)
- Attending faculty review sessions
- Making or sharing flash cards
- Reviewing old syllabi and notes
- Making cassette tapes of review material to study during commuting time
- Playing Trivial Pursuit–style games with facts and questions
- Getting away from home for an extended period to avoid distractions and to immerse yourself in studying

Study Groups

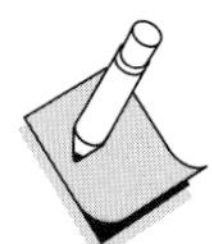

Balance individual and group study.

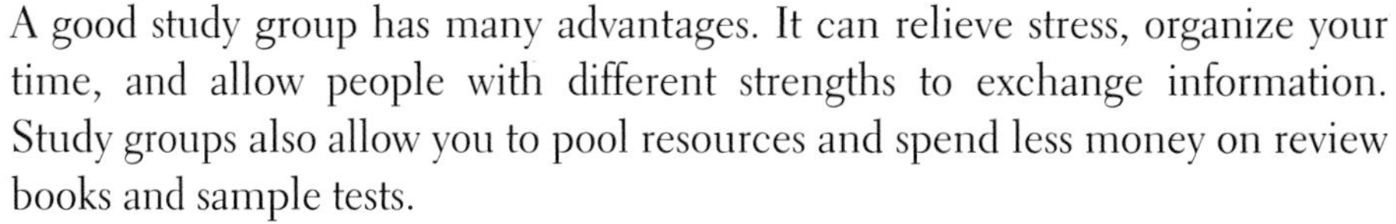

A good study group has many advantages. It can relieve stress, organize your time, and allow people with different strengths to exchange information. Study groups also allow you to pool resources and spend less money on review books and sample tests.

There are, however, potential problems associated with study groups. Above all, it is difficult to study with people who have different goals and study paces. Avoid study groups that tend to socialize more than study. If you choose not to belong to a study group, it may be a good idea to find a support group or a study partner with whom to keep pace and share study ideas. It is always beneficial to get different perspectives from other students.

Mnemonics and Memorizing

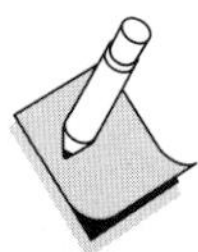

Developing good mnemonics takes time and work. Quiz yourself periodically. Do not simply reread highlighted material.

Mnemonics are memory aids that work by linking isolated facts or abstract ideas to acronyms, pictures, patterns, rhymes, and stories—information that the mind tends to store well.[11] The best mnemonics are your own, and developing them takes work. The first step to creating a mnemonic lies in understanding the information to be memorized. Play around with the information, and look for unique features that help you remember it. Effective mnemonics should link the topic with the facts in as specific and unambiguous a manner as possible. Keep the information fresh by quizzing yourself periodically with flash cards, in study groups, and so on. Do not make the common mistake of simply rereading highlighted review material. The material might start to look familiar, but that does not mean you will be able to remember it in another context during the exam. Strive to gain an understanding rather than relying on rote memorization.

Review Sessions

Faculty review sessions can also be of use. Review sessions that are geared specifically toward the USMLE Step 1 tend to be more helpful than general review sessions. By contrast, open "question and answer" sessions tend to be inefficient and not worth the time. Focus on reviews given by faculty who are knowledgeable in the content and testing format of the USMLE Step 1.

Commercial Courses

Commercial preparation courses can be helpful for some students, but they are expensive and require significant time commitment. The data also show that such courses have a limited impact on Step 1 scores.[12] However, this may reflect the fact that students who take such courses are concerned about their readiness to take the exam. Nevertheless, commercial courses are often an effective organizing tool for students who feel overwhelmed by the sheer volume of material involved in preparing for Step 1. Note, however, that multiple-week courses may be quite intense and may thus leave limited time for independent study.

▶ STUDY MATERIALS

Quality and Cost Considerations

Although an ever-increasing number of review books and software are now available on the market, the quality of such material is highly variable. Some common problems are as follows:

- Certain review books are too detailed to allow for review in a reasonable amount of time or cover subtopics that are not emphasized on the exam.
- Many sample question books were originally written years ago and have not been adequately updated to reflect recent trends.
- Many sample question books use poorly written questions or contain factual errors in their explanations.
- Explanations for sample questions vary in quality.

Basic Science Review Books

If a given review book is not working for you, stop using it no matter how highly rated it may be or how much it costs.

In selecting review books, be sure to weigh different opinions against each other, read the reviews and ratings in Section IV of this guide, examine the books closely in the bookstore, and choose carefully. You are investing not only money but also your limited study time. Do not worry about finding the "perfect" book, as many subjects simply do not have one, and different students prefer different styles.

There are two types of review books: those that are stand-alone titles and those that are part of a series. Books in a series generally have the same style, and you must decide if that style works for you. However, a given style is not optimal for every subject. For example, charts and diagrams may be the best approach for physiology and biochemistry, whereas tables and outlines may be preferable for microbiology.

You should also find out which books are up to date. Some new editions represent major improvements, whereas others contain only cursory changes. Take into consideration how a book reflects the format of the USMLE Step 1.

Practice Tests

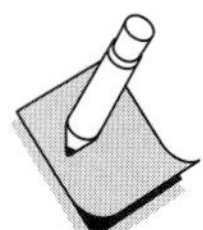

Most practice exams are shorter and less clinical than the real thing.

Taking practice tests provides valuable information about potential strengths and weaknesses in your fund of knowledge and test-taking skills. Some students use practice examinations simply as a means of breaking up the monotony of studying and adding variety to their study schedule, whereas other students rely almost solely on practice tests. Your best preview of the computerized exam can be found in the practice exams on the USMLE CD-ROM. Some students also recommend using computerized test simulation programs. In addition, students report that many current practice-exam books have questions that are, on average, shorter and less clinically oriented than the current USMLE Step 1.

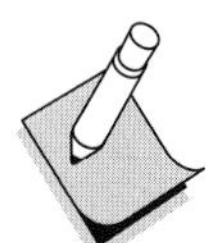

Use practice tests to identify concepts and areas of weakness, not just facts that you missed.

After taking a practice test, try to identify concepts and areas of weakness, not just the facts that you missed. Do not panic if you miss a lot of questions on a practice examination; instead, use the experience you have gained to motivate your study and prioritize those areas in which you need the most work. Use quality practice examinations to improve your test-taking skills. Analyze your ability to pace yourself.

Clinical Review Books

Keep your eye out for more clinically oriented review books; purchase them early and begin to use them. A number of students are turning to Step 2 books, pathophysiology books, and case-based reviews to prepare for the clinical vignettes. Examples of such books include:

- *First Aid for the® Wards* (McGraw-Hill)
- *First Aid Clerkship* series (McGraw-Hill)
- *Blueprints* clinical series (Lippincott Williams & Wilkins)
- *PreTest Physical Diagnosis* (McGraw-Hill)
- *Washington Manual* (Lippincott Williams & Wilkins)
- Various USMLE Step 2 review books

Texts, Syllabi, and Notes

Limit your use of texts and syllabi for Step 1 review. Many textbooks are too detailed for high-yield review and include material that is generally not tested on the USMLE Step 1 (e.g., drug dosages, complex chemical structures). Syllabi, although familiar, are inconsistent and frequently reflect the emphasis of individual faculty, which often does not correspond to that of the USMLE Step 1. Syllabi also tend to be less organized than top-rated books and generally contain fewer diagrams and study questions.

▶ GENERAL STUDY STRATEGIES

The USMLE Step 1 was created according to an integrated outline that organizes basic science material in a multidisciplinary approach. Broad-based knowledge is now more important than it was in the exams of previous years. The exam is designed to test basic science material and its application to clinical situations. Approximately three-quarters of the questions include clinical vignettes, although some are brief. Some useful studying guidelines are as follows:

Familiarize yourself with the commonly tested normal laboratory values.

- Be familiar with the CBT tutorial. This will give you 15 minutes of extra break time.
- Use computerized practice tests in addition to paper exams.
- Consider doing a simulated test at a Prometric center.
- Practice taking 50 questions in one-hour bursts.
- Be familiar with the Windows environment.
- Consider scheduling a light rotation for your first clinical block in case you get a test date later than you expected.

Practice questions that include case histories or descriptive vignettes are critical in preparing for the clinical slant of the USMLE Step 1. The normal lab values provided on the computerized test are difficult to use and access. For quick reference, see the table of high-yield laboratory values on the inside back cover of this book.

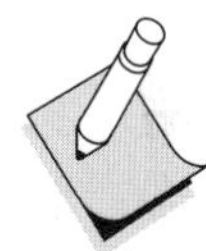

Practice questions that include case histories or descriptive vignettes are critical for Step 1 preparation.

▶ TEST-TAKING STRATEGIES

Your test performance will be influenced by both your fund of knowledge and your test-taking skills. You can strengthen your performance by considering each of these factors. Test-taking skills and strategies should be developed and perfected well in advance of the test date so that you can concentrate on the test itself. We suggest that you try the following strategies to see if they might work for you.

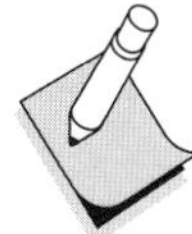

Practice and perfect test-taking skills and strategies well before the test date.

Pacing

You have seven hours to complete 350 questions. Note that each one-hour block contains 50 questions. This works out to about 72 seconds per question.

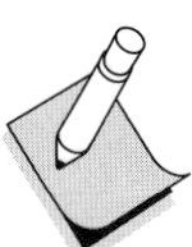

Time management is an important skill for exam success.

NBME officials note that time was not an issue for most takers of the CBT field test. However, pacing errors have in the past been detrimental to the performance of even highly prepared examinees. The bottom line is to keep one eye on the clock at all times!

Dealing with Each Question

There are several established techniques for efficiently approaching multiple-choice questions; see what works for you. One technique begins with identifying each question as easy, workable, or impossible. Your goal should be to answer all easy questions, resolve all workable questions in a reasonable amount of time, and make quick and intelligent guesses on all impossible questions. Most students read the stem, think of the answer, and turn immediately to the choices. A second technique is to first skim the answer choices and the last sentence of the question and then read through the passage quickly, extracting only relevant information to answer the question. Try a variety of techniques on practice exams and see what works best for you.

Difficult Questions

Do not dwell excessively on questions that you are on the verge of "figuring out." Make your best guess and move on.

Because of the exam's clinical emphasis, you may find that many of the questions on the Step 1 exam appear workable but take more time than is available to you. It can be tempting to dwell on such questions because you feel you are on the verge of "figuring it out," but resist this temptation and budget your time. Answer difficult questions with your best guess, mark them for review, and come back to them if you have time after you have completed the rest of the questions in the block. This will keep you from inadvertently leaving any questions blank in your efforts to "beat the clock."

Another reason for not dwelling too long on any one question is that certain questions may be **experimental** or may be **incorrectly phrased.** Moreover, not all questions are scored. Some questions serve as "embedded pretest items" that do not count toward your overall score.[11] In fact, anywhere from 10% to 20% of exam questions have been designated as experimental on past exams.

Remember that some questions may be experimental.

Guessing

There is **no penalty** for wrong answers. Thus, no test block should be left with unanswered questions. A hunch is probably better than a random guess. If you have to guess, we suggest selecting an answer you recognize over one that is totally unfamiliar to you.

Changing Your Answer

The conventional wisdom is not to change answers that you have already marked unless there is a convincing and logical reason to do so—in other words, go with your "first hunch." However, studies show that if you change your answer, you are twice as likely to change it from an incorrect answer to a correct one than vice versa. So if you have a strong "second hunch," go for it!

Your first hunch is not always correct.

Fourth-Quarter Effect (Avoiding Burnout)

Pacing and endurance are important. Practice helps develop both. Fewer and fewer examinees are leaving the examination session early. Use any extra time you might have at the end of each block to return to marked questions or to recheck your answers; you cannot add the extra time to any remaining blocks of questions or to your break time. Do not be too casual in your review or you may overlook serious mistakes. Remember your goals, and keep in mind the effort you have devoted to studying compared with the small additional effort you will need to maintain focus and concentration throughout the examination. Never give up. If you begin to feel frustrated, try taking a 30-second breather.

Do not terminate the block too early. Carefully review your answers if possible.

▶ CLINICAL VIGNETTE STRATEGIES

In recent years, the USMLE Step 1 has become increasingly clinically oriented. Students polled from 2003 exams reported that nearly 80% of the questions were presented as clinical vignettes. This change mirrors the trend in medical education toward introducing students to clinical problem solving during the basic science years. The increasing clinical emphasis on Step 1 may be challenging to those students who attend schools with a more traditional curriculum.

What Is a Clinical Vignette?

Be prepared to read fast and think on your feet!

A clinical vignette is a short (usually paragraph-long) description of a patient, including demographics, presenting symptoms, signs, and other information concerning the patient. Sometimes this paragraph is followed by a brief listing of important physical findings and/or laboratory results. The task of assimilating all this information and answering the associated question in the span of one minute can be intimidating. So be prepared to read quickly and think on your feet. Remember that the question is often indirectly asking something you already know.

Strategy

Step 1 vignettes usually describe diseases or disorders in their most classic presentation.

Remember that the Step 1 vignettes usually describe diseases or disorders in their most classic presentation. Look for buzzwords or cardinal signs (e.g., malar rash for SLE or nuchal rigidity for meningitis) in the narrative history. Be aware, however, that the question may contain classic signs and symptoms instead of mere buzzwords. Sometimes the data from labs and the physical exam will help you confirm or reject possible diagnoses, thereby helping you rule answer choices in or out. In some cases, they will be a dead giveaway for the diagnosis.

Sometimes making a diagnosis is not necessary at all.

Making a diagnosis from the history and data is often not the final answer. Not infrequently, the diagnosis is divulged at the end of the vignette, after you have just struggled through the narrative to come up with a diagnosis of your own. The question might then ask about a related aspect of the diagnosed disease.

One strategy that many students suggest is to skim the questions and answer choices before reading a vignette, especially if the vignette is lengthy. This focuses your attention on the relevant information and reduces the time spent on that vignette. Sometimes you may not need much of the information in the vignette to answer the question.

▶ TESTING AGENCIES

- **National Board of Medical Examiners (NBME)**
  Department of Licensing Examination Services
  3750 Market Street
  Philadelphia, PA 19104-3102
  (215) 590-9700
  Fax: (215) 590-9457
  E-mail: webmail@nbme.org
  www.nbme.org

- **Educational Commission for Foreign Medical Graduates (ECFMG)**
  3624 Market Street
  Philadelphia, PA 19104-2685
  (215) 386-5900
  Fax: (215) 386-9196
  E-mail: info@ecfmg.org
  www.ecfmg.org

- **Federation of State Medical Boards (FSMB)**
  P.O. Box 619850
  Dallas, TX 75261-9850
  (817) 868-4000
  Fax: (817) 868-4099
  E-mail: usmle@fsmb.org
  www.fsmb.org

- **USMLE Secretariat**
  3750 Market Street
  Philadelphia, PA 19104-3190
  (215) 590-9700
  E-mail: webmail@nbme.org
  www.usmle.org

▶ REFERENCES

1. Bidese, Catherine M., *U.S. Medical Licensure Statistics and Current Licensure Requirements 1995*, Chicago, American Medical Association, 1995.
2. National Board of Medical Examiners, *2002 USMLE Bulletin of Information*, Philadelphia, 2001.
3. National Board of Medical Examiners, *Bulletin of Information and Description of National Board Examinations, 1991*, Philadelphia, 1990.
4. Federation of State Medical Boards and National Board of Medical Examiners, *USMLE: 1993 Step 1 General Instructions, Content Outline, and Sample Items*, Philadelphia, 1992.
5. Pohl, Charles A., Robeson, Mary R., Hojat, Mohammadreza, and Veloski, J. Jon, "Sooner or Later? USMLE Step 1 Performance and Test Administration Date at the End of the Second Year," *Academic Medicine*, 2002, Vol. 77, No. 10, pp. S17–S19.
6. Case, Susan M., and Swanson, David B., "Validity of NBME Part I and Part II Scores for Selection of Residents in Orthopaedic Surgery, Dermatology, and Preventive Medicine," *Academic Medicine*, February Supplement 1993, Vol. 68, No. 2, pp. S51–S56.
7. Holtman, Matthew C., Swanson, David B., Ripkey, Douglas R., and Case, Susan M., "Using Basic Science Subject Tests to Identify Students at Risk for Failing Step 1," *Academic Medicine*, 2001, Vol. 76, No. 10, pp. S48–S51.
8. Basco, William T., Jr., Way, David P., Gilbert, Gregory E., and Hudson, Andy, "Undergraduate Institutional MCAT Scores as Predictors of USMLE Step 1 Performance," *Academic Medicine*, 2002, Vol. 77, No. 10, pp. S13–S16.
9. "Report on 1995 Examinations," *National Board Examiner*, Winter 1997, Vol. 44, No. 1, pp. 1–4.
10. O'Donnell, M. J., Obenshain, S. Scott, and Erdmann, James B., "I: Background Essential to the Proper Use of Results of Step 1 and Step 2 of the USMLE," *Academic Medicine*, October 1993, Vol. 68, No. 10, pp. 734–739.
11. Robinson, Adam, *What Smart Students Know*, New York, Crown Publishers, 1993.
12. Thadani, Raj A., Swanson, David B., and Galbraith, Robert M., "A Preliminary Analysis of Different Approaches to Preparing for the USMLE Step 1," *Academic Medicine*, 2000, Vol. 75, No. 10, pp. S40–S42.

NOTES

SECTION I SUPPLEMENT

Special Situations

▶ FIRST AID FOR THE INTERNATIONAL MEDICAL GRADUATE

"International medical graduate" (IMG) is the term now used to describe any student or graduate of a non-U.S., non-Canadian, non–Puerto Rican medical school, regardless of whether he or she is a U.S. citizen. The old term "foreign medical graduate" (FMG) was replaced because it was misleading when applied to U.S. citizens attending medical schools outside the United States.

The IMG's Steps to Licensure in the United States

If you are an IMG, you must go through the following steps (not necessarily in this order) to become licensed to practice in the United States. You must complete these steps even if you are already a practicing physician and have completed a residency program in your own country.

- Complete the basic sciences program of your medical school (equivalent to the first two years of U.S. medical school).
- Take the USMLE Step 1. You can do this while still in school or after graduating, but in either case your medical school must certify that you completed the basic sciences portion of your school's curriculum before taking the USMLE Step 1.
- Complete the clinical clerkship program of your medical school (equivalent to the third and fourth years of U.S. medical school).
- Take the USMLE Step 2 Clinical Knowledge (CK) exam. If you are still in medical school, you must have completed two years of school.
- Take the Step 2 Clinical Skills (CS) exam.
- Graduate with your medical degree.
- Then, send the ECFMG a copy of your degree and transcript, which they will verify with your medical school.
- Obtain an ECFMG certificate. To do this, candidates must accomplish the following:
  - Graduate from a medical school that is listed in the International Medical Education Directory (IMED). The list can be accessed at www.ecfmg.org.
  - Pass Step 1, the Step 2 CK, and the Step 2 CS within a seven-year period.
  - Have your medical credentials verified by the ECFMG.
- The standard certificate is usually sent two weeks after all the above requirements have been fulfilled. You must have a valid certificate before entering an accredited residency program, although you may begin the application process before you receive your certification.
- Apply for residency positions in your field of interest, either directly or through the Electronic Residency Application Service (ERAS) and the National Residency Matching Program ("the Match"). To be entered into the Match, you need to have passed all the examinations necessary for ECFMG certification (i.e., Step 1, the Step 2 CK, and the Step 2 CS) by the rank order list deadline (February 27, 2008, for the 2008 Match). If you do not pass these exams by the deadline, you will be withdrawn from the Match.

More detailed information can be found in the 2008 edition of the ECFMG Information Booklet, *available at www.ecfmg.org/pubshome.html.*

Applicants may apply online for the USMLE Step 2 CK or Step 2 CS or request an extension of the USMLE eligibility period at www.ecfmg.org/usmle/index.html or www.ecfmg.org/usmle/step2cs/index.html.

- Obtain a visa that will allow you to enter and work in the United States if you are not already a U.S. citizen or a green-card holder (permanent resident).
- If required for IMGs by the state in which your residency is located, obtain an educational/training/limited medical license. Your residency program may assist you with this application. Note that medical licensing is the prerogative of each individual state, not of the federal government, and that states vary with respect to their laws about licensing (although all 50 states recognize the USMLE).
- In order to begin your residency program, make sure your scores are valid.
- Once you have the ECFMG certification, take the USMLE Step 3 during your residency, and then obtain a full medical license. Once you have a license in any state, you are permitted to practice in federal institutions such as VA hospitals and Indian Health Service facilities in any state. This can open the door to "moonlighting" opportunities and possibilities for an H1B visa application. For details on individual state rules, write to the licensing board in the state in question or contact the FSMB.
- Complete your residency and then take the appropriate specialty board exams in order to become board certified (e.g., in internal medicine or surgery). If you already have a specialty certification in your home country (e.g., in surgery or cardiology), some specialty boards may grant you six months' or one year's credit toward your total residency time.
- Currently, many residency programs are accepting applications through ERAS. For more information, see *First Aid for the Match* or contact:

  ECFMG/ERAS Program
  P.O. Box 11746
  Philadelphia, PA 19101-0746
  (215) 386-5900
  e-mail: eras-support@ecfmg.org
  www.ecfmg.org/eras

The USMLE and the IMG

The USMLE is a series of standardized exams that give IMGs a level playing field. It is the same exam series taken by U.S. graduates even though it is administered by the ECFMG rather than by the NBME. This means that passing marks for IMGs for Step 1, the Step 2 CK, and the Step 2 CS are determined by a statistical process that is based on the scores of U.S. medical students. For example, to pass Step 1, you will probably have to score higher than the bottom 8–10% of U.S. and Canadian graduates.

Timing of the USMLE

For an IMG, the timing of a complete application is critical. It is extremely important that you send in your application early if you are to garner the maximum number of interview calls. A rough guide would be to complete all exam requirements by August of the year in which you wish to apply. This would translate into sending both your score sheets and your ECFMG certificate with your application.

In terms of USMLE exam order, arguments can be made for taking the Step 1 or the Step 2 CK exam first. For example, you may consider taking the Step 2 CK exam first if you have just graduated from medical school and the clinical topics are still fresh in your mind. However, keep in mind that there is substantial overlap between Step 1 and Step 2 CK topics in areas such as pharmacology, pathophysiology, and biostatistics. You might therefore consider taking the Step 1 and Step 2 CK exams close together to take advantage of this overlap in your test preparation.

USMLE Step 1 and the IMG

What Is the USMLE Step 1? It is a computerized test of the basic medical sciences that consists of 350 multiple-choice questions divided into seven blocks.

Content. Step 1 includes test items in the following content areas:

- Anatomy
- Behavioral sciences
- Biochemistry
- Microbiology and immunology
- Pathology
- Pharmacology
- Physiology
- Interdisciplinary topics such as nutrition, genetics, and aging

Significance of the Test. Step 1 is required for the ECFMG certificate as well as for registration for the Step 2 CS. Since most U.S. graduates apply to residency with their Step 1 scores only, it may be the only objective tool available with which to compare IMGs with U.S. graduates.

Official Web Sites. www.usmle.org and www.ecfmg.org/usmle.

Eligibility. Both students and graduates from medical schools that are listed in IMED are eligible to take the test. Students must have completed at least two years of medical school by the beginning of the eligibility period selected.

Eligibility Period. A three-month period of your choice.

Fee. The fee for Step 1 is $695 plus an international test delivery surcharge (if you choose a testing region other than the United States or Canada).

Retaking the Exam. In the event that you failed the test, you can reapply and select an eligibility period that begins at least 60 days after the last attempt. You cannot take the same Step more than three times in any 12-month period. You cannot retake the exam if you passed. The minimum score to pass the exam is 75 on a two-digit scale. To pass, you must answer roughly 60–65% of the questions correctly.

Statistics. In 2006, only 71% of ECFMG candidates passed Step 1 on their first attempt, compared with 92% of U.S. and Canadian medical students and graduates. Of note, 1994–1995 data showed that USFMGs (U.S. citizens attending non-U.S. medical schools) performed 0.4 SD lower than IMGs (non-U.S. citizens attending non-U.S. medical schools). Although their overall scores were lower, USFMGs performed better than IMGs on behavioral sciences. In general, students from non-U.S. medical schools perform worst in behavioral science and biochemistry (1.9 and 1.5 SDs below U.S. students) and comparatively better in gross anatomy and pathology (0.7 and 0.9 SD below U.S. students). Although derived from data collected in 1994–1995, these data may help you focus your studying efforts.

Tips. Although few if any students feel totally prepared to take Step 1, IMGs in particular require serious study and preparation in order to reach their full potential on this exam. It is also imperative that IMGs do their best on Step 1, as a poor score on Step 1 is a distinct disadvantage in applying for most residencies. Remember that if you pass Step 1, you cannot retake it in an attempt to improve your score. Your goal should thus be to beat the mean, because you can then assert with confidence that you have done better than average for U.S. students. Good Step 1 scores will also lend credibility to your residency application and help you get into highly competitive specialties such as radiology, orthopedics, and dermatology.

Commercial Review Courses. Do commercial review courses help improve your scores? Reports vary, and such courses can be expensive. Many IMGs decide to try the USMLE on their own and then consider a review course only if they fail. Just keep in mind that many states require that you pass the USMLE within three attempts. (For more information on review courses, see Section IV.)

USMLE Step 2 CK and the IMG

What Is the Step 2 CK? It is a computerized test of the clinical sciences consisting of 368 multiple-choice questions divided into eight blocks. It can be taken at Prometric centers in the United States and several other countries.

Content. The Step 2 CK includes test items in the following content areas:

- Internal medicine
- Obstetrics and gynecology
- Pediatrics
- Preventive medicine
- Psychiatry
- Surgery
- Other areas relevant to the provision of care under supervision

Significance of the Test. The Step 2 CK is required for the ECFMG certificate. It reflects the level of clinical knowledge of the applicant. It tests clinical subjects, primarily internal medicine. Other areas that are tested are surgery, obstetrics and gynecology, pediatrics, orthopedics, psychiatry, ENT, ophthalmology, and medical ethics.

Official Web Sites. www.usmle.org and www.ecfmg.org/usmle.

Eligibility. Students and graduates from medical schools that are listed in IMED are eligible to take the Step 2 CK. Students must have completed at least two years of medical school. This means that students must have completed the basic medical science component of the medical school curriculum by the beginning of the eligibility period selected.

Eligibility Period. A three-month period of your choice.

Fee. The fee for the Step 2 CK is $695 plus an international test delivery surcharge (if you choose a testing region other than the United States or Canada).

Retaking the Exam. In the event that you fail the Step 2 CK, you can reapply and select an eligibility period that begins at least 60 days after the last attempt. You cannot take the same Step more than three times in any 12-month period. You cannot retake the exam if you passed.

Statistics. In 2005–2006, 85% of ECFMG candidates passed Step 2 on their first attempt, compared with 98% of U.S. and Canadian candidates.

Tips. It's better to take the Step 2 CK after your internal medicine rotation because most of the questions on the exam give clinical scenarios and ask you to make medical diagnoses and clinical decisions. In addition, because this is a clinical sciences exam, cultural and geographic considerations play a greater role than is the case with Step 1. For example, if your medical education gave you ample exposure to malaria, brucellosis, and malnutrition but little to alcohol withdrawal, child abuse, and cholesterol screening, you must work to familiarize yourself with topics that are more heavily emphasized in U.S. medicine. You must also have a basic understanding of the legal and social aspects of U.S. medicine, because you will be asked questions about communicating with and advising patients.

USMLE Step 2 CS and the IMG

What Is the Step 2 CS? The Step 2 CS is a test of clinical and communication skills administered as a one-day, eight-hour exam. It includes 10 to 12 encounters with standardized patients (15 minutes each, with 10 minutes to write a note after each encounter). Test results are valid indefinitely.

Content. The Step 2 CS tests the ability to communicate in English as well as interpersonal skills, data-gathering skills, the ability to perform a physical exam, and the ability to formulate a brief note, a differential diagnosis, and a list of diagnostic tests. The areas that are covered in the exam are as follows:

- Internal medicine
- Surgery
- Obstetrics and gynecology
- Pediatrics
- Psychiatry
- Family medicine

Unlike the USMLE Step 1, Step 2 CK, or Step 3, there are no numerical grades for the Step 2 CS—it's simply either a "pass" or a "fail." To pass, a candidate must attain a passing performance in **each** of the following three components:

- Integrated Clinical Encounter (ICE): includes Data Gathering, Physical Exam, and the Patient Note
- Spoken English Proficiency (SEP)
- Communication and Interpersonal Skills (CIS)

According to the NBME, the most common component failed by IMGs on the Step 2 CS is the CIS component.

Significance of the Test. The Step 2 CS is required for the ECFMG certificate. It has eliminated the Test of English as a Foreign Language (TOEFL) as a requirement for ECFMG certification.

Official Web Site. www.ecfmg.org/usmle/step2cs.

Eligibility. Students must have completed at least two years of medical school in order to take the test. That means students must have completed the basic medical science component of the medical school curriculum at the time they apply for the exam.

Fee. The fee for the Step 2 CS is $1200.

Scheduling. You must schedule the Step 2 CS within **four months** of the date indicated on your notification of registration. You must take the exam within 12 months of the date indicated on your notification of registration. It is generally advisable to take the Step 2 CS as soon as possible in the year before your Match, as often the results either come in late or arrive too late to allow you to retake the test and pass it before the Match.

Retaking the Exam. There is no limit to the number of attempts you can make to pass the Step 2 CS. However, you cannot retake the exam within 60 days of a failed attempt, and you cannot take it more than three times in a 12-month period.

Test Site Locations. The Step 2 CS is currently administered at the following five locations:

- Philadelphia, PA
- Atlanta, GA
- Los Angeles, CA
- Chicago, IL
- Houston, TX

For more information about the Step 2 CS exam, please refer to *First Aid for the Step 2 CS.*

USMLE Step 3 and the IMG

What Is the USMLE Step 3? It is a two-day computerized test in clinical medicine consisting of 480 multiple-choice questions and nine computer-based case simulations (CCS). The exam aims at testing your knowledge and its application to patient care and clinical decision making (i.e., this exam tests if you can safely practice medicine independently and without supervision).

Significance of the Test. Taking Step 3 before residency is critical for IMGs seeking an H1B visa and is also a bonus that can be added to the residency application. Step 3 is also required to obtain a full medical license in the United States and can be taken during residency for this purpose.

Official Web Site. www.usmle.org.

Fee. The fee for Step 3 is $655 (the total application fee can vary among states).

Eligibility. Most states require that applicants have completed one, two, or three years of postgraduate training (residency) before they apply for Step 3 and permanent state licensure. The exceptions are the 13 states mentioned below, which allow IMGs to take Step 3 at the beginning of or even before residency. So if you don't fulfill the prerequisites to taking Step 3 in your state of choice, simply use the name of one of the 13 states in your Step 3 application. You can take the exam in any state you choose regardless of the state that you mentioned on your application. Once you pass Step 3, it will be recognized by all states. Basic eligibility requirements for the USMLE Step 3 are as follows:

- Obtaining an MD or DO degree (or its equivalent) by the application deadline.
- Obtaining an ECFMG certificate if you are a graduate of a foreign medical school or are successfully completing a "fifth pathway" program (at a date no later than the application deadline).
- Meeting the requirements imposed by the individual state licensing authority to which you are applying to take Step 3. Please refer to www.fsmb.org for more information.

The following states do not have postgraduate training as an eligibility requirement to apply for Step 3:

- Arkansas
- California
- Connecticut
- Florida
- Louisiana
- Maryland
- Nebraska*
- New York
- South Dakota
- Texas
- Utah*
- Washington
- West Virginia

* Requires that IMGs obtain a "valid indefinite" ECFMG certificate.

The Step 3 exam is not available outside the United States. Applications can be found online at www.fsmb.org and must be submitted to the FSMB.

Residencies and the IMG

It is becoming increasingly difficult for IMGs to obtain residencies in the United States given the rising concern about an oversupply of physicians in this country. Official bodies such as the Council on Graduate Medical Education (COGME) have recommended that the total number of residency slots be reduced. Furthermore, changes in immigration law are likely to make it much harder for noncitizens or legal residents of the United States to remain in the country after completing a residency.

In the residency Match, the number of U.S.-citizen IMG applications has been stable for the past few years, while the percentage accepted has slowly increased. For non-U.S.-citizen IMGs, applications fell from 7977 in 1999 to 5554 in 2005, while the percentage accepted significantly increased (see Table 5). This decrease in the total number of IMGs applying for the Match may be attributed to several factors:

- A decrease in the Step 2 CS passing rate to 80%.
- Increased difficulty obtaining U.S. visas.
- Increased expenses associated with the USMLE exams, ERAS, and travel to the United States.
- An increase in the number of IMGs who are withdrawing from the Match to sign a separate "pre-Match" contract with programs.

More information about residency programs can be obtained at www.ama-assn.org.

TABLE 5. IMGs in the Match.

Applicants	2005	2006	2007
U.S.-citizen IMGs	2,091	2,435	2,694
% U.S.-citizen IMGs accepted	55	51	50
Non-U.S.-citizen IMGs	5,554	6,442	6,992
% non-U.S.-citizen IMGs accepted	56	49	46
U.S. graduates (non-IMGs)	14,719	15,008	15,206
% U.S. graduates accepted	94	94	93

The Match and the IMG

Given the growing number of IMG candidates with strong applications, you should bear in mind that good USMLE scores are not the only way to gain a competitive edge. However, USMLE Step 1 and Step 2 CK scores continue to be used as the initial screening mechanism when candidates are being considered for interviews.

Based on accumulated IMG Match experiences over recent years, here are a few pointers to help IMGs maximize their chances for a residency interview.

The IMG Checklist

- **Apply early.** Programs offer a limited number of interviews and often select candidates on a first-come, first-served basis. Because of this, you should aim to complete the entire process of applying for the ERAS token, registering with the Association of American Medical Colleges (AAMC), mailing necessary documents to ERAS, and completing the ERAS application before September (see Figure 5). Community programs usually send out interview offers earlier than do university and university-affiliated programs.
- **U.S. clinical experience helps.** Externships and observerships in an American hospital setting have emerged as an important credential on an IMG application. Externships are like short-term medical school internships and offer hands-on clinical experience. Observerships, also called "shadowing," involve following a physician and observing how he or she manages patients. Externships are considered superior to observerships, but having either of them is always better than having none. Some programs require students to have participated in an externship or observership before applying. It is best to gain such an experience before or at the time you apply to various programs so that you can mention it on your ERAS application. If such an experience or opportunity comes up after you apply, be sure to inform the programs accordingly.

FIGURE 5. **IMG Timeline for Application.**

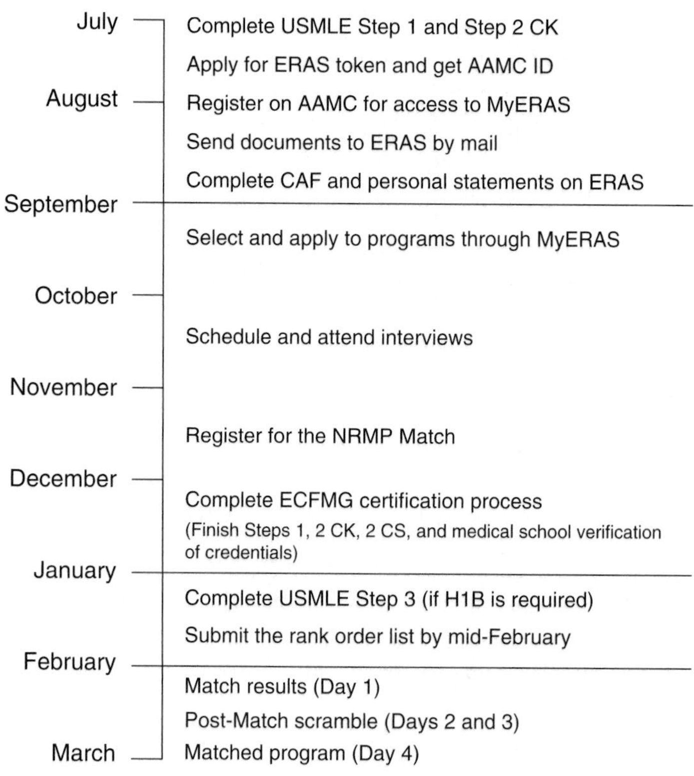

- **Clinical research helps.** University programs are attracted to candidates who show a strong interest in clinical research and academics. They may even relax their application criteria for individuals with unique backgrounds and strong research experience. Publications in well-known journals are an added bonus.
- **Time the Step 2 CS well.** ECFMG has published the new Step 2 CS score-reporting schedule for the years 2007–2008 at http://ecfmg.org/announce.htm#reportsched. Most program directors would like to see a passing score on Step 1, Step 2 CK, and Step 2 CS before they rank an IMG on their rank order list in mid-February. There have been too many instances in which candidates have relinquished a position on the rank order list—and have thus lost a potential match—either because of delayed CS results or because they have been unable to retake the exam on time following a failure. It is difficult to predict a result on the Step 2 CS, since the grading process is not very transparent. Therefore, it is advisable to take the Step 2 CS as early as possible in the application year.
- **U.S. letters of recommendation (LORs) help.** LORs from clinicians practicing in the United States carry more weight than recommendations from home countries.
- **Step up the Step 3.** If H1B visa sponsorship is desired, aim to have Step 3 results by January of the Match year. In addition to the visa advantage you

will gain, an early and good Step 3 score may benefit IMGs who have been away from clinical medicine for a while as well as those who have low scores on Step 1 and Step 2 CK.

- **Verify medical credentials in a timely manner.** Do not overlook the medical school credential verification process. The ECFMG certificate arrives only after credentials have been verified and after you have passed Step 1, Step 2 CK, and Step 2 CS, so you should keep track of the process and keep checking with ECFMG from time to time about your status.
- **Schedule interviews with pre-Matches in mind.** Schedule interviews with your favorite programs first. This will leave you better prepared to make a decision in the event that you are offered a pre-Match position.

Visa Options for the IMG

If you are living outside the United States, you will need to apply for a visa that will allow you lawful entry into the United States in order to take the Step 2 CS and/or do your interviews for residency. A B1 or B2 visitor visa may be issued by the U.S. consulate in your country. Citizens of some countries may have to undergo an additional security check that could take up to six months. Upon your entry into the United States, either the B1 or, more commonly, the B2 will be issued on your I-94. Both visas allow you a limited period within which to stay in the United States (two to six months) in order to take the exam. If the given period is not sufficient, you may apply for an extension before the expiration of your I-94.

Documents that are recommended to facilitate this process include the following:

- The Step 2 CS admission permit and a letter from the ECFMG (which explains why the applicant must enter the United States)
- Your medical diploma
- Transcripts from your medical school
- Your USMLE score sheets
- A sponsor letter or affidavit of support stating that you (if you are sponsoring yourself) or your sponsor will bear the expense of your trip and that you have sufficient funds to meet that expense
- An alien status affidavit

Individuals from certain countries may be allowed to enter the United States for up to 90 days without a visa under the Visa Waiver Program. See http://uscis.gov.

As an IMG, you need a visa to work or train in the United States unless you are a U.S. citizen or a permanent resident (i.e., hold a green card). Two types of visas enable you to accept a residency appointment in the United States: J1 and H1B. Most sponsoring residency programs (SRPs) prefer a J1 visa. Above all, this is because SRPs are authorized by the Department of Homeland Security (DHS) to issue a Form DS-2019 directly to an IMG. By contrast, SRPs must complete considerable paperwork, including an application to the Immigration and Labor Department, to apply to the DHS for an H1B visa on behalf of an IMG.

The J1 Visa

Also known as the Exchange Visitor Program, the J1 visa was introduced to give IMGs in diverse specialties the chance to use their training experience in the United States to improve conditions in their home countries. As mentioned above, the DHS authorizes most SRPs to issue Form DS-2019 in the same manner that I-20s are issued to regular international students in the United States.

To enable an SRP to issue a DS-2019, you must obtain a certificate from the ECFMG indicating that you are eligible to participate in a residency program in the United States. First, however, you must ask the Ministry of Health in your country to issue a statement indicating that your country needs physicians with the skills you propose to acquire from a U.S. residency program. This statement, which must bear the seal of your country's government and must be signed by a duly designated government official, is intended to satisfy the U.S. Secretary of Health and Human Services (HHS) that there is such a need. The Health Ministry in your country should send this statement to the ECFMG (or they may allow you to mail it to the ECFMG).

How can you find out if the government of your country will issue such a statement? In many countries, the Ministry of Health maintains a list of medical specialties in which there is a need for further training abroad. You can also consult seniors in your medical school. A word of caution: If you are applying for a residency in internal medicine and internists are not in short supply in your country, it may help to indicate an intention to pursue a subspecialty after completing your residency training.

The text of your statement of need should read as follows:

> Name of applicant for visa: ___________. There currently exists in ___________ (your country) a need for qualified medical practitioners in the specialty of ___________. (Name of applicant for visa) has filed a written assurance with the government of this country that he/she will return to ___________ (your country) upon completion of training in the United States and intends to enter the practice of medicine in the specialty for which training is being sought.
>
> Stamp (or seal and signature) of issuing official of named country. Dated ___________

To facilitate the issuing of such a statement by the Ministry of Health in your country, you should submit a certified copy of the agreement or a contract from your SRP in the United States. The agreement or contract must be signed by you and the residency program official responsible for the training.

Armed with Form DS-2019, you should then go to the U.S. consulate closest to the residential address indicated in your passport. As for other nonimmigrant visas, you must show that you have a genuine nonimmigrant intent to return to your home country. You must also show that all your expenses will be paid.

When you enter the United States, bring your Form DS-2019 along with your visa. You are usually admitted to the United States for the length of the J1 program, designated as "D/S," or duration of status. The duration of your program is indicated on the DS-2019.

In the wake of the terrorist attacks of September 11, 2001, a number of new regulations have been introduced to improve the monitoring of exchange visitors during their time in the United States. All SRPs and students are currently required to register with the Student and Exchange Visitor Program (SEVP) via the Student and Exchange Visitor Information System (SEVIS). SEVIS allows the DHS to maintain up-to-date information (e.g., enrollment status, current address) on exchange visitors. SEVIS Form DS-2019 is used for visa applications, admission, and change of status. Procedural details for this new legislation are still being hammered out, so contact your SRP or check http://uscis.gov for the most current information.

Duration of Participation. The duration of a resident's participation in a program of graduate medical education or training is limited to the time normally required to complete such a program. If you would like to get an idea of the typical training time for the various medical subspecialties, you may consult the *Directory of Medical Specialties*, published by Marquis Who's Who for the American Board of Medical Specialties. The authority charged with determining the duration of time required by an individual IMG is the State Department. The maximum amount of time for participation in a training program is ordinarily limited to seven years unless the IMG has demonstrated to the satisfaction of the ECFMG and the State Department that his or her home country has an exceptional need for the specialty in which he or she will receive further training. An extension of stay may be granted in the event that an IMG needs to repeat a year of clinical medical training or needs time for training or education to take an exam required for board certification.

Requirements after Entry into the United States. Each year, all IMGs participating in a residency program on a J1 visa must furnish the Attorney General of the United States with an affidavit (Form I-644) attesting that they are in good standing in the program of graduate medical education or training in which they are participating and that they will return to their home countries upon completion of the education or training for which they came to the United States.

Restrictions under the J1 Visa. No later than two years after the date of entry into the United States, an IMG participating in a residency program on a J1 visa is allowed one opportunity to change his or her designated program of graduate medical education or training if his or her director approves that change.

The J1 visa includes a condition called the "two-year foreign residence requirement." The relevant section of the Immigration and Nationality Act states:

> Any exchange visitor physician coming to the United States on or after January 10, 1977, for the purpose of receiving graduate medical education or training is automatically subject to the two-year home-country physical presence requirement of section 212(e) of the Immigration and Nationality Act, as amended. Such physicians are not eligible to be considered for section 212(e) waivers on the basis of "No Objection" statements issued by their governments.

The law thus requires that a J1 visa holder, upon completion of the training program, leave the United States and reside in his or her home country for a period of at least two years. Currently, the American Medical Association (AMA) is advocating that this period be extended to five years.

An IMG on a J1 visa is ordinarily not allowed to change from a J1 to most other types of visas or (in most cases) to change from J1 to permanent residence while in the United States until he or she has fulfilled the "foreign residence requirement." The purpose of the foreign residence requirement is to ensure that an IMG uses the training he or she obtained in the United States for the benefit of his or her home country. The U.S. government may, however, waive the two-year foreign residence requirement under the following circumstances:

- If you as an IMG can prove that returning to your country would result in "exceptional hardship" to you or to members of your immediate family who are U.S. citizens or permanent residents;
- If you as an IMG can demonstrate a "well-founded fear of persecution" due to race, religion, or political opinions if forced to return to your country;
- If you obtain a "no objection" statement from your government; or
- If you are sponsored by an "interested governmental agency" or a designated state Department of Health in the United States.

Applying for a J1 Visa Waiver. IMGs who have sought a waiver on the basis of the last alternative have found it beneficial to approach the following potentially "interested government agencies":

- **The Department of Health and Human Services.** Recently, HHS has expanded its role in reviewing J1 waiver applications. HHS's considerations for a waiver have classically been as follows: (1) the program or activity in which the IMG is engaged is "of high priority and of national or international significance in an area of interest" to HHS; (2) the IMG must be an "integral" part of the program or activity "so that the loss of his/her services would necessitate discontinuance of the program or a major phase of it"; and (3) the IMG "must possess outstanding qualifications, training, and experience well beyond the usually expected accomplishments at the graduate, postgraduate, and residency levels and must clearly demonstrate the capability to make original and significant contributions to the program." Under these criteria, HHS waivers are granted to physicians working in high-level biomedical research.

New rules will also allow HHS to review J1 waiver applications from community health centers, rural hospitals, and other health care providers. In the past, the U.S. Department of Agriculture (USDA) served as the interested federal government agency that reviewed waiver applications to allow foreign doctors to serve in rural underserved communities outside Appalachia, while the Appalachian Regional Commission (ARC) played that role for Appalachian communities. The USDA is no longer handling applications for J1 waivers. HHS will now review waiver applications for primary care practitioners and psychiatrists who have completed residency training within one year of application to practice in designated Health Professional Shortage Areas (HPSAs), Medically Underserved Areas and Populations (MUA/Ps), and Mental Health Professional Shortage Areas (MHPSAs). HHS waiver applications should be mailed to Joyce E. Jones, Executive Secretary, Exchange Visitor Waiver Review Board, Room 639-H, Hubert H. Humphrey Building, Department of Health and Human Services, 200 Independence Avenue, S.W., Washington, D.C. 20201; phone (202) 690-6174.

- **The Department of Veterans Affairs.** With more than 170 health care facilities located in various parts of the United States, the VA is a major employer of physicians in this country. In addition, many VA hospitals are affiliated with university medical centers. The VA sponsors IMGs working in research, patient care (regardless of specialty), and teaching. The waiver applicant may engage in teaching and research in conjunction with clinical duties. The VA's latest guidelines (issued on June 22, 1994) provide that it will act as an interested government agency only when the loss of an IMG's services would necessitate the discontinuance of a program or a major phase of it and when recruitment efforts have failed to locate a U.S. physician to fill the position.

  The procedure for obtaining a VA sponsorship for a J1 waiver is as follows: (1) the IMG should deal directly with the Human Resources Department at the local VA facility; and (2) the facility must request that the VA's chief medical director sponsor the IMG for a waiver. The waiver request should include the following documentation: (1) a letter from the director of the local facility describing the program, the IMG's immigration status, the health care needs of the facility, and the facility's recruitment efforts; (2) recruitment efforts, including copies of all job advertisements run within the preceding year; and (3) copies of the IMG's licenses, test results, board certifications, IAP-66 or SEVIS DS-2019 forms, and the like. The VA contact person in Washington, D.C., should be contacted by the local medical facility rather than by IMGs or their attorneys.

- **The Appalachian Regional Commission.** ARC sponsors physicians in certain places in the eastern and southern United States—namely, in Alabama, Georgia, Kentucky, Maryland, Mississippi, New York, North Carolina, Ohio, Pennsylvania, South Carolina, Tennessee, Virginia, and West Virginia. Since 1992, ARC has sponsored approximately 200 primary care IMGs annually in counties within its jurisdiction that have been designated as HPSAs by HHS.

  In accordance with its February 1994 revision of its J1 waiver policies, ARC requires that waiver requests initially be submitted to the ARC contact person in the state of intended employment. Contact information for each state can be found on the ARC Web site (www.arc.gov). If the state concurs, a letter from the state's governor recommending the waiver must be addressed to Anne B. Pope, the new federal cochair of ARC. The waiver request should include the following: (1) a letter from the facility to Ms. Pope stating the proposed dates of employment, the IMG's medical specialty, the address of the practice location, an assertion that the IMG will practice primary care for at least 40 hours per week in the HPSA, and details as to why the facility needs the services of the IMG; (2) a J1 Visa Data Sheet; (3) the ARC federal cochair's J1 Visa Waiver Policy and the J1 Visa Waiver Policy Affidavit and Agreement with the notarized signature of the IMG; (4) a contract of at least three years' duration; (5) evidence of the IMG's qualifications, including a résumé, medical diplomas and licenses, and IAP-66 or SEVIS DS-2019 forms; and (6) evidence of unsuccessful attempts to recruit qualified U.S. physicians within the preceding six months. Copies of advertisements, copies of résumés received, and reasons for rejection must also be included. ARC will not sponsor IMGs who have been out of status for six months or longer.

  Requests for ARC waivers are then processed in Washington, D.C. (ARC, 1666 Connecticut Avenue, N.W., Washington, D.C. 20009). ARC is usually able to forward a letter confirming that a waiver has been recommended to the requesting facility or attorney within 30 days of the request.

- **The Department of Agriculture.** At the time of publication, the USDA is no longer sponsoring J1 waivers. The scope of the HHS J1 waiver program has been expanded to fill the gap.

- **State Departments of Public Health.** There is no application form for a state-sponsored J1 waiver. However, regulations specify that an application must include the following documents: (1) a letter from the state Department of Public Health identifying the physician and specifying that it would be in the public interest to grant him or her a J1 waiver; (2) an employment contract that is valid for a minimum of three years and that states the name and address of the facility that will employ the physician and the geographic areas in which he or she will practice medicine; (3) evidence that these geographic areas are located within HPSAs; (4) a statement by the physician agreeing to the contractual requirements; (5) copies of all IAP-66 or SEVIS DS-2019 forms; and (6) a completed U.S. Information Agency (USIA) Data Sheet. Applications are numbered in the order in which they are received, since only 30 physicians per year may be granted waivers in a particular state under the Conrad State 30 program. Individual states may elect to participate or not to participate in this program. At the time of publication, nonparticipating states included Idaho, Oklahoma, and Wyoming, while Texas had suspended its J1 waiver program pending new legislation.

The H1B Visa

Since 1991, the law has allowed medical residency programs to sponsor foreign-born medical residents for H1B visas. There are no restrictions on changing the H1B visa to any other kind of visa, including permanent resident status (green card), through employer sponsorship or through close relatives who are U.S. citizens or permanent residents. It is advisable for SRPs to apply for H1B visas as soon as possible in the official year (beginning October 1) when the new quota officially opens up.

According to the Web site www.immihelp.com, as of October 17, 2000, the following beneficiaries of approved H1B petitions are exempt from the H1B annual cap:

- Beneficiaries who are in J1 nonimmigrant status in order to receive graduate medical education or training, and who have obtained a waiver of the two-year home residency requirement;
- Beneficiaries who are employed at, or who have received an offer of employment at, an institution of higher education or a related or affiliated nonprofit entity;
- Beneficiaries who are employed by, or who have received an offer of employment from, a nonprofit research organization;
- Beneficiaries who are employed by, or who have received an offer of employment from, a governmental research organization;
- Beneficiaries who are currently maintaining, or who have held within the last six years, H1B status, and are ineligible for another full six-year stay as an H1B; and
- Beneficiaries who have been counted once toward the numerical limit and are the beneficiary of multiple petitions.

H1B visas are intended for "professionals" in a "specialty occupation." This means that an IMG intending to pursue a residency program in the United States with an H1B visa needs to clear all three USMLE Steps before becoming eligible for the H1B. The ECFMG administers Steps 1 and 2, whereas Step 3 is conducted by the individual states. You will need to contact the FSMB or the medical board of the state where you intend to take Step 3 for details (see p. 34, USMLE Step 3 and the IMG).

H1B Application. An application for an H1B visa is filed not by the IMG but rather by his or her employment sponsor—in your case, by the SRP in the United States. If an SRP is willing to do so, you will be told about it at the time of your interview for the residency program.

Before filing an H1B application with the DHS, an SRP must file an application with the U.S. Department of Labor affirming that the SRP will pay at least the normal salary for your job that a U.S. professional would earn. After receiving approval from the Labor Department, your SRP should be ready to file the H1B application with the DHS. The SRP's supporting letter is the most important part of the H1B application package; it must describe the job duties to make it clear that the physician is needed in a "specialty occupation" (resident) under the prevalent legal definition of that term.

Most SRPs prefer to issue a SEVIS Form DS-2019 for a J1 visa rather than file papers for an H1B visa because of the burden of paperwork and the attorney costs involved in securing approval of an H1B visa application. Even so, a sizable number of SRPs are willing to go through the trouble, particularly if an IMG is an excellent candidate or if the SRP concerned finds it difficult to fill all the available residency slots (although this is becoming rarer with continuing cuts in residency slots). If an SRP is unwilling to file for an H1B visa because of attorney costs, you could suggest that you would be willing to bear the burden of such costs. The entire process of getting an H1B visa can take anywhere from 10 to 20 weeks.

H1B Premium Processing Service. According to the Web site www.myvisa.com, the DHS offers the opportunity to obtain processing of an H1B visa application within 15 calendar days. Within 15 days of receiving Form I-907, the DHS will mail you a notice of approval, request for evidence, intent to deny, or notice of investigation for fraud or misrepresentation. If the notice requires the submission of additional evidence or indicates an intent to deny, a new 15-day period will begin upon delivery to the DHS of a complete response to the request for evidence or notice of intent to deny. The fee for this service is $1000. With this service, the total time needed to obtain an H1B visa has become significantly shorter than that required for the J1.

Although an H1B visa can be stamped by any U.S. consulate abroad, it is advisable that you have it stamped at the U.S. consulate where you first applied for a visitor visa to travel to the United States for interviews.

A Final Word

IMGs should also be aware of a new program called the National Security Entry-Exit Registration System, which aims to tighten up homeland security by keeping closer tabs on nonimmigrants residing in or entering the United States on temporary visas.

Male citizens or nationals of specific countries who are already residing in the United States may be required to report to a designated DHS office for registration, which includes being fingerprinted, photographed, and interviewed under oath. The official list of countries includes Bangladesh, Egypt, Indonesia, Jordan, Kuwait, Pakistan, Saudi Arabia, Afghanistan, Algeria, Bahrain, Eritrea, Lebanon, Morocco, North Korea, Oman, Qatar, Somalia, Tunisia, the United Arab Emirates, Yemen, Iran, Iraq, Libya, Sudan, and Syria. Different registration deadlines and criteria have been assigned to citizens of the abovementioned countries, so please refer to http://uscis.gov for details.

If you are entering the United States, you may be registered at the port of entry if you are (1) a citizen or national of Iran, Iraq, Libya, Sudan, or Syria; (2) a nonimmigrant who has been designated by the State Department; or (3) any other nonimmigrant identified by immigration officers at airports, seaports, and land ports of entry in accordance with new regulation 8 CFR 264.1(f)(2). If you will be staying in the United States for more than 30 days, you will then be required to register in person at a DHS district office within 30 days for an interview and will be required to reregister annually.

Once you are registered, certain special procedures will apply. If you leave the United States for any reason, you must appear in person before a DHS inspecting officer at a preapproved airport, seaport, or land port and leave the United States from that port on the same day. If you change your address, employment, or school, you must report to the DHS in writing within 10 days using Form AR-11 SR. If any of these regulations are not followed, you may be considered out of status and subject to arrest, detention, fines, and/or removal from the United States, and any further application for immigration may be affected.

For the most up-to-date information regarding policies and procedures, please consult http://uscis.gov.

Summary

Despite some significant obstacles, a number of viable methods are available to IMGs who seek visas to pursue a residency program or eventually practice medicine in the United States. There is no doubt that the best alternative for an IMG is to obtain an H1B visa to pursue a medical residency. However, in cases where an IMG joins a residency program with a J1 visa, there are some possibilities for obtaining waivers of the two-year foreign residency requirement, particularly for those who are willing to make a commitment to perform primary care medicine in medically underserved areas.

Resources for the IMG

- **ECFMG**
  3624 Market Street
  Philadelphia, PA 19104-2685
  (215) 386-5900
  Fax: (215) 386-9196
  www.ecfmg.org

  The ECFMG telephone number is answered only between 9:00 A.M. and 12:30 P.M. and between 1:30 P.M. and 5:00 P.M. Monday through Friday EST. The ECFMG often takes a long time to answer the phone, which is frequently busy at peak times of the year, and then gives you a long voice-mail message—so it is better to write or fax early than to rely on a last-minute phone call. Do not contact the NBME, as all IMG exam matters are conducted by the ECFMG. The ECFMG also publishes an information booklet on ECFMG certification and the USMLE program, which gives details on the dates and locations of forthcoming USMLE and English tests for IMGs together with application forms. It is free of charge and is also available from the public affairs offices of U.S. embassies and consulates worldwide as well as from Overseas Educational Advisory Centers. You may order single copies of the handbook by calling (215) 386-5900, preferably on weekends or between 6 P.M. and 6 A.M. Philadelphia time, or by faxing to (215) 387-9963. Requests for multiple copies must be made by fax or mail on organizational letterhead. The full text of the booklet is also available on the ECFMG's Web site at www.ecfmg.org.

- **FSMB**
  P.O. Box 619850
  Dallas, TX 75261-9850
  (817) 868-4000
  Fax: (817) 868-4099
  www.fsmb.org

  The FSMB has a number of publications available, including *The Exchange, Section I*, which gives detailed information on examination and licensing requirements in all U.S. jurisdictions. The cost is $30. (Texas residents must add 8.25% state sales tax.) To obtain these publications, submit the online order form. Payment options include Visa or MasterCard. Alternatively, write to Federation Publications at the above address. All orders must be prepaid with a personal check drawn on a U.S. bank, a cashier's check, or a money order payable to the federation. Foreign orders must be accompanied by an international money order or the equivalent, payable in U.S. dollars through a U.S. bank or a U.S. affiliate of a foreign bank. For Step 3 inquiries, the telephone number is (817) 868-4041. You may e-mail the FSMB at usmle@fsmb.org or write to Examination Services at the address above.

- Immigration information for IMGs is available from the sites of Siskind Susser, a firm of attorneys specializing in immigration law: www.visalaw.com/IMG/resources.html.
- Another source of immigration information can be found on the Web site of the law offices of Carl Shusterman, a Los Angeles attorney specializing in medical immigration law: www.shusterman.com.
- The AMA has dedicated a portion of its Web site to information on IMG demographics, residencies, immigration, and the like: www.ama-assn.org/ama/pub/category/17.html.
- International Medical Placement Ltd., a U.S. company specializing in recruiting foreign physicians to work in the United States, has a site at www.intlmedicalplacement.com.
- Two more useful Web sites are www.myvisa.com and www.immihelp. com.
- *First Aid for the International Medical Graduate*, 2nd ed., by Keshav Chander (2002; 313 pages; ISBN 0071385320), is an excellent resource written by a successful IMG. The book includes interviews with successful IMGs and students gearing up for the USMLE, complete "getting settled" information for new residents, and tips for dealing with possible social and cultural transition difficulties. The book provides useful advice on the U.S. curriculum, the health care delivery system, and ethical issues—and the differences IMGs should expect. Dr. Chander points out the weaknesses often found in IMG hopefuls and suggests ways to improve their performance on standardized tests as well as on academic and clinical evaluations. As a bonus, the guide contains information on how to get good fellowships after residency. The bottom line is that this is a reassuring guide that can help IMGs boost their confidence and proficiency. A great "first of its kind" that will empower IMGs with information that they need to succeed.

Other books that may be useful and of interest to IMGs are as follows:

- *International Medical Graduates in U.S. Hospitals: A Guide for Directors and Applicants*, by Faroque A. Khan and Lawrence G. Smith (1995; ISBN 094312641X).
- *Insider's Guide for the International Medical Graduate to Obtain a Medical Residency in the U.S.A.*, by Ahmad Hakemi (1999; ISBN 1929803001).

What Is the COMLEX Level 1?

In 1995, the National Board of Osteopathic Medical Examiners (NBOME) introduced a new assessment tool called the Comprehensive Osteopathic Medical Licensing Examination, or COMLEX-USA. As with the former NBOME examination series, the COMLEX-USA is administered over three levels. In 1995, only Level 3 was administered, but by 1998 all three levels had been implemented. The COMLEX-USA is now the only exam offered to osteopathic students. One goal of this changeover is to have all 50 states recognize this examination as equivalent to the USMLE. Currently, the COMLEX-USA exam sequence is accepted for licensure in all 50 states.

The COMLEX-USA series assesses osteopathic medical knowledge and clinical skills using clinical presentations and physician tasks. A description of the COMLEX-USA Written Examination Blueprints for each level, which outline the various clinical presentations and physician tasks that examinees will encounter, is given on the NBOME Web site. Another stated goal of the COMLEX-USA Level 1 is to create a more primary care–oriented exam that integrates osteopathic principles into clinical situations. As of July 1, 2004, the NBOME has initiated the administration of a Performance Evaluation/Clinical Skills component of the COMLEX-USA designated Level 2-PE, which candidates must pass in order to be eligible for the COMLEX Level 3.

To be eligible to take the COMLEX-USA Level 1, you must have satisfactorily completed at least one-half of your sophomore year in an American Osteopathic Association (AOA)–approved medical school. In addition, you must obtain verification that you are in good standing at your medical school via approval of your dean. Applications may be downloaded from the NBOME Web site.

For all three levels of the COMLEX-USA, raw scores are converted to a percentile score and a score ranging from 5 to 800. For Levels 1 and 2, a score of 400 is required to pass; for Level 3, a score of 350 is needed. COMLEX-USA scores are usually mailed eight weeks after the test date. The mean score is always 500. From 2002 through October 2005, the standard deviation for Level 1 was 79.

If you pass a COMLEX-USA examination, you are not allowed to retake it to improve your grade. If you fail, there is no specific limit to the number of times you can retake it in order to pass. Level 2 and 3 exams must be passed in sequential order within seven years of passing Level 1.

What Is the Structure of the COMLEX Level 1?

The final paper-and-pencil COMLEX Level 1 examination was administered on October 11–12, 2005. In 2006, the NBOME began delivering the COMLEX Level 1 by computer. This conversion to a computer-based examination reduced the test duration from two days to one day, decreased the total number of questions from about 800 to 400, and decreased the total testing time from 16 hours to 8 hours.

The computer-based COMLEX Level 1 examination consists of multiple-choice questions in the same format as that of the old paper-and-pencil COMLEX Level 1 examination. Most of the questions are in one-best-answer format, but a small number are matching-type questions. Some one-best-answer questions are bundled together around a common question stem that usually takes the form of a clinical scenario. New question formats may gradually be introduced, but candidates will be notified if this occurs.

Questions are grouped into six sections of 50 questions each in a manner similar to the USMLE. Reviewing and changing answers may be done only in the current section. A "review page" is presented for each block in order to advise test takers of questions completed, questions marked for further review, and incomplete questions for which no answer has been given.

Only three optional breaks are permitted during the test session. These breaks are offered after the first two sections of the morning or afternoon session have been completed. The first optional 10-minute break is offered in the morning session after completion of section 2. The second optional 10-minute break is offered in the afternoon session after completion of section 6. These two blocks count against the total exam time. A 40-minute lunch break is also optional, but it will not count against the total exam time. This break may be taken after completion of section 4. This is an important departure from the USMLE. More information about the computer-based COMLEX-USA examinations can be obtained from www.nbome.org.

What Is the Difference Between the USMLE and the COMLEX-USA?

Although the COMLEX-USA and the USMLE are similar in scope, content, and emphasis, some differences are worth noting. For example, the COMLEX-USA Level 1 tests osteopathic principles in addition to basic science materials but does not emphasize lab techniques. In addition, although both exams often require that you apply and integrate knowledge over several areas of basic science to answer a given question, many students who took both tests in 2004 reported that the questions differed somewhat in style. Students reported, for example, that USMLE questions generally required that the test taker reason and draw from the information given (often a two-step process), whereas those on the COMLEX-USA exam tended to be more straightforward. Furthermore, USMLE questions were on average found to be considerably longer than those on the COMLEX-USA.

Students also commented that the COMLEX-USA utilized "buzzwords," although limited in their use (e.g., "rose spots" in typhoid fever), whereas the USMLE avoided buzzwords in favor of descriptions of clinical findings or symptoms (e.g., rose-colored papules on the abdomen rather than rose spots).

Finally, the 2004 USMLE had many more photographs than did the COMLEX-USA. In general, the overall impression was that the USMLE was a more "thought-provoking" exam, while the COMLEX-USA was more of a "knowledge-based" exam.

Who Should Take Both the USMLE and the COMLEX-USA?

Aside from facing the COMLEX-USA Level 1, you must decide if you will also take the USMLE Step 1. We recommend that you consider taking both the USMLE and the COMLEX-USA under the following circumstances:

- **If you are applying to allopathic residencies.** Although there is growing acceptance of COMLEX-USA certification on the part of allopathic residencies, some allopathic programs prefer or even require passage of the USMLE Step 1. These include many academic programs, programs in competitive specialties (e.g., orthopedics, ophthalmology, or dermatology), and programs in competitive geographic areas (such as California). Fourth-year doctor of osteopathy (DO) students who have already matched may be a good source of information about which programs and specialties look for USMLE scores. It is also a good idea to contact program directors at the institutions you are interested in to ask about their policy regarding the COMLEX-USA versus the USMLE.
- **If you are unsure about your postgraduate training plans.** Successful passage of both the COMLEX-USA Level 1 and the USMLE Step 1 is certain to provide you with the greatest possible range of options when you are applying for internship and residency training.

The clinical coursework that some DO students receive during the summer of their third year (as opposed to their starting clerkships) is considered helpful in integrating basic science knowledge for the COMLEX-USA or the USMLE.

How Do I Prepare for the COMLEX-USA Level 1?

Student experience suggests that you should start studying for the COMLEX-USA four to six months before the test is given, as an early start will allow you to spend up to a month on each subject. The recommendations made in Section I regarding study and testing methods, strategies, and resources, as well as the books suggested in Section IV for the USMLE Step 1, hold true for the COMLEX-USA as well.

Another important source of information is in the *Examination Guidelines and Sample Exam*, a booklet that discusses the breakdown of each subject while also providing sample questions and corresponding answers. Many students, however, felt that this breakdown provided only a general guideline and was not representative of the level of difficulty of the actual COMLEX-USA. The sample questions did not provide examples of clinical vignettes, which made up approximately 25% of the exam. You will receive this publication with registration materials for the COMLEX-USA Level 1 exam, but you can also receive a copy and additional information by writing:

NBOME
8765 W. Higgins Road, Suite 200
Chicago, IL 60631-4174
(773) 714-0622
Fax: (773) 714-0631

or by visiting the NBOME Web page at www.nbome.org.

Level 1 Practice Items is a new feature offered by the NBOME. It contains about 200 COMLEX-USA Level 1 items and answers. It is important to note that items in this booklet have been used in previous exams. The booklet costs $8 and can be purchased via the NBOME Web site.

The 2007 COMLEX-USA exam consisted of 50 questions per section. There were eight sections, with one hour dedicated to each section for an examination total of eight hours. Each multiple-choice question accompanied a small case (about one to two sentences long).

In 2007, students reported an emphasis in certain areas. For example:

- There was an increased emphasis on upper limb anatomy/brachial plexus.
- Specific topics were repeatedly tested on the exam. These included cardiovascular physiology and pathology, acid-base physiology, diabetes, benign prostatic hyperplasia, sexually transmitted diseases, measles, and rubella. Thyroid and adrenal function, neurology (head injury), specific drug treatments for bacterial infection, migraines/cluster headaches, and drug mechanisms also received heavy emphasis.
- Behavioral science questions were based on psychiatry.
- High-yield osteopathic manipulative technique (OMT) topics on the 2007 exam included an extremely heavy emphasis on the sympathetic and parasympathetic innervations of viscera and nerve roots, rib mechanics/diagnosis, and basic craniosacral theory.

Since topics that were repeatedly tested appeared in all four booklets, students found it useful to review them in between the two test days. It is important to understand that the topics emphasized on the 2007 exam may not be stressed on the 2008 exam. However, some topics are heavily tested each year, so it may be beneficial to have a solid foundation of the above-mentioned topics.

The National Board of Podiatric Medical Examiners (NBPME) tests are designed to assess whether a candidate possesses the knowledge required to practice as a minimally competent entry-level podiatrist. The NBPME examinations are used as part of the licensing process governing the practice of podiatric medicine. The NBPME exam is recognized by all 50 states and the District of Columbia, the U.S. Army, the U.S. Navy, and the Canadian provinces of Alberta, British Columbia, and Ontario. Individual states use the examination scores differently; therefore, doctor of podiatric medicine (DPM) candidates should refer to the *NBPME Bulletin of Information: 2007 Examinations.*

The NBPME Part I is generally taken after the completion of the second year of podiatric medical education. Unlike the USMLE Step 1, there is no behavioral science section, nor is biomechanics tested on the NBPME Part I. The exam samples seven basic science disciplines: general anatomy (10%); lower extremity anatomy (22%); biochemistry (10%); physiology (12%); medical microbiology and immunology (15%); pathology (15%); and pharmacology (16%). A detailed outline of topics and subtopics covered on the exam can be found in the *NBPME Bulletin of Information,* available on the NBPME Web site.

Your NBPME Appointment

In early spring, your college registrar will have you fill out an application for the NBPME Part I. After your application and registration fees are received, you will be mailed the *NBPME Bulletin of Information: 2007 Examinations.* The exam will be offered at an independent location in each city with a podiatric medical school (New York, Philadelphia, Miami, Cleveland, Chicago, Des Moines, Phoenix, and San Francisco). You may take the exam at any of these locations regardless of which school you attend. However, you must designate on your application which testing location you desire. Specific instructions about exam dates and registration deadlines can be found in the *NBPME Bulletin.*

Exam Format

The NBPME Part I is a written exam of 150 questions. The test consists entirely of multiple-choice questions with four answer choices. Examinees have three hours in which to take the exam and are given scratch paper and a calculator, both of which must be turned in at the end of the exam. Some questions on the exam will be "trial questions." These questions are evaluated as future board questions but are not counted in your score.

Interpreting Your Score

Three to four weeks following the exam date, test takers will receive their scores by mail. NBPME scores are reported as pass/fail, with a scaled score of at least 75 needed to pass. Eighty-five percent of first-time test takers pass the NBPME Part I. Failing candidates receive a report with one score between 55 and 74 in addition to diagnostic messages intended to help identify strengths or weaknesses in specific content areas. If you fail the NBPME Part I, you must retake the entire examination at a later date. There is no limit to the number of times you can retake the exam.

Preparation for the NBPME Part I

Students suggest that you begin studying for the NBPME Part I at least three months prior to the test date. The suggestions made in Section I regarding study and testing methods for the USMLE Step 1 can be applied to the NBPME as well. This book should, however, be used as a supplement and not as the sole source of information. Keep in mind that you need only a passing score. Neither you nor your school or future residency will ever see your actual numerical score. Competing with colleagues should not be an issue, and study groups are beneficial to many.

A potential study method that helps many students is to copy the outline of the material to be tested from the *NBPME Bulletin*. Check off each topic during your study, because doing so will ensure that you have engaged each topic. If you are pressed for time, prioritize subjects on the basis of their weight on the exam. Approximately 22% of the NBPME Part I focuses on lower extremity anatomy. In this area, students should rely on the notes and material that they received from their class. Remember, lower extremity anatomy is the podiatric physician's specialty—so everything about it is important. Do not forget to study osteology. Keep your old tests and look through old lower extremity class exams, since each of the podiatric colleges submits questions from its own exams. This strategy will give you an understanding of the types of questions that may be asked. On the NBPME Part I, you will see some of the same classic lower extremity anatomy questions you were tested on in school.

The NBPME, like the USMLE, requires that you apply and integrate knowledge over several areas of basic science in order to answer the questions. Students report that many questions emphasize clinical presentations; however, the facts in this book are very useful in helping students recall the various diseases and organisms. DPM candidates should expand on the high-yield pharmacology section and study antifungal drugs and treatments for *Pseudomonas*, methicillin-resistant S. *aureus*, candidiasis, and erythrasma. The high-yield section focusing on pathology is very useful; however, additional emphasis on diabetes mellitus and all its secondary manifestations, particularly peripheral neuropathy, should not be overlooked. Students should also focus on renal physiology and drug elimination, the biochemistry of gout, and neurophysiology, all of which have been noted to be important topics on the NBPME Part I exam.

A sample set of questions is found in the *NBPME Bulletin of Information: 2007 Examinations*. These samples are similar in difficulty to actual board questions. If you do not receive an *NBPME Bulletin* or if you have any questions regarding registration, fees, test centers, authorization forms, or score reports, please contact your college registrar or:

NBPME
P.O. Box 510
Bellefonte, PA 16823
(814) 357-0487
E-mail: NBPMEOfc@aol.com

or visit the NBPME Web page at www.nbpme.info.

▶ FIRST AID FOR THE STUDENT WITH A DISABILITY

The USMLE provides accommodations for students with documented disabilities. The basis for such accommodations is the Americans with Disabilities Act (ADA) of 1990. The ADA defines a disability as "a significant limitation in one or more major life activities." This includes both "observable/physical" disabilities (e.g., blindness, hearing loss, narcolepsy) and "hidden/mental disabilities" (e.g., attention-deficit hyperactivity disorder, chronic fatigue syndrome, learning disabilities).

To provide appropriate support, the administrators of the USMLE must be informed of both the nature and the severity of an examinee's disability. Such documentation is required for an examinee to receive testing accommodations. Accommodations include extra time on tests, low-stimulation environments, extra or extended breaks, and zoom text.

Who Can Apply for Accommodations?

Students or graduates of a school in the United States or Canada that is accredited by the Liaison Committee on Medical Education (LCME) or the AOA may apply for test accommodations directly from the NBME. Requests are granted only if they meet the ADA definition of a disability. If you are a disabled student or a disabled graduate of a foreign medical school, you must contact the ECFMG (see below).

Who Is Not Eligible for Accommodations?

Individuals who do not meet the ADA definition of disabled are not eligible for test accommodations. Difficulties not eligible for test accommodations include test anxiety, slow reading without an identified underlying cognitive deficit, English as a second language, and learning difficulties that have not been diagnosed as a medically recognized disability.

Understanding the Need for Documentation

Although most learning-disabled medical students are all too familiar with the often exhausting process of providing documentation of their disability, you should realize that **applying for USMLE accommodation is different from these previous experiences.** This is because the NBME determines whether an individual is disabled solely on the basis of the guidelines set by the ADA. Previous accommodation does not in itself justify provision of an accommodation, so be sure to review the NBME guidelines carefully.

Getting the Information

The first step in applying for USMLE special accommodations is to contact the NBME and obtain a guidelines and questionnaire booklet. This can be obtained by calling or writing to:

Testing Coordinator
Office of Test Accommodations
National Board of Medical Examiners
3750 Market Street
Philadelphia, PA 19104-3102
(215) 590-9700

Internet access to this information is also available at www.nbme.org. This information is also relevant for IMGs, since the information is the same as that sent by the ECFMG.

Foreign graduates should contact the ECFMG to obtain information on special accommodations by calling or writing to:

ECFMG
3624 Market Street
Philadelphia, PA 19104-2685
(215) 386-5900

When you get this information, take some time to read it carefully. The guidelines are clear and explicit about what you need to do to obtain accommodations.

NOTES

SECTION II

High-Yield General Principles

"There comes a time when for every addition of knowledge you forget something that you knew before. It is of the highest importance, therefore, not to have useless facts elbowing out the useful ones."
—Sir Arthur Conan Doyle, A *Study in Scarlet*

"Never regard study as a duty, but as the enviable opportunity to learn."
—Albert Einstein

"Live as if you were to die tomorrow. Learn as if you were to live forever."
—Gandhi

HOW TO USE THE DATABASE

The 2008 edition of *First Aid for the USMLE Step 1* contains a revised and expanded database of basic science material that student authors and faculty have identified as high yield for board reviews. The information is presented in a partially organ-based format. Hence, Section II is devoted to pathology, the foundational principles of behavioral science, biochemistry, embryology, microbiology and immunology, and pharmacology. Section III focuses on organ systems, with subsections covering the embryology, anatomy and histology, physiology, pathology, and pharmacology relevant to each. Each subsection is then divided into smaller topic areas containing related facts. Individual facts are generally presented in a three-column format, with the **Title** of the fact in the first column, the **Description** of the fact in the second column, and the **Mnemonic** or **Special Note** in the third column. Some facts do not have a mnemonic and are presented in a two-column format. Others are presented in list or tabular form in order to emphasize key associations.

The database structure used in Sections II and III is useful for reviewing material already learned. These sections are **not** ideal for learning complex or highly conceptual material for the first time. At the beginning of each subsection, we list supplementary high-yield clinical vignettes and topics that have appeared on recent exams in order to help focus your review.

The database of high-yield facts is not comprehensive. Use it to complement your core study material and not as your primary study source. The facts and notes have been condensed and edited to emphasize the essential material, and as a result each entry is "incomplete." Work with the material, add your own notes and mnemonics, and recognize that not all memory techniques work for all students.

We update the database of high-yield facts annually to keep current with new trends in boards content as well as to expand our database of information. However, we must note that inevitably many other very high yield entries and topics are not yet included in our database.

We actively encourage medical students and faculty to submit entries and mnemonics so that we may enhance the database for future students. We also solicit recommendations of alternate tools for study that may be useful in preparing for the examination, such as diagrams, charts, and computer-based tutorials (see How to Contribute, p. xv).

Disclaimer

The entries in this section reflect student opinions of what is high yield. Owing to the diverse sources of material, no attempt has been made to trace or reference the origins of entries individually. We have regarded mnemonics as essentially in the public domain. All errors and omissions will gladly be corrected if brought to the attention of the authors, either through the publisher or directly by e-mail.

HIGH-YIELD PRINCIPLES IN

Behavioral Science

"It's psychosomatic. You need a lobotomy. I'll get a saw."
—Calvin, "Calvin & Hobbes"

A heterogeneous mix of epidemiology, biostatistics, ethics, psychology, sociology, and more falls under this heading. Many medical students do not study this discipline diligently because the material is felt to be "easy" or "common sense." In our opinion, this is a missed opportunity.

Behavioral science questions may seem less concrete than questions from other disciplines, requiring an awareness of the social aspects of medicine. For example: If a patient does or says something, what should you do or say in response? These so-called "quote" questions now constitute much of the behavioral science section, and we have included several examples in the high-yield clinical vignettes. Medical ethics and medical law are also appearing with increasing frequency. In addition, the key aspects of the doctor-patient relationship (e.g., communication skills, open-ended questions, facilitation, silence) are high yield, as are biostatistics and epidemiology. Make sure you can apply biostatistical concepts such as specificity and predictive values in a problem-solving format.

BEHAVIORAL SCIENCE—HIGH-YIELD CLINICAL VIGNETTES

Vignette	Question	Answer
■ Woman with anxiety about a gynecologic exam is told to relax and to imagine going through the steps of the exam.	What process does this exemplify?	Systematic desensitization.
■ 65-year-old man is diagnosed with incurable metastatic pancreatic adenocarcinoma. His family asks you, the doctor, not to tell the patient.	What do you do?	Assess whether telling the patient will negatively affect his health. If not, tell him.
■ Man admitted for chest pain is medicated for ventricular tachycardia. The next day he jumps out of bed and does 50 push-ups to show the nurses he has not had a heart attack.	What defense mechanism is he using?	Denial.
■ You find yourself attracted to your 26-year-old patient.	What do you say?	Nothing! The tone of the interview must be very professional; it is not acceptable to have any sort of romantic relationship with patients. If you feel your actions may be misinterpreted, invite a chaperone into the room.
■ Large group of people is followed over 10 years. Every 2 years, it is determined who develops heart disease and who does not.	What type of study is this?	Cohort study.
■ Girl can groom herself, can hop on one foot, and has an imaginary friend.	How old is she?	Four years old.
■ Man has flashbacks about his girlfriend's death 2 months ago following a hit-and-run accident. He often cries and wishes for the death of the culprit.	What is the diagnosis?	Normal bereavement.
■ 36-year-old woman with a strong family history of breast cancer refuses a mammogram because she heard it hurts.	What do you do?	Discuss the risks and benefits of not having a mammogram. Each patient must give her own informed consent to each procedure; if the patient refuses, you must abide by her wishes.

4-year-old girl complains of a burning feeling in her genitalia; otherwise, she behaves and sleeps normally. A smear of the discharge shows N. *gonorrhoeae*.	How was she infected?	Sexual abuse.
72-year-old man insists on stopping treatment for his heart condition because it makes him feel "funny."	What do you do?	Although you want to encourage the patient to take his medication, the patient has the final say in his own treatment regimen. You should investigate the "funny" feeling and determine if there are drugs available that don't elicit this particular side effect.
During a particular stage of sleep, man has variable blood pressure and EEG together with penile tumescence.	What stage of sleep is he in?	REM sleep.
A certain screening test has a 2% false-negative rate.	What is the sensitivity of the test?	Sensitivity is 98%.
The prevalence of influenza in population A is 2 times the prevalence of influenza in population B. The incidence is the same in populations A and B.	What can be assumed about the disease course in population A versus population B?	The disease duration is 2 times longer in population A.

Types of studies

Study type	Design	Measures/example
Case-control study Observational and retrospective	Compares a group of people with disease to a group without. Asks, "What happened?"	**Odds ratio** (OR). "Patients with COPD had higher odds of a history of smoking than those without COPD."
Cohort study Observational and prospective	Compares a group with a given risk factor to a group without to assess whether the risk factor ↑ the likelihood of disease. Asks, "What will happen?"	**Relative risk** (RR). "Smokers had a higher risk of developing COPD than did nonsmokers."
Cross-sectional study Observational	Collects data from a group of people to assess frequency of disease (and related risk factors) at a particular point in time. Asks, "What is happening?"	**Disease prevalence.** Can show risk factor association with disease, but does not establish causality.
Twin concordance study	Compares the frequency with which both monozygotic twins or both dizygotic twins develop a disease.	Measures heritability.
Adoption study	Compares siblings raised by biologic vs. adoptive parents.	Measures heritability and influence of environmental factors.

Clinical trial

Experimental study involving humans. Compares therapeutic benefits of 2 or more treatments, or of treatment and placebo. Highest-quality study when randomized, controlled, and double-blinded.

	Study sample	Purpose
Phase I	Small number of patients, usually healthy volunteers.	Assesses safety, toxicity, and pharmacokinetics.
Phase II	Small number of patients with disease of interest.	Assesses treatment efficacy, optimal dosing, and adverse effects.
Phase III	Large number of patients randomly assigned either to the treatment under investigation or to the best available treatment (or placebo).	Compares the new treatment to the current standard of care. Is more convincing if double-blinded (i.e., neither patient nor doctor knows if the patient is in the treatment or control group).

Meta-analysis	Pools data from several studies to come to an overall conclusion. Achieves greater statistical power and integrates results of similar studies. Highest echelon of clinical evidence.	May be limited by quality of individual studies or bias in study selection.

Prevalence vs. incidence	$$\text{Prevalence} = \frac{\text{total cases in population at a given time}}{\text{total population at risk}}$$	
	$$\text{Incidence} = \frac{\text{new cases in population over a given time period}}{\text{total population at risk during that time}}$$	**Incidence** is new **incidents.**
	Prevalence ≅ incidence × disease duration. Prevalence > incidence for chronic diseases (e.g., diabetes). Prevalence = incidence for acute disease (e.g., common cold).	When calculating incidence, don't forget that people previously positive for a disease are no longer considered at risk.
Evaluation of diagnostic tests	Uses 2 × 2 table comparing test results with the actual presence of disease.	Disease (⊕ / ⊖) vs. Test (⊕ / ⊖): Test ⊕: a | b Test ⊖: c | d
Sensitivity	Proportion of all people with disease who test positive. Value approaching 1 is desirable for ruling **out** disease and indicates a low false-negative rate. Used for screening in diseases with low prevalence.	= a / (a + c) = 1 – false-negative rate **SNOUT** = **S**e**N**sitivity rules **OUT.**
Specificity	Proportion of all people without disease who test negative. Value approaching 1 is desirable for ruling **in** disease and indicates a low false-positive rate. Used as a confirmatory test after a positive screening test. Example: HIV testing. Screen with ELISA (sensitive, high false-positive rate, low threshold); confirm with Western blot (specific, high false-negative rate, high threshold).	= d / (d + b) = 1 – false-positive rate **SPIN** = **SP**ecificity rules **IN.**
Positive predictive value (PPV)	Proportion of positive test results that are true positive. Probability that person actually has the disease given a positive test result. (Note: If the prevalence of a disease in a population is low, even tests with high specificity or high sensitivity will have low positive predictive values!)	= a / (a + b)
Negative predictive value (NPV)	Proportion of negative test results that are true negative. Probability that person actually is disease free given a negative test result.	= d / (c+ d)

Odds ratio vs. relative risk

Odds ratio (OR) for case control studies — Odds of having disease in exposed group divided by odds of having disease in unexposed group. Approximates relative risk if prevalence of disease is not too high.

Relative risk (RR) for cohort studies — Relative probability of getting a disease in the exposed group compared to the unexposed group. Calculated as percent with disease in exposed group divided by percent with disease in unexposed group.

Attributable risk — The difference in risk between exposed and unexposed groups, or the proportion of disease occurrences that are a result of the exposure (e.g., smoking causes one-third of cases of pneumonia).

$$\text{Odds ratio} = \frac{a/b}{c/d} = \frac{ad}{bc}$$

$$\text{Relative risk} = \frac{a/(a+b)}{c/(c+d)}$$

$$\text{Attributable risk} = \frac{a}{a+b} - \frac{c}{c+d}$$

		Disease ⊕	Disease ⊖
Risk factor	⊕	a	b
	⊖	c	d

Precision vs. accuracy

Precision is:

1. The consistency and reproducibility of a test (reliability)
2. The absence of random variation in a test

Accuracy is the trueness of test measurements (validity).

Random error—reduced precision in a test.

Systematic error—reduced accuracy in a test.

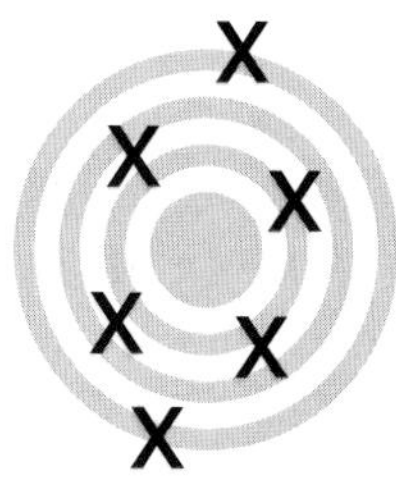

Accuracy

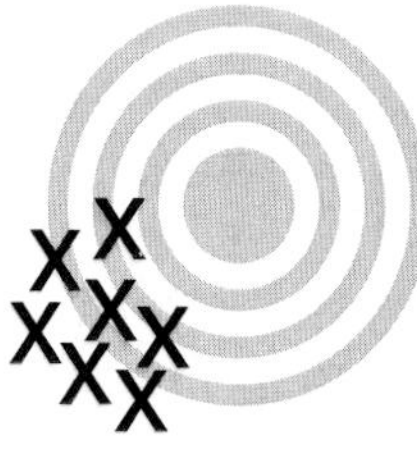

Precision

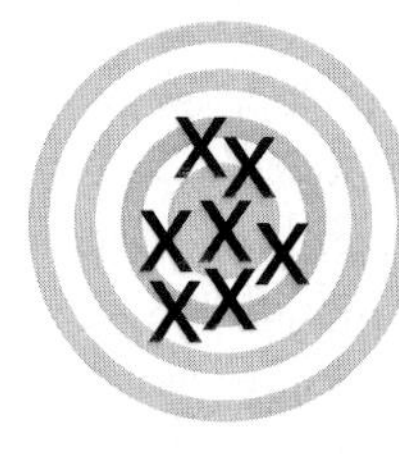

Accuracy and precision

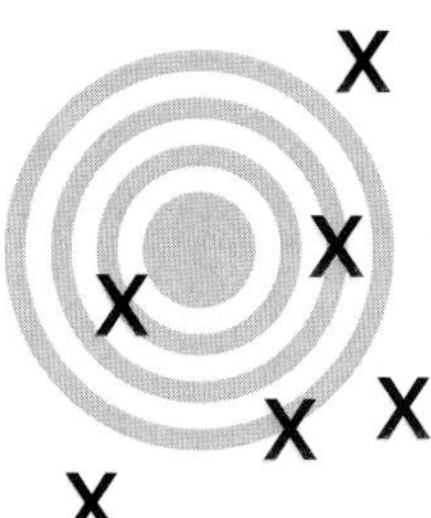

No accuracy, no precision

Bias

Occurs when 1 outcome is systematically favored over another. Systematic errors.

1. **Selection bias**—nonrandom assignment to study group
2. **Recall bias**—knowledge of presence of disorder alters recall by subjects
3. **Sampling bias**—subjects are not representative relative to general population; therefore, results are not generalizable
4. **Late-look bias**—information gathered at an inappropriate time
5. **Procedure bias**—subjects in different groups are not treated the same—e.g., more attention is paid to treatment group, stimulating greater compliance

Ways to reduce bias:

1. Blind studies (double blind is better)
2. Placebo responses
3. Crossover studies (each subject acts as own control)
4. Randomization

Statistical distribution

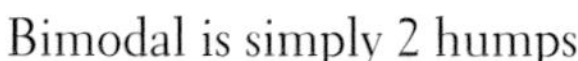

Terms that describe statistical distributions:

Normal ≈ Gaussian ≈ bell-shaped (mean = median = mode).

Bimodal is simply 2 humps.

Positive skew—mean > median > mode. Asymmetry with tail on right.

Negative skew—mean < median < mode. Asymmetry with tail on left.

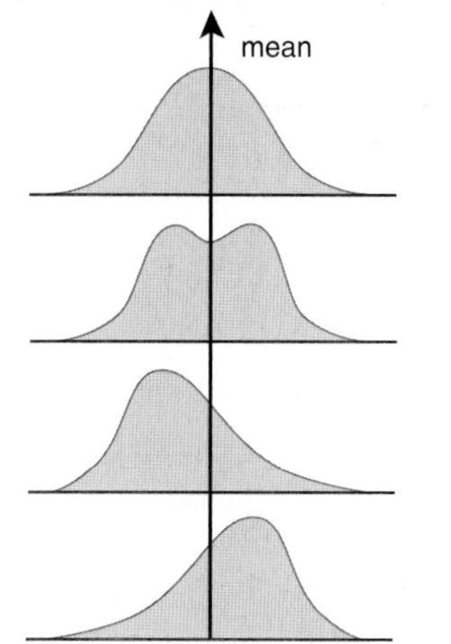

Statistical hypotheses

Null (H_0) — Hypothesis of no difference (e.g., there is no association between the disease and the risk factor in the population).

Alternative (H_1) — Hypothesis that there is some difference (e.g., there is some association between the disease and the risk factor in the population).

Study results \ Reality	H_1	H_0
H_1	Power $(1 - \beta)$	α
H_0	β	

Error types

Type I error (α) — Stating that there **is** an effect or difference when none exists (to mistakenly accept the experimental hypothesis and reject the null hypothesis). p = probability of making a type I error. p is judged against α, a preset level of significance (usually $< .05$).

If $p < .05$, then there is less than a 5% chance that the data will show something that is not really there.
α = you "saw" a difference that did not exist—for example, convicting an innocent man.

Type II error (β) — Stating that there **is not** an effect or difference when one exists (to fail to reject the null hypothesis when in fact H_0 is false).
β is the probability of making a type II error.

β = you did not "see" a difference that does exist—for example, setting a guilty man free.

Power $(1 - \beta)$

Probability of rejecting null hypothesis when it is in fact false, or the likelihood of finding a difference if one in fact exists. It depends on:

1. Total number of end points experienced by population
2. Difference in compliance between treatment groups (differences in the mean values between groups)
3. Size of expected effect

If you ↑ sample size, you ↑ power. There is power in numbers.
Power = $1 - \beta$.

Standard deviation vs. standard error

n = sample size.
σ = standard deviation.
SEM = standard error of the mean.
SEM = $\sigma/\sqrt{n}$.
Therefore, SEM < σ and SEM decreases as n increases.

Normal (Gaussian) distribution:

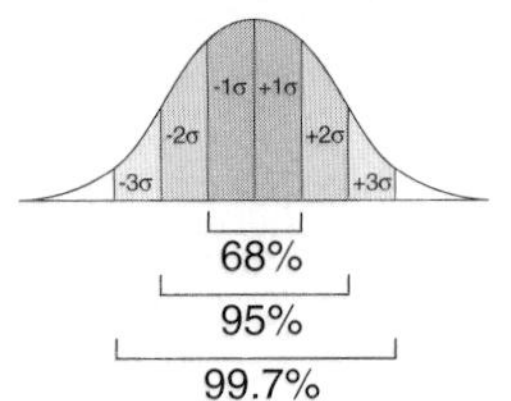

Confidence interval

Range of values in which a specified probability of the means of repeated samples would be expected to fall.
CI = confidence interval.
CI = range from [mean – Z(SEM)] to [mean + Z(SEM)].
The 95% CI (corresponding to *p* = .05) is often used. For the 95% CI, Z = 1.96.

If the 95% CI for a mean difference between 2 variables includes 0, then there is no significant difference and H_0 is not rejected. If the 95% CI for odds ratio or relative risk includes 1, H_0 is not rejected.

***t*-test vs. ANOVA vs. χ^2**

t-test checks difference between the **means** of 2 groups.
ANOVA checks difference between the means of 3 or more groups.
χ^2 checks difference between 2 or more percentages or proportions of categorical outcomes (not mean values).

Mr. **T** is **mean.**

ANOVA = **AN**alysis **O**f **VA**riance of 3 or more variables.
χ^2 = compare percentages (%) or proportions.

Correlation coefficient (r)

r is always between −1 and +1. The closer the absolute value of r is to 1, the stronger the correlation between the two variables.
Coefficient of determination = r^2 (value that is usually reported).

Disease prevention

1°—prevent disease occurrence (e.g., vaccination).
2°—early detection of disease (e.g., Pap smear).
3°—reduce disability from disease (e.g., exogenous insulin for diabetes).

PDR:
Prevent
Detect
Reduce disability

Important prevention measures

Risk factor	Services
Diabetes	Eye, foot exams; urine tests
Drug use	Hepatitis immunizations; HIV, TB tests
Alcoholism	Influenza, pneumococcal immunizations; TB test
Overweight	Blood sugar tests for diabetes
Homeless, recent immigrant, inmate	TB test
High-risk sexual behavior	HIV, hepatitis B, syphilis, gonorrhea, chlamydia tests

Reportable diseases	Only some infectious diseases are reportable in all states, including AIDS, chickenpox, gonorrhea, hepatitis A and B, measles, mumps, rubella, salmonella, shigella, syphilis, and TB. Other diseases (including HIV) vary by state.	**Hep, Hep, Hep, H**ooray, the **SSSMMART Chick** is **Go**ne! **Hep** B **Hep** A **Hep** C **H**IV **S**almonella **S**higella **S**yphilis **M**easles **M**umps **A**IDS **R**ubella **T**uberculosis **Chick**enpox **Go**norrhea

Leading causes of death in the United States by age

Infants	Congenital anomalies, short gestation/low birth weight, sudden infant death syndrome, maternal complications of pregnancy, respiratory distress syndrome.
Age 1–14	Injuries, cancer, congenital anomalies, homicide, heart disease.
Age 15–24	Injuries, homicide, suicide, cancer, heart disease.
Age 25–64	Cancer, heart disease, injuries, suicide, stroke.
Age 65+	Heart disease, cancer, stroke, COPD, pneumonia, influenza.

Medicare and Medicaid	Medicare and Medicaid are federal programs that originated from amendments to the Social Security Act. Medicare Part A = hospital; Part B = doctor bills. Medicaid is federal and state assistance for very low income people.	MedicarE is for Elderly. MedicaiD is for Destitute.

▶ BEHAVIORAL SCIENCE–ETHICS

Core ethical principles

Autonomy	Obligation to respect patients as individuals and to honor their preferences in medical care.
Beneficence	Physicians have a special ethical (fiduciary) duty to act in the patient's best interest. May conflict with autonomy. If the patient can make an informed decision, ultimately the patient has the right to decide.
Nonmaleficence	"Do no harm." However, if the benefits of an intervention outweigh the risks, a patient may make an informed decision to proceed (most surgeries fall into this category).
Justice	To treat persons fairly.

Informed consent	Legally requires: 1. Discussion of pertinent information 2. Patient's agreement to the plan of care 3. Freedom from coercion	Patients must understand the risks, benefits, and alternatives, which include no intervention.

▶ BEHAVIORAL SCIENCE–ETHICS *(continued)*

Exceptions to informed consent	1. Patient lacks decision-making capacity or is legally incompetent 2. Implied consent in an emergency 3. Therapeutic privilege—withholding information when disclosure would severely harm the patient or undermine informed decision-making capacity 4. Waiver—patient waives the right of informed consent	
Consent for minors	Parental consent must be obtained unless minor is married or otherwise emancipated.	
Decision-making capacity	1. Patient makes and communicates a choice 2. Patient is informed 3. Decision remains stable over time 4. Decision is consistent with patient's values and goals 5. Decision is not a result of delusions or hallucinations	The patient's family cannot require that a doctor withhold information from the patient.
Oral advance directive	Incapacitated patient's prior oral statements commonly used as guide. Problems arise from variance in interpretation. If patient was informed, directive is specific, patient made a choice, and decision was repeated over time, the oral directive is more valid.	
Written advance directive	Living will—describes treatments the patient wishes to receive or not receive if he/she becomes incapacitated and cannot communicate about treatment decisions. Usually, patient directs physician to withhold or withdraw life-sustaining treatment if he/she develops a terminal disease or enters a persistent vegetative state. Durable power of attorney—patient designates a surrogate to make medical decisions in the event that he/she loses decision-making capacity. Patient may also specify decisions in clinical situations. Surrogate retains power unless revoked by patient. More flexible than a living will.	
Confidentiality	Confidentiality respects patient privacy and autonomy. Disclosing information to family and friends should be guided by what the patient would want. The patient may waive the right to confidentiality (e.g., insurance companies).	
Exceptions to confidentiality	1. Potential harm to others is serious 2. Likelihood of harm to self is great 3. No alternative means exist to warn or to protect those at risk 4. Physicians can take steps to prevent harm Examples include: 1. Infectious diseases—physicians may have a duty to warn public officials and identifiable people at risk 2. The Tarasoff decision—law requiring physician to directly inform and protect potential victim from harm; may involve breach of confidentiality 3. Child and/or elder abuse 4. Impaired automobile drivers 5. Suicidal/homicidal patients—physicians may hold patients involuntarily for a period of time	

Malpractice	Civil suit under negligence requires: 1. Physician had a duty to the patient (**D**uty) 2. Physician breached that duty (**D**ereliction) 3. Patient suffers harm (**D**amage) 4. The breach of the duty was what caused the harm (**D**irect) The most common factor leading to litigation is poor communication between physician and patient.	The **4 D's.** Unlike a criminal suit, in which the burden of proof is "beyond a reasonable doubt," the burden of proof in a malpractice suit is "more likely than not."
Good Samaritan law	Relieves health care workers, as well as laypersons in some instances, from liability in certain emergency situations with the objective of encouraging health care workers to offer assistance.	

Ethical situations

Situation	Appropriate response
Patient is noncompliant.	Work to improve the physician-patient relationship.
Patient has difficulty taking medications.	Provide written instructions; attempt to simplify treatment regimens.
Family members ask for information about patient's prognosis.	Avoid discussing issues with relatives without the permission of the patient.
A 17-year-old girl is pregnant and requests an abortion.	Many states require parental notification or consent for minors for an abortion. Parental consent is **not** required for emergency situations, treatment of STDs, medical care during pregnancy, and management of drug addiction.
A terminally ill patient requests physician assistance in ending his life.	In the overwhelming majority of states, refuse involvement in any form of physician-assisted suicide. Physicians may, however, prescribe medically appropriate analgesics that coincidentally shorten the patient's life.
Patient states that he finds you attractive.	Ask direct, closed-ended questions and use a chaperone if necessary. Romantic relationships with patients are **never** appropriate.
Patient refuses a necessary procedure or desires an unnecessary one.	Attempt to understand why the patient wants/does not want the procedure. Address the underlying concerns. Avoid performing unnecessary procedures.
Patient is angry about the amount of time he spent in the waiting room.	Apologize to the patient for any inconvenience. Stay away from efforts to explain the delay.
Patient is upset with the way he was treated by another doctor.	Suggest that the patient speak directly to that physician regarding his/her concerns. If the problem is with a member of the office staff, tell the patient you will speak to that individual.
A child wishes to know more about his illness.	Ask what the parents have told the child about his illness. Parents of a child decide what information can be relayed about the illness.
Patient continues to smoke, believing that cigarettes are good for him.	Ask how the patient feels about his/her smoking. Offer advice on cessation if the patient seems willing to make an effort to quit.
Minor (under age 18) requests condoms.	Physicians can provide counsel and contraceptives to minors without a parent's knowledge or consent.

Apgar score

A 10-point scale evaluated at 1 minute and 5 minutes.

	0 points	1 point	2 points
Appearance	Blue	Trunk pink	All pink
Pulse	None	< 100/min	> 100/min
Grimace	None	Grimace	Grimace + cough
Activity	Limp	Some	Active
Respiration	None	Irregular	Regular

Low birth weight

Defined as < 2500 g. Associated with greater incidence of physical and emotional problems. Caused by prematurity or intrauterine growth retardation. Complications include infections, respiratory distress syndrome, necrotizing enterocolitis, intraventricular hemorrhage, and persistent fetal circulation.

Developmental milestones

Approximate age	Motor milestone	Cognitive/social milestone
Infant		
Birth–3 mo	Rooting reflex	
3 mo	Holds head up, Moro reflex disappears	Social smile
4–5 mo	Rolls front to back, sits when propped	Recognizes people
7–9 mo	Sits alone, crawls	Stranger anxiety, orients to voice
12–14 mo	Upgoing Babinski disappears	
15 mo	Walks	Few words, separation anxiety
Toddler		
12–24 mo	Climbs stairs, stacks 3 blocks	Object permanence; 200 words and 2-word sentences at age 2
18–24 mo	Stacks 6 blocks	Rapprochement
24–48 mo		Parallel play
24–36 mo		Core gender identity
Preschool		
30–36 mo	Stacks 9 blocks (number of blocks stacked = age in years × 3)	Toilet training ("**pee** at age **3**").
3 yrs	Rides tricycle (rides **3**-cycle at age **3**); copies line or circle drawing	900 words and complete sentences
4 yrs	Simple drawings (stick figure), hops on 1 foot	Cooperative play, imaginary friends, grooms self, brushes teeth
School age		
6–11 yrs		Reads; understands death Development of conscience (superego), same-sex friends, identification with same-sex parent
Adolescence (puberty)		
11 yrs (girls) 13 yrs (boys)		Abstract reasoning (formal operations), formation of personality

Changes in the elderly	1. Sexual changes: Men—slower erection/ejaculation, longer refractory period Women—vaginal shortening, thinning, and dryness 2. Sleep patterns— ↓ REM sleep, ↓ slow-wave sleep, ↑ sleep latency, ↑ awakenings during the night 3. Common medical conditions—arthritis, hypertension, heart disease, osteoporosis 4. Psychiatric disorders (excluding comorbidities) are found at a lower prevalence among the healthy elderly than at other life stages 5. ↑ suicide rate (males 65–74 years of age have the highest suicide rate in the United States) 6. ↓ vision, hearing, immune response, bladder control 7. ↓ renal, pulmonary, GI function 8. ↓ muscle mass, ↑ fat	Sexual interest does not ↓. Intelligence does not ↓.
Tanner stages of sexual development	1. Childhood 2. Pubic hair begins to develop (adrenarche), ↑ size of testes, breast tissue elevation 3. ↑ pubic hair, darkens, becomes curly, ↑ penis size/length 4. ↑ penis width, darker scrotal skin, development of glans, raised areolae 5. Adult; areolae are no longer raised	
Grief	Normal bereavement characterized by shock, denial, guilt, and somatic symptoms. Typically lasts 6 months to 1 year. May experience illusions. Pathologic grief includes excessively intense or prolonged grief or grief that is delayed, inhibited, or denied. May experience depressive symptoms, delusions, and hallucinations.	
Kübler-Ross grief stages	**D**enial, **A**nger, **B**argaining, **G**rieving, **A**cceptance. Stages do not necessarily occur in this order, and > 1 stage can be present at once.	**D**eath **A**rrives **B**ringing **G**rave **A**djustments.

▶ BEHAVIORAL SCIENCE—PHYSIOLOGY

Stress effects	Stress induces production of free fatty acids, 17-OH corticosteroids, lipids, cholesterol, catecholamines; affects water absorption, muscular tonicity, gastrocolic reflex, and mucosal circulation.
Sexual dysfunction	Differential diagnosis includes: 1. Drugs (e.g., antihypertensives, neuroleptics, SSRIs, ethanol) 2. Diseases (e.g., depression, diabetes) 3. Psychological (e.g., performance anxiety)

▶ BEHAVIORAL SCIENCE–PHYSIOLOGY *(continued)*

Body-mass index (BMI)

BMI is a measure of weight adjusted for height.

$$BMI = \frac{\text{weight in kg}}{(\text{height in meters})^2}$$

< 18.5 underweight;
18.5–24.9 normal;
25.0–29.9 overweight;
> 30.0 obese.

Sleep stages

Stage (% of total sleep time in young adults)	Description	EEG waveform
	Awake (eyes open), alert, active mental concentration	Beta (highest frequency, lowest amplitude)
	Awake (eyes closed)	Alpha
1 (5%)	Light sleep	Theta
2 (45%)	Deeper sleep	Sleep spindles and K complexes
3–4 (25%)	Deepest, non-REM sleep; sleepwalking; night terrors; bedwetting (slow-wave sleep)	Delta (lowest frequency, highest amplitude)
REM (25%)	Dreaming, loss of motor tone, possibly a memory processing function, erections, ↑ brain O_2 use	Beta
		At night, **BATS Drink Blood.**

1. Serotonergic predominance of raphe nucleus key to initiating sleep
2. NE reduces REM sleep
3. Extraocular movements during REM due to activity of PPRF (paramedian pontine reticular formation/conjugate gaze center)
4. REM sleep having the same EEG pattern as while awake and alert has spawned the terms "paradoxical sleep" and "desynchronized sleep"
5. Benzodiazepines shorten stage 4 sleep; thus useful for night terrors and sleepwalking
6. Imipramine is used to treat enuresis because it ↓ stage 4 sleep

---

REM sleep

↑ and variable pulse, REM, ↑ and variable blood pressure, penile/clitoral tumescence. Occurs every 90 minutes; duration ↑ through the night. ACh is the principal neurotransmitter involved in REM sleep. REM sleep ↓ with age.

REM sleep is like sex: ↑ pulse, penile/clitoral tumescence, ↓ with age.

Narcolepsy

Disordered regulation of sleep-wake cycles. May include hypnagogic (just before sleep) or hypnopompic (just before awakening) hallucinations. The patient's nocturnal and narcoleptic sleep episodes start off with REM sleep. **Cataplexy** (loss of all muscle tone following a strong emotional stimulus) in some patients. Strong genetic component. Treat with stimulants (e.g., amphetamines).

HIGH-YIELD PRINCIPLES IN

Biochemistry

"Biochemistry is the study of carbon compounds that crawl."

—Mike Adams

"World, world, O world!
But that thy strange mutations make us hate thee,
Life would not yield to age."

—William Shakespeare, *King Lear*, Act IV, Scene I

This high-yield material includes molecular biology, genetics, cell biology, and principles of metabolism (especially vitamins, cofactors, minerals, and single-enzyme-deficiency diseases). When studying metabolic pathways, emphasize important regulatory steps and enzyme deficiencies that result in disease. For example, understanding the defect in Lesch-Nyhan syndrome and its clinical consequences is higher yield than memorizing every intermediate in the purine salvage pathway. Do not spend time on hard-core organic chemistry, mechanisms, and physical chemistry. Detailed chemical structures are infrequently tested. Familiarity with the latest biochemical techniques that have medical relevance—such as enzyme-linked immunosorbent assay (ELISA), immunoelectrophoresis, Southern blotting, and PCR—is useful. Beware if you placed out of your medical school's biochemistry class, for the emphasis of the test differs from that of many undergraduate courses. Review the related biochemistry when studying pharmacology or genetic diseases as a way to reinforce and integrate the material.

BIOCHEMISTRY—HIGH-YIELD CLINICAL VIGNETTES

Vignette	Question	Answer
Full-term neonate of an uneventful delivery becomes mentally retarded and hyperactive and has a musty odor.	What is the diagnosis?	PKU.
Stressed executive comes home from work, consumes 7 or 8 martinis in rapid succession before dinner, and becomes hypoglycemic.	What is the mechanism?	NADH ↑ prevents gluconeogenesis by shunting pyruvate and oxaloacetate to lactate and malate.
2-year-old girl has an ↑ in abdominal girth, failure to thrive, and skin and hair depigmentation.	What is the diagnosis?	Kwashiorkor.
Alcoholic develops a rash, diarrhea, and altered mental status.	What is the vitamin deficiency?	Vitamin B_3 (pellagra).
51-year-old man has black spots in his sclera and has noted that his urine turns black upon standing.	What is the diagnosis?	Alkaptonuria.
25-year-old man complains of severe chest pain and has xanthomas of his Achilles tendons.	What is the disease, and where is the defect?	Familial hypercholesterolemia; LDL receptor.
Woman complains of intense muscle cramps and darkened urine after exercise.	What is the diagnosis?	McArdle's disease.
2 parents with albinism have a son who is normal.	What genetic mechanism could explain why the son is not affected?	Locus heterogeneity.
40-year-old man has chronic pancreatitis with pancreatic insufficiency.	What vitamins are likely deficient?	A, D, E, and K.
Child exhibits weakness and enlarged calves.	What is the disease, and how it is inherited?	Duchenne's muscular dystrophy; X-linked recessive.

Vitamins

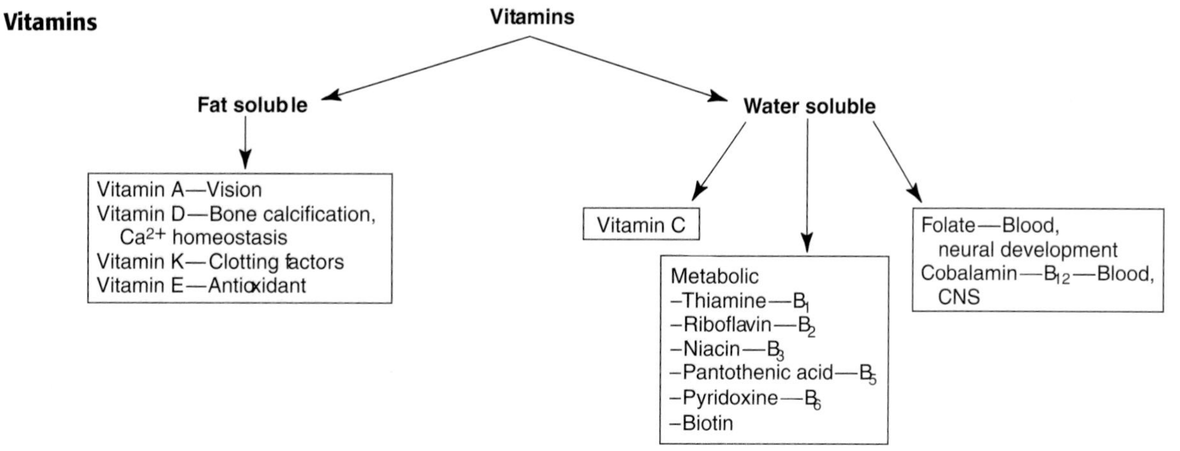

Vitamins: fat soluble	A, D, E, K. Absorption dependent on gut (ileum) and pancreas. Toxicity more common than for water-soluble vitamins, because these accumulate in fat.	Malabsorption syndromes (steatorrhea), such as cystic fibrosis and sprue, or mineral oil intake can cause fat-soluble vitamin deficiencies.
Vitamins: water soluble	B_1 (thiamine: TPP) B_2 (riboflavin: FAD, FMN) B_3 (niacin: NAD^+) B_5 (pantothenic acid: CoA) B_6 (pyridoxine: PLP) B_{12} (cobalamin) C (ascorbic acid) Biotin Folate	All wash out easily from body except B_{12} and folate (stored in liver). B-complex deficiencies often result in dermatitis, glossitis, and diarrhea.
Vitamin A (retinol)		
Deficiency	Night blindness, dry skin.	**Retinol** is vitamin **A,** so think **Retin-A** (used topically for wrinkles and acne). Found in leafy vegetables.
Function	Constituent of visual pigments (retinal).	
Excess	Arthralgias, fatigue, headaches, skin changes, sore throat, alopecia.	
Vitamin B_1 (thiamine)		
Deficiency	Beriberi and Wernicke-Korsakoff syndrome. Seen in alcoholism and malnutrition.	Spell beriberi as **Ber1Ber1.** Dry beriberi—polyneuritis, symmetrical muscle wasting. Wet beriberi—high-output cardiac failure (dilated cardiomyopathy), edema.
Function	In thiamine pyrophosphate, a cofactor for oxidative decarboxylation of α-ketoacids (pyruvate, α-ketoglutarate) and branched-chain AA dehydrogenase, and a cofactor for transketolase in the HMP shunt.	

Vitamin B_2 (riboflavin)		
Deficiency	Angular stomatitis (inflammation of oral mucous linings), Cheilosis (inflammation of lips), Corneal vascularization.	The **2 C's.** **F**AD and **F**MN are derived from riboFlavin (B_2 = 2 ATP).
Function	Cofactor in oxidation and reduction (e.g., $FADH_2$).	
Vitamin B_3 (niacin)		
Deficiency	Niacin is made by the body from tryptophan. Synthesis requires B_6. Pellagra can be caused by Hartnup disease (↓ tryptophan absorption), malignant carcinoid syndrome (↑ tryptophan metabolism), and INH (↓ vitamin B_6).	Pellagra's symptoms are the **3 D's: D**iarrhea, **D**ermatitis, **D**ementia (also beefy glossitis). **N**AD derived from **N**iacin (B_3 = **3** ATP).
Function	Constituent of NAD^+, $NADP^+$ (used in redox reactions). Derived from tryptophan using vitamin B_6.	
Vitamin B_5 (pantothenate)		
Deficiency	Dermatitis, enteritis, alopecia, adrenal insufficiency.	
Function	Constituent of CoA (a cofactor for acyl transfers) and component of fatty acid synthase.	Pantothen-**A** is in Co-**A**.
Vitamin B_6 (pyridoxine)		
Deficiency	Convulsions, hyperirritability (deficiency inducible by INH and oral contraceptives), peripheral neuropathy.	
Function	Converted to pyridoxal phosphate, a cofactor used in transamination (e.g., ALT and AST), decarboxylation reactions, glycogen phosphorylase, and heme synthesis. Required for the synthesis of niacin from tryptophan.	
Vitamin B_{12} (cobalamin)		
Deficiency	Macrocytic, megaloblastic anemia; neurologic symptoms (optic neuropathy, subacute combined degeneration, paresthesia); glossitis.	Found only in animal products. Vitamin B_{12} deficiency is usually caused by malabsorption (sprue, enteritis, *Diphyllobothrium latum*), lack of intrinsic factor (pernicious anemia, gastric bypass surgery), or absence of terminal ileum (Crohn's disease). Use Schilling test to detect the etiology of the deficiency. Abnormal myelin is seen in B_{12} deficiency, possibly due to ↓ methionine or ↑ methylmalonic acid (from metabolism of accumulated methylmalonyl-CoA).
Function	Cofactor for homocysteine methyltransferase (transfers CH_3 groups as methylcobalamin) and methylmalonyl-CoA mutase. Stored primarily in the liver. Very large reserve pool (several years). Synthesized only by microorganisms.	

$$\text{Homocysteine + N-methyl THF} \xrightarrow{B_{12}} \text{Methionine + THF}$$

$$\text{Methylmalonyl-CoA} \xrightarrow{B_{12}} \text{Succinyl-CoA}$$

Folic acid		
Deficiency	Most common vitamin deficiency in the United States. Macrocytic, megaloblastic anemia (often no neurologic symptoms, as opposed to vitamin B_{12} deficiency).	**FOL**ate from **FOL**iage. Eat green leaves (because folic acid is not stored very long). Supplemental folic acid in early pregnancy reduces neural tube defects.
Function	Coenzyme (THF) for 1-carbon transfer; involved in methylation reactions. Important for the synthesis of nitrogenous bases in DNA and RNA.	
Biotin		
Deficiency	Dermatitis, enteritis. Caused by antibiotic use, excessive ingestion of raw eggs.	"**AVID**in in egg whites **AVID**ly binds biotin."
Function	Cofactor for carboxylations: 1. Pyruvate → oxaloacetate 2. Acetyl-CoA → malonyl-CoA 3. Propionyl-CoA → methylmalonyl-CoA	
Vitamin C (ascorbic acid)		
Deficiency	Scurvy—swollen gums, bruising, anemia, poor wound healing.	British sailors carried limes to prevent scurvy (origin of the word "limey").
Function	Necessary for hydroxylation of proline and lysine in collagen synthesis. Facilitates iron absorption by keeping iron in Fe^{2+} reduced state (more absorbable). Necessary as a cofactor for dopamine β-hydroxylase, which converts dopamine to NE.	
Vitamin D	D_2 = ergocalciferol, consumed in milk. D_3 = cholecalciferol, formed in sun-exposed skin. 25-OH D_3 = storage form. 1,25 $(OH)_2$ D_3 (calcitriol) = active form.	Remember that drinking milk (fortified with vitamin D) is good for bones.
Deficiency	Rickets in children (bending bones), osteomalacia in adults (soft bones), and hypocalcemic tetany.	
Function	↑ intestinal absorption of calcium and phosphate.	
Excess	Hypercalcemia, loss of appetite, stupor. Seen in sarcoidosis, a disease where the epithelioid macrophages convert vitamin D into its active form.	
Vitamin E		
Deficiency	↑ fragility of erythrocytes, neurodysfunction.	Vitamin **E** is for **E**rythrocytes.
Function	Antioxidant (protects erythrocytes from hemolysis).	

Vitamin K

Deficiency — Neonatal hemorrhage with ↑ PT and ↑ aPTT but normal bleeding time, because neonates have sterile intestines and are unable to synthesize vitamin K.

Function — Catalyzes γ-carboxylation of glutamic acid residues on various proteins concerned with blood clotting. Synthesized by intestinal flora. Therefore, vitamin K deficiency can occur after the prolonged use of broad-spectrum antibiotics.

K for **K**oagulation. Note that the vitamin K–dependent clotting factors are II, VII, IX, X, and protein C and S. Warfarin is a vitamin K antagonist.

Neonates are given vitamin K injection at birth to prevent hemorrhage.

Zinc deficiency

Delayed wound healing, hypogonadism, ↓ adult hair (axillary, facial, pubic); may predispose to alcoholic cirrhosis.

Ethanol metabolism

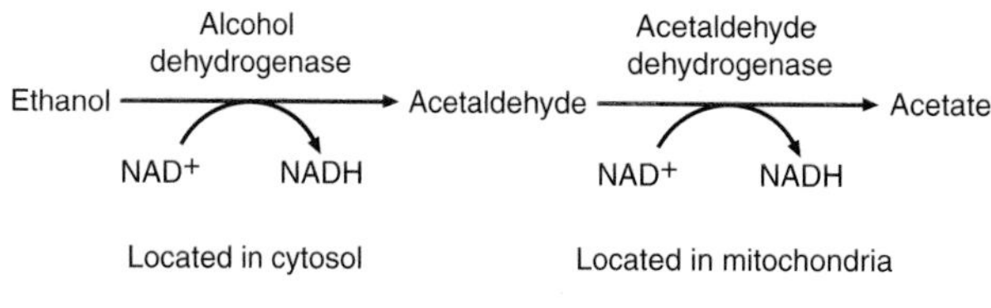

NAD^+ is the limiting reagent.

Alcohol dehydrogenase operates via zero-order kinetics.

Fomepizole inhibits alcohol dehydrogenase.

Disulfiram (Antabuse) inhibits acetaldehyde dehydrogenase (acetaldehyde accumulates, contributing to hangover symptoms).

Ethanol hypoglycemia

Ethanol metabolism ↑ $NADH/NAD^+$ ratio in liver, causing diversion of pyruvate to lactate and OAA to malate, thereby inhibiting gluconeogenesis and leading to hypoglycemia. This altered $NADH/NAD^+$ ratio is responsible for the hepatic fatty change (hepatocellular steatosis) seen in chronic alcoholics (shunting away from glycolysis and toward fatty acid synthesis, which normalizes the ratio).

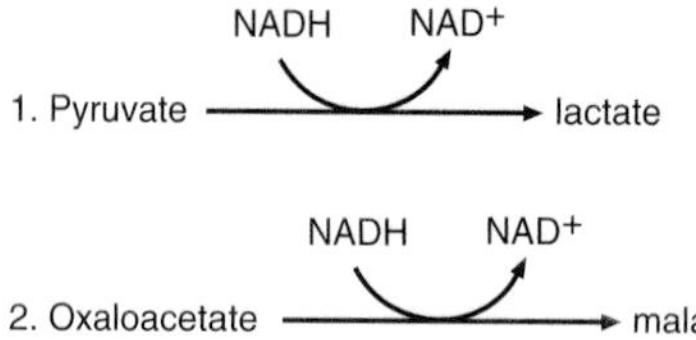

Kwashiorkor vs. marasmus

Kwashiorkor—protein malnutrition resulting in skin lesions, edema, liver malfunction (fatty change). Clinical picture is small child with swollen belly.

Marasmus—energy malnutrition resulting in tissue and muscle wasting, loss of subcutaneous fat, and variable edema.

Kwashiorkor results from a protein-deficient **MEAL**:

- **M**alnutrition
- **E**dema
- **A**nemia
- **L**iver (fatty)

Chromatin structure	Negatively charged DNA loops twice around histone octamer (2 each of the positively charged H2A, H2B, H3, and H4) to form nucleosome bead.	Think of beads on a string.
	H1 ties nucleosomes together in a string (30-nm fiber).	H1 is the only histone that is not in the nucleosome core.
	In mitosis, DNA condenses to form mitotic chromosomes.	
Heterochromatin	Condensed, transcriptionally inactive.	
Euchromatin	Less condensed, transcriptionally active.	*Eu* = true, "truly transcribed."

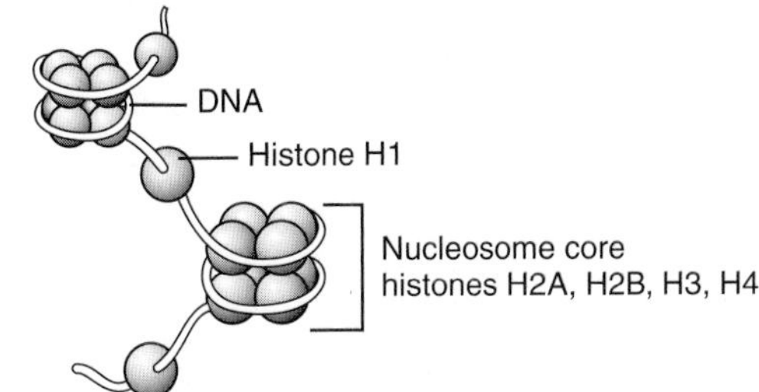

Nucleotides	Purines (**A**, **G**) have 2 rings. Pyrimidines (**C**, **T**, **U**) have 1 ring. Guanine has a ketone. Thymine has a methyl. Deamination of cytosine makes uracil.	**PUR**e **A**s **G**old: **PUR**ines.
	Uracil found in RNA; thymine in DNA.	**CUT** the **PY** (pie): **PY**rimidines.
	G-C bond (3 H-bonds) stronger than A-T bond (2 H-bonds). ↑ G-C content → ↑ melting temperature.	**THY**mine has a me**THY**l.

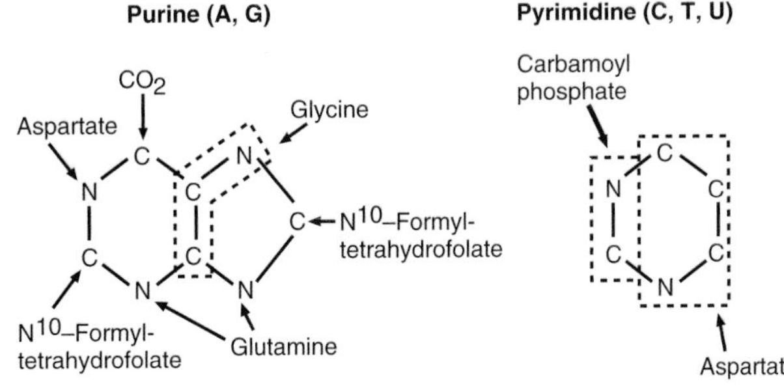

Nucleotides (base + ribose + phosphate) are linked by 3′-5′ phosphodiester bond.

Nucleoside = base + ribose.

Amino acids necessary for purine synthesis:
- Glycine
- Aspartate
- Glutamine

De novo nucleotide synthesis:
- Purines are made from IMP precursor.
- Pyrimidines are made from orotate precursor, with PRPP added later.
- Ribonucleotides are synthesized first and are converted to deoxyribonucleotides by ribonucleotide reductase.

Transition vs. transversion

Transition	Substituting purine for purine or pyrimidine for pyrimidine.	TransItion = **I**dentical type.
Transversion	Substituting purine for pyrimidine or vice versa.	Trans**V**ersion = con**V**ersion between types.

Genetic code features

Unambiguous	Each codon specifies only 1 amino acid.	
Degenerate/redundant	More than 1 codon may code for the same amino acid.	Methionine encoded by only 1 codon (AUG).
Commaless, nonoverlapping	Read from a fixed starting point as a continuous sequence of bases.	Some viruses are an exception.
Universal	Genetic code is conserved throughout evolution.	Exceptions include mitochondria, archaebacteria, *Mycoplasma*, and some yeasts.

Mutations in DNA

Silent	Same aa, often base change in 3rd position of codon (tRNA wobble).	Severity of damage: nonsense > missense > silent.
Missense	Changed aa (conservative—new aa is similar in chemical structure).	
Nonsense	Change resulting in early **stop** codon.	**Stop** the **nonsense**!
Frame shift	Change resulting in misreading of all nucleotides downstream, usually resulting in a truncated protein.	

DNA replication

Eukaryotes	Eukaryotic genome has multiple origins of replication. Replication begins at a consensus sequence of AT-rich base pairs.	Eukaryotic DNA replication is more complicated than the prokaryotic process but uses many enzymes analogous to those below.
Prokaryotes	Single origin of replication—continuous bidirectional DNA synthesis on leading strand and discontinuous (Okazaki fragments) on lagging strand.	DNA replication is semiconservative.
Replication fork	Y-shaped region along DNA template where leading and lagging strands are synthesized.	
Helicase	Unwinds DNA template at replication fork. Single-stranded binding (SSB) protein prevents strands from reannealing.	
DNA topoisomerases	Create a nick in the helix to relieve supercoils. DNA gyrase is a specific prokaryotic topoisomerase.	Fluoroquinolones inhibit DNA gyrase.
Primase	Makes an RNA primer on which DNA polymerase III can initiate replication.	
DNA polymerase III	Elongates the chain by adding deoxynucleotides to the 3′ end (leading strand). Elongates lagging strand until it reaches primer of preceding fragment. 3′ → 5′ exonuclease activity "proofreads" each added nucleotide.	DNA polymerase III has 5′ → 3′ synthesis and proofreads with 3′ → 5′ exonuclease. DNA polymerase I and III are prokaryotic.
DNA polymerase I	Degrades RNA primer and fills in the gap with DNA.	DNA polymerase I excises RNA primer with 5′ → 3′ exonuclease.
DNA ligase	Seals.	

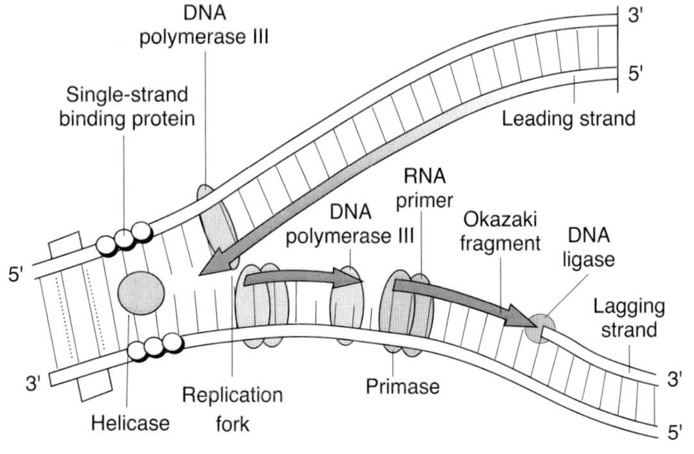

DNA repair		
Single strand		
Nucleotide excision repair	Specific endonucleases release the oligonucleotide-containing damaged bases; DNA polymerase and ligase fill and reseal the gap, respectively.	Mutated in **xeroderma pigmentosum** (dry skin with melanoma and other cancers, "children of the night"), which prevents repair of thymidine dimers.
Base excision repair	Specific glycosylases recognize and remove damaged bases, AP endonuclease cuts DNA at apyrimidinic site, empty sugar is removed, and the gap is filled and resealed.	
Mismatch repair	Unmethylated, newly synthesized string is recognized, mismatched nucleotides are removed, and the gap is filled and resealed.	Mutated in **hereditary nonpolyposis colorectal cancer** (HNPCC).
Double strand		
Nonhomologous end joining	Brings together two ends of DNA fragments. No requirement for homology.	
DNA/RNA/protein synthesis direction	DNA and RNA are both synthesized **5′ → 3′**. Remember that the 5′ of the incoming nucleotide bears the triphosphate (energy source for bond). The 3′ hydroxyl of the nascent chain is the target.	mRNA is read 5′ to 3′. Protein synthesis is N to C.
Types of RNA	Of mRNA, rRNA, and tRNA: **m**RNA is the longest type. **r**RNA is the most abundant type. **t**RNA is the smallest type.	**M**assive, **R**ampant, **T**iny.
Start and stop codons		
mRNA initiation codons	AUG (or rarely GUG).	**AUG** in**AUG**urates protein synthesis.
Eukaryotes	Codes for methionine, which may be removed before translation is completed.	
Prokaryotes	Codes for formyl-methionine (f-Met).	
mRNA stop codons	UGA, UAA, UAG.	**UGA** = **U G**o **A**way. **UAA** = **U A**re **A**way. **UAG** = **U A**re **G**one.
Regulation of gene expression		
Promoter	Site where RNA polymerase and multiple other transcription factors bind to DNA upstream from gene locus (AT-rich upstream sequence with TATA and CAAT boxes).	Promoter mutation commonly results in dramatic ↓ in amount of gene transcribed.
Enhancer	Stretch of DNA that alters gene expression by binding transcription factors. May be located close to, far from, or even within (in an intron) the gene whose expression it regulates.	
Silencer	Site where negative regulators (repressors) bind.	

Functional organization of the gene

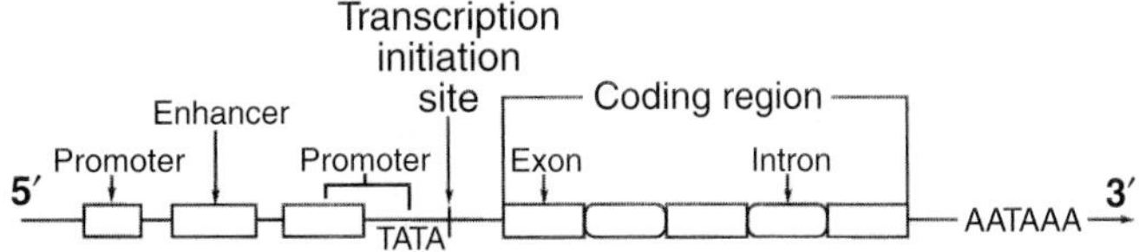

RNA polymerases Eukaryotes	RNA polymerase I makes **r**RNA. RNA polymerase II makes **m**RNA. RNA polymerase III makes **t**RNA. No proofreading function, but can initiate chains. RNA polymerase II opens DNA at promoter site. α-amanitin inhibits RNA polymerase II.	I, II, and III are numbered as their products are used in protein synthesis. α-amanitin is found in death cap mushrooms.
Prokaryotes	RNA polymerase (multisubunit complex) makes all 3 kinds of RNA.	
RNA processing (eukaryotes) 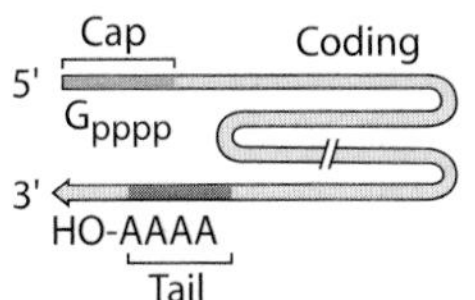	Occurs in nucleus. After transcription: 1. Capping on 5′ end (7-methylguanosine) 2. Polyadenylation on 3′ end (≈ 200 A's) 3. Splicing out of introns Initial transcript is called heterogeneous nuclear RNA (hnRNA). Capped and tailed transcript is called mRNA.	Only processed RNA is transported out of the nucleus. AAUAAA = polyadenylation signal. Poly-A polymerase does not require a template.

Splicing of pre-mRNA

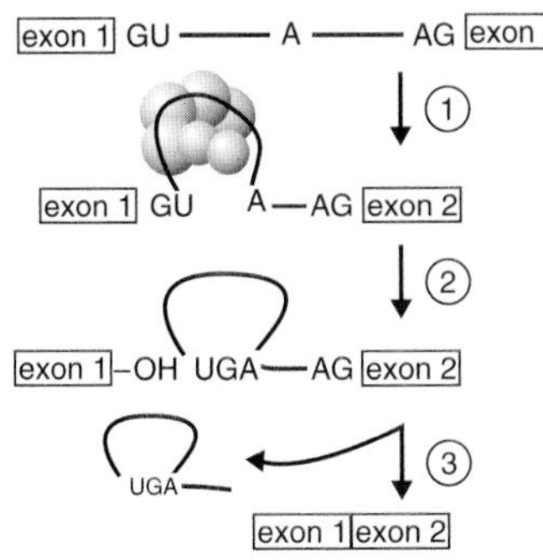

Pre-mRNA splicing occurs in eukaryotes.
1—Primary transcript combines with snRNPs and other proteins to form spliceosome.
2—Lariat-shaped intermediate is generated.
3—Lariat is released to remove intron precisely and join 2 exons.

Introns vs. exons

Exons contain the actual genetic information coding for protein.
Introns are intervening noncoding segments of DNA.

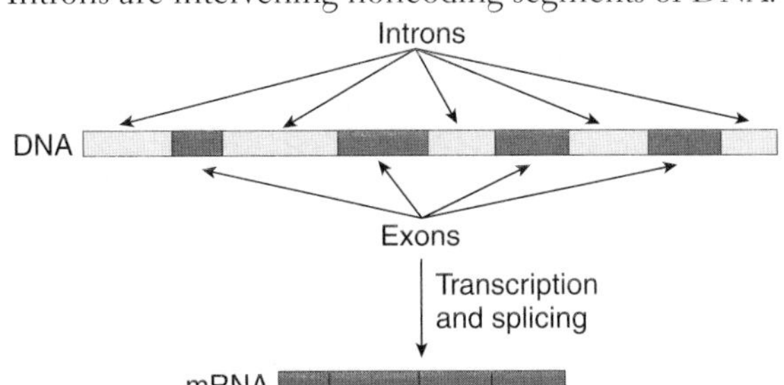

INtrons stay **IN** the nucleus, whereas **EX**ons **EX**it and are **EX**pressed.

Different exons can be combined by **alternative splicing** to make unique proteins in different tissues (e.g., β-thalassemia mutations).

tRNA

Structure	75–90 nucleotides, 2° structure, cloverleaf form, anticodon end is opposite 3′ aminoacyl end. All tRNAs, both eukaryotic and prokaryotic, have CCA at 3′ end along with a high percentage of chemically modified bases. The amino acid is covalently bound to the 3′ end of the tRNA.	
Charging	Aminoacyl-tRNA synthetase (1 per aa, uses ATP) scrutinizes aa before and after it binds to tRNA. If incorrect, bond is hydrolyzed by synthetase. The aa-tRNA bond has energy for formation of peptide bond. A mischarged tRNA reads usual codon but inserts wrong amino acid.	Aminoacyl-tRNA synthetase and binding of charged tRNA to the codon are responsible for accuracy of amino acid selection.

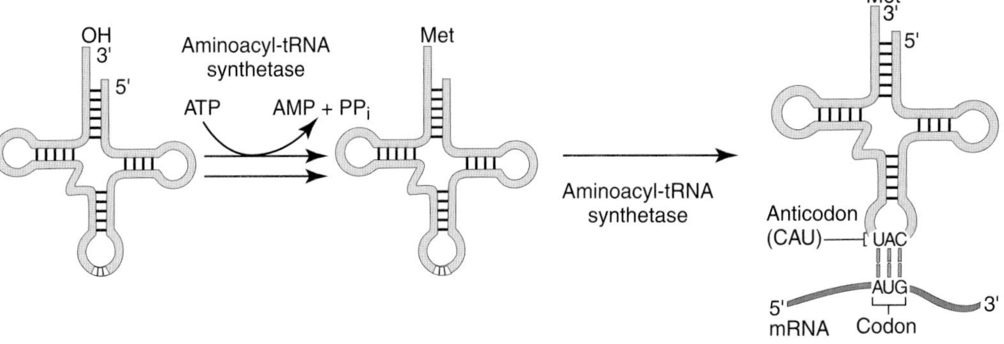

tRNA wobble

Accurate base pairing is required only in the first 2 nucleotide positions of an mRNA codon, so codons differing in the 3rd "wobble" position may code for the same tRNA/amino acid.

Protein synthesis

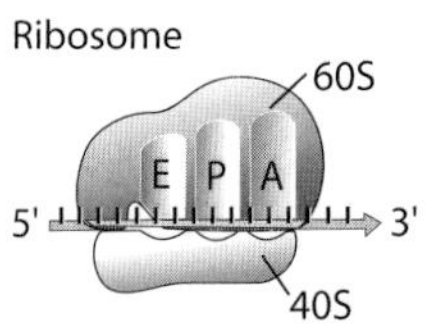

Initiation	Activated by GTP hydrolysis, initiation factors (eIFs) help assemble the 40S ribosomal subunit with the initiator tRNA and are released when the mRNA and the ribosomal subunit assemble with the complex.	Eukaryotes—80S → 60S + 40S (Even). Prokaryotes—70S → 50S + 30S (odd). ATP—tRNA **A**ctivation (charging).
Elongation	1. Aminoacyl-tRNA binds to A site except for initiator methionine 2. Peptidyltransferase catalyzes peptide bond formation, transfers growing polypeptide to amino acid in A site 3. Ribosome advances 3 nucleotides toward 3′ end of RNA, moving peptidyl RNA to P site (translocation)	**G**TP—tRNA **G**ripping and **G**oing places (translocation). **A** site = incoming **A**minoacyl tRNA. **P** site = accommodates growing **P**eptide.
Termination	Completed protein is released from ribosome through simple hydrolysis and dissociates.	**E** site = holds **E**mpty tRNA as it **E**xits.

Energy requirements of translation

tRNA aminoacylation	ATP → AMP (2 phosphoanhydride bonds)
Loading tRNA onto ribosome	GTP → GDP
Translocation	GTP → GDP
Total energy expenditure	4 high-energy phosphoanhydride bonds

Posttranslational modifications

Trimming	Removal of N- or C-terminal propeptides from zymogens to generate mature proteins.
Covalent alterations	Phosphorylation, glycosylation, and hydroxylation.
Proteasomal degradation	Attachment of ubiquitin to defective proteins to tag them for breakdown.

▶ BIOCHEMISTRY—CELLULAR

Enzyme regulation methods Enzyme concentration alteration (synthesis and/or destruction), covalent modification (e.g., phosphorylation), proteolytic modification (zymogen), allosteric regulation (e.g., feedback inhibition), pH, temperature, and transcriptional regulation (e.g., steroid hormones).

Cell cycle phases

Checkpoints control transitions between phases; regulated by cyclins, CDKs, and tumor suppressors

Mitosis (shortest phase): prophase-metaphase-anaphase-telophase. G_1 and G_0 are of variable duration.

CDKs—constitutive and inactive.

Cyclins—phase specific, activate CDKs.

Cyclin-CDK complexes must be both activated and inactivated for cell cycle to progress.

Rb and p53 tumor suppressors normally inhibit G_1-to-S progression; mutations in these genes result in unrestrained growth.

G stands for Gap or Growth; S for Synthesis.

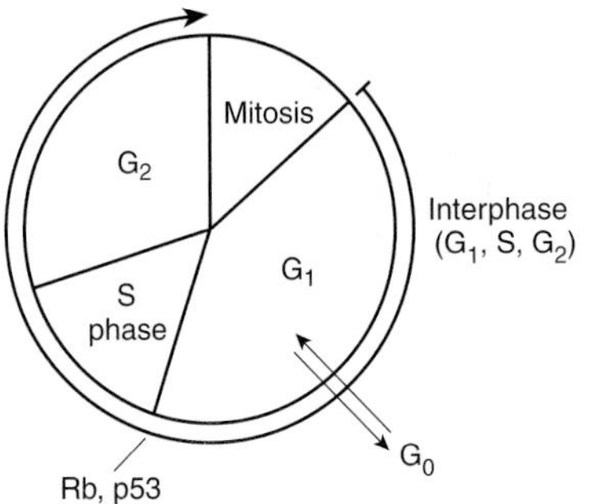

Permanent cells	Remain in G_0, regenerate from stem cells.	Neurons, skeletal and cardiac muscle cells, and RBCs remain in G_0.
Stable (quiescent) cells	Enter G_1 from G_0 when stimulated.	Hepatocytes, lymphocytes.
Labile cells	Never go to G_0, divide rapidly with a short G_1.	Bone marrow, gut epithelium, skin, hair follicles.

Rough endoplasmic reticulum (RER)

RER is the site of synthesis of secretory (exported) proteins and of N-linked oligosaccharide addition to many proteins.

Nissl bodies (in neurons)—synthesize enzymes (e.g., ChAT) and peptide neurotransmitters.

Free ribosomes—unattached to any membrane; site of synthesis of cytosolic and organellar proteins.

Mucus-secreting goblet cells of the small intestine and antibody-secreting plasma cells are rich in RER.

Smooth endoplasmic reticulum (SER)	SER is the site of steroid synthesis and detoxification of drugs and poisons.	Liver hepatocytes and steroid hormone–producing cells of the adrenal cortex are rich in SER.
Functions of Golgi apparatus	1. Distribution center of proteins and lipids from ER to the plasma membrane, lysosomes, and secretory vesicles 2. Modifies N-oligosaccharides on asparagine 3. Adds O-oligosaccharides to serine and threonine residues 4. Addition of mannose-6-phosphate to specific lysosomal proteins, which targets the protein to the lysosome 5. Proteoglycan assembly from proteoglycan core proteins 6. Sulfation of sugars in proteoglycans and of selected tyrosine on proteins	**I-cell disease**—failure of addition of mannose-6-phosphate to lysosome proteins; enzymes are secreted outside the cell instead of being targeted to the lysosome. Characterized by coarse facial features, clouded corneas, restricted joint movement, and high plasma levels of lysosomal enzymes. Often fatal in childhood. **Vesicular trafficking proteins:** COPI: retrograde, Golgi → ER. COPII: anterograde, RER → cis-Golgi. Clathrin: trans-Golgi → lysosomes, plasma membrane → endosomes (receptor-mediated endocytosis).

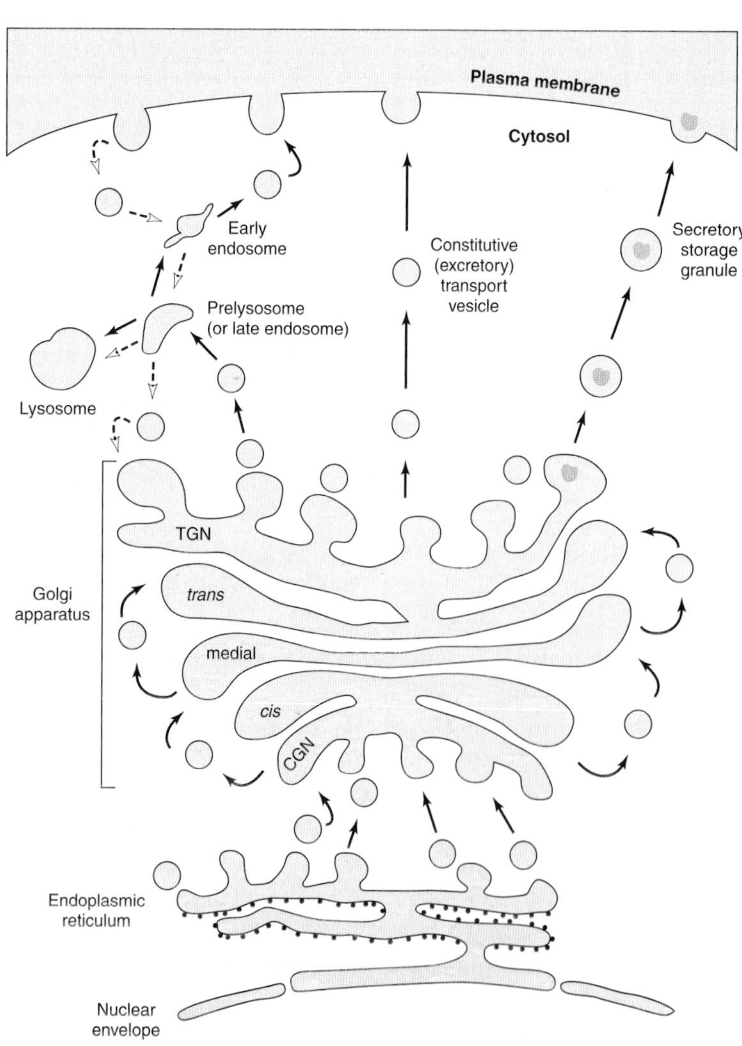

(Reproduced, with permission, from Murray RK et al. *Harper's Illustrated Biochemistry,* 27th ed. New York: McGraw-Hill, 2005, Fig. 45-2.)

Microtubule

Cylindrical structure composed of a helical array of polymerized dimers of α- and β-tubulin. Each dimer has 2 GTP bound. Incorporated into flagella, cilia, mitotic spindles. Grows slowly, collapses quickly. Microtubules are also involved in slow axoplasmic transport in neurons.

Drugs that act on microtubules:
1. Mebendazole/thiabendazole (antihelminthic)
2. Paclitaxel (Taxol) (anti–breast cancer)
3. Griseofulvin (antifungal)
4. Vincristine/vinblastine (anti-cancer)
5. Colchicine (anti-gout)

Chédiak-Higashi syndrome is due to a microtubule polymerization defect resulting in ↓ phagocytosis.

Cilia structure

9 + 2 arrangement of microtubules.
Dynein is an ATPase that links peripheral 9 doublets and causes bending of cilium by differential sliding of doublets.

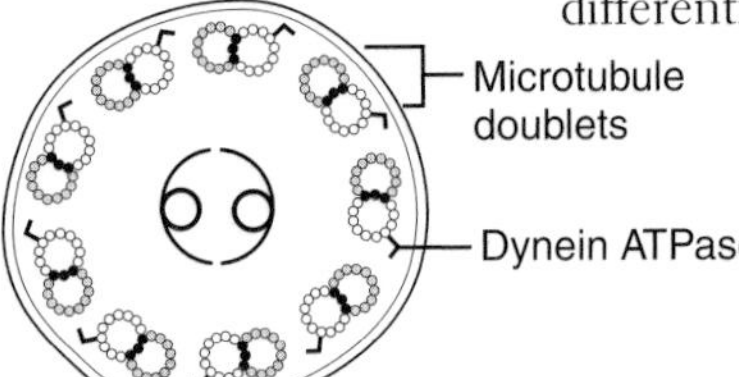

Molecular motors:
Dynein = retrograde to microtubule (+ → −).
Kinesin = anterograde to microtubule (− → +).

Kartagener's syndrome

Immotile cilia due to a dynein arm defect. Results in male and female infertility (sperm immotile), bronchiectasis, and recurrent sinusitis (bacteria and particles not pushed out); associated with situs inversus.

Cytoskeletal elements

Actin and myosin	Microvilli, muscle contraction, cytokinesis, adhering junctions.
Microtubule	Cilia, flagella, mitotic spindle, neurons, centrioles.
Intermediate filaments	Vimentin, desmin, cytokeratin, glial fibrillary acid proteins (GFAP), neurofilaments.

Plasma membrane composition

Asymmetric fluid bilayer.
Contains cholesterol (~50%), phospholipids (~50%), sphingolipids, glycolipids, and proteins.
High cholesterol or long saturated fatty acid content → ↑ melting temperature, ↓ fluidity.

Phosphatidylcholine (lecithin) function

Major component of RBC membranes, of myelin, bile, and surfactant (DPPC—dipalmitoyl phosphatidylcholine).
Used in esterification of cholesterol (LCAT is lecithin-cholesterol acyltransferase).

Immunohistochemical stains

Stain	Cell type
Vimentin	Connective tissue
Desmin	Muscle
Cytokeratin	Epithelial cells
GFAP	Neuroglia
Neurofilaments	Neurons

Sodium pump

Na^+-K^+ ATPase is located in the plasma membrane with ATP site on cytoplasmic side. For each ATP consumed, 3 Na^+ go out and 2 K^+ come in. During cycle, pump is phosphorylated.

Ouabain inhibits by binding to K^+ site.
Cardiac glycosides (digoxin and digitoxin from foxglove) also inhibit the Na^+-K^+ ATPase, causing ↑ cardiac contractility.

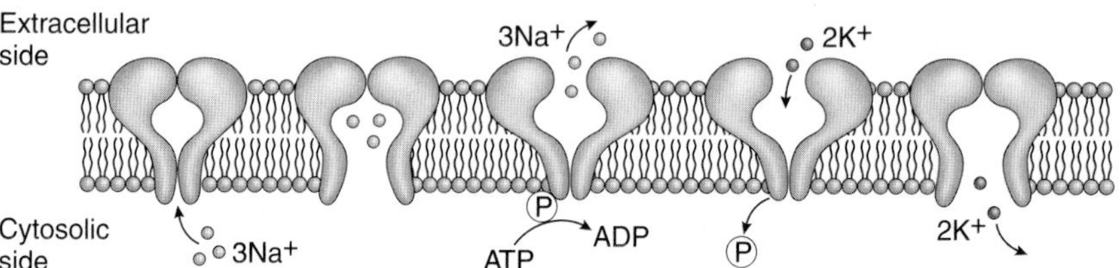

Collagen

Most abundant protein in the human body. Extensively modified.
Organizes and strengthens extracellular matrix.

Be (**S**o **T**otally) **C**ool, **R**ead **B**ooks.

Type I (90%)—**B**one, **S**kin, **T**endon, dentin, fascia, cornea, late wound repair.

Type **I**: B**ONE**.

Type II—**C**artilage (including hyaline), vitreous body, nucleus pulposus.

Type **II**: car**TWO**lage.

Type III (**R**eticulin)—skin, blood vessels, uterus, fetal tissue, granulation tissue.

Type IV—**B**asement membrane or basal lamina.

Type **IV**: Under the **floor** (basement membrane).

Collagen synthesis and structure

Inside fibroblasts

1. Synthesis (RER) — Translation of collagen α chains (**preprocollagen**)—usually Gly-X-Y polypeptide (X and Y are proline, hydroxyproline, or hydroxylysine).
2. Hydroxylation (ER) — Hydroxylation of specific proline and lysine residues (requires **vitamin C**).
3. Glycosylation (ER) — Glycosylation of pro-α-chain lysine residues and formation of **procollagen** (triple helix of 3 collagen α chains).
4. Exocytosis — Exocytosis of procollagen into extracellular space.

Outside fibroblasts

5. Proteolytic processing — Cleavage of terminal regions of procollagen transforms it into insoluble **tropocollagen.**
6. Cross-linking — Reinforcement of many staggered tropocollagen molecules by covalent lysine-hydroxylysine cross-linkage (by lysyl oxidase) to make **collagen fibrils.**

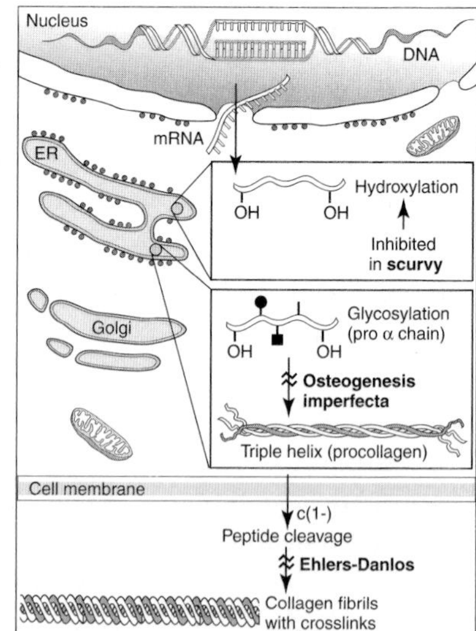

Ehlers-Danlos syndrome

Faulty collagen synthesis causing:
1. Hyperextensible skin
2. Tendency to bleed (easy bruising)
3. Hypermobile joints

10 types. Inheritance varies. Associated with berry aneurysms.

Type III collagen is most frequently affected (resulting in blood vessel instability).

Osteogenesis imperfecta	Variety of gene defects; all result in abnormal collagen synthesis. Most common form is autosomal-dominant with abnormal collagen type I. 1. **Multiple fractures** occurring with minimal trauma (brittle bone disease), which may occur during the birth process 2. **Blue sclerae** due to the translucency of the connective tissue over the choroid 3. Hearing loss (abnormal middle ear bones) 4. Dental imperfections due to lack of dentin	May be confused with child abuse. Type II is fatal in utero or in the neonatal period. Incidence is 1:10,000.
Elastin	Stretchy protein within lungs, large arteries, elastic ligaments, vocal cords, ligamenta flava (connect vertebrae). Rich in proline and glycine, nonglycosylated forms. Tropoelastin with fibrillin scaffolding. Relaxed and stretched conformations. α_1-antitrypsin inhibits elastase.	Marfan's syndrome is caused by a defect in fibrillin. Emphysema can be caused by excess elastase activity.

▶ BIOCHEMISTRY–METABOLISM

Metabolism sites

Mitochondria	Fatty acid oxidation (β-oxidation), acetyl-CoA production, Krebs cycle, oxidative phosphorylation.	
Cytoplasm	Glycolysis, fatty acid synthesis, HMP shunt, protein synthesis (RER), steroid synthesis (SER).	
Both	**H**eme synthesis, **U**rea cycle, **G**luconeogenesis.	**HUG**s take **two.**

Rate-determining enzymes of metabolic processes

Process	**Enzyme**
De novo pyrimidine synthesis	Aspartate transcarbamylase (ATCase)
De novo purine synthesis	Glutamine-PRPP amidotransferase
Glycolysis	Phosphofructokinase-1 (PFK-1)
Gluconeogenesis	Pyruvate carboxylase
TCA cycle	Isocitrate dehydrogenase
Glycogen synthesis	Glycogen synthase
Glycogenolysis	Glycogen phosphorylase
HMP shunt	Glucose-6-phosphate dehydrogenase (G6PD)
Fatty acid synthesis	Acetyl-CoA carboxylase (ACC)
Fatty acid oxidation	Carnitine acyltransferase I
Ketogenesis	HMG-CoA synthase
Cholesterol synthesis	HMG-CoA reductase
Heme synthesis	ALA synthase
Urea cycle	Carbamoyl phosphate synthase I

Summary of pathways

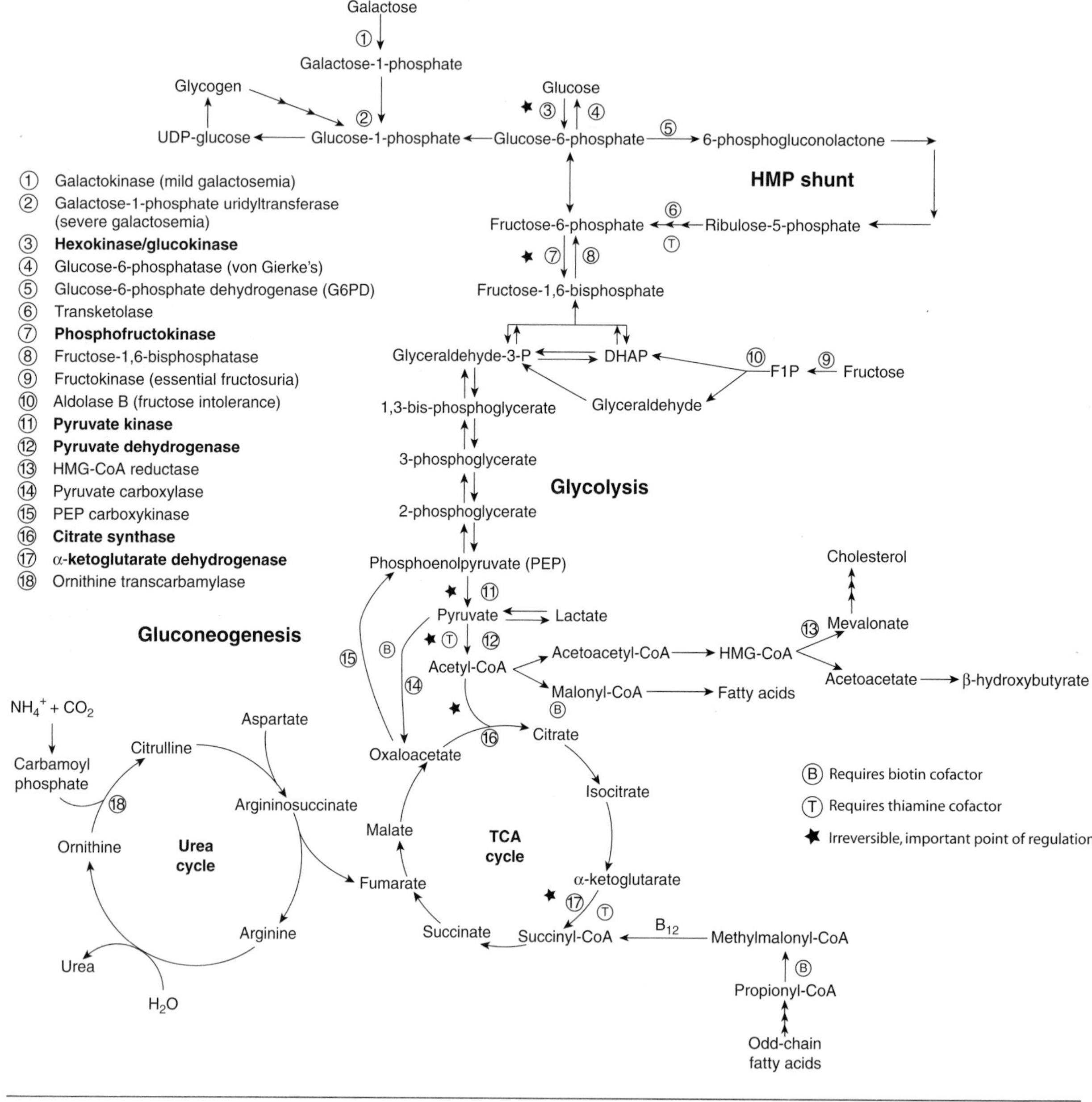

ATP

Aerobic metabolism of glucose produces 32 ATP via malate-aspartate shuttle (heart and liver), 30 ATP via glycerol-3-phosphate shuttle (muscle).
Anaerobic glycolysis produces only 2 net ATP per glucose molecule.
ATP hydrolysis can be coupled to energetically unfavorable reactions.

Base (adenine)
Ribose
Triphosphate moiety

(Reproduced, with permission, from Murray RK et al. *Harper's Illustrated Biochemistry,* 27th ed. New York: McGraw-Hill, 2005, Fig. 11-4.)

Activated carriers

Phosphoryl (ATP).
Electrons (NADH, NADPH, $FADH_2$).
Acyl (coenzyme A, lipoamide).
CO_2 (biotin).
1-carbon units (tetrahydrofolates).
CH_3 groups (SAM).
Aldehydes (TPP).

***S*-adenosyl-methionine**

ATP + methionine → **SAM.**
SAM transfers methyl units.
Regeneration of methionine (and thus SAM) is dependent on vitamin B_{12} and folate.

SAM the methyl donor man.

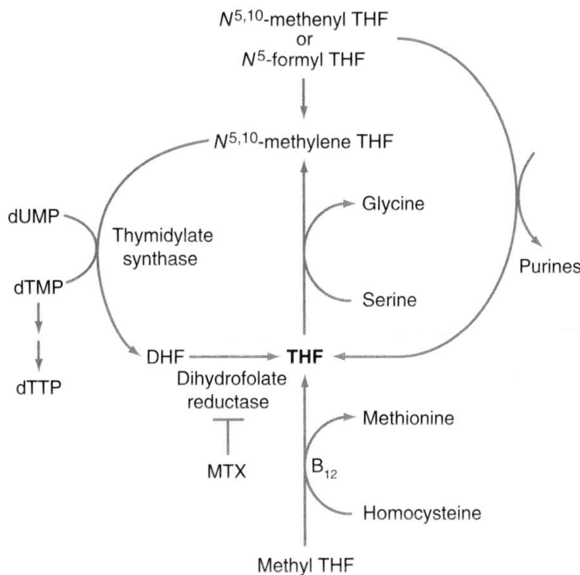

(Reproduced, with permission, from Kasper DL et al. *Harrison's Principles of Internal Medicine,* 16th ed. New York: McGraw-Hill, 2004.)

Universal electron acceptors	Nicotinamides (**NAD^+**, **$NADP^+$**) and flavin nucleotides (**FAD^+**).	NADPH is a product of the HMP shunt.
	NAD^+ is generally used in **catabolic** processes to carry reducing equivalents away as NADH.	
	NADPH is used in **anabolic** processes (steroid and fatty acid synthesis) as a supply of reducing equivalents.	NADPH is used in: 1. Anabolic processes 2. Respiratory burst 3. P-450

Oxygen-dependent respiratory burst

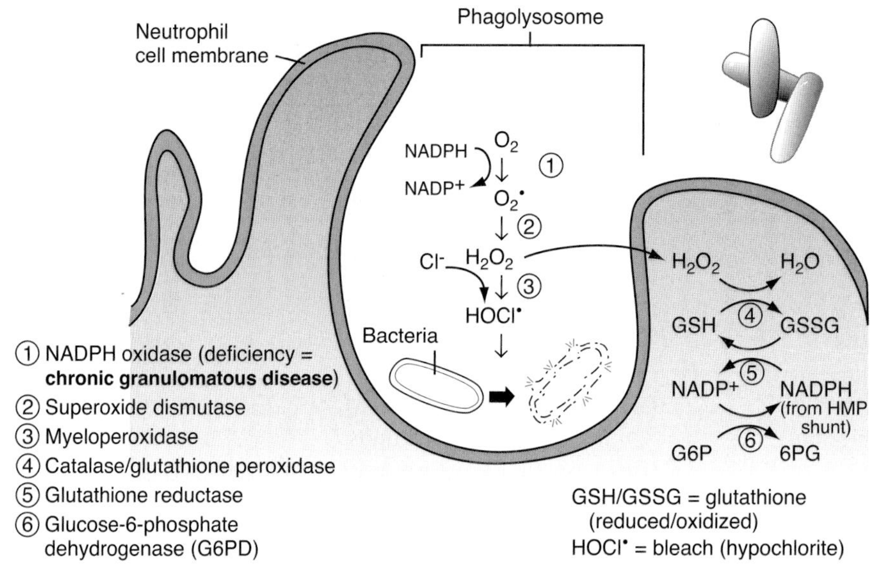

Hexokinase vs. glucokinase

Hexokinase (ubiquitous)	High affinity (low K_m), low capacity (low V_{max}), uninduced by insulin.	Feedback inhibited by glucose-6-phosphate.
Glucokinase (liver and β cells of pancreas)	Low affinity (high K_m), high capacity (high V_{max}), induced by insulin.	No direct feedback inhibition. Phosphorylates excess glucose (e.g., after a meal) to sequester it in the liver.

Glycolysis regulation, key enzymes

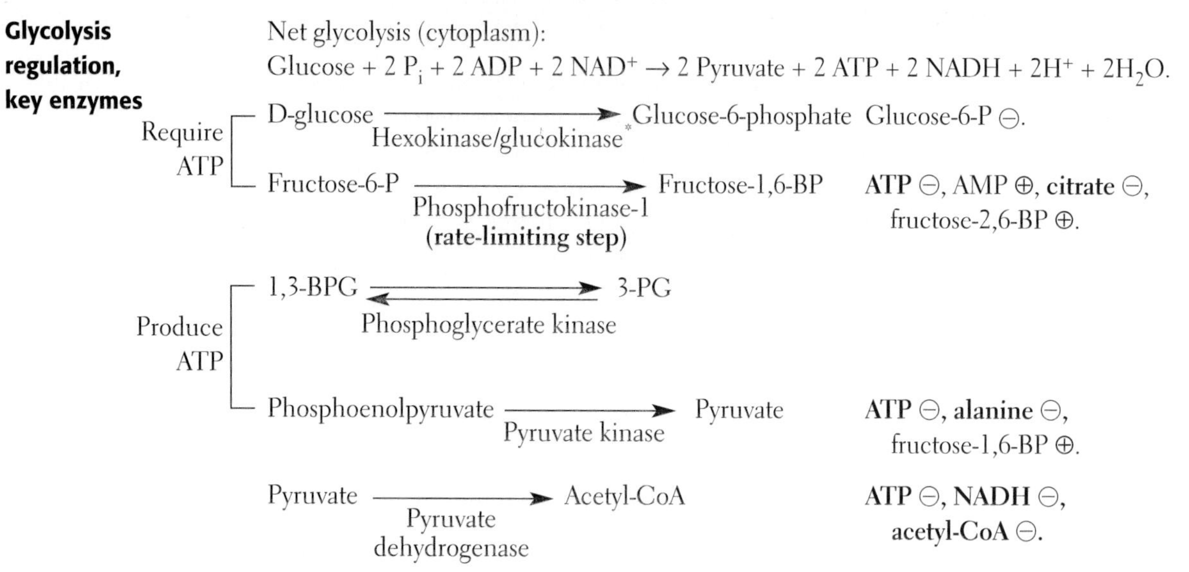

* Glucokinase in liver; hexokinase in all other tissues.

Regulation by F2,6BP

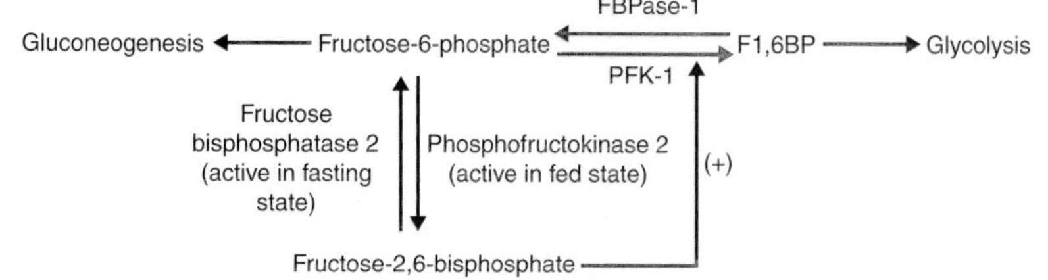

F2,6BP is the most potent activator of phosphofructokinase (overrides inhibition by ATP and citrate) and is a potent regulator of glycolysis and gluconeogenesis.

Glycolytic enzyme deficiency

Associated with **hemolytic anemia** by decreasing activity of Na^+-K^+ ATPase, leading to RBC swelling and lysis.
Due to deficiencies in pyruvate kinase (95%), phosphoglucose isomerase (4%), and other glycolytic enzymes.

RBCs metabolize glucose anaerobically (no mitochondria) and thus depend solely on glycolysis.

Pyruvate dehydrogenase complex

The complex contains 3 enzymes that require 5 cofactors (the first 4 B vitamins plus lipoic acid):

1. Pyrophosphate (B_1, thiamine; TPP)
2. FAD (B_2, riboflavin)
3. NAD (B_3, niacin)
4. CoA (B_5, pantothenate)
5. Lipoic acid

Reaction: pyruvate + NAD^+ + CoA → acetyl-CoA + CO_2 + NADH.

Activated by exercise:
↑ NAD^+/NADH ratio
↑ ADP
↑ Ca^{2+}

The complex is similar to the α-ketoglutarate dehydrogenase complex (same cofactors, similar substrate and action).

Arsenic inhibits lipoic acid:
Vomiting
Rice water stools
Garlic breath

Pyruvate dehydrogenase deficiency

Causes backup of substrate (pyruvate and alanine), resulting in lactic acidosis. Can be congenital or acquired (as in alcoholics due to B_1 deficiency).
Findings: neurologic defects.
Treatment: ↑ intake of ketogenic nutrients (e.g., high fat content or ↑ lysine and leucine).

Lysine and Leucine—the only purely ketogenic amino acids.

Pyruvate metabolism

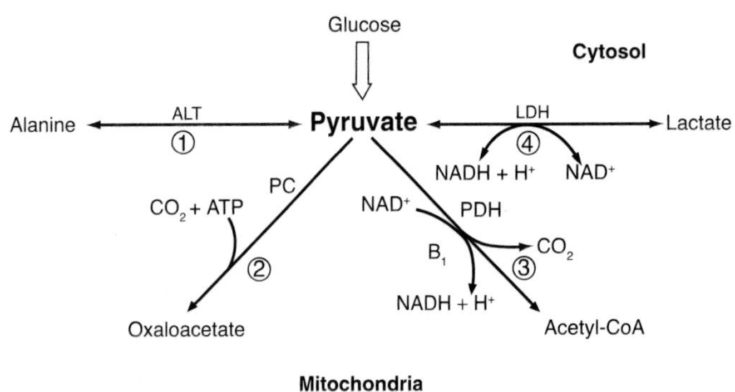

Functions of different pyruvate metabolic pathways:

1. Alanine carries amino groups to the liver from muscle
2. Oxaloacetate can replenish TCA cycle or be used in gluconeogenesis
3. Transition from glycolysis to the TCA cycle
4. End of anaerobic glycolysis (major pathway in RBCs, leukocytes, kidney medulla, lens, testes, and cornea)

Cori cycle

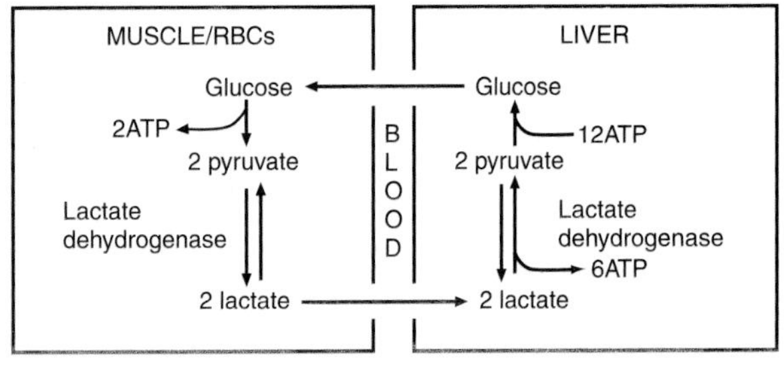

The Cori cycle allows lactate generated during anaerobic metabolism to undergo hepatic gluconeogenesis and become a source of glucose for muscle/RBCs. This comes at the cost of a net loss of 4 ATP/cycle.
Shifts metabolic burden to the liver.

TCA cycle (mitochondria)

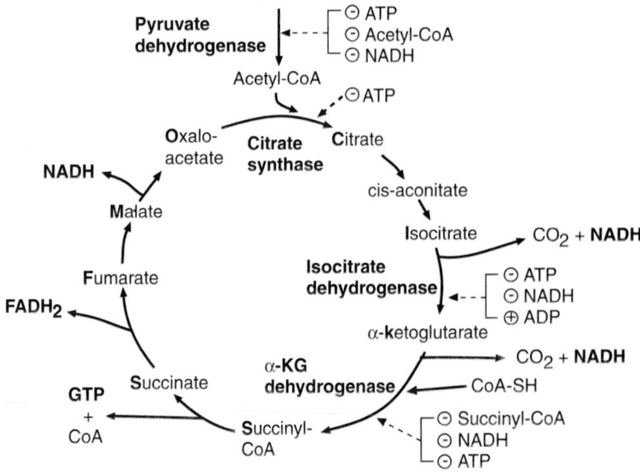

Produces 3 NADH, 1 $FADH_2$, 2 CO_2, 1 GTP per acetyl-CoA = 12 ATP/acetyl-CoA (2× everything per glucose).

α-ketoglutarate dehydrogenase complex requires same cofactors as the pyruvate dehydrogenase complex (B_1, B_2, B_3, B_5, lipoic acid).

Citrate Is Krebs' Starting Substrate For Making Oxaloacetate.

Electron transport chain and oxidative phosphorylation

NADH electrons from glycolysis enter mitochondria via malate-aspartate or glycerol-3-phosphate shuttle.

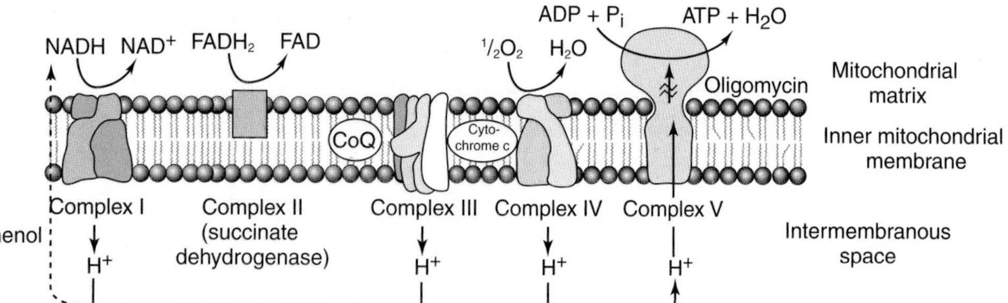

Electron transport chain — 1 NADH → 3 ATP; 1 $FADH_2$ → 2 ATP.

Oxidative phosphorylation poisons

Electron transport inhibitors	Directly inhibit electron transport, causing a ↓ proton gradient and block of ATP synthesis.	Rotenone, CN^-, antimycin A, CO.
ATPase inhibitors	Directly inhibit mitochondrial ATPase, causing an ↑ proton gradient, but no ATP is produced because electron transport stops.	Oligomycin.
Uncoupling agents	↑ permeability of membrane, causing a ↓ proton gradient and ↑ O_2 consumption. ATP synthesis stops, but electron transport continues.	2,4-DNP, aspirin, and thermogenin in brown fat.

Gluconeogenesis, irreversible enzymes

Pyruvate carboxylase	In mitochondria. Pyruvate → oxaloacetate. Gluconeogenesis goes through oxaloacetate (vs. glycolysis)	Requires biotin, ATP. Activated by acetyl-CoA.
PEP carboxykinase	In cytosol. Oxaloacetate → phosphoenolpyruvate.	Requires GTP.
Fructose-1,6-bisphosphatase	In cytosol. Fructose-1,6-bisphosphate → fructose-6-P.	
Glucose-6-phosphatase	In ER. Glucose-6-P → glucose.	**P**athway **P**roduces **F**resh **G**lucose.

Above enzymes found only in **liver, kidney, intestinal epithelium.** Muscle cannot participate in gluconeogenesis.

Deficiency of the key gluconeogenic enzymes causes hypoglycemia.

Odd-chain fatty acids yield 1 propionyl-CoA during metabolism, which can enter the TCA cycle, undergo gluconeogenesis, and serve as a glucose source. Even-chain fatty acids cannot produce new glucose, since they yield only acetyl-CoA equivalents.

Pentose phosphate pathway (HMP shunt)

Produces NADPH, which is required for fatty acid and steroid biosynthesis and for glutathione reduction inside RBCs. All reactions of this pathway occur in the cytoplasm. No ATP is used or produced.

Sites: lactating mammary glands, liver, adrenal cortex (sites of fatty acid or steroid synthesis), and RBCs.

Reactions	Key enzymes	Products
Oxidative (irreversible)	Glucose-6-phosphate dehydrogenase	NADPH (for fatty acid and steroid synthesis, glutathione reduction, and cytochrome P-450)
Nonoxidative (reversible)	Transketolases (require thiamine)	Ribose-5-phosphate (for nucleotide synthesis), G3P, F6P (glycolytic intermediates)

Glucose-6-phosphate dehydrogenase deficiency

G6PD is a rate-limiting enzyme in HMP shunt (which yields NADPH). NADPH is necessary to keep glutathione reduced, which in turn detoxifies free radicals and peroxides. ↓ NADPH in RBCs leads to **hemolytic anemia** due to poor RBC defense against oxidizing agents (fava beans, sulfonamides, primaquine) and antituberculosis drugs.

G6PD deficiency is more prevalent among blacks.

Heinz bodies—altered Hemoglobin precipitates within RBCs. Bite cells result from the phagocytic removal of Heinz bodies from macrophages.

X-linked recessive disorder.

↑ malarial resistance.

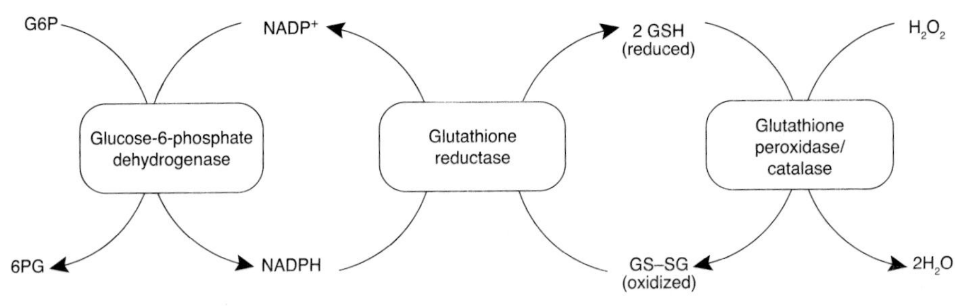

Disorders of fructose metabolism

Fructose intolerance	Hereditary deficiency of **aldolase B** (recessive). Fructose-1-phosphate accumulates, causing a ↓ in available phosphate, which results in inhibition of glycogenolysis and gluconeogenesis. Symptoms: hypoglycemia, jaundice, cirrhosis, vomiting. Treatment: must ↓ intake of both fructose and sucrose (glucose + fructose).
Essential fructosuria	Involves a defect in **fructokinase** and is a benign, asymptomatic condition, since fructose does not enter cells. Symptoms: fructose appears in blood and urine.

Disorders of fructose metabolism cause milder symptoms than analogous disorders of galactose metabolism.

FRUCTOSE METABOLISM (LIVER)

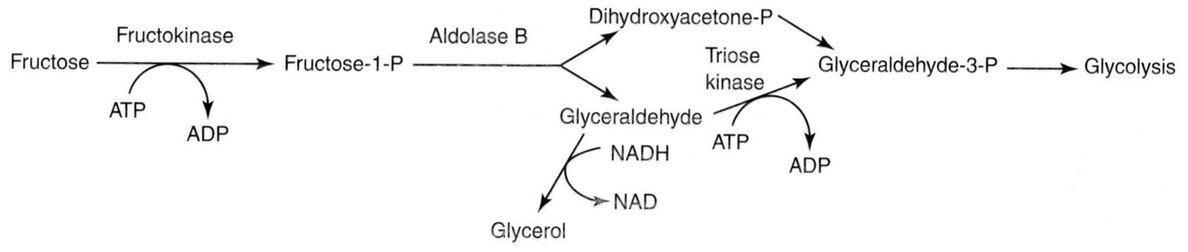

Disorders of galactose metabolism

Galactosemia	Absence of **galactose-1-phosphate uridyltransferase.** Autosomal recessive. Damage is caused by accumulation of toxic substances (including galactitol) rather than absence of an essential compound. Symptoms: cataracts, hepatosplenomegaly, mental retardation. Treatment: exclude galactose and lactose (galactose + glucose) from diet.
Galactokinase deficiency	Causes galactosemia and galactosuria, galactitol accumulation if galactose is present in diet.

GALACTOSE METABOLISM

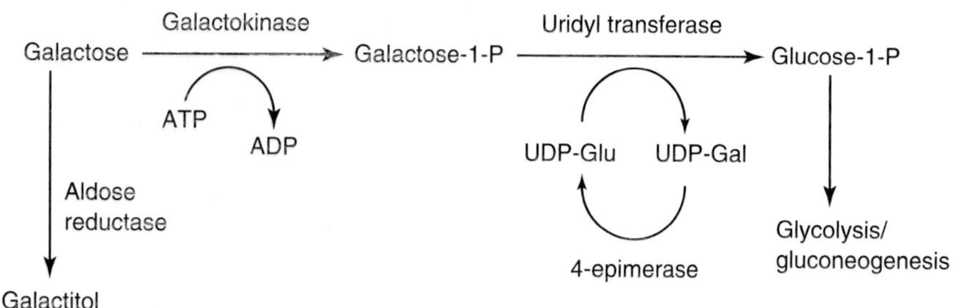

Lactase deficiency	Age-dependent and/or hereditary lactose intolerance (blacks, Asians) due to loss of brush-border enzyme. Symptoms: bloating, cramps, osmotic diarrhea. Treatment: avoid milk or add lactase pills to diet.

Amino acids

Essential

Only L-form amino acids are found in proteins.
Ketogenic: Leu, Lys.
Glucogenic/ketogenic: Ile, Phe, Tyr, Thr.
Glucogenic: Met, Val, Arg, His.

Ketogenic amino acids form ketone bodies.
Arg and His are required during periods of growth.

Acidic

Asp and Glu (negatively charged at body pH).

Basic

Arg, Lys, and His.
Arg is most basic.
His has no charge at body pH.

Arg and Lys are ↑ in histones, which bind negatively charged DNA.

Transport of ammonium by alanine and glutamine

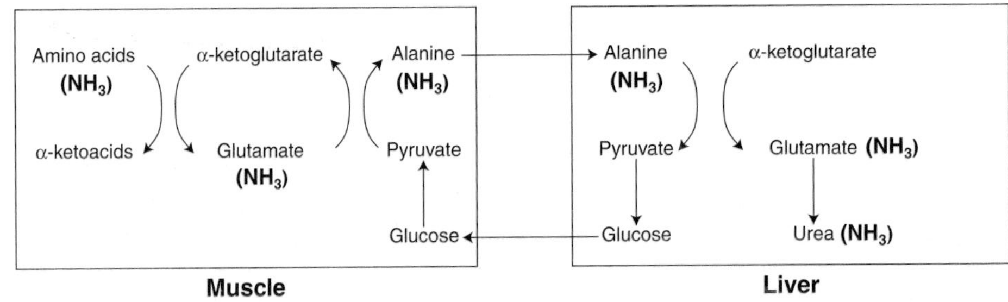

Hyperammonemia

Can be acquired (e.g., liver disease) or hereditary (e.g., ornithine transcarbamoylase deficiency).
Excess NH_4^+ depletes α-ketoglutarate, leading to inhibition of TCA cycle.
Treatment: benzoate or phenylbutyrate to lower serum ammonia levels.

Ammonia intoxication: tremor, slurring of speech, somnolence, vomiting, cerebral edema, blurring of vision.

Urea cycle

The urea cycle does not itself degrade amino acids into amino groups. Instead, it functions to excrete excess nitrogen (NH_4^+) generated by amino acid catabolism.

Ordinarily, **C**areless **C**rappers **A**re **A**lso **F**rivolous **A**bout **U**rination.

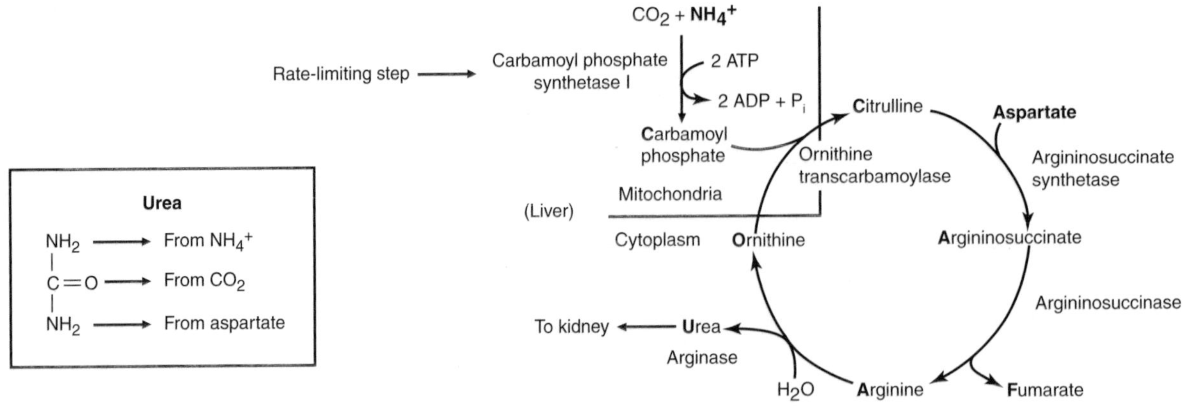

Amino acid derivatives

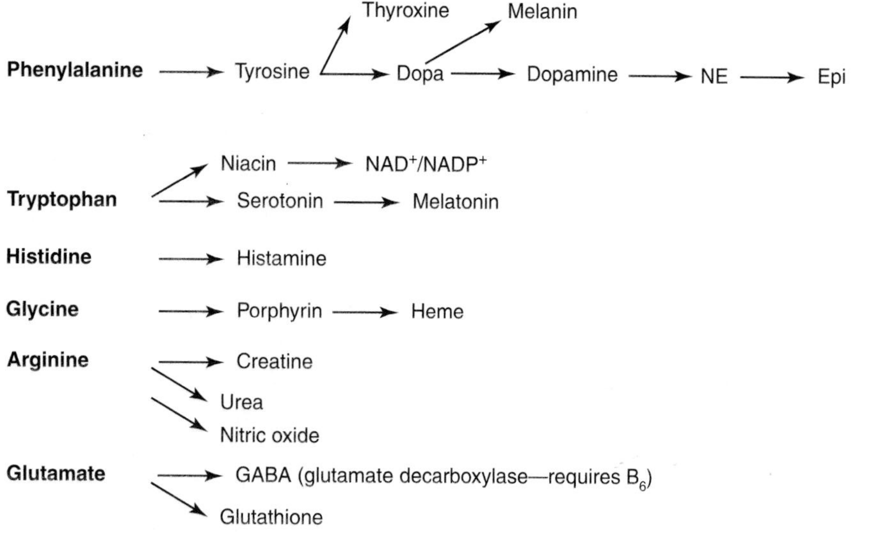

Phenylketonuria

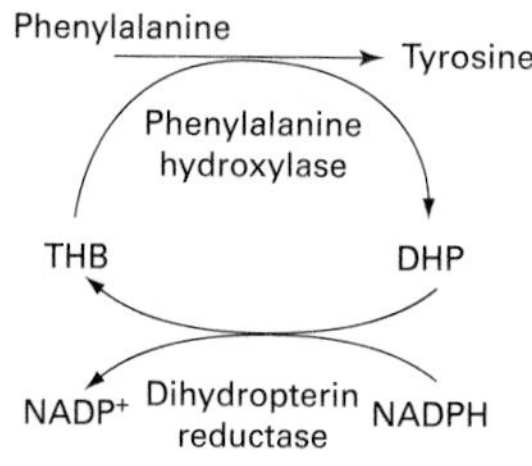

Normally, phenylalanine is converted into tyrosine (nonessential AA). In PKU, there is ↓ phenylalanine hydroxylase or ↓ tetrahydrobiopterin cofactor. Tyrosine becomes essential and phenylalanine builds up, leading to excess phenylketones in urine.

Findings: mental retardation, growth retardation, fair skin, eczema, musty body odor.

Treatment: ↓ **phenylalanine** (contained in aspartame, e.g., NutraSweet) and ↑ **tyrosine** in diet.

Screened for at birth.

Phenylketones—phenylacetate, phenyllactate, and phenylpyruvate.

Autosomal-recessive disease. Incidence ≈ 1:10,000.

Disorder of **aromatic** amino acid metabolism → musty body **odor**.

Alkaptonuria (ochronosis)

Congenital deficiency of **homogentisic acid oxidase** in the degradative pathway of tyrosine. Resulting alkapton bodies cause urine to turn black on standing. Also, the connective tissue is dark. Benign disease. May have debilitating arthralgias.

Albinism

Congenital deficiency of either of the following:

1. Tyrosinase (inability to synthesize melanin from tyrosine)—autosomal recessive
2. Defective tyrosine transporters (↓ amounts of tyrosine and thus melanin)

Can result from a lack of migration of neural crest cells.

Lack of melanin results in an ↑ risk of skin cancer.

Variable inheritance due to locus heterogeneity.

Homocystinuria	3 forms (all autosomal recessive): 1. Cystathionine synthase deficiency (treatment: ↓ Met and ↑ Cys, and ↑ B_{12} and folate in diet) 2. ↓ affinity of cystathionine synthase for pyridoxal phosphate (treatment: ↑↑ vitamin B_6 in diet) 3. Homocysteine methyltransferase deficiency	All forms result in excess homocysteine, and cysteine becomes essential. Can cause mental retardation, osteoporosis, tall stature, kyphosis, lens subluxation (downward and inward), and atherosclerosis (stroke and MI).
Cystinuria	Common (1:7000) inherited defect of renal tubular amino acid transporter for cysteine, ornithine, lysine, and arginine in the PCT of the kidneys. Excess cystine in urine can lead to the precipitation of **cystine kidney stones** (staghorn calculi).	Treat with acetazolamide to alkalinize the urine. Cystine is made of 2 cysteines connected by a disulfide bond.
Maple syrup urine disease	Blocked degradation of **branched** amino acids (Ile, Val, Leu) due to ↓ α-ketoacid dehydrogenase. Causes ↑ α-ketoacids in the blood, especially Leu. Causes severe CNS defects, mental retardation, and death.	Urine smells like maple syrup. **I** Love **V**ermont maple syrup.

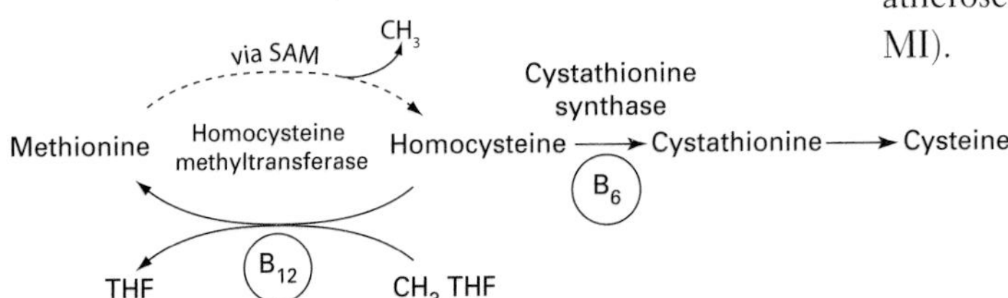

Purine salvage deficiencies

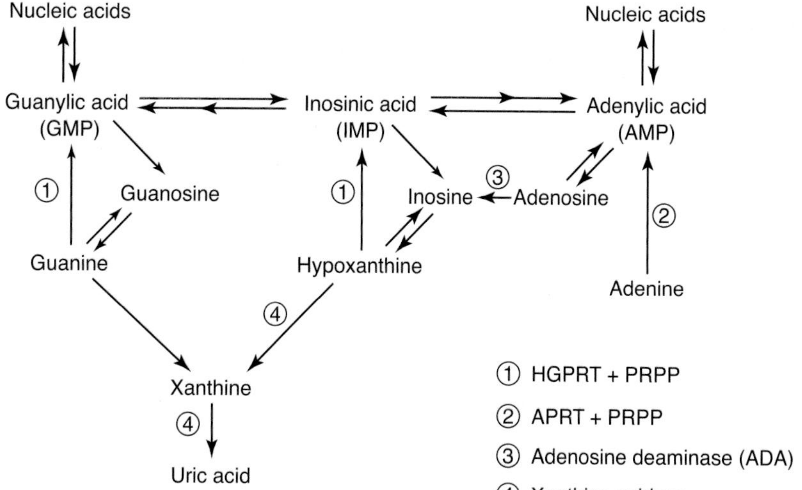

Adenosine deaminase deficiency	ADA deficiency can cause SCID. Excess ATP and dATP imbalances nucleotide pool via feedback inhibition of ribonucleotide reductase. This prevents DNA synthesis and thus ↓ lymphocyte count. 1st disease to be treated by experimental human gene therapy.	SCID—severe combined (T and B) immunodeficiency disease. **SCID** happens to **kids** (i.e., "bubble boy").
Lesch-Nyhan syndrome	Purine salvage problem owing to absence of **HGPRT**, which converts hypoxanthine to IMP and guanine to GMP. X-linked recessive. Results in excess uric acid production. Findings: retardation, self-mutilation, aggression, hyperuricemia, gout, and choreoathetosis.	**H**e's **G**ot **P**urine **R**ecovery **T**rouble.

Metabolic fuel use

Exercise	As distances ↑, ATP is obtained from additional sources.	1 g protein or carbohydrate = 4 kcal. 1 g fat = 9 kcal.
100-meter sprint (seconds)	Stored ATP, creatine phosphate, anaerobic glycolysis.	
1000-meter run (minutes)	Above + oxidative phosphorylation.	
Marathon (hours)	Glycogen and FFA oxidation; glucose conserved for final sprinting.	
Fasting and starvation	Priorities are to supply sufficient glucose to brain and RBCs and to preserve protein.	
Days 1–3	Blood glucose level maintained by: 1. Hepatic glycogenolysis and glucose release 2. Adipose release of FFA 3. Muscle and liver shifting fuel use from glucose to FFA 4. Hepatic gluconeogenesis from peripheral tissue lactate and alanine, and from adipose tissue glycerol and propionyl-CoA from odd-chain FFA metabolism (the only triacylglycerol components that can contribute to gluconeogenesis)	
After day 3	Muscle protein loss is maintained by hepatic formation of ketone bodies, supplying the brain and heart.	
After several weeks	Ketone bodies become main source of energy for brain, so less muscle protein is degraded than during days 1–3. Survival time is determined by amount of fat stores. After this is depleted, vital protein degradation accelerates, leading to organ failure and death.	

Insulin

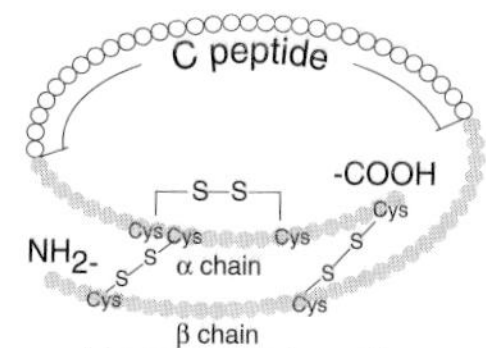

Human proinsulin

Made in β cells of pancreas in response to ATP from glucose metabolism acting on K^+ channels and depolarizing cells. Required for adipose and skeletal muscle uptake of glucose.

GLUT2 receptors are found in β cells and GLUT4 in **muscle and fat.** Insulin inhibits glucagon release by α cells of pancreas.

Serum C-peptide is not present with exogenous insulin intake (proinsulin → insulin + C-peptide).

Anabolic effects of insulin:

1. ↑ glucose transport
2. ↑ glycogen synthesis and storage
3. ↑ triglyceride synthesis and storage
4. ↑ Na^+ retention (kidneys)
5. ↑ protein synthesis (muscles)
6. ↑ cellular uptake of K^+

Insulin moves glucose **In**to cells.

BRICK L (don't need insulin for glucose uptake):

- **B**rain
- **R**BCs
- **I**ntestine
- **C**ornea
- **K**idney
- **L**iver

GLUT1: RBCs, brain.

GLUT2 (bidirectional): β islet cells, liver, kidney.

GLUT4 (insulin responsive): adipose tissue, skeletal muscle.

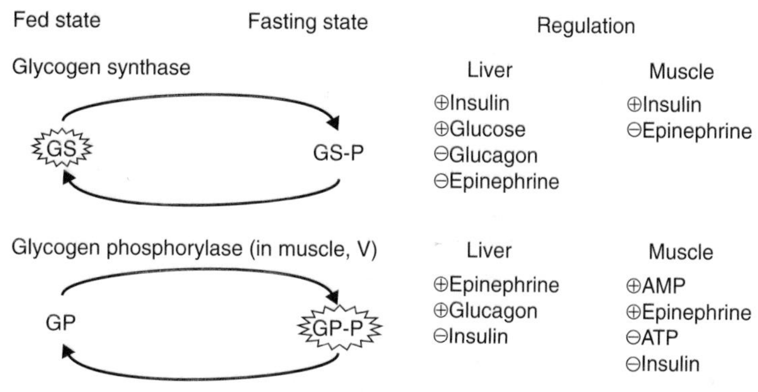

Insulin dephosphorylates (↓ cAMP → ↓ PKA).
Glucagon phosphorylates (↑ cAMP→ ↑ PKA).

Glycogen

Branches have α (1,6) bonds; linkages have α (1,4) bonds.

Skeletal muscle — Glycogen undergoes glycogenolysis to form glucose, which is rapidly metabolized during exercise.

Hepatocytes — Glycogen is stored and undergoes glycogenolysis to maintain blood sugar at appropriate levels.

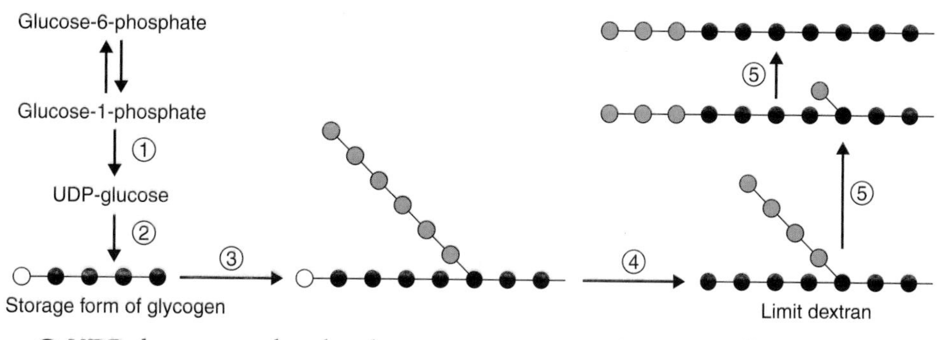

① UDP-glucose pyrophosphorylase
② Glycogen synthase
③ Branching enzyme
④ Glycogen phosphorylase
⑤ Debranching enzyme

Note: A small amount of glycogen is degraded in lysosomes by α-1,4-glucosidase

Glycogen storage diseases	12 types, all resulting in abnormal glycogen metabolism and an accumulation of glycogen within cells.		Very Poor Carbohydrate Metabolism.
Disease	**Findings**	**Deficient enzyme**	**Comments**
Von Gierke's disease (type I)	Severe fasting hypoglycemia, ↑↑ glycogen in liver, ↑ blood lactate, hepatomegaly	Glucose-6-phosphatase	
Pompe's disease (type II)	Cardiomegaly and systemic findings leading to early death	Lysosomal α-1,4-glucosidase (acid maltase)	Pompe's trashes the Pump (heart, liver, and muscle).
Cori's disease (type III)	Milder form of type I with normal blood lactate levels	Debranching enzyme α-1,6-glucosidase	Gluconeogenesis is intact.
McArdle's disease (type V)	↑ glycogen in muscle, but cannot break it down, leading to painful muscle cramps, myoglobinuria with strenuous exercise	Skeletal muscle glycogen phosphorylase	McArdle's = Muscle.

Glycogenolysis/glycogen synthesis

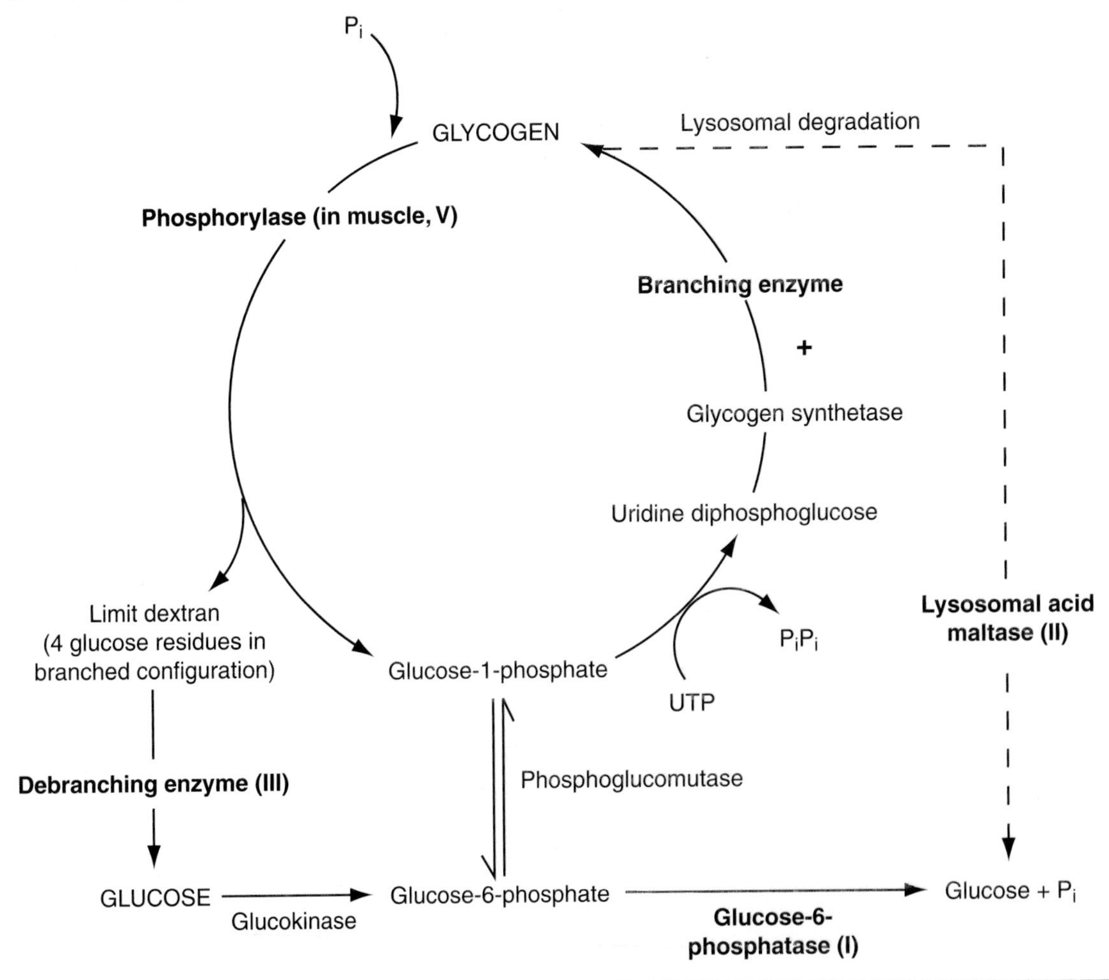

Lysosomal storage diseases Each is caused by a deficiency in one of the many lysosomal enzymes.

Disease	Findings	Deficient enzyme	Accumulated substrate	Inheritance
Sphingolipidoses				
Fabry's disease	Peripheral neuropathy of hands/feet, angiokeratomas, cardiovascular/renal disease	α-galactosidase A	Ceramide trihexoside	**XR**
Gaucher's disease (most common)	Hepatosplenomegaly, aseptic necrosis of femur, bone crises, Gaucher's cells (macrophages that look like crumpled tissue paper)	β-glucocerebrosidase	Glucocerebroside	AR
Niemann-Pick disease	Progressive neurodegeneration, hepatosplenomegaly, cherry-red spot (on macula), foam cells	Sphingomyelinase	Sphingomyelin	AR
Tay-Sachs disease	Progressive neurodegeneration, developmental delay, cherry-red spot, lysosomes with onion skin	Hexosaminidase A	GM_2 ganglioside	AR
Krabbe's disease	Peripheral neuropathy, developmental delay, optic atrophy, globoid cells	Galactocerebrosidase	Galactocerebroside	AR
Metachromatic leukodystrophy	Central and peripheral demyelination with ataxia, dementia	Arylsulfatase A	Cerebroside sulfate	AR
Mucopolysaccharidoses				
Hurler's syndrome	Developmental delay, gargoylism, airway obstruction, corneal clouding, hepatosplenomegaly	α-L-iduronidase	Heparan sulfate, dermatan sulfate	AR
Hunter's syndrome	Mild Hurler's + aggressive behavior, no corneal clouding	Iduronate sulfatase	Heparan sulfate, dermatan sulfate	**XR**

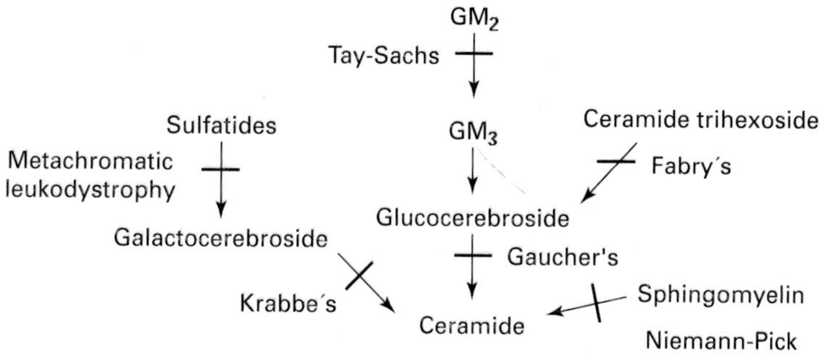

No man picks (**Niemann-Pick**) his nose with his **sphinger** (**sphingo**myelinase).

Tay-Sa**X** (**Tay-Sachs**) lacks he**X**osaminidase.

Hunters aim for the **X** (**X**-linked recessive).

↑ incidence of Tay-Sachs, Niemann-Pick, and some forms of Gaucher's disease in Ashkenazi Jews.

Fatty acid metabolism sites

SYtrate = **SY**nthesis.
CARnitine = **CAR**nage of fatty acids.

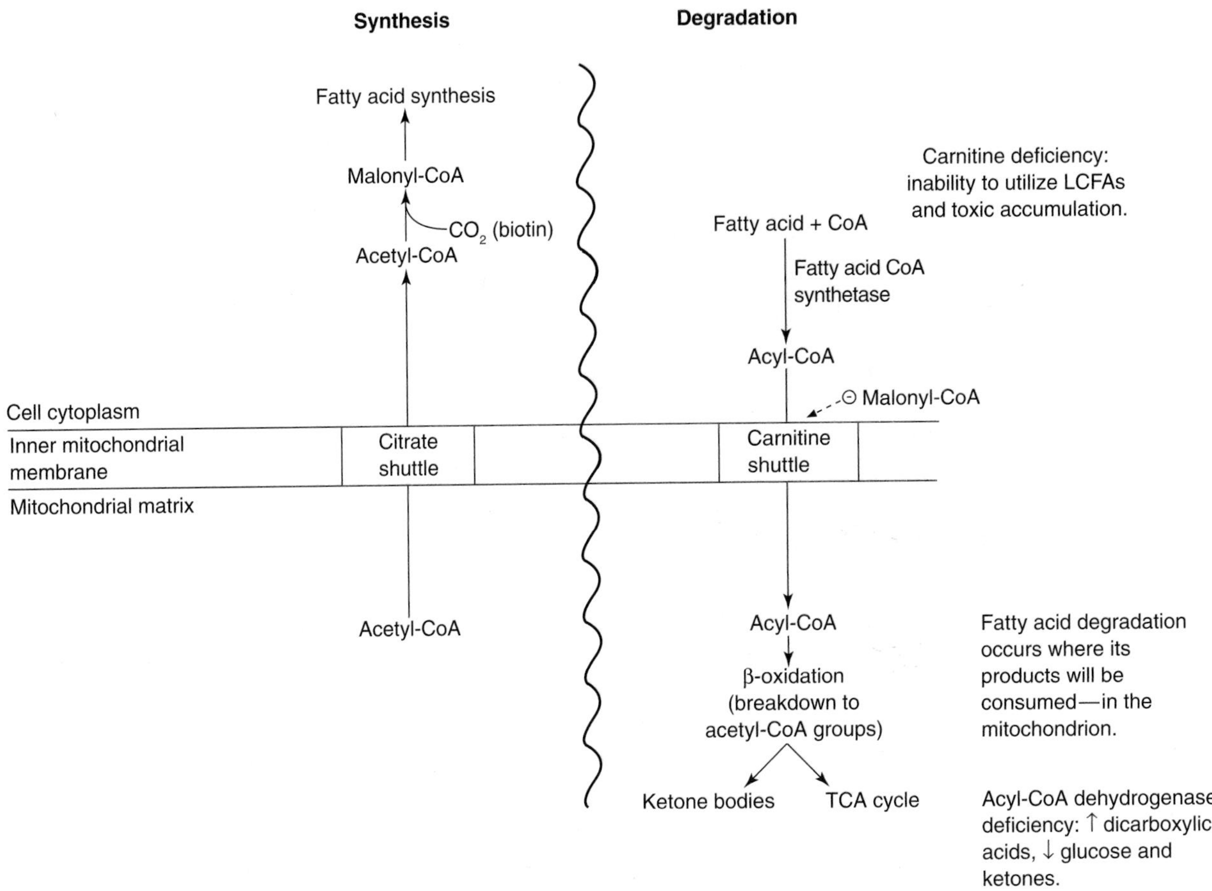

Ketone bodies	In liver, fatty acid and amino acids are metabolized to **acetoacetate** and **β-hydroxybutyrate** (to be used in muscle and brain). In prolonged starvation and diabetic ketoacidosis, oxaloacetate is depleted for gluconeogenesis. In alcoholism, excess NADH shunts oxaloacetate to malate. Both processes stall the TCA cycle, which shunts glucose and FFA to ketone bodies. Excreted in urine. Made from HMG-CoA. Ketone bodies are metabolized by the brain to 2 molecules of acetyl-CoA.	Breath smells like acetone (fruity odor). Urine test for ketones does not detect β-hydroxybutyrate (favored by high redox state).
Cholesterol synthesis	Rate-limiting step is catalyzed by **HMG-CoA reductase,** which converts HMG-CoA to mevalonate. ⅔ of plasma cholesterol is esterified by lecithin-cholesterol acyltransferase (LCAT).	Statins (e.g., lovastatin) inhibit HMG-CoA reductase.

Essential fatty acids	Linoleic and linolenic acids. Arachidonic acid, if linoleic acid is absent.	Eicosanoids are dependent on essential fatty acids.

Lipoproteins

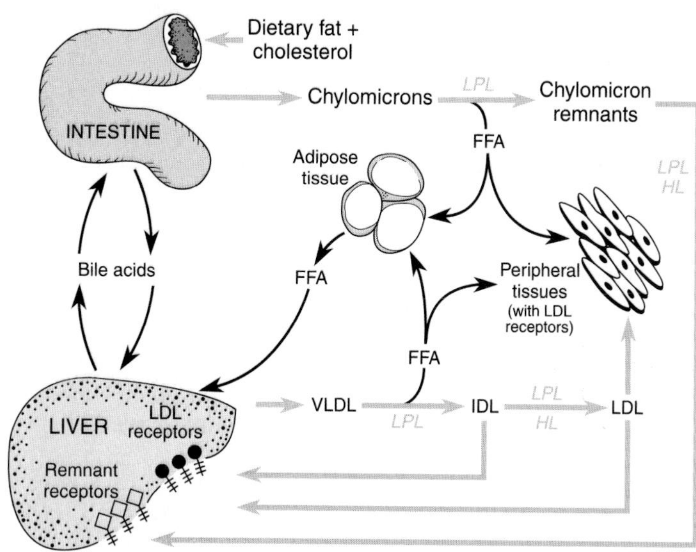

(Reproduced, with permission, from Brunton LL et al. *Goodman & Gilman's The Pharmacological Basis of Therapeutics,* 11th ed. New York: McGraw-Hill, 2005, Fig. 35-1.)

Pancreatic lipase—degradation of dietary TG in small intestine.
Lipoprotein lipase (LPL)—degradation of TG circulating in chylomicrons and VLDLs.
Hepatic TG lipase (HL)—degradation of TG remaining in IDL.
Hormone-sensitive lipase—degradation of TG stored in adipocytes.
Lecithin-cholesterol acyltransferase (LCAT)—catalyzes esterification of cholesterol.
Cholesterol ester transfer protein (CETP)—mediates transfer of cholesterol esters to other lipoprotein particles.

Major apolipoproteins	A-I—**A**ctivates LCAT. B-100—**B**inds to LDL receptor, mediates VLDL secretion. C-II—**C**ofactor for lipoprotein lipase. B-48—Mediates chylomicron secretion. E—Mediates **E**xtra (remnant) uptake.

Lipoprotein functions

Lipoproteins are composed of varying proportions of cholesterol, triglycerides, and phospholipids.

LDL and HDL carry most cholesterol. LDL transports cholesterol from liver to tissue; HDL transports it from periphery to liver.

HDL is **H**ealthy.
LDL is **L**ousy.

	Function and route	Apolipoproteins
Chylomicron	Delivers dietary triglycerides to peripheral tissues. Delivers cholesterol to liver in the form of chylomicron remnants, which are mostly depleted of their triacylglycerols. Secreted by intestinal epithelial cells. Excess causes pancreatitis, lipemia retinalis, and eruptive xanthomas.	B-48, A-IV, C-II, and E
VLDL	Delivers hepatic triglycerides to peripheral tissues. Secreted by liver. Excess causes pancreatitis.	B-100, C-II, and E
IDL	Formed in the degradation of VLDL. Delivers triglycerides and cholesterol to liver, where they are degraded to LDL.	B-100 and E
LDL	Delivers hepatic cholesterol to peripheral tissues. Formed by lipoprotein lipase modification of VLDL in the peripheral tissue. Taken up by target cells via receptor-mediated endocytosis. Excess causes atherosclerosis, xanthomas, and arcus corneae.	B-100
HDL	Mediates centripetal transport of cholesterol (reverse cholesterol transport, from periphery to liver). Acts as a repository for apoC and apoE (which are needed for chylomicron and VLDL metabolism). Secreted from both liver and intestine.	

Familial dyslipidemias

Type	Increased	Elevated blood levels	Pathophysiology
I—hyperchylomicronemia	Chylomicrons	TG, cholesterol	Lipoprotein lipase deficiency or altered apolipoprotein C-II
IIa—hypercholesterolemia	LDL	Cholesterol	↓ LDL receptors
IV—hypertriglyceridemia	VLDL	TG	Hepatic overproduction of VLDL

Heme synthesis

Underproduction of heme causes microcytic hypochromic anemia. Accumulation of intermediates causes porphyrias.

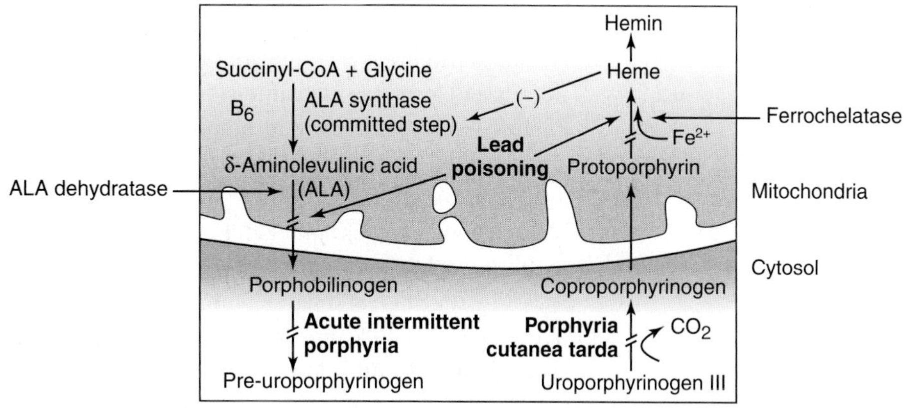

Porphyrias

	Affected enzyme	Accumulated substrate in urine	
Lead poisoning	Ferrochelatase and ALA dehydratase	Coproporphyrin and δ-ALA	
Acute intermittent porphyria	Porphobilinogen deaminase	Porphobilinogen and δ-ALA	Symptoms = 5 **P**'s: Painful abdomen, Pink urine, Polyneuropathy, Psychological disturbances, Precipitated by drugs
Porphyria cutanea tarda	Uroporphyrinogen decarboxylase	Uroporphyrin (tea-colored)	

Heme catabolism

Heme is scavenged from RBCs and Fe^{2+} is reused. Heme → biliverdin → bilirubin (sparingly water soluble, toxic to CNS, transported by albumin). Bilirubin is removed from blood by liver, conjugated with glucuronate, and excreted in bile. Some urobilinogen, an intestinal intermediate, is reabsorbed into blood and excreted as urobilin into urine. Biliverdin gives bruises their blue-green color. Jaundiced newborns are exposed to UV light, which converts bilirubin to urine-soluble products.

Hemoglobin 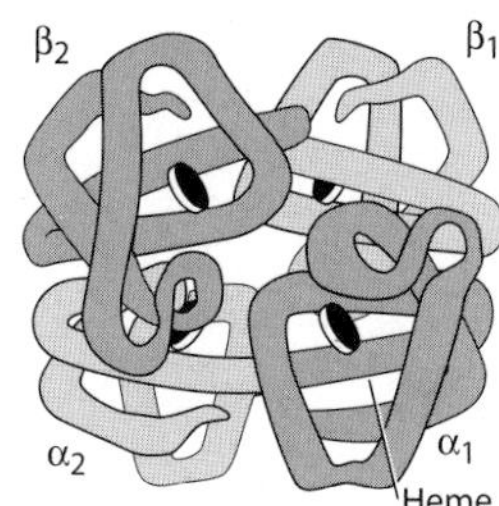	Hemoglobin is composed of 4 polypeptide subunits (2 α and 2 β) and exists in 2 forms: 1. T (taut) form has low affinity for O_2. 2. R (relaxed) form has high affinity for O_2 (300×). Hemoglobin exhibits positive cooperativity and negative allostery (accounts for the sigmoid-shaped O_2 dissociation curve for hemoglobin), unlike myoglobin.	Fetal hemoglobin (2α and 2γ subunits) has lower affinity for 2,3-BPG than adult hemoglobin (HbA) and thus has higher affinity for O_2.
	↑ Cl^-, H^+, CO_2, 2,3-BPG, and temperature favor T form over **R** form (shifts dissociation curve to right, leading to ↑ O_2 unloading).	When you're **R**elaxed, you do your job better (carry O_2).
CO_2 transport in blood	CO_2 that is transported in blood and not bound to hemoglobin is primarily in bicarbonate form. CO_2 (primarily as carbamate) binds to amino acids in globin chain at N terminus, but not to heme. CO_2 binding favors T (taut) form of hemoglobin, promoting O_2 unloading (negative allosteric regulation).	CO_2 must be transported from tissue to lungs, the reverse of O_2.
Hemoglobin modifications	Lead to tissue hypoxia from ↓ O_2 saturation and ↓ O_2 content.	
Methemoglobin	Oxidized form of hemoglobin (ferric, Fe^{3+}) that does not bind O_2 as readily, but has ↑ affinity for CN^-. Iron in hemoglobin is normally in a reduced state (ferrous, Fe^{2+}). To treat cyanide poisoning, use nitrites to oxidize hemoglobin to methemoglobin, which binds cyanide, allowing cytochrome oxidase to function. Use thiosulfate to bind this cyanide, forming thiocyanate, which is renally excreted.	**METH**emoglobinemia can be treated with **METH**ylene blue.
Carboxyhemoglobin	Form of hemoglobin bound to CO in place of O_2.	CO has 200× greater affinity than O_2 for hemoglobin.

Genetic terms	
Codominance	Neither of 2 alleles is dominant (e.g., blood groups).
Variable expression	Nature and severity of the phenotype varies from 1 individual to another.
Incomplete penetrance	Not all individuals with a mutant genotype show the mutant phenotype.
Pleiotropy	1 gene has > 1 effect on an individual's phenotype.
Imprinting	Differences in phenotype depend on whether the mutation is of maternal or paternal origin (e.g., AngelMan's syndrome [Maternal], Prader-Willi syndrome [Paternal]).
Anticipation	Severity of disease worsens or age of onset of disease is earlier in succeeding generations (e.g., Huntington's disease).
Loss of heterozygosity	If a patient inherits or develops a mutation in a tumor suppressor gene, the complementary allele must be deleted/mutated before cancer develops. This is not true of oncogenes.
Dominant negative mutation	Exerts a **dominant effect.** A heterozygote produces a nonfunctional altered protein that also prevents the normal gene product from functioning.
Linkage disequilibrium	Tendency for certain alleles at 2 linked loci to occur together more often than expected by chance. Measured in a population, not in a family, and often varies in different populations.
Mosaicism	Occurs when cells in the body have different genetic makeup (e.g., lyonization—random X inactivation in females).
Locus heterogeneity	Mutations at different loci can produce the same phenotype (e.g., albinism).
Heteroplasmy	Presence of both normal and mutated mtDNA, resulting in variable expression in mitochondrial inherited diseases.
Uniparental disomy	Offspring receives 2 copies of a chromosome from 1 parent and no copies from the other parent.

Hardy-Weinberg population genetics

If a population is in Hardy-Weinberg equilibrium, then:

Disease prevalence: $p^2 + 2pq + q^2 = 1$

Allele prevalence: $p + q = 1$

p and q are separate alleles; 2pq = heterozygote prevalence. The prevalence of an X-linked recessive disease in males = q and in females = q^2.

Hardy-Weinberg law assumes:

1. There is no mutation occurring at the locus
2. There is no selection for any of the genotypes at the locus
3. Mating is completely random
4. There is no migration into or out of the population being considered

Imprinting	At a single locus, only 1 allele is active; the other is inactive (imprinted/inactivated by methylation). Deletion of the active allele → disease.	Can also occur as a result of uniparental disomy.
Prader-Willi syndrome	Deletion of normally active paternal allele.	Mental retardation, obesity, hypogonadism, hypotonia.
Angelman's syndrome	Deletion of normally active maternal allele.	Mental retardation, seizures, ataxia, inappropriate laughter (happy puppet).

Modes of inheritance

Autosomal dominant 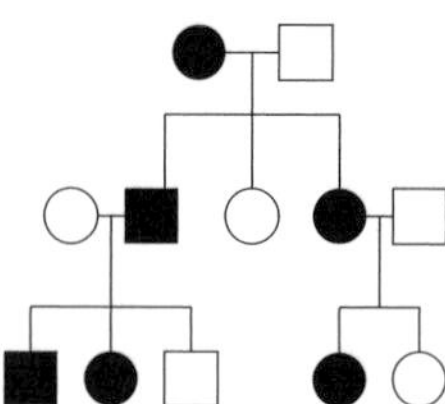	Often due to defects in structural genes. Many generations, both male and female, affected.	Often pleiotropic and, in many cases, present clinically after puberty. Family history crucial to diagnosis.
Autosomal recessive 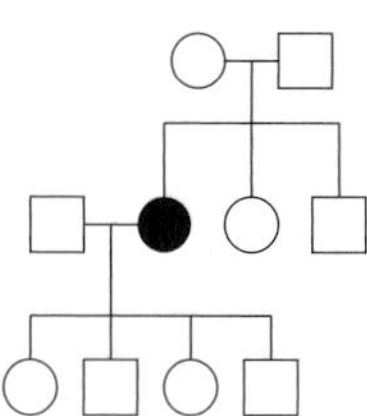	25% of offspring from 2 carrier parents are affected. Often due to enzyme deficiencies. Usually seen in only 1 generation.	Commonly more severe than dominant disorders; patients often present in childhood.
X-linked recessive 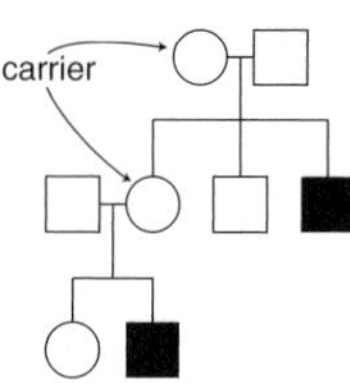	Sons of heterozygous mothers have a 50% chance of being affected. No male-to-male transmission.	Commonly more severe in males. Heterozygous females may be affected.
X-linked dominant 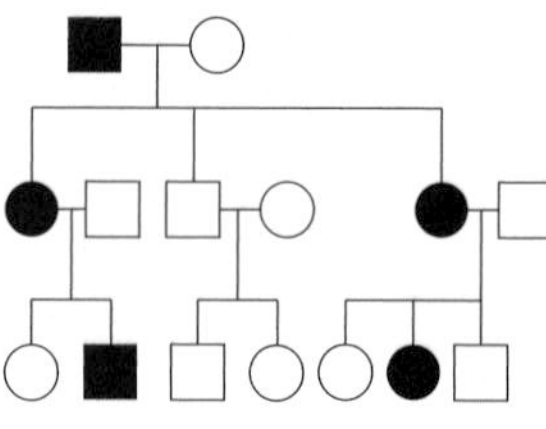	Transmitted through both parents. Either male or female offspring of the affected mother may be affected, while **all** female offspring of the affected father are diseased.	Hypophosphatemic rickets.
Mitochondrial inheritance 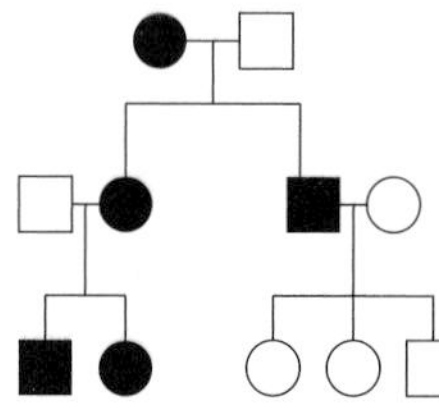	Transmitted only through mother. All offspring of affected females may show signs of disease.	Leber's hereditary optic neuropathy; mitochondrial myopathies. Variable expression in population due to heteroplasmy.

Autosomal-dominant diseases

Adult polycystic kidney disease	**Always bilateral,** massive enlargement of kidneys due to multiple large cysts. Patients present with pain, hematuria, hypertension, progressive renal failure. 90% of cases are due to mutation in *APKD1* (chromosome 16). Associated with polycystic liver disease, **berry aneurysms,** mitral valve prolapse. Juvenile form is recessive.
Familial hypercholesterolemia (hyperlipidemia type IIA)	Elevated LDL owing to defective or absent LDL receptor. Heterozygotes (1:500) have cholesterol ≈ 300 mg/dL. Homozygotes (very rare) have cholesterol ≈ 700+ mg/dL, severe atherosclerotic disease early in life, and tendon xanthomas (classically in the Achilles tendon); MI may develop before age 20.
Marfan's syndrome	Fibrillin gene mutation → connective tissue disorders. Skeletal abnormalities—tall with long extremities, pectus excavatum, hyperextensive joints, and long, tapering fingers and toes (arachnodactyly; see Figure 110). Cardiovascular—cystic medial necrosis of aorta → aortic incompetence and dissecting aortic aneurysms. Floppy mitral valve. Ocular—subluxation of lenses.
Neurofibromatosis type 1 (von Recklinghausen's disease)	Findings: café-au-lait spots, neural tumors, Lisch nodules (pigmented iris hamartomas). Also marked by skeletal disorders (e.g., scoliosis), optic pathway gliomas, pheochromocytoma, and ↑ tumor susceptibility. On long arm of chromosome **17; 17** letters in von Recklinghausen.
Neurofibromatosis type 2	Bilateral acoustic neuroma, juvenile cataracts. *NF2* gene on chromosome **22;** type **2** = **22.**
Tuberous sclerosis	Findings: facial lesions (adenoma sebaceum), hypopigmented "ash leaf spots" on skin, cortical and retinal hamartomas, seizures, mental retardation, renal cysts and renal angiomyolipomas, cardiac rhabdomyomas, ↑ incidence of astrocytomas. Incomplete penetrance, variable presentation.
von Hippel–Lindau disease	Findings: hemangioblastomas of retina/cerebellum/medulla; about half of affected individuals develop multiple bilateral renal cell carcinomas and other tumors. Associated with deletion of *VHL* gene (tumor suppressor) on chromosome 3 (3p). Von Hippel–Lindau = **3** words for chromosome **3.**
Huntington's disease	Findings: depression, progressive dementia, choreiform movements, caudate atrophy, and ↓ levels of GABA and ACh in the brain. Symptoms manifest in affected individuals between the ages of 20 and 50. Gene located on chromosome **4;** triplet repeat disorder. "Hunting **4** food."
Familial adenomatous polyposis	Colon becomes covered with adenomatous polyps after puberty. Progresses to colon cancer unless resected. Deletion on chromosome **5 (APC gene); 5** letters in "polyp."
Hereditary spherocytosis	Spheroid erythrocytes; hemolytic anemia; ↑ MCHC. Splenectomy is curative.
Achondroplasia	Autosomal-dominant cell-signaling defect of fibroblast growth factor (FGF) receptor 3. Results in dwarfism; short limbs, but head and trunk are normal size. Associated with advanced paternal age.

Autosomal-recessive diseases	Cystic fibrosis, albinism, α_1-antitrypsin deficiency, phenylketonuria, thalassemias, sickle cell anemias, glycogen storage diseases, mucopolysaccharidoses (except Hunter's), sphingolipidoses (except Fabry's), infant polycystic kidney disease, hemochromatosis.

Cystic fibrosis	Autosomal-recessive defect in *CFTR* gene on chromosome 7, commonly deletion of Phe 508. CFTR channel actively secretes Cl^- in lungs and GI tract and actively reabsorbs Cl^- from sweat. Defective Cl^- channel → secretion of abnormally thick mucus that plugs lungs, pancreas, and liver → recurrent pulmonary infections (*Pseudomonas* species and *S. aureus*), chronic bronchitis, bronchiectasis, pancreatic insufficiency (malabsorption and steatorrhea), meconium ileus in newborns. ↑ concentration of Cl^- ions in sweat test is diagnostic.	Infertility in males due to bilateral absence of vas deferens. Fat-soluble vitamin deficiencies (A, D, E, K). Can present as failure to thrive in infancy. Most common lethal genetic disease of Caucasians. Treatment: *N*-acetylcysteine to loosen mucous plugs.
X-linked recessive disorders	**B**ruton's agammaglobulinemia, **W**iskott-Aldrich syndrome, **F**ragile X, **G**6PD deficiency, **O**cular albinism, **L**esch-Nyhan syndrome, **D**uchenne's muscular dystrophy, **H**emophilia A and B, **F**abry's disease, **H**unter's syndrome. Female carriers of X-linked recessive disorders are rarely affected because of random inactivation of X chromosomes in each cell.	**B**e **W**ise, **F**ool's **GOLD H**eeds **F**alse **H**ope.
Muscular dystrophies		
Duchenne's (X-linked)	Frame-shift mutation → deletion of dystrophin gene → accelerated muscle breakdown. Onset before 5 years of age. Weakness begins in pelvic girdle muscles and progresses superiorly. Pseudohypertrophy of calf muscles due to fibrofatty replacement of muscle; cardiac myopathy. The use of Gowers' maneuver, requiring assistance of the upper extremities to stand up, is characteristic (indicates proximal lower limb weakness).	**D**uchenne's = **D**eleted **D**ystrophin. Diagnose muscular dystrophies by ↑ CPK and muscle biopsy.
Becker's	Mutated dystrophin gene is less severe than Duchenne's.	
Fragile X syndrome	X-linked defect affecting the methylation and expression of the *FMR1* gene. Associated with chromosomal breakage. The 2nd most common cause of genetic mental retardation (the most common cause is Down syndrome). Associated with macro-orchidism (enlarged testes), long face with a large jaw, large everted ears, and autism.	Triplet repeat disorder $(CGG)_n$ that may show genetic anticipation (germline expansion in females). Fragile **X** = e**X**tra-large testes, jaw, ears.
Trinucleotide repeat expansion diseases	**Hunting**ton's disease, **my**otonic dystrophy, **Fried**reich's ataxia, fragile **X** syndrome. May show anticipation (disease severity ↑ and age of onset ↓ in successive generations).	**Try** (**tri**nucleotide) **hunting** for **my fried** eggs (**X**).

Autosomal trisomies

Disorder	Down syndrome	Edwards' syndrome	Patau's syndrome
Trisomy	21 (**D**rinking age = 21)	18 (**E**lection age = 18)	13 (**P**uberty = 13)
Incidence	1:700; **most common chromosomal disorder**	1:8000	1:15,000
↑ with maternal age	Yes	Yes	Yes
Genetics	95% meiotic nondisjunction; 4% robertsonian translocation; 1% mosaicism (nonmaternal)	—	—
Prenatal screening	↑ α-fetoprotein, ↓ β-hCG, ↑ nuchal translucency	—	—
Other disease risks	ALL, Alzheimer's > age 35	—	—
Life expectancy	45–50 years	< 1 year	< 1 year
Mental retardation	Yes, **most common cause**	Severe	Severe
Head	Flat facial profile, prominent epicanthal folds	Prominent occiput, micrognathia (small jaw), low-set ears	Microphthalmia, microcephaly, cleft lip/palate
Congenital heart defects	Yes, especially septum primum–type ASD due to endocardial cushion defects	Yes	Yes
Hands	Simian crease (see Image 111)	Clenched hands	Polydactyly
Feet	Gap between first 2 toes	Rocker-bottom feet	Rocker-bottom feet

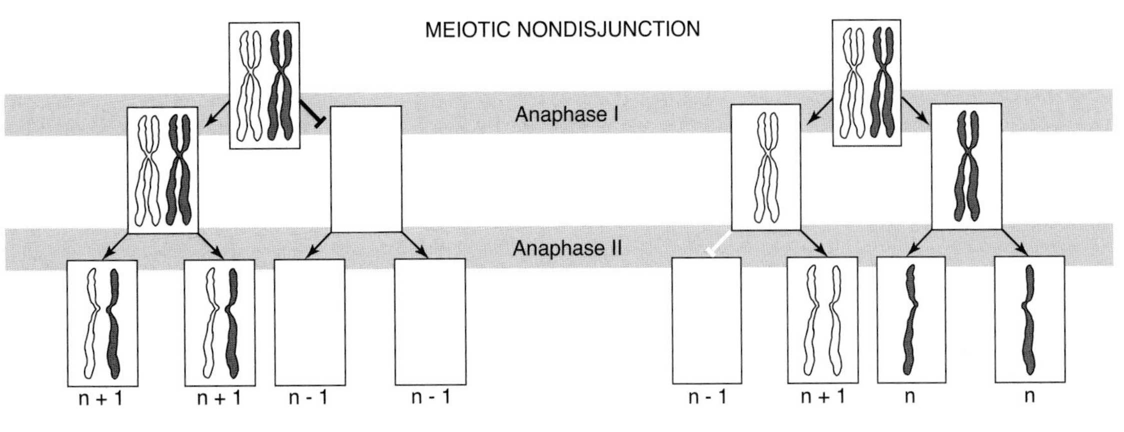

Chromosomal inversions		
Pericentric	Involves centromere; proceeds through meiosis.	
Paracentric	Does not involve centromere; does not proceed through meiosis.	
Cri-du-chat syndrome	Congenital deletion of short arm of chromosome 5 (46,XX or XY, 5p–). Findings: microcephaly, severe mental retardation, high-pitched crying/mewing, epicanthal folds, cardiac abnormalities.	*Cri du chat* = cry of the cat.
22q11 syndromes	**C**left palate, **A**bnormal facies, **T**hymic aplasia → T-cell deficiency, **C**ardiac defects, **H**ypocalcemia 2° to parathyroid aplasia, microdeletion at chromosome **22**q11. Variable presentation as DiGeorge syndrome (thymic, parathyroid, and cardiac defects) or velocardiofacial syndrome (palate, facial, and cardiac defects).	CATCH-22.

HIGH-YIELD PRINCIPLES IN

Embryology

"Zygote. This cell, formed by the union of an ovum and a sperm, represents the beginning of a human being."

—Keith Moore and Vid Persaud,
Before We Are Born

Embryology is traditionally one of the higher-yield areas within anatomy. This topic can be crammed closer to the exam date. Many questions focus on underlying mechanisms of congenital malformations (e.g., failure of fusion of the maxillary and medial nasal processes leading to cleft lip).

Fetal landmarks

Day 0	Fertilization by sperm forming zygote, initiating embryogenesis.
Within week 1	Implantation (as a blastocyst).
Within week 2	Bilaminar disk (epiblast, hypoblast).
Within week 3	Gastrulation. Primitive streak, notochord, and neural plate begin to form.
Weeks 3–8	Neural tube formed. Organogenesis. Extremely susceptible to teratogens.
Week 4	Heart begins to beat. Upper and lower limb buds begin to form.
Week 8	Fetal movement; fetus looks like a baby.
Week 10	Genitalia have male/female characteristics.
Alar plate (dorsal)	Sensory
Basal plate (ventral)	Motor

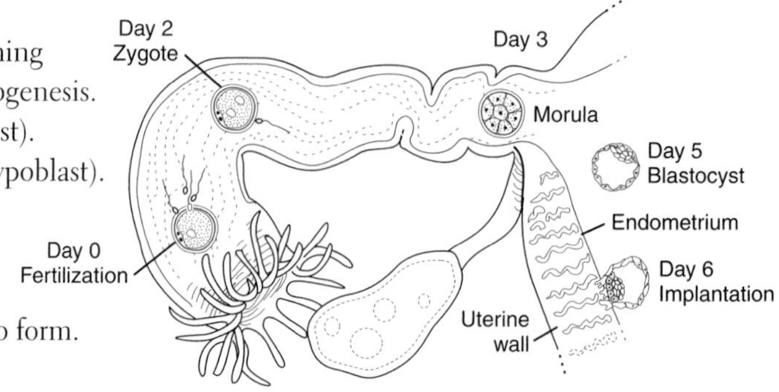

Day 2 Zygote
Day 3
Morula
Day 5 Blastocyst
Endometrium
Day 0 Fertilization
Day 6 Implantation
Uterine wall

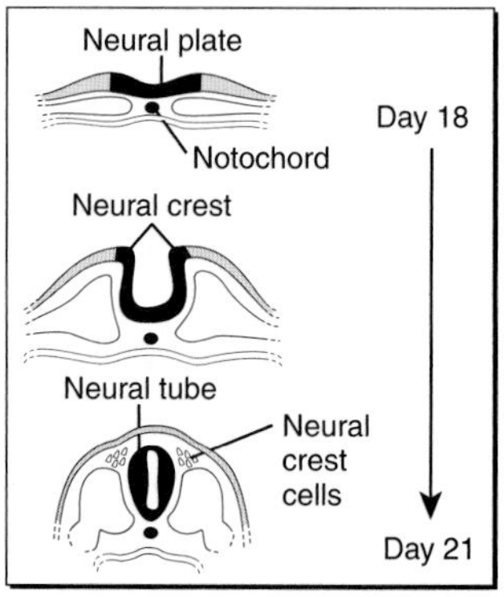

Neural plate
Notochord
Day 18
Neural crest
Neural tube
Neural crest cells
Day 21

Early development

Rule of 2's for 2nd week	2 germ layers (bilaminar disk): epiblast, hypoblast. 2 cavities: amniotic cavity, yolk sac. 2 components to placenta: cytotrophoblast, syncytiotrophoblast.	The epiblast (precursor to ectoderm) invaginates to form primitive streak. Cells from the primitive streak give rise to both intraembryonic mesoderm and endoderm.
Rule of 3's for 3rd week	3 germ layers (gastrula): ectoderm, mesoderm, endoderm.	
Rule of 4's for 4th week	4 heart chambers. 4 limb buds grow.	

Embryologic derivatives

Ectoderm	
Surface ectoderm	Adenohypophysis; lens of eye; epithelial linings of skin, ear, eye, and nose; epidermis.
Neuroectoderm	Neurohypophysis, CNS neurons, oligodendrocytes, astrocytes, ependymal cells, pineal gland.
Neural crest	ANS, dorsal root ganglia, melanocytes, chromaffin cells of adrenal medulla, enterochromaffin cells, pia and arachnoid, celiac ganglion, Schwann cells, odontoblasts, parafollicular (C) cells of thyroid, laryngeal cartilage, bones of the skull.
Endoderm	Gut tube epithelium and derivatives (e.g., lungs, liver, pancreas, thymus, parathyroid, thyroid follicular cells).
Mesoderm	Dura mater, connective tissue, muscle, bone, cardiovascular structures, lymphatics, blood, urogenital structures, serous linings of body cavities (e.g., peritoneal), spleen, adrenal cortex, kidneys. Notochord induces ectoderm to form neuroectoderm (neural plate). Its postnatal derivative is the nucleus pulposus of the intervertebral disk. Mesodermal defects = **VACTERL:** **V**ertebral defect, **A**nal atresia, **C**ardiac defects, **T**racheo-**E**sophageal fistula, **R**enal defects, **L**imb defects (bone and muscle).

Teratogens

Most susceptible in 3rd–8th weeks (organogenesis) of pregnancy.

Examples	Effects on fetus
Alcohol	(See the discussion of fetal alcohol syndrome below)
ACE inhibitors	Renal damage
Cocaine	Abnormal fetal development and fetal addiction
Diethylstilbestrol (DES)	Vaginal clear cell adenocarcinoma
Iodide	Congenital goiter or hypothyroidism
Vitamin A	Extremely high risk for birth defects
Thalidomide	Limb defects ("flipper" limbs)
Tobacco	Preterm labor, placental problems, attention-deficit hyperactivity disorder (ADHD)
Warfarin, x-rays, anticonvulsants	Multiple anomalies

Fetal infections can also cause congenital malformations. (Other medications contraindicated in pregnancy are shown in the pharmacology section.)

Fetal alcohol syndrome

Leading cause of congenital malformations in the United States. Newborns of mothers who consumed significant amounts of alcohol during pregnancy have an ↑ incidence of congenital abnormalities, including pre- and postnatal developmental retardation, microcephaly, facial abnormalities, limb dislocation, and heart and lung fistulas. Mechanism may include inhibition of cell migration.

Twinning

Monozygotic

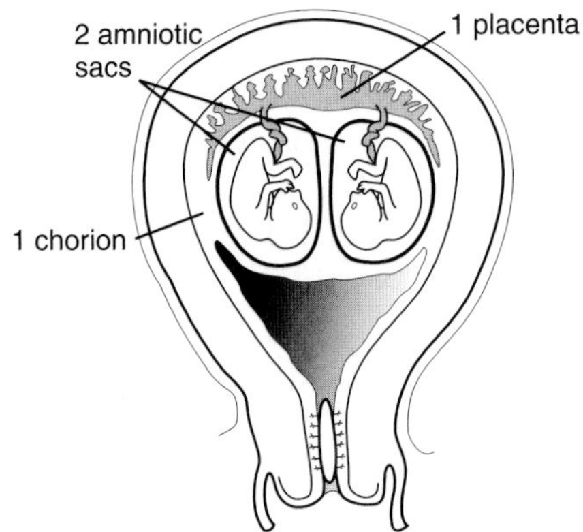

1 zygote splits evenly to develop 2 amniotic sacs with a single common chorion and placenta.

Dizygotic (fraternal) or monozygotic

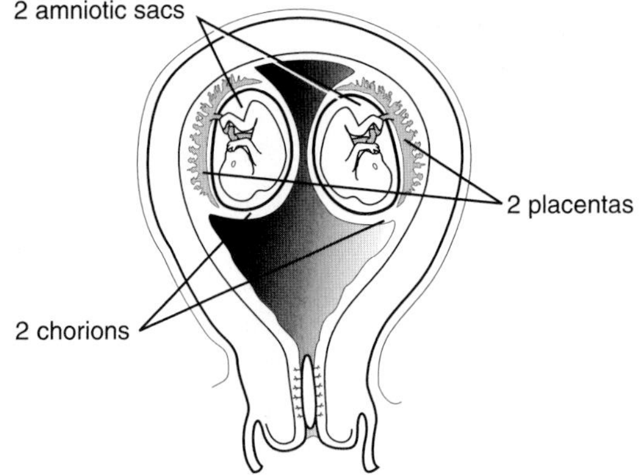

Monozygotes that split early develop 2 placentas (separate/fused), chorions, and amniotic sacs.

Dizygotes develop individual placentas, chorions, and amniotic sacs.

Placental development	1° site of nutrient and gas exchange between mother and fetus.
Fetal component	Cytotrophoblast composes the inner layer of chorionic villi. Syncytiotrophoblast is the outer layer and secretes hCG.
Maternal component	Decidua basalis derived from the endometrium.

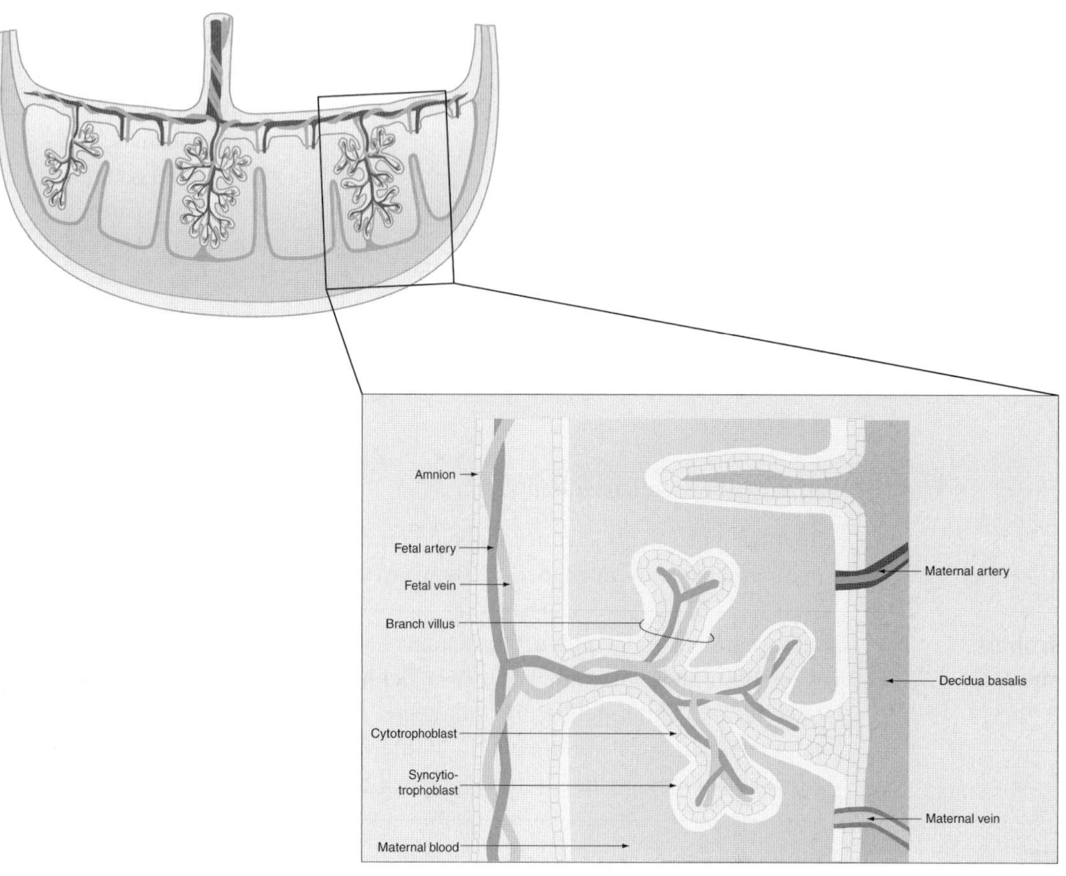

Umbilical cord	Contains 2 umbilical arteries, which return deoxygenated blood from fetal internal iliac arteries, and 1 umbilical vein, which supplies oxygenated blood from the placenta to the fetus.	Single umbilical artery is associated with congenital and chromosomal anomalies.
	Urachus removes nitrogenous waste from fetal bladder (like a urethra).	Urachus connects fetal bladder with allantois. Umbilical arteries and veins are derived from the allantois.

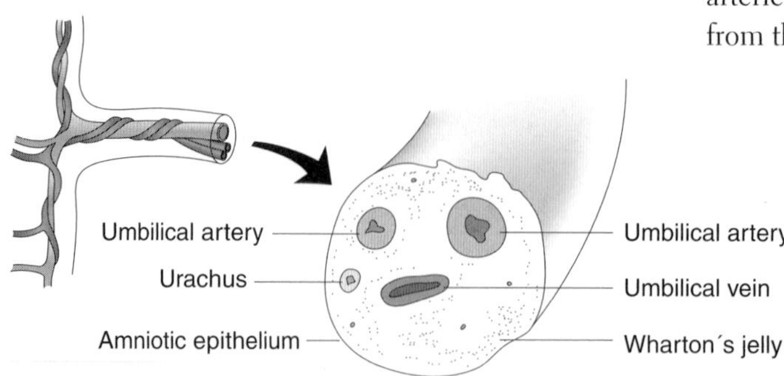

Heart embryology

Embryonic structure	Gives rise to
Truncus arteriosus (TA)	Ascending aorta and pulmonary trunk
Bulbus cordis	Smooth parts of left and right ventricle
Primitive ventricle	Trabeculated parts of left and right ventricle
Primitive atria	Trabeculated left and right atrium
Left horn of sinus venosus (SV)	Coronary sinus
Right horn of SV	Smooth part of right atrium
Right common cardinal vein and right anterior cardinal vein	SVC

Interventricular septum development

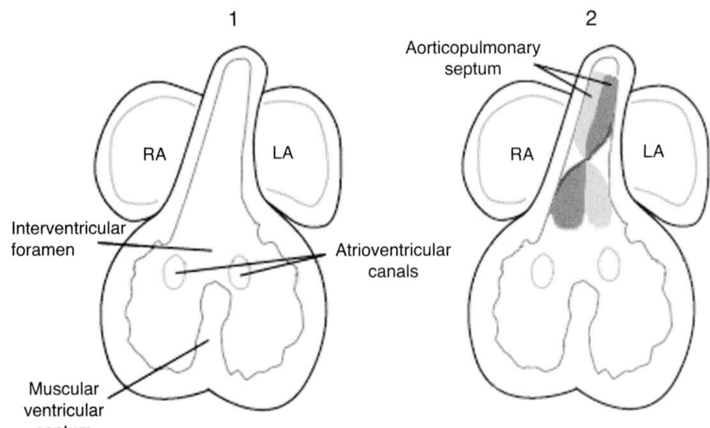

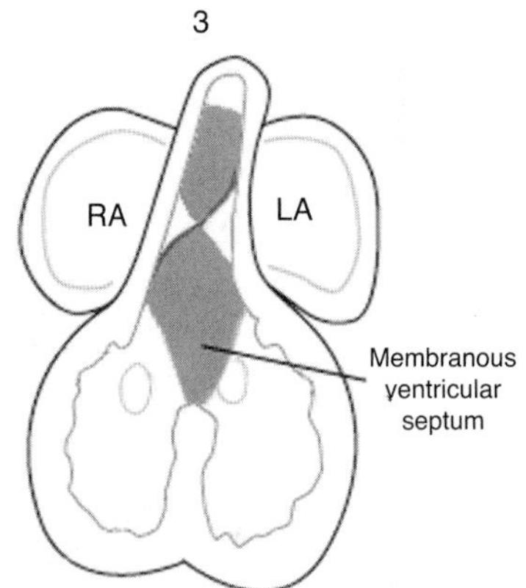

1. Muscular ventricular septum forms. Opening is called the interventricular foramen.
2. The aorticopulmonary septum divides the TA into the aortic and pulmonary trunks.
3. The aorticopulmonary septum meets and fuses with the muscular ventricular septum to form the membranous interventricular septum, closing the interventricular foramen.

Interatrial septum development

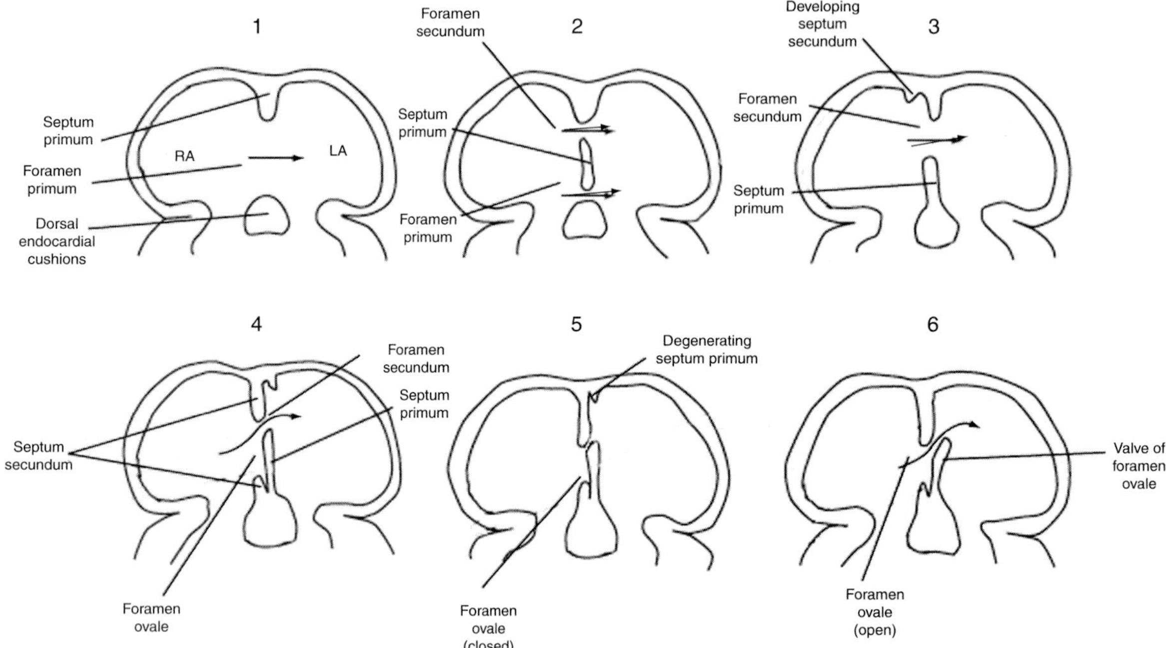

1. Foramen primum narrows as the septum primum grows toward the endocardial cushions.
2. Perforations in the septum primum form the foramen secundum as the foramen primum disappears.
3. The foramen secundum maintains the right-to-left shunt as the septum secundum begins to grow.
4. The septum secundum contains a permanent opening called the foramen ovale.
5. The foramen secundum enlarges and the upper part of the septum primum degenerates.
6. The remaining portion of the septum primum is now called the valve of the foramen ovale.

Fetal erythropoiesis

Fetal erythropoiesis occurs in:

1. **Y**olk sac (3–8 wk)
2. **L**iver (6–30 wk)
3. **S**pleen (9–28 wk)
4. **B**one marrow (28 wk onward)

Young **L**iver **S**ynthesizes **B**lood.

Fetal hemoglobin = $\alpha_2\gamma_2$.
Adult hemoglobin = $\alpha_2\beta_2$.

Fetal circulation	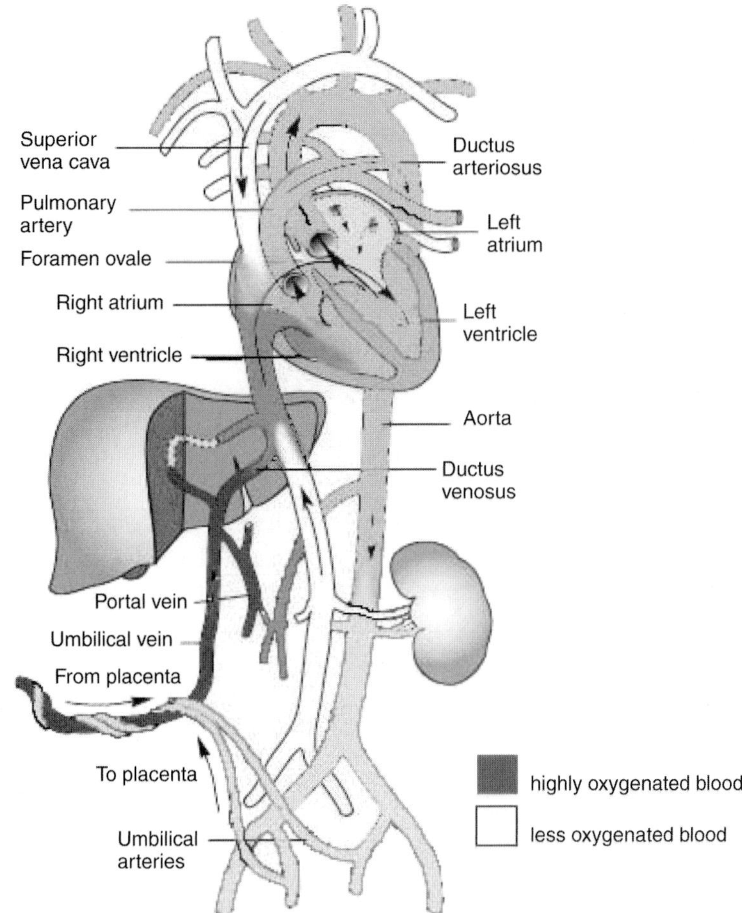 (Adapted, with permission, from Ganong WF. *Review of Medical Physiology,* 19th ed. Stamford, CT: Appleton & Lange, 1999: 600.)	Blood in umbilical vein is ≈ 80% saturated with O_2. Umbilical arteries have low O_2 saturation. 3 important shunts: 1. Blood entering the fetus through the umbilical vein is conducted via the **ductus venosus** into the IVC. 2. Most oxygenated blood reaching the heart via the IVC is diverted through the **foramen ovale** and pumped out the aorta to the head and body. 3. Deoxygenated blood from the SVC is expelled into the pulmonary artery and **ductus arteriosus** to the lower body of the fetus. At birth, infant takes a breath; ↓ resistance in pulmonary vasculature causes ↑ left atrial pressure vs. right atrial pressure; foramen ovale closes (now called fossa ovalis); ↑ in O_2 leads to ↓ in prostaglandins, causing closure of ductus arteriosus. Indomethacin helps close PDA. Prostaglandins keep PDA open.
Fetal-postnatal derivatives	1. Umbilical vein—ligamentum teres hepatis 2. UmbiLical arteries—**mediaL** umbilical ligaments 3. Ductus arteriosus—ligamentum arteriosum 4. Ductus venosus—ligamentum venosum 5. Foramen ovale—fossa ovalis 6. Alla**N**tois—urachus—**mediaN** umbilical ligament 7. Notochord—nucleus pulposus of intervertebral disk	Contained in falciform ligament. The urachus is the part of the allantoic duct between the bladder and the umbilicus. Urachal cyst or sinus is a remnant.

Aortic arch derivatives 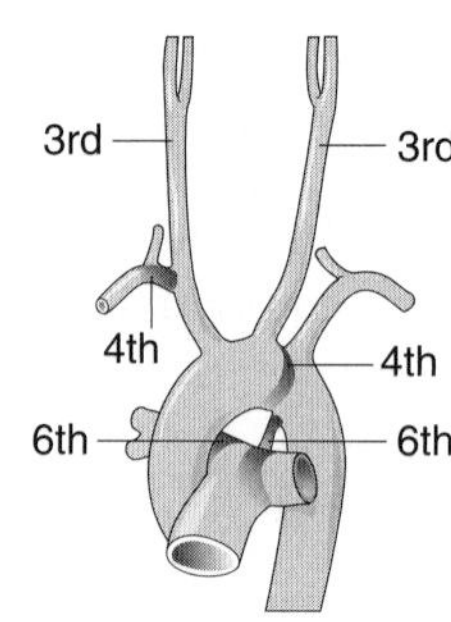	1st—part of **MAX**illary artery. 2nd—**S**tapedial artery and hyoid artery. 3rd—common **C**arotid artery and proximal part of internal carotid artery. 4th—on left, aortic arch; on right, proximal part of right subclavian artery. 6th—proximal part of pulmonary arteries and (on left only) ductus arteriosus.	1st arch is **MAX**imal. **S**econd = **S**tapedial. **C** is 3rd letter of alphabet. 4th arch (4 limbs) = systemic. 6th arch = pulmonary and the pulmonary-to-systemic shunt (ductus arteriosus).
Branchial apparatus 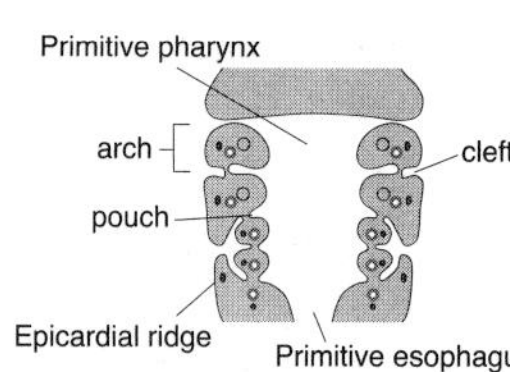	Composed of branchial clefts, arches, and pouches. Branchial clefts are derived from ectoderm. Branchial arches are derived from mesoderm and neural crests. Branchial pouches are derived from endoderm.	**CAP** covers outside from inside (**C**lefts = ectoderm, **A**rches = mesoderm, **P**ouches = endoderm). Clefts are also called grooves. Branchial apparatus is also called pharyngeal apparatus.
Branchial arch 1 derivatives	Meckel's cartilage: **M**andible, **M**alleus, incus, spheno**M**andibular ligament. Muscles: **M**uscles of **M**astication (temporalis, **M**asseter, lateral and **M**edial pterygoids), **M**ylohyoid, anterior belly of digastric, tensor tympani, tensor veli palatini, anterior ⅔ of tongue. Nerve: CN V_2 and CN V_3.	
Branchial arch 2 derivatives	Reichert's cartilage: **S**tapes, **S**tyloid process, lesser horn of hyoid, **S**tylohyoid ligament. Muscles: muscles of facial expression, **S**tapedius, **S**tylohyoid, posterior belly of digastric. Nerve: CN VII.	
Branchial arch 3 derivatives	Cartilage: greater horn of hyoid. Muscle: stylopharyngeus. Nerve: CN IX.	Think of pharynx: stylo**pharyngeus** innervated by glosso**pharyngeal** nerve.
Branchial arches 4–6 derivatives	Cartilages: thyroid, cricoid, arytenoids, corniculate, cuneiform. Muscles (4th arch): most pharyngeal constrictors, cricothyroid, levator veli palatini. Muscles (6th arch): all intrinsic muscles of larynx **except cricothyroid.** Nerve: 4th arch—CN X (superior laryngeal branch); 6th arch—CN X (recurrent laryngeal branch).	Arches 3 and 4 form posterior ⅓ of tongue. Arch 5 makes no major developmental contributions.

Branchial arch innervation

Arch 1 derivatives supplied by CN V_2 and V_3.
Arch 2 derivatives supplied by CN VII.
Arch 3 derivatives supplied by CN IX.
Arch 4 and 6 derivatives supplied by CN X.
These CNs are the only ones with both sensory and motor components.

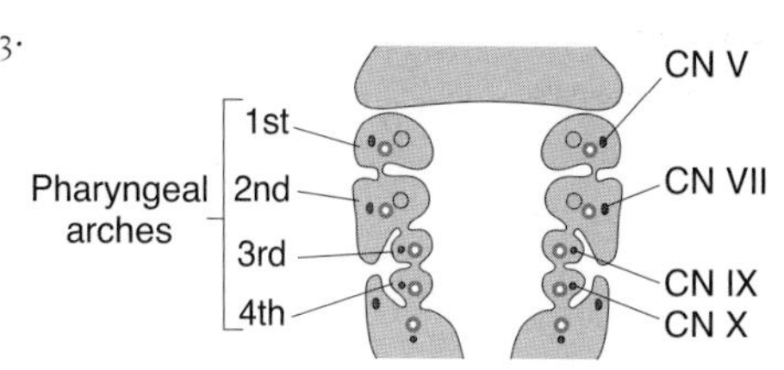

Branchial cleft derivatives

1st cleft develops into external auditory meatus.
2nd through 4th clefts form temporary cervical sinuses, which are obliterated by proliferation of 2nd arch mesenchyme.

Branchial pouch derivatives

1st pouch develops into middle ear cavity, eustachian tube, mastoid air cells.
2nd pouch develops into epithelial lining of palatine tonsil.
3rd pouch (dorsal wings) develops into **inferior** parathyroids.
3rd pouch (ventral wings) develops into thymus.
4th pouch (dorsal wings) develops into **superior** parathyroids.

1st pouch contributes to endoderm-lined structures of ear.
3rd pouch contributes to 3 structures (thymus, left and right inferior parathyroids).
Aberrant development of 3rd and 4th pouches → DiGeorge syndrome → leads to T-cell deficiency (thymic aplasia) and hypocalcemia (failure of parathyroid development).

Ear development

Bones	Muscles (innervation)	Origin	Miscellaneous
Malleus/incus	Tensor tyMpani (V_3)	1st arch	
Stapes	Stapedius (VII)	2nd arch	
		1st cleft	External auditory meatus
		1st branchial membrane	Tympanic membrane

Tongue development

1st branchial arch forms anterior ²⁄₃ (thus sensation via CN V_3, taste via CN VII).
3rd and 4th arches form posterior ¹⁄₃ (thus sensation and taste mainly via CN IX, extreme posterior via CN X).
Motor innervation is via CN XII.
Muscles of the tongue are derived from occipital myotomes.

Taste is CN VII, IX, X (solitary nucleus); pain is CN V_3, IX, X; motor is CN XII.

X
X X
Taste/sensation via IX
Arches 3, 4
Foramen cecum
Taste via VII
Arch 1
Sensation via V_3

Thyroid development

Thyroid diverticulum arises from floor of primitive pharynx, descends into neck. Connected to tongue by thyroglossal duct, which normally disappears but may persist as pyramidal lobe of thyroid. Foramen cecum is normal remnant of thyroglossal duct. Most common ectopic thyroid tissue site is the tongue.

Thyroglossal duct cyst in midline neck and will move with swallowing (vs. persistent cervical sinus leading to branchial cyst in lateral neck).

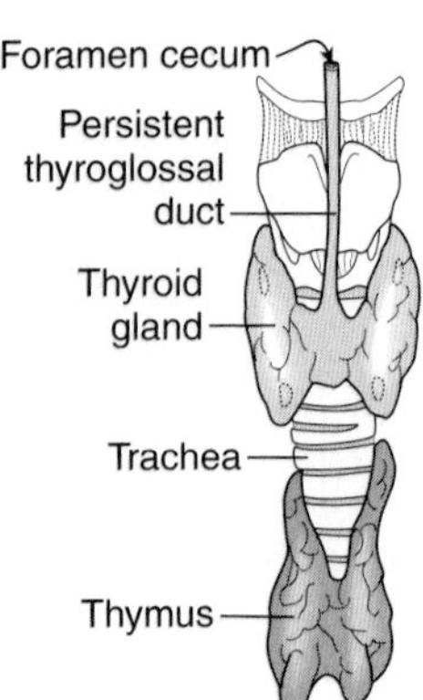

Cleft lip and cleft palate

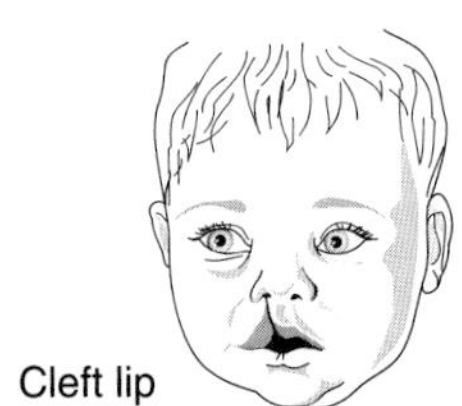

Cleft lip—failure of fusion of the maxillary and medial nasal processes (formation of 1° palate).

Cleft palate—failure of fusion of the lateral palatine processes, the nasal septum, and/or the median palatine process (formation of 2° palate).

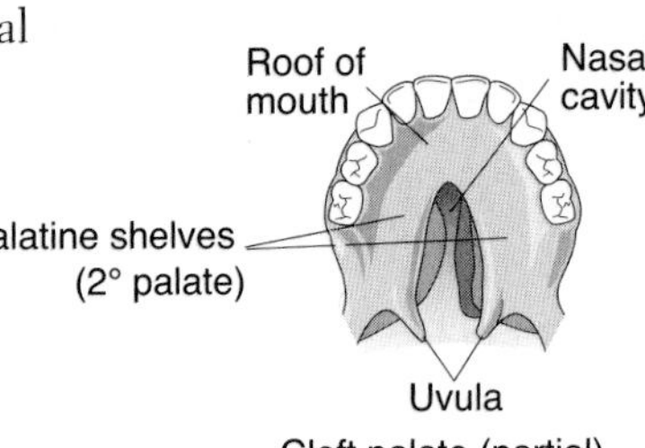

Cleft palate (partial)

Diaphragm embryology

Diaphragm is derived from:

1. **S**eptum transversum
2. **P**leuroperitoneal folds
3. **B**ody wall
4. **D**orsal mesentery of esophagus

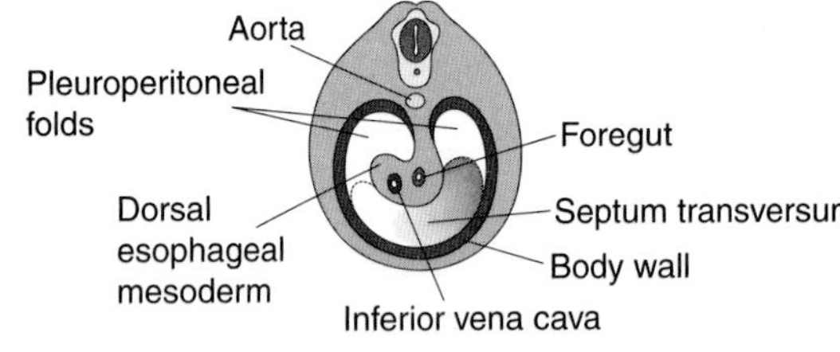

Several **P**arts **B**uild **D**iaphragm.

Diaphragm descends during development but maintains innervation from above C3–C5. "**C3, 4, 5** keeps the diaphragm alive."

Abdominal contents may herniate into the thorax because of incomplete development (diaphragmatic hernia) → hypoplasia of thoracic organs due to space compression.

Pancreas and spleen embryology

Pancreas is derived from the foregut. Ventral pancreatic bud becomes pancreatic head, uncinate process (lower half of head), and main pancreatic duct. Dorsal pancreatic bud becomes everything else (body, tail, isthmus, and accessory pancreatic duct).

Annular pancreas—ventral pancreatic bud abnormally encircles 2nd part of duodenum; forms a ring of pancreatic tissue that may cause duodenal narrowing.

Spleen arises from dorsal mesentery but is supplied by artery of foregut.

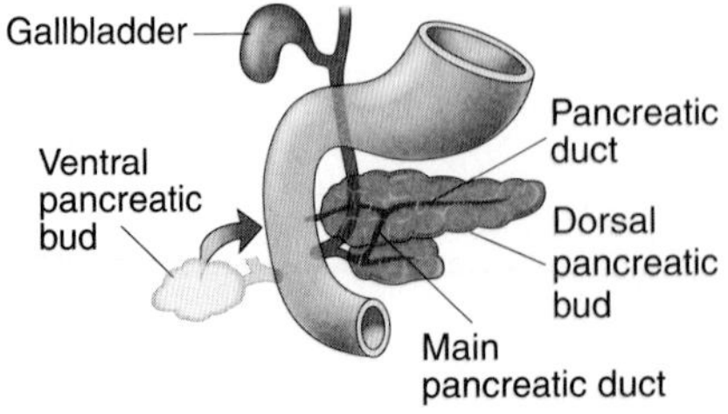

GI embryology

1. Foregut—pharynx to duodenum
2. Midgut—duodenum to transverse colon
3. Hindgut—distal transverse colon to rectum

Gastroschisis—failure of lateral body folds to fuse → extrusion of abdominal contents through abdominal folds.

Omphalocele—persistence of herniation of abdominal contents into umbilical cord.

Kidney embryology

1. Pronephros—week 4; then degenerates
2. Mesonephros—functions as interim kidney for 1st trimester; later contributes to male genital system
3. Metanephros—permanent
4. Urogenital sinus—develops into bladder, urethra, allantois

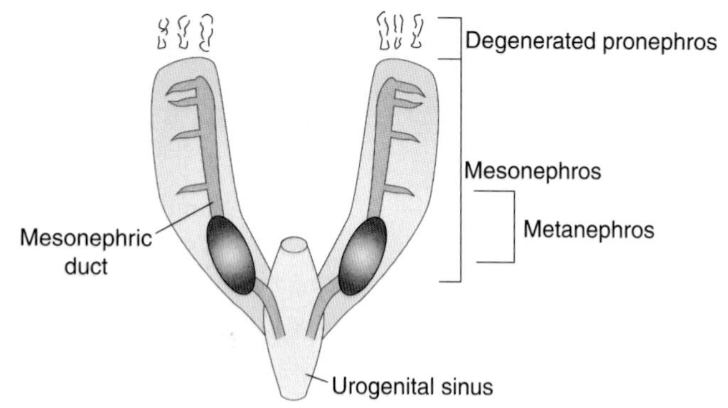

Genital embryology

Female	Default development. Mesonephric duct disappears and paramesonephric duct develops.	
Male	*SRY* gene on Y chromosome codes for testis-determining factor. Müllerian inhibiting substance secreted by testes suppresses development of paramesonephric ducts. ↑ androgens → development of mesonephric ducts.	
Mesonephric (wolffian) duct	Develops into male internal structures (except prostate)—**S**eminal vesicles, **E**pididymis, **E**jaculatory duct, and **D**uctus deferens.	SEED.
Paramesonephric (müllerian) duct	Develops into fallopian tube, uterus, and part of vagina.	

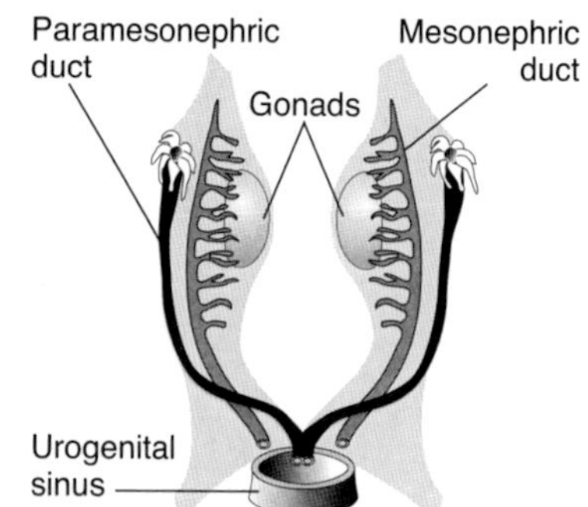

Male/female genital homologues

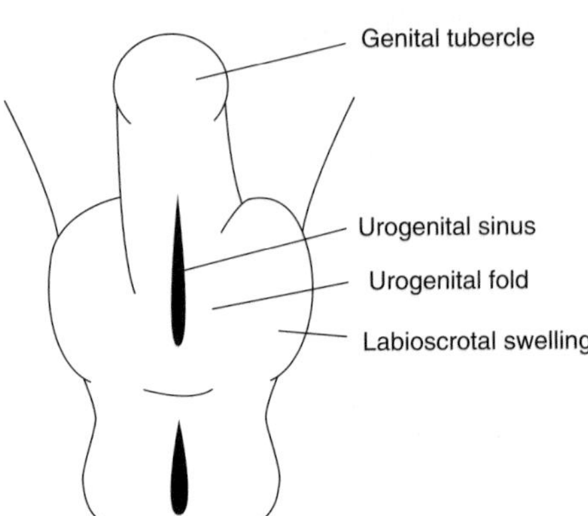

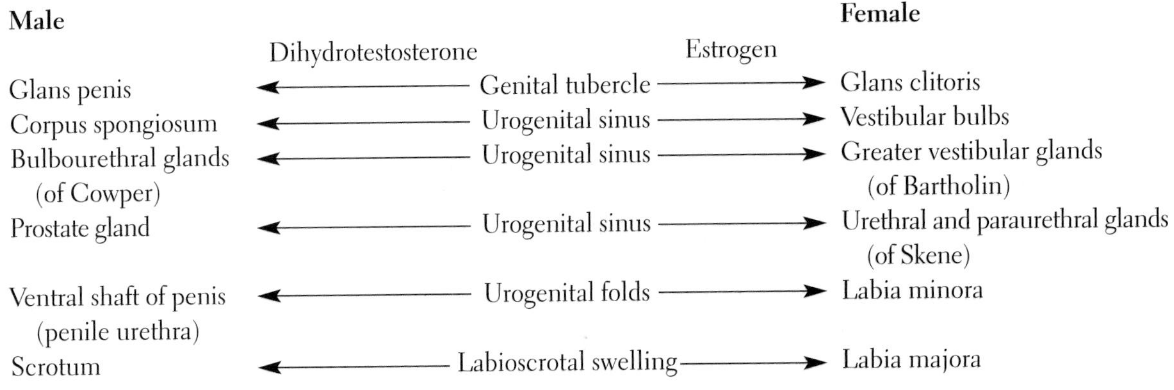

Male	Dihydrotestosterone ←		Estrogen →	Female
Glans penis	←	Genital tubercle	→	Glans clitoris
Corpus spongiosum	←	Urogenital sinus	→	Vestibular bulbs
Bulbourethral glands (of Cowper)	←	Urogenital sinus	→	Greater vestibular glands (of Bartholin)
Prostate gland	←	Urogenital sinus	→	Urethral and paraurethral glands (of Skene)
Ventral shaft of penis (penile urethra)	←	Urogenital folds	→	Labia minora
Scrotum	←	Labioscrotal swelling	→	Labia majora

HIGH-YIELD PRINCIPLES IN

Microbiology

"What lies behind us and what lies ahead of us are tiny matters compared to what lives within us."

—Oliver Wendell Holmes

This high-yield material covers the basic concepts of microbiology. The emphasis in previous examinations has been approximately 40% bacteriology (20% basic, 20% quasi-clinical), 25% immunology, 25% virology (10% basic, 15% quasi-clinical), 5% parasitology, and 5% mycology. Learning the distinguishing characteristics, target organs, and method of spread of—as well as relevant laboratory tests for—major pathogens can improve your score substantially.

MICROBIOLOGY—HIGH-YIELD CLINICAL VIGNETTES

Vignette	Question	Answer
Alcoholic vomits gastric contents and develops foul-smelling sputum.	What organisms are most likely?	Anaerobes.
Middle-age male presents with acute-onset monoarticular joint pain and bilateral Bell's palsy.	What is the likely disease, and how did he get it?	Lyme disease; bite from *Ixodes* tick.
UA of patient shows WBC casts.	What is the diagnosis?	Pyelonephritis.
Patient presents with "rose gardener's" scenario (thorn prick with ulcers along lymphatic drainage).	What is the infectious bug?	*Sporothrix schenckii.*
25-year-old medical student has a burning feeling in his gut after meals. Biopsy of gastric mucosa shows gram-negative rods.	What is the likely organism?	*Helicobacter pylori.*
32-year-old male has "cauliflower" skin lesions. Tissue biopsy shows broad-based budding yeasts.	What is the likely organism?	*Blastomyces.*
Breast-feeding woman suddenly develops redness and swelling of her right breast. On examination, it is found to be a fluctuant mass.	What is the diagnosis?	Mastitis caused by S. *aureus.*
20-year-old college student presents with lymphadenopathy, fever, and hepatosplenomegaly. His serum agglutinates sheep RBCs.	What cell is infected?	B cell (EBV; infectious mononucleosis).
3 hours after eating custard at a picnic, a whole family began to vomit. After 10 hours, they were better.	What is the organism?	*S. aureus* (produces preformed enterotoxin).
Infant becomes flaccid after eating honey.	What organism is implicated, and what is the mechanism of action?	*Clostridium botulinum;* inhibited release of ACh.
Man presents with squamous cell carcinoma of the penis.	He had exposure to what virus?	HPV.
Patient develops endocarditis 3 weeks after receiving a prosthetic heart valve.	What organism is suspected?	*S. epidermidis.*

55-year-old man who is a smoker and a heavy drinker presents with a new cough and flulike symptoms. Gram stain shows no organisms; silver stain of sputum shows gram-negative rods.	What is the diagnosis?	*Legionella* pneumonia.
After taking clindamycin, patient develops toxic megacolon and diarrhea.	What is the mechanism of diarrhea?	*Clostridium difficile* overgrowth.
25-year-old man presents with 3 days of fever, chills, and a painful, swollen knee.	What is the diagnosis, and what is the causative agent?	Septic arthritis; N. *gonorrhoeae.*
19-year-old female college student presents with vaginal itching and a thick, curdy discharge.	What is the causative agent?	*Candida albicans.*
30-year-old woman returns from a camping trip and complains of watery diarrhea and cramps.	What is the causative agent?	*Giardia lamblia.*

Bacterial structures

Structure	Function	Chemical composition
Peptidoglycan	Gives rigid support, protects against osmotic pressure.	Sugar backbone with cross-linked peptide side chains.
Cell wall/cell membrane (gram positives)	Major surface antigen.	Peptidoglycan for support. Teichoic acid induces TNF and IL-1.
Outer membrane (gram negatives)	Site of endotoxin (lipopolysaccharide); major surface antigen.	Lipid A induces TNF and IL-1; polysaccharide is the antigen.
Plasma membrane	Site of oxidative and transport enzymes.	Lipoprotein bilayer.
Ribosome	Protein synthesis.	50S and 30S subunits.
Periplasm	Space between the cytoplasmic membrane and outer membrane in gram-negative bacteria.	Contains many hydrolytic enzymes, including β-lactamases.
Capsule	Protects against phagocytosis.	Polysaccharide (except *Bacillus anthracis*, which contains D-glutamate).
Pilus/fimbria	Mediates adherence of bacteria to cell surface; sex pilus forms attachment between 2 bacteria during conjugation.	Glycoprotein.
Flagellum	Motility.	Protein.
Spore	Provides resistance to dehydration, heat, and chemicals.	Keratin-like coat; dipicolinic acid.
Plasmid	Contains a variety of genes for antibiotic resistance, enzymes, and toxins.	DNA.
Glycocalyx	Mediates adherence to surfaces, especially foreign surfaces (e.g., indwelling catheters).	Polysaccharide.

Bacteria with unusual cell membranes/walls

Mycoplasma	Contain sterols and have no cell wall.
Mycobacteria	Contain mycolic acid. High lipid content.

Cell walls

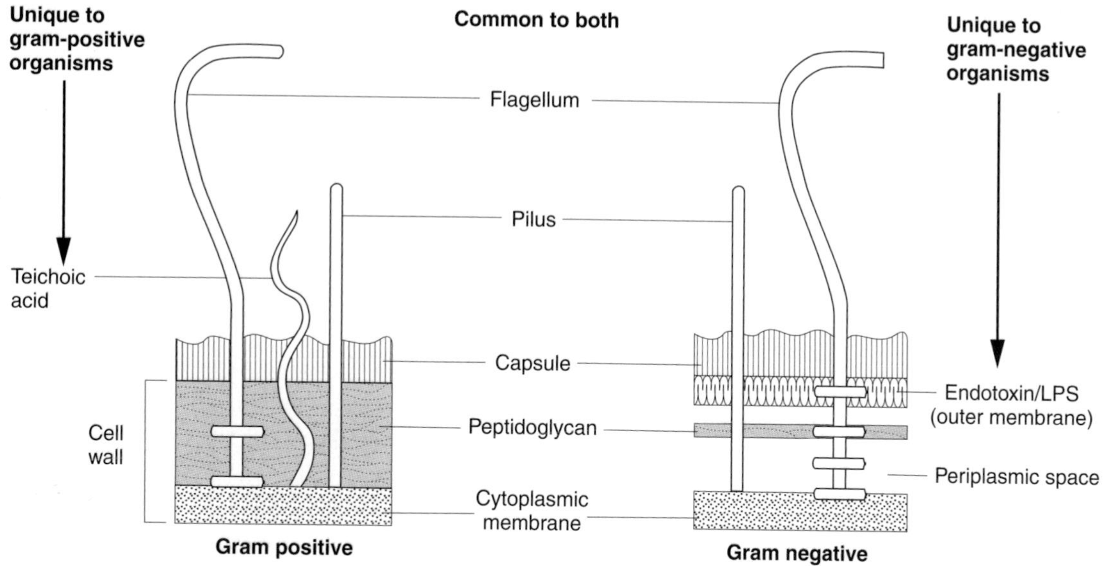

(Adapted, with permission, from Levinson W, Jawetz E. *Medical Microbiology and Immunology: Examination and Board Review,* 9th ed. New York: McGraw-Hill, 2006: 7.)

Gram stain limitations

These bugs do not Gram stain well:

Treponema (too thin to be visualized).

Rickettsia (intracellular parasite).

Mycobacteria (high-lipid-content cell wall requires acid-fast stain).

Mycoplasma (no cell wall).

Legionella pneumophila (primarily intracellular).

Chlamydia (intracellular parasite; lacks muramic acid in cell wall).

These **R**ascals **M**ay **M**icroscopically **L**ack **C**olor.

Treponemes—darkfield microscopy and fluorescent antibody staining.

Mycobacteria—acid fast.

Legionella—silver stain.

Bacterial growth curve

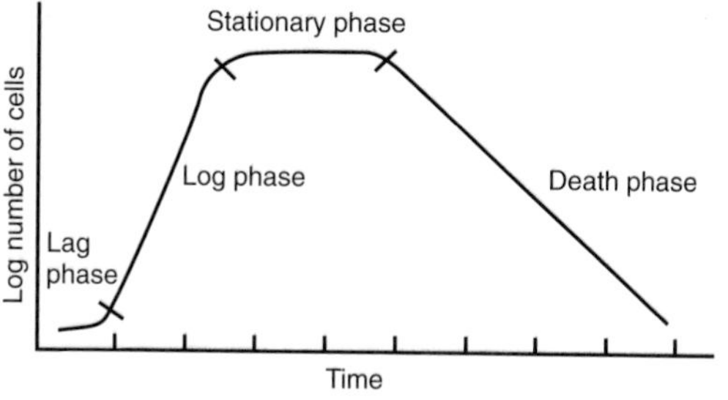

(Adapted, with permission, from Levinson W. *Medical Microbiology and Immunology: Examination and Board Review,* 9th ed. New York: McGraw-Hill, 2006: 15.)

Lag—metabolic activity without division.

Log—rapid cell division.

Stationary—nutrient depletion slows growth. Spore formation in some bacteria.

Death—prolonged nutrient depletion and buildup of waste products lead to death.

Main features of exotoxins and endotoxins

Property	Exotoxin	Endotoxin
Source	Certain species of some gram-positive and gram-negative bacteria	Outer cell membrane of most gram-negative bacteria and *Listeria*
Secreted from cell	Yes	No
Chemistry	Polypeptide	Lipopolysaccharide
Location of genes	Plasmid or bacteriophage	Bacterial chromosome
Toxicity	High (fatal dose on the order of 1 μg)	Low (fatal dose on the order of hundreds of micrograms)
Clinical effects	Various effects (see text)	Fever, shock
Mode of action	Various modes (see text)	Includes TNF and IL-1
Antigenicity	Induces high-titer antibodies called antitoxins	Poorly antigenic
Vaccines	Toxoids used as vaccines	No toxoids formed and no vaccine available
Heat stability	Destroyed rapidly at 60°C (except staphylococcal enterotoxin)	Stable at 100°C for 1 hour
Typical diseases	Tetanus, botulism, diphtheria	Meningococcemia, sepsis by gram-negative rods

(Adapted, with permission, from Levinson W. *Medical Microbiology and Immunology: Examination and Board Review,* 8th ed. New York: McGraw-Hill, 2004: 39.)

Bacterial virulence factors	These promote evasion of host immune response.
S. aureus protein A	Binds Fc region of Ig.
IgA protease	Enzyme that cleaves IgA. Polysaccharide capsules also inhibit phagocytosis. Secreted by *S. pneumoniae, H. influenzae,* and *Neisseria.*
Group A streptococcal M protein	Helps prevent phagocytosis.

Bugs with exotoxins	
Superantigens	Bind directly to MHC II and T-cell receptor simultaneously, activating large numbers of T cells to stimulate release of IFN-γ and IL-2.
S. aureus	TSST-1 superantigen causes toxic shock syndrome (fever, rash, shock). Other *S. aureus* toxins include enterotoxins that cause food poisoning as well as exfoliatin, which causes staphylococcal scalded skin syndrome.
S. pyogenes	Scarlet fever–erythrogenic toxin causes toxic shock–like syndrome.
ADP ribosylating A-B toxins	Interfere with host cell function. B (binding) component binds to a receptor on surface of host cell, enabling endocytosis. A (active) component then attaches an ADP-ribosyl to a host cell protein (ADP ribosylation), altering protein function.
Corynebacterium diphtheriae	Inactivates elongation factor (EF-2) (similar to *Pseudomonas* exotoxin A); causes pharyngitis and "pseudomembrane" in throat.
Vibrio cholerae	ADP ribosylation of G protein stimulates adenylyl cyclase; ↑ pumping of Cl^- into gut and ↓ Na^+ absorption. H_2O moves into gut lumen; causes voluminous rice-water diarrhea.
E. coli	Heat-labile toxin stimulates **A**denylate cyclase. Heat-stable toxin stimulates **G**uanylate cyclase. Both cause watery diarrhea. "Labile like the **A**ir, stable like the **G**round."
Bordetella pertussis	Increases cAMP by inhibiting $G\alpha_i$; causes whooping cough; inhibits chemokine receptor, causing lymphocytosis.
Other toxins	
Clostridium perfringens	α toxin causes gas gangrene; get double zone of hemolysis on blood agar.
C. tetani	Blocks the release of inhibitory neurotransmitters GABA and glycine; causes "lockjaw."
C. botulinum	Blocks the release of acetylcholine; causes anticholinergic symptoms, CNS paralysis, especially cranial nerves; spores found in canned food, honey (causes floppy baby).
Bacillus anthracis	1 toxin in the toxin complex is an adenylate cyclase.
Shigella	Shiga toxin (also produced by *E. coli* O157:H7) cleaves host cell rRNA; also enhances cytokine release, causing HUS.
S. pyogenes	Streptolysin O is a hemolysin; antigen for ASO antibody, which is used in the diagnosis of rheumatic fever.

Endotoxin

A lipopolysaccharide found in cell wall of gram-negative bacteria.

N-dotoxin is an integral part of gram-**N**egative cell wall. Endotoxin is heat stable.

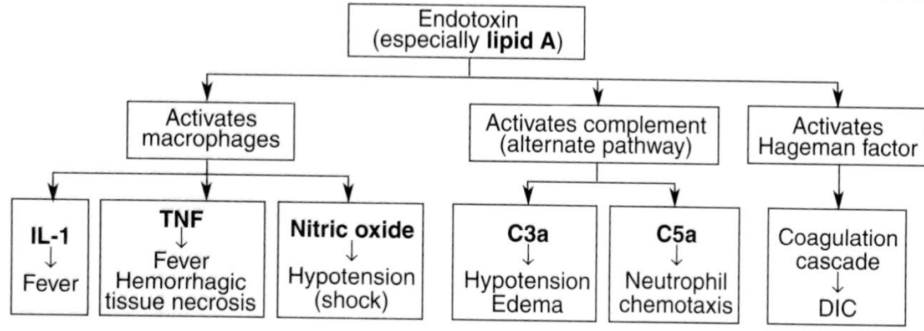

(Adapted, with permission, from Levinson W, Jawetz E. *Medical Microbiology and Immunology: Examination and Board Review*, 6th ed. New York: McGraw-Hill, 2000: 39.)

Fermentation patterns of *Neisseria*	The pathogenic *Neisseria* species are differentiated on the basis of sugar fermentation (see Color Image 4).	MeninGococci ferment Maltose and Glucose. Gonococci ferment Glucose.
Pigment-producing bacteria	*S. aureus*—yellow pigment. *Pseudomonas* ***aeruginosa***—blue-**green** pigment. *Serratia marcescens*—red pigment.	*Aureus* (Latin) = gold. **AERUG**ula is **green.** *Serratia marcescens*—think red maraschino cherries!

Gram-positive lab algorithm

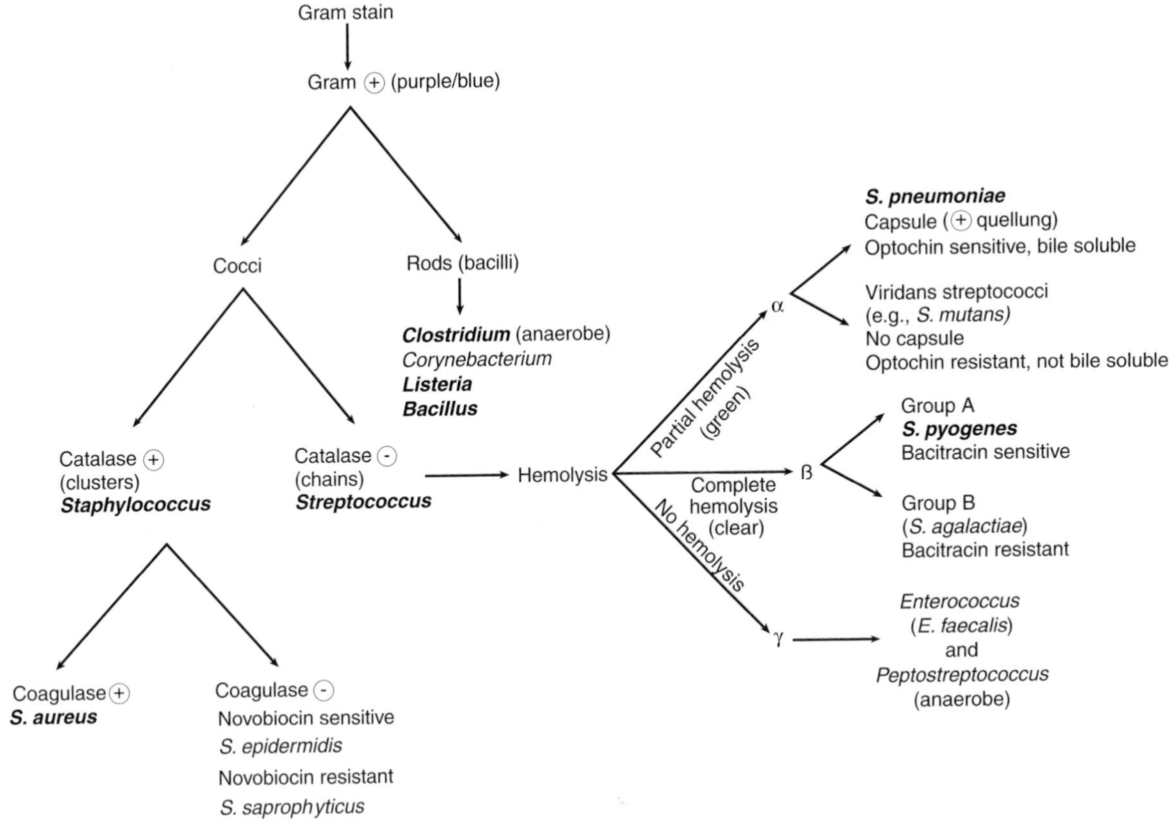

Important pathogens are in **bold type.**
Note: *Enterococcus* is either α- or γ-hemolytic.

Identification of gram-positive bacteria

Staphylococci	NOvobiocin—*Saprophyticus* is Resistant; *Epidermidis* is Sensitive.	NO StRES.
Streptococci	Optochin—*Viridans* is Resistant; *Pneumoniae* is Sensitive.	OVRPS (overpass).
	Bacitracin—group **B** strep are Resistant; group **A** strep are Sensitive.	B-BRAS.

Gram-negative lab algorithm

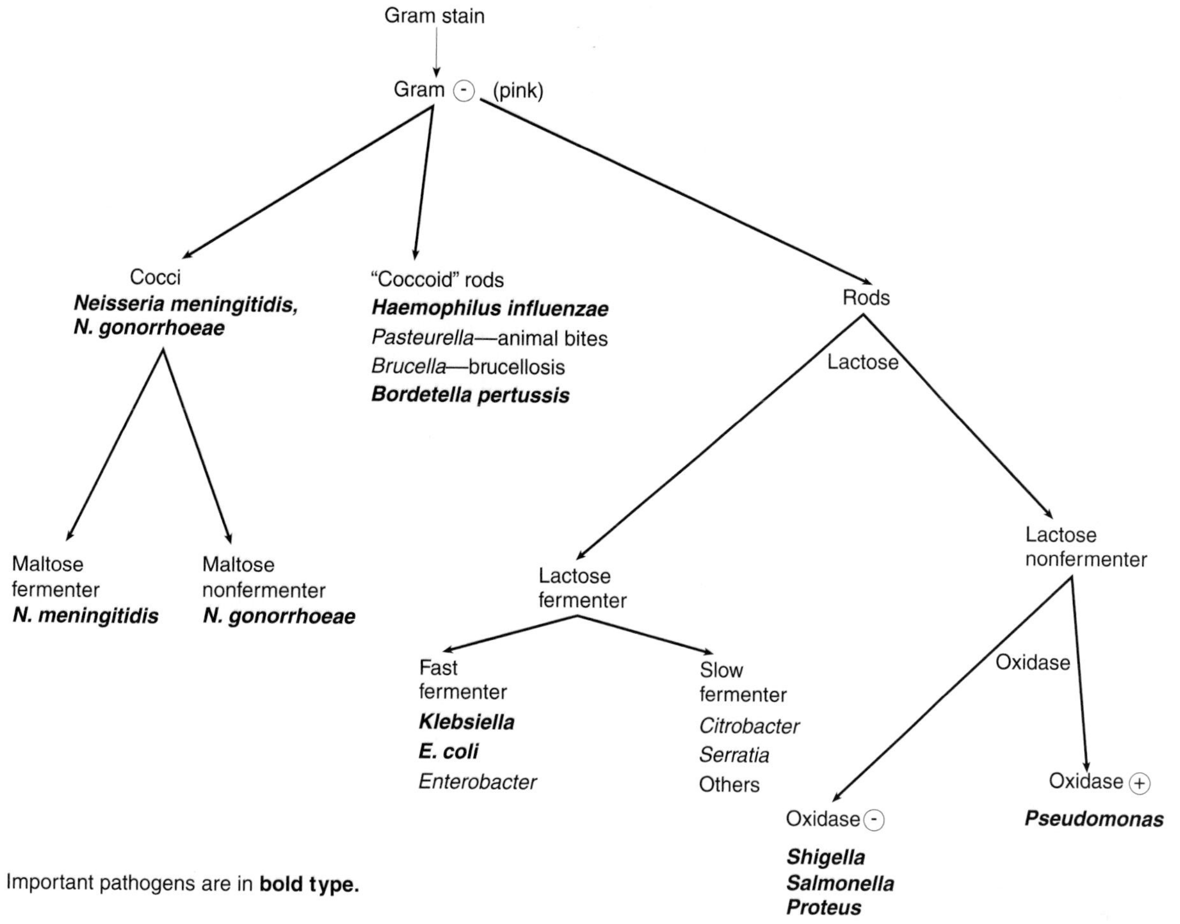

Special culture requirements

Bug	Media used for isolation
H. influenzae	Chocolate agar with factors V (NAD) and X (hematin)
N. gonorrhoeae	Thayer-Martin media
B. pertussis	Bordet-Gengou (potato) agar
C. diphtheriae	Tellurite plate, Löffler's media
M. tuberculosis	Löwenstein-Jensen agar
Lactose-fermenting enterics	Pink colonies on MacConkey's agar
Legionella	Charcoal yeast extract agar buffered with ↑ iron and cysteine
Fungi	Sabouraud's agar

Stains

Congo red	Amyloid; apple-green birefringence in polarized light (because of β-pleated sheets).
Giemsa's	*Borrelia, Plasmodium,* trypanosomes, *Chlamydia.*
PAS (periodic acid-Schiff)	Stains glycogen, mucopolysaccharides; used to diagnose Whipple's disease.
Ziehl-Neelsen	Acid-fast bacteria.
India ink	*Cryptococcus neoformans.*
Silver stain	Fungi, *Legionella.*

▶ MICROBIOLOGY—CLINICAL BACTERIOLOGY *(continued)*

Bacterial genetics	
Transformation	DNA taken up directly from environment by competent prokaryotic and eukaryotic cells. Any DNA can be used.
Conjugation	
$F^+ \times F^-$	F^+ plasmid contains genes required for conjugation process. Bacteria without this plasmid are termed F^-. Plasmid is replicated and transferred through pilus from F^+ cell. Plasmid DNA only; no transfer of chromosomal genes.
Hfr × F^-	F^+ plasmid can become incorporated into bacterial chromosomal DNA, termed Hfr cell. Replication of incorporated plasmid DNA may include some flanking chromosomal DNA. Transfer of plasmid and chromosomal genes.
Transduction	
Generalized	Lytic phage infects bacterium, leading to cleavage of bacterial DNA and synthesis of viral proteins. Parts of bacterial chromosomal DNA may become packaged in viral capsid. Phage infects another bacterium, transferring these genes.
Specialized	Lysogenic phage infects bacterium; viral DNA incorporated into bacterial chromosome. When phage DNA is excised, flanking bacterial genes may be excised with it. DNA is packaged into phage viral capsid and can infect another bacterium.
Transposition	Segment of DNA that can "jump" (excision and reincorporation) from one location to another, can transfer genes from plasmid to chromosome and vice versa. When excision occurs, may include some flanking chromosomal DNA, which can be incorporated into a plasmid and transferred to another bacterium.

Lysogeny	Genetic code for a bacterial toxin encoded in a lysogenic phage. Shig**A**-like toxin **B**otulinum toxin (certain strains) **C**holera toxin **D**iphtheria toxin **E**rythrogenic toxin of *Streptococcus pyogenes*	ABCDE.

▶ MICROBIOLOGY—BACTERIOLOGY

Obligate aerobes	Use an O_2-dependent system to generate ATP. Examples include **N**ocardia, *Pseudomonas aeruginosa*, **M**ycobacterium tuberculosis, and **B**acillus. *M. tuberculosis* has a predilection for the apices of the lung, which have the highest PO_2.	**N**agging **P**ests **M**ust **B**reathe. *P.* ***AER**uginosa* is an **AER**obe seen in burn wounds, nosocomial pneumonia, and pneumonias in cystic fibrosis patients.
Obligate anaerobes	Examples include *Actinomyces*. ***B**acteroides*, and ***C**lostridium*. They lack catalase and/or superoxide dismutase and are thus susceptible to oxidative damage. Generally foul smelling (short-chain fatty acids), are difficult to culture, and produce gas in tissue (CO_2 and H_2).	Anaerobes know their **ABC**s. Anaerobes are normal flora in GI tract, pathogenic elsewhere. AminO_2glycosides are ineffective against anaerobes because these antibiotics require O_2 to enter into bacterial cell.

Intracellular bugs		
Obligate intracellular	*Rickettsia*, *Chlamydia*. Can't make own ATP.	Stay inside (cells) when it is **R**eally **C**old.
Facultative intracellular	*Salmonella*, *Neisseria*, *Brucella*, *Mycobacterium*, *Listeria*, *Francisella*, *Legionella*, *Yersinia*.	Some **N**asty **B**ugs **M**ay **L**ive Facultative**LY**.
Encapsulated bacteria	Positive **quellung** reaction—if encapsulated bug is present, capsule **swells** when specific anticapsular antisera are added. Examples are *Streptococcus pneumoniae*, *Haemophilus influenzae* (especially B serotype), *Neisseria meningitidis*, and *Klebsiella pneumoniae*. Their polysaccharide capsule is an antiphagocytic virulence factor.	**Quellung** = capsular "**swellung.**" Capsule serves as antigen in vaccines (Pneumovax, *H. influenzae* B, meningococcal vaccines). Conjugation with protein ↑ immunogenicity and T-cell-dependent response.
Spores: bacterial	Only certain gram-positive rods form spores when nutrients are limited (at end of stationary phase). Spores are highly resistant to destruction by heat and chemicals. Have dipicolinic acid in their core. Have no metabolic activity. Must autoclave to kill spores (as is done to surgical equipment).	Gram-positive spores found in soil: *Bacillus anthracis*, *Clostridium perfringens*, *C. tetani*. Other spore formers include *B. cereus*, *C. botulinum*.
Urease-positive bugs	*H. pylori*, *Proteus*, *Klebsiella*, *Ureaplasma*.	
α-hemolytic bacteria	Form green ring around colonies on blood agar. Include the following organisms: 1. *Streptococcus pneumoniae* (catalase negative and optochin sensitive) (see Color Image 1) 2. Viridans streptococci (catalase negative and optochin resistant)	
β-hemolytic bacteria	Form clear area of hemolysis on blood agar. Include the following organisms: 1. *Staphylococcus aureus* (catalase and coagulase positive) 2. *Streptococcus pyogenes*—group A strep (catalase negative and bacitracin sensitive) 3. *Streptococcus agalactiae*—group B strep (catalase negative and bacitracin resistant) 4. *Listeria monocytogenes* (tumbling motility, meningitis in newborns, unpasteurized milk)	
Catalase/coagulase (gram-positive cocci)	Catalase degrades H_2O_2, an antimicrobial product of PMNs. H_2O_2 is a substrate for myeloperoxidase. Staphylococci make catalase, whereas streptococci do not. *S. aureus* makes coagulase, whereas *S. epidermidis* and *S. saprophyticus* do not.	**Staph** make catalase because they have more "**staff.**" Bad staph (*aureus*, because *epidermidis* is skin flora) make coagulase and toxins.

▶ MICROBIOLOGY–BACTERIOLOGY *(continued)*

Staphylococcus aureus 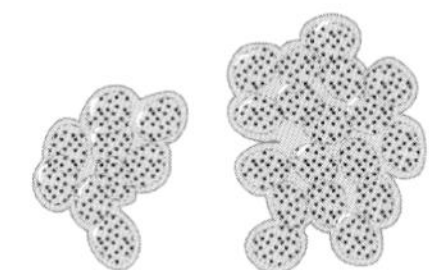	Protein A (virulence factor) binds Fc-IgG, inhibiting complement fixation and phagocytosis. Causes: 1. Inflammatory disease—skin infections, organ abscesses, pneumonia 2. Toxin-mediated disease—toxic shock syndrome (TSST-1 toxin), scalded skin syndrome (exfoliative toxin), rapid-onset food poisoning (enterotoxins) (see Color Image 3) 3. MRSA (methicillin-resistant S. *aureus*) infection—important cause of serious nosocomial and community-acquired infections. Resistant to β-lactams due to altered penicillin-binding protein.	TSST is a superantigen that binds to MHC II and T-cell receptor, resulting in polyclonal T-cell activation. S. *aureus* food poisoning is due to ingestion of preformed toxin. Causes acute bacterial endocarditis, osteomyelitis.
***Streptococcus pyogenes* (group A β-hemolytic streptococci) sequelae**	Causes: 1. Pyogenic—pharyngitis, cellulitis, impetigo 2. Toxigenic—scarlet fever, toxic shock syndrome 3. Immunologic—rheumatic fever, acute glomerulonephritis Bacitracin sensitive. Antibodies to **M protein** enhance host defenses against S. *pyogenes* but can give rise to rheumatic fever. ASO titer detects recent S. *pyogenes* infection.	**PH**aryngitis gives you rheumatic "**PH**ever" and glomerulone**PH**ritis. No "**rheum**" for **SPECC**ulation: **S**ubcutaneous nodules, **P**olyarthritis, **E**rythema marginatum, **C**horea, **C**arditis.
Streptococcus pneumoniae	Most common cause of: **M**eningitis **O**titis media (in children) **P**neumonia **S**inusitis Encapsulated. IgA protease.	S. *pneumoniae* **MOPS** are **M**ost **OP**tochin **S**ensitive. Pneumococcus is associated with "rusty" sputum, sepsis in sickle cell anemia and splenectomy.
Group B streptococci	Bacitracin resistant, β-hemolytic; cause pneumonia, meningitis, and sepsis, mainly in babies.	
Enterococci 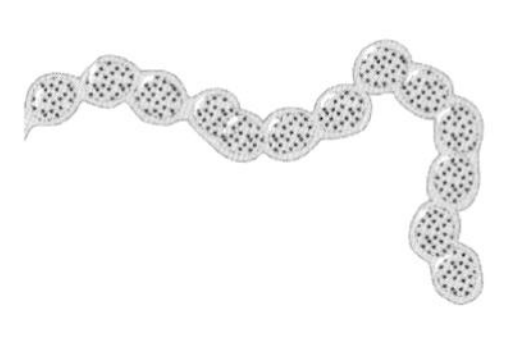	Enterococci (*Enterococcus faecalis* and *E. faecium*) are penicillin G resistant and cause UTI and subacute endocarditis. Lancefield group D includes the enterococci and the nonenterococcal group D streptococci. Lancefield grouping is based on differences in the C carbohydrate on the bacterial cell wall. Variable hemolysis. VRE (vancomycin-resistant enterococci) are an important cause of nosocomial infection.	Enterococci, hardier than nonenterococcal group D, can thus grow in 6.5% NaCl (lab test). *Entero* = intestine, *faecalis* = feces, *strepto* = twisted (chains), *coccus* = berry.
Staphylococcus epidermidis	Infects prosthetic devices and catheters. Component of normal skin flora; contaminates blood cultures.	

Viridans group streptococci	Viridans streptococci are α-hemolytic. They are normal flora of the oropharynx and cause dental caries (*Streptococcus mutans*) and subacute bacterial endocarditis (*S. sanguis*). Resistant to optochin, differentiating them from *S. pneumoniae*, which is α-hemolytic but is optochin sensitive.	*Sanguis* (Latin) = blood. There is lots of blood in the heart (endocarditis). Viridans group strep live in the mouth because they are not afraid **of-the-chin** (**op-to-chin** resistant).
Clostridia (with exotoxins)	Gram-positive, spore-forming, obligate anaerobic bacilli. *Clostridium tetani* produces an exotoxin causing tetanus.	**TET**anus is **TET**anic paralysis (blocks glycine release [inhibitory neurotransmitter]) from Renshaw cells in spinal cord.
	C. botulinum produces a preformed, heat-labile toxin that inhibits ACh release at the neuromuscular junction, causing botulism. In adults, disease is caused by ingestion of preformed toxin. In babies, ingestion of bacterial spores in honey causes disease.	***BOT****ulinum* is from bad **BOT**tles of food and honey (causes a flaccid paralysis).
	C. perfringens produces α toxin (lecithinase) that can cause myonecrosis (gas gangrene) and hemolysis.	***PERF****ringens* **PERF**orates a gangrenous leg.
	C. difficile produces a cytotoxin, an exotoxin that kills enterocytes, causing pseudomembranous colitis. Often 2° to antibiotic use, especially clindamycin or ampicillin.	***DI****fficile* causes **DI**arrhea. Treat with metronidazole.
Diphtheria (and exotoxin)	Caused by *Corynebacterium diphtheriae* via exotoxin encoded by β-prophage. Potent exotoxin inhibits protein synthesis via ADP ribosylation of EF-2. Symptoms include pseudomembranous pharyngitis (grayish-white membrane) with lymphadenopathy. Lab diagnosis based on gram-positive rods with metachromatic granules.	*Coryne* = club shaped. Grows on tellurite agar. **ABCDEFG:** **A**DP ribosylation **B**eta-prophage ***C****orynebacterium* ***D****iphtheriae* **E**longation **F**actor 2 **G**ranules
Anthrax	Caused by *Bacillus anthracis*, a gram-positive, spore-forming rod that produces anthrax toxin. The only bacterium with a protein capsule. Contact → malignant pustule (painless ulcer); can progress to bacteremia and death. Inhalation of spores → flulike symptoms that rapidly progress to fever, pulmonary hemorrhage, mediastinitis, and shock.	Black skin lesions—vesicular papules covered by black eschar. Woolsorters' disease—inhalation of spores from contaminated wool.

Listeria monocytogenes

Acquired by ingestion of unpasteurized milk/cheese or by vaginal transmission during birth. Form "actin rockets" by which they move from cell to cell.

Can cause amnionitis, septicemia, and spontaneous abortion in pregnant women; granulomatosis infantiseptica; neonatal meningitis; meningitis in immunocompromised patients; mild gastroenteritis in healthy individuals.

Actinomyces* vs. *Nocardia

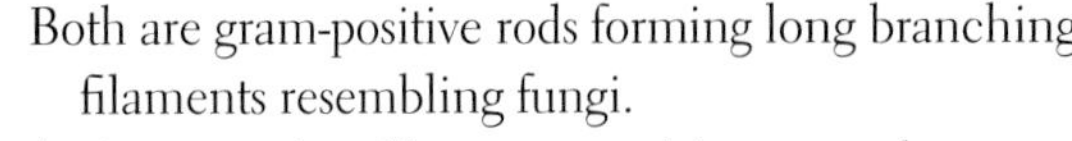

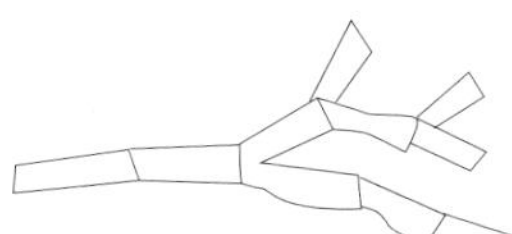

Both are gram-positive rods forming long branching filaments resembling fungi.

Actinomyces israelii, a gram-positive anaerobe, causes oral/facial abscesses that may drain through sinus tracts in skin. Normal oral flora.

Nocardia asteroides, a gram-positive and also a weakly acid-fast aerobe in soil, causes pulmonary infection in immunocompromised patients.

A. israelii forms yellow "sulfur granules" in sinus tracts.

SNAP:
Sulfa for
Nocardia;
Actinomyces use
Penicillin

Penicillin and gram-negative bugs

Gram-negative bugs are resistant to benzylpenicillin G but may be susceptible to penicillin derivatives such as ampicillin. The gram-negative outer membrane layer inhibits entry of penicillin G and vancomycin.

Neisseria

Gram-negative cocci. Both ferment glucose and produce IgA proteases.

Gonococci	Meningococci
No polysaccharide capsule	Polysaccharide capsule
No maltose fermentation	Maltose fermentation
No vaccine	Vaccine
Sexually transmitted	Respiratory and oral secretions
Causes gonorrhea, septic arthritis, neonatal conjunctivitis, PID	Causes meningococcemia and meningitis, Waterhouse-Friderichsen syndrome

Haemophilus influenzae

HaEMOPhilus causes **E**piglottitis, **M**eningitis, **O**titis media, and **P**neumonia. Small gram-negative (coccobacillary) rod. Aerosol transmission. Most invasive disease caused by capsular type B. Produces IgA protease. Culture on **chocolate agar** requires factors **V** (NAD) and **X** (hematin) for growth. Treat meningitis with ceftriaxone. Rifampin prophylaxis in close contacts. Does not cause the flu (influenza virus does).

When a child has "flu," mom goes to five (**V**) and dime (**X**) store to buy some **chocolate.**
Vaccine contains type B capsular polysaccharide conjugated to diphtheria toxoid or other protein. Given between 2 and 18 months of age.

Enterobacteriaceae

Diverse family including *E. coli, Salmonella, Shigella, Klebsiella, Enterobacter, Serratia, Proteus.*

All species have somatic (O) antigen (which is the polysaccharide of endotoxin). The capsular (K) antigen is related to the virulence of the bug. The flagellar (H) antigen is found in motile species. All ferment glucose and are oxidase negative.

Think **COFFE**e:
Capsular
O antigen
Flagellar antigen
Ferment glucose
Enterobacteriaceae

Klebsiella	Pneumonia in alcoholics and diabetics. Red currant jelly sputum. Also cause of nosocomial UTIs.	3 A's: **A**spiration pneumonia **A**bscess in lungs **A**lcoholics
Lactose-fermenting enteric bacteria	These bacteria grow pink colonies on MacConkey's agar. Examples include *Klebsiella, E. coli, Enterobacter,* and *Citrobacter.*	Lactose is **KEE.** Test with MacCon**KEE**'s agar.
Salmonella* vs. *Shigella	Both are non–lactose fermenters; both invade intestinal mucosa and can cause bloody diarrhea. ***Salmonella*** have flagella and can disseminate hematogenously. Only *Salmonella* produce H_2S. Symptoms of salmonellosis may be prolonged with antibiotic treatments, and there is typically a monocytic response. *Shigella* is more virulent (10^1 organisms) than *Salmonella* (10^5 organisms). *Salmonella typhi* causes typhoid fever—fever, diarrhea, headache, rose spots on abdomen. Can remain in gallbladder chronically.	**Salmon swim** (motile and disseminate). Most species of *Salmonella* have an animal reservoir; *Shigella* do not have flagella but can propel themselves while within a cell by actin polymerization. Transmission is via "Food, Fingers, Feces, and Flies."
Yersinia enterocolitica	Usually transmitted from pet feces (e.g., puppies), contaminated milk, or pork. Outbreaks are common in day-care centers. Can mimic Crohn's or appendicitis.	
Bugs causing food poisoning	*Vibrio parahaemolyticus* and *V. vulnificus* in contaminated seafood. *V. vulnificus* can also cause wound infections from contact with contaminated water or shellfish. *Bacillus cereus* in reheated rice. *S. aureus* in meats, mayonnaise, custard. *Clostridium perfringens* in reheated meat dishes. *C. botulinum* in improperly canned foods (bulging cans). *E. coli* O157:H7 in undercooked meat. *Salmonella* in poultry, meat, and eggs.	*S. aureus* and *B. cereus* food poisoning starts quickly and ends quickly. "Food poisoning from reheated rice? **Be serious!**" (***B. cereus***).

Bugs causing diarrhea

Type	Species	Findings
Bloody diarrhea	*Campylobacter*	Comma- or S-shaped organisms; growth at 42°C; oxidase positive
	Salmonella	Lactose negative; flagellar motility
	Shigella	Lactose negative; very low ID_{50}; produces Shiga toxin
	Enterohemorrhagic *E. coli*	O157:H7; can cause HUS; makes Shiga-like toxin
	Enteroinvasive *E. coli*	Invades colonic mucosa
	Yersinia enterocolitica	Day-care outbreaks, pseudoappendicitis
	C. difficile (can cause both watery and bloody diarrhea)	Pseudomembranous colitis
	Entamoeba histolytica	Protozoan
Watery diarrhea	Enterotoxigenic *E. coli*	Traveler's diarrhea; produces ST and LT toxins
	Vibrio cholerae	Comma-shaped organisms; rice-water diarrhea
	C. perfringens	Also causes gas gangrene
	Protozoa	*Giardia*, *Cryptosporidium* (in immunocompromised)
	Viruses	Rotavirus, adenovirus, Norwalk virus (norovirus)

---

cAMP inducers

1. *Vibrio cholerae* toxin permanently activates G_s, causing rice-water diarrhea.
2. Pertussis toxin permanently disables G_i, causing whooping cough.
3. *E. coli*—heat-labile toxin.
4. *Bacillus anthracis* toxin includes edema factor, a bacterial adenylate cyclase (↑ cAMP).

Cholera, pertussis, and *E. coli* toxins act via ADP ribosylation to permanently activate adenylate cyclase (↑ cAMP), while the anthrax edema factor is itself an adenylate cyclase.

Cholera turns the "on" on.
Pertussis turns the "off" off.
Pertussis toxin also promotes lymphocytosis by inhibiting chemokine receptors.

Legionella pneumophila

Legionnaires' disease = severe pneumonia. Pontiac fever = mild influenza.

Gram-negative rod. Gram stains poorly—use silver stain. Grow on charcoal yeast extract culture with iron and cysteine. Aerosol transmission from environmental water source habitat. No person-to-person transmission. Treat with erythromycin.

Think of a French legionnaire (soldier) with his silver helmet, sitting around a campfire (charcoal) with his iron dagger—he is no **sissy** (**cysteine**).

Pseudomonas aeruginosa	***PSEUDOmonas*** is associated with wound and burn infections, **P**neumonia (especially in cystic fibrosis), **S**epsis (black lesions on skin), **E**xternal otitis (swimmer's ear), **U**TI, **D**rug use and **D**iabetic **O**steomyelitis, and hot tub folliculitis. Aerobic gram-negative rod. Non–lactose fermenting, oxidase positive. Produces pyocyanin (blue-green) pigment; has a grapelike odor. Water source. Produces endotoxin (fever, shock) and exotoxin A (inactivates EF-2). Treat with aminoglycoside plus extended-spectrum penicillin (e.g., piperacillin, ticarcillin).	**AER**uginosa—**AER**obic. Think water connection and blue-green pigment. Think *Pseudomonas* in burn victims.

Helicobacter pylori

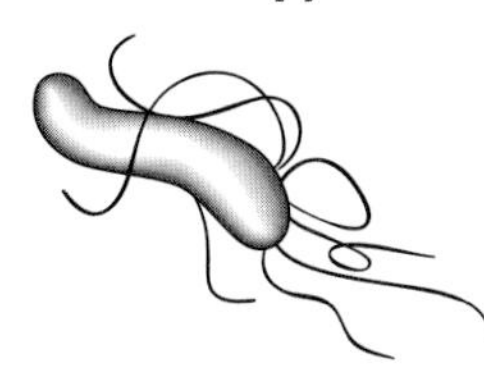

Causes gastritis and up to 90% of duodenal ulcers. Risk factor for peptic ulcer, gastric adenocarcinoma, and lymphoma. Gram-negative rod. Urease positive (e.g., urease breath test). Creates alkaline environment. Treat with triple therapy: (1) bismuth (Pepto-Bismol), metronidazole, and either tetracycline or amoxicillin; or (2) (more costly) metronidazole, omeprazole, and clarithromycin.

Zoonotic bacteria

Species	Disease	Transmission and source	
Bartonella henselae	Cat scratch fever	Cat scratch	**B**ig **B**ad **B**ugs **F**rom **Y**our **P**et.
Borrelia burgdorferi	Lyme disease	Tick bite; *Ixodes* ticks that live on deer and mice	
Brucella spp.	Brucellosis/Undulant fever	Dairy products, contact with animals	**Un**pasteurized dairy products give you **Un**dulant fever.
Francisella tularensis	Tularemia	Tick bite; rabbits, deer	
Yersinia pestis	Plague	Flea bite; rodents, especially prairie dogs	
Pasteurella multocida	Cellulitis	Animal bite; cats, dogs	

Gardnerella vaginalis

A pleomorphic, gram-variable rod that causes vaginosis—off-white/gray vaginal discharge with fishy smell; nonpainful. *Mobiluncus*, an anaerobe, is also involved. Sexually transmitted. Treat with metronidazole. Clue cells, or vaginal epithelial cells covered with bacteria, are visible under the microscope (see Color Image 13).

1° and 2° tuberculosis

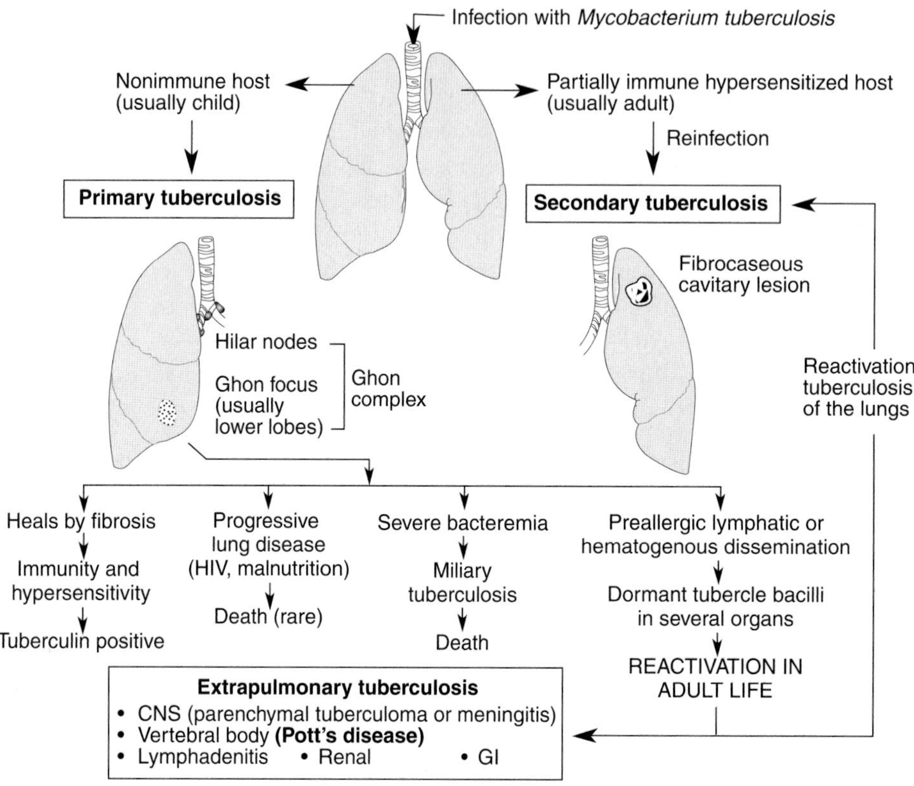

(Adapted, with permission, from Chandrasoma P, Taylor CR. *Concise Pathology,* 3rd ed. Stamford, CT: Appleton & Lange, 1998: 523.)

PPD+ if current infection, past exposure, or BCG vaccinated.
PPD– if no infection or anergic (steroids, malnutrition, immunocompromise, sarcoidosis).

Ghon complex	TB granulomas (Ghon focus) with lobar and perihilar lymph node involvement. Reflects 1° infection or exposure.	
Mycobacteria	*Mycobacterium tuberculosis* (TB, often resistant to multiple drugs). *M. kansasii* (pulmonary TB-like symptoms). *M. scrofulaceum* (cervical lymphadenitis in kids). *M. avium–intracellulare* (often resistant to multiple drugs; causes disseminated disease in AIDS). All mycobacteria are acid-fast organisms.	TB symptoms include fever, night sweats, weight loss, and hemoptysis (see Color Image 2).

Leprosy (Hansen's disease)

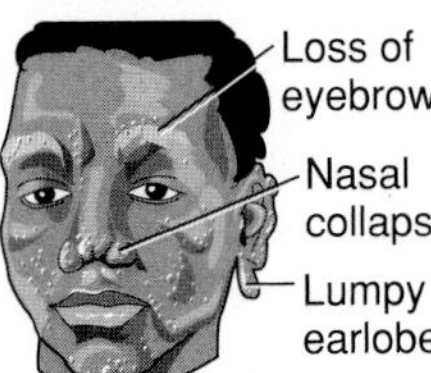

"Leonine facies" of lepromatous leprosy

Caused by *Mycobacterium leprae*, an acid-fast bacillus that likes cool temperatures (infects skin and superficial nerves) and cannot be grown in vitro. Reservoir in United States: armadillos.

Treatment: long-term oral dapsone; toxicity is hemolysis and methemoglobinemia.

Alternate treatments include rifampin and combination of clofazimine and dapsone.

Hansen's disease has 2 forms: lepromatous and tuberculoid; lepromatous is worse (failed cell-mediated immunity); tuberculoid is self-limited.

LEpromatous = **LE**thal.

Rickettsiae

Rickettsiae are obligate intracellular parasites that need CoA and NAD. All except *Coxiella* are transmitted by an arthropod vector and cause headache, fever, and rash; *Coxiella* is an atypical rickettsia because it is transmitted by aerosol and causes pneumonia.

Tetracycline is the treatment of choice for most rickettsial infections.

Classic triad—headache, fever, rash (vasculitis).

Rickettsial diseases and vectors

Rocky Mountain spotted fever (tick)—*Rickettsia rickettsii.*

Endemic typhus (fleas)—*R. typhi.*

Epidemic typhus (human body louse)—*R. prowazekii.*

Ehrlichiosis (tick)—*Ehrlichia.*

Q fever (inhaled aerosols)—*Coxiella burnetii.*

Treatment for all: tetracycline.

Rickettsial rash starts on hands and feet; typhus rash starts centrally and spreads out: "**R**ickettsia on the w**R**ists, **T**yphus on the **T**runk."

Q fever is **Q**ueer because it has no rash, has no vector, and has negative Weil-Felix, and its causative organism can survive outside for a long time and does not have *Rickettsia* as its genus name.

Rocky Mountain spotted fever

Caused by *Rickettsia rickettsii.*

Symptoms: rash on palms and soles (migrating to wrists, ankles, then trunk), headache, fever.

Endemic to East Coast (in spite of name).

Palm and sole rash is seen in Rocky Mountain spotted fever, syphilis, and coxsackievirus A infection (hand, foot, and mouth disease).

Weil-Felix reaction

Weil-Felix reaction assays for antirickettsial antibodies, which cross-react with *Proteus* antigen. Weil-Felix is usually positive for typhus and Rocky Mountain spotted fever but negative for Q fever.

Chlamydiae	Chlamydiae cannot make their own ATP. They are obligate intracellular parasites that cause mucosal infections. 2 forms: 1. Elementary body (small, dense), which **E**nters cell via endocytosis 2. Initial or **R**eticulate body, which **R**eplicates in cell by fission *Chlamydia trachomatis* causes reactive arthritis, conjunctivitis, nongonococcal urethritis, and pelvic inflammatory disease (PID). *C. pneumoniae* and *C. psittaci* cause atypical pneumonia; transmitted by aerosol. Treatment: erythromycin or tetracycline.	*Chlamys* = cloak (intracellular). *Chlamydia psittaci*—notable for an avian reservoir. The chlamydial cell wall is unusual in that it lacks muramic acid. Lab diagnosis: cytoplasmic inclusions seen on Giemsa or fluorescent antibody–stained smear.

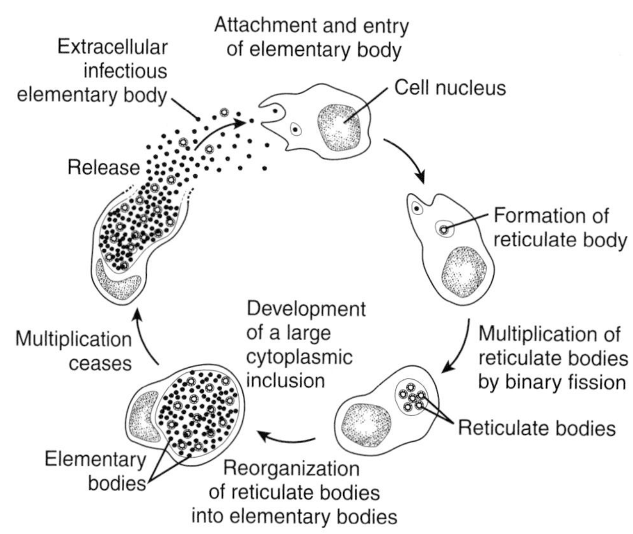

***Chlamydia trachomatis* serotypes**	Types A, B, and C—chronic infection, cause blindness in Africa. Types D–K—urethritis/PID, ectopic pregnancy, neonatal pneumonia, or neonatal conjunctivitis. Types L1, L2, and L3—lymphogranuloma venereum (acute lymphadenitis—positive Frei test).	**ABC** = **A**frica/**B**lindness/ **C**hronic infection. **L**1–3 = **L**ymphogranuloma venereum. D–K = everything else. Neonatal disease can be acquired during passage through infected birth canal. Treat with oral erythromycin.
Spirochetes 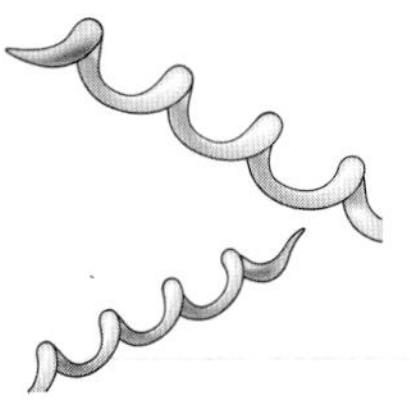	The spirochetes are spiral-shaped bacteria with axial filaments and include ***B****orrelia* (big size), ***L****eptospira*, and ***T****reponema*. Only *Borrelia* can be visualized using aniline dyes (Wright's or Giemsa stain) in light microscopy. *Treponema* is visualized by dark-field microscopy.	**BLT. B** is **B**ig.

Leptospira interrogans 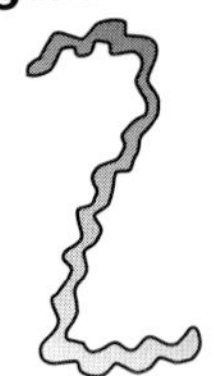	Question mark–shaped bacteria found in water contaminated with animal urine. Leptospirosis includes flulike symptoms, fever, headache, abdominal pain, and jaundice. Most prevalent in the tropics. Weil's disease (icterohemorrhagic leptospirosis)—severe form with jaundice and azotemia from liver and kidney dysfunction; fever, hemorrhage, and anemia.	
Lyme disease	Caused by *Borrelia burgdorferi*, which is transmitted by the tick *Ixodes*. Classic symptom is erythema chronicum migrans, an expanding "bull's eye" red rash with central clearing. Also affects joints, CNS, and heart. Mice are important reservoirs. Deer required for tick life cycle. Treat with doxycycline. Named after Lyme, Connecticut; disease is common in northeastern United States. Transmission is most common in summer months.	3 stages of Lyme disease: Stage 1—erythema chronicum migrans, flulike symptoms. Stage 2—neurologic and cardiac manifestations. Stage 3—chronic monoarthritis, and migratory polyarthritis. **BAKE** a Key **Lyme** pie: **B**ell's palsy, **A**rthritis, **K**ardiac block, **E**rythema migrans.
Treponemal disease	Treponemes are spirochetes. *Treponema pallidum* causes syphilis. *T. pertenue* causes yaws (a tropical infection that is not an STD, although VDRL test is positive).	
Syphilis	Caused by spirochete *Treponema pallidum*.	Treat with penicillin G.
1° syphilis	Presents with painless chancre (localized disease).	
2° syphilis	Disseminated disease with constitutional symptoms, maculopapular rash (palms and soles), condylomata lata. Many treponemes are present in chancres of 1° and 2° syphilis.	**S**econdary syphilis = **S**ystemic.
3° syphilis	Gummas, aortitis, neurosyphilis (tabes dorsalis), Argyll Robertson pupil (see Color Image 12).	Signs: broad-based ataxia, positive Romberg, Charcot joints, stroke without hypertension.
Congenital syphilis	Saber shins, saddle nose, CN VIII deafness, Hutchinson's teeth.	
Argyll Robertson pupil	Argyll Robertson pupil constricts with accommodation but is not reactive to light. Associated with 3° syphilis.	"Prostitute's pupil"—accommodates but does not react.
VDRL vs. FTA-ABS	FTA-ABS is specific for treponemes, turns positive earliest in disease, and remains positive longest. **VDRL / FTA / Interpretation** + / + / Active infection + / – / Probably false positive – / + / Successfully treated	**FTA-ABS** = **F**ind **T**he **A**ntibody-**ABS**olutely: 1. Most specific 2. Earliest positive 3. Remains positive the longest

▶ MICROBIOLOGY–BACTERIOLOGY *(continued)*

VDRL false positives	VDRL detects nonspecific antibody that reacts with beef cardiolipin. Used for diagnosis of syphilis, but many biologic false positives, including viral infection (mononucleosis, hepatitis), some drugs, rheumatic fever, SLE, and leprosy.	**VDRL:** **V**iruses (mono, hepatitis) **D**rugs **R**heumatic fever **L**upus and leprosy
Mycoplasma pneumoniae 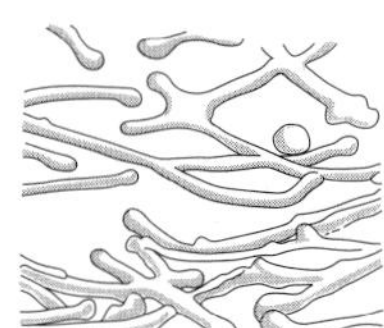	Classic cause of atypical "walking" pneumonia (insidious onset, headache, nonproductive cough, diffuse interstitial infiltrate). X-ray looks worse than patient. High titer of cold agglutinins (IgM). Grown on Eaton's agar. Treatment: tetracycline or erythromycin (bugs are penicillin resistant because they have no cell wall).	No cell wall. Not seen on gram stain. Only bacterial membrane containing cholesterol. Mycoplasmal pneumonia is more common in patients < 30 years of age. Frequent outbreaks in military recruits and prisons.

▶ MICROBIOLOGY–MYCOLOGY

Spores: fungal	Most fungal spores are asexual. Both coccidioidomycosis and histoplasmosis are transmitted by inhalation of asexual spores.	Conidia—asexual fungal spores (e.g., blastoconidia, arthroconidia).
Candida albicans	Systemic or superficial fungal infection (budding yeast with pseudohyphae in culture at 20°C; germ tube formation at 37°C). Thrush esophagitis in immunocompromised patients, endocarditis in IV drug users, vaginitis (post-antibiotic), diaper rash. Transmission occurs by inhalation of spores. No person-to-person spread. Treatment: nystatin for superficial infection; amphotericin B for serious systemic infection.	*Alba* = **white.**

Systemic mycoses

Disease	Endemic location and pathologic features	Notes
Histoplasmosis	Mississippi and Ohio river valleys. Causes pneumonia.	Bird or bat droppings; intracellular (tiny yeast inside macrophages).

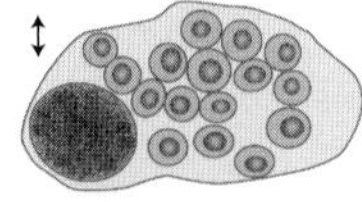

Disease	Endemic location and pathologic features	Notes
Blastomycosis	States east of Mississippi River and Central America. Causes inflammatory lung disease and can disseminate to skin and bone. Forms granulomatous nodules.	**B**ig, **B**road-**B**ased **B**udding. **Cold = Mold. Heat = Yeast.** Culture on Sabouraud's agar.

5–15 μm

Broad-base budding

Disease	Endemic location and pathologic features	Notes
Coccidioidomycosis	Southwestern United States, California. Causes pneumonia and meningitis; can disseminate to bone and skin.	San Joaquin Valley or desert (desert bumps) "valley fever" (see Color Image 7).

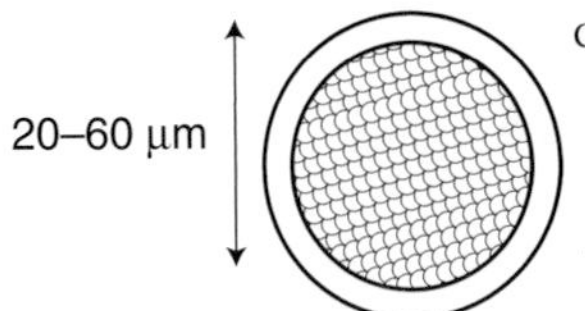

Disease	Endemic location and pathologic features	Notes
Paracoccidioidomycosis	Rural Latin America.	"Captain's wheel" appearance.

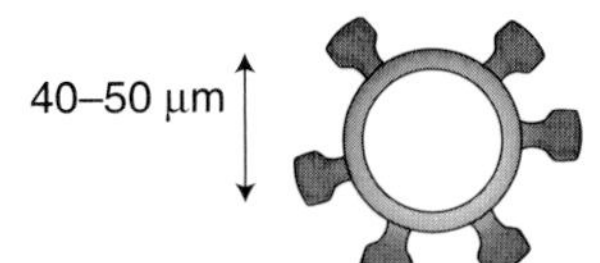

All of the above are caused by **dimorphic** fungi, which are mold in soil (at lower temperature) and yeast in tissue (at higher/body temperature: 37°C) except coccidioidomycosis, which is a spherule in tissue. All can cause pneumonia and can disseminate. Treat with fluconazole or ketoconazole for local infection; amphotericin B for systemic infection. Systemic mycoses can mimic TB (granuloma formation).

Cutaneous mycoses

Tinea versicolor	Caused by *Malassezia furfur*. Occurs in hot, humid weather. Treat with topical miconazole, selenium sulfide (Selsun). "Spaghetti and meatball" appearance on KOH prep.

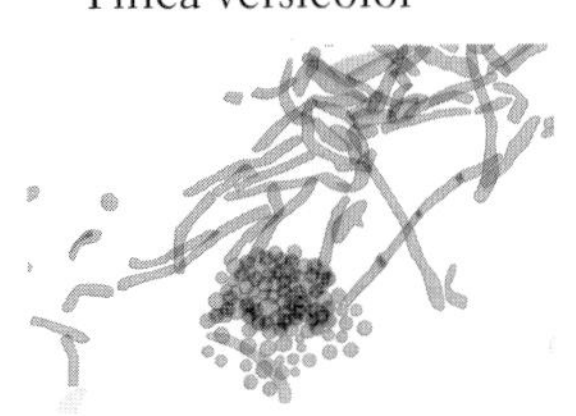

Tinea pedis, cruris, corporis, capitis	Pruritic lesions with central clearing resembling a ring, caused by dermatophytes (*Microsporum*, *Trichophyton*, and *Epidermophyton*). See mold hyphae in KOH prep, not dimorphic. Pets are a reservoir for *Microsporum* and can be treated with topical azoles.

Opportunistic fungal infections

Candida albicans	Thrush in immunocompromised (neonates, steroids, diabetes, AIDS), vulvovaginitis (high pH, diabetes, use of antibiotics), disseminated candidiasis (to any organ), chronic mucocutaneous candidiasis (see Color Image 9). Germ tube test is diagnostic.
Aspergillus fumigatus	Allergic bronchopulmonary aspergillosis, lung cavity aspergilloma ("fungus ball"), invasive aspergillosis, especially in immunocompromised individuals and those with chronic granulomatous disease. **Mold** with septate hyphae that branch at a V-shaped (45°) angle. Not dimorphic.
Cryptococcus neoformans	Cryptococcal meningitis, cryptococcosis. Heavily encapsulated **yeast.** Not dimorphic. Found in soil, pigeon droppings. Culture on Sabouraud's agar. Stains with India ink. Latex agglutination test detects polysaccharide capsular antigen (see Color Image 8). "Soap bubble" lesions in brain.
Mucor and *Rhizopus* spp.	Mucormycosis. **Mold** with irregular nonseptate hyphae branching at wide angles (≥ 90°). Disease mostly in ketoacidotic diabetic and leukemic patients. Fungi also proliferate in the walls of blood vessels and cause infarction and necrosis of distal tissue. Rhinocerebral, frontal lobe abscesses.

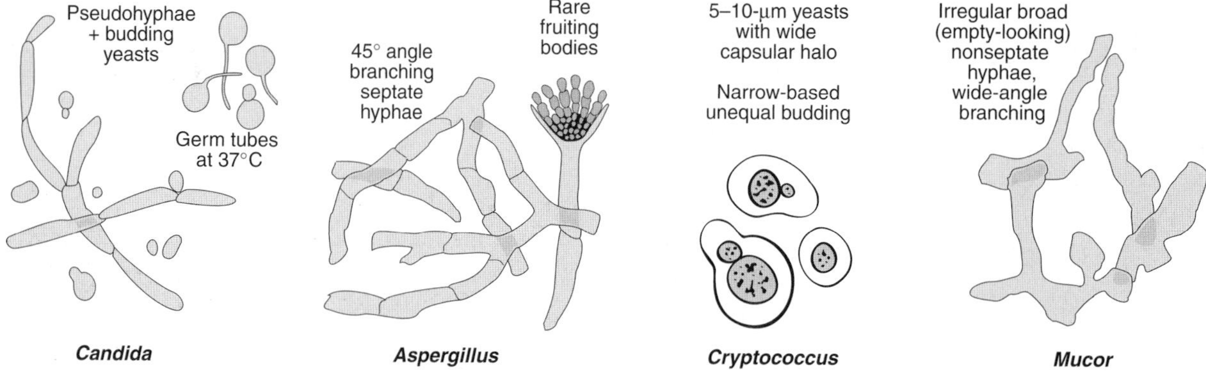

***Pneumocystis jiroveci* (formerly *carinii*)**

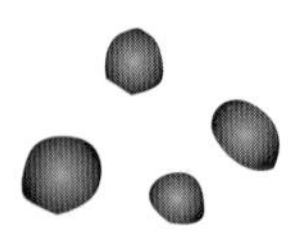

Causes diffuse interstitial pneumonia (PCP). Yeast (originally classified as protozoan). Inhaled. Most infections asymptomatic. Immunosuppression (e.g., AIDS) predisposes to disease. Diffuse, bilateral CXR appearance. Diagnosed by lung biopsy or lavage. Identified by methenamine silver stain of lung tissue. Treat with TMP-SMX, pentamidine, dapsone. Start prophylaxis when CD4 drops < 200 cells/mL in HIV patients (see Color Image 17).

Sporothrix schenckii

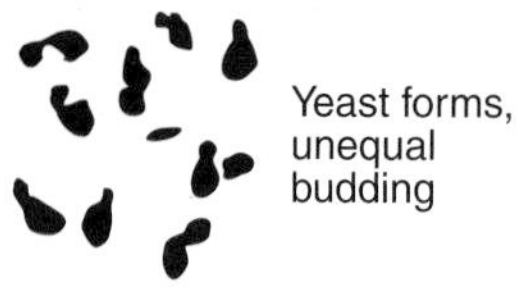

Sporotrichosis. Dimorphic fungus that lives on vegetation. When traumatically introduced into the skin, typically by a thorn ("rose gardener's" disease), causes local pustule or ulcer with nodules along draining lymphatics (ascending lymphangitis). Little systemic illness. Cigar-shaped budding yeast visible in pus. Treat with itraconazole or potassium iodide.

Medically important protozoa—single-celled organisms

Organism	Disease	Transmission	Diagnosis	Treatment
Giardia lamblia (see Color Image 5) Trophozoite Cyst	Giardiasis: bloating, flatulence, foul-smelling diarrhea (often seen in campers/hikers)	Cysts in water	Trophozoites or cysts in stool	Metronidazole
Trichomonas vaginalis (see Color Image 10)	Vaginitis: foul-smelling, greenish discharge; itching and burning	Sexual	Trophozoites (motile) on wet mount	Metronidazole
Trypanosoma cruzi RBC Blood smear	Chagas' disease (dilated cardiomyopathy, megacolon, megaesophagus); predominantly in South America	Reduviid bug	Blood smear	Nifurtimox
Trypanosoma *T. gambiense* *T. rhodesiense*	African sleeping sickness	Tsetse fly	Blood smear	Suramin for blood-borne disease or melarsoprol for CNS penetration
Leishmania donovani	Visceral leishmaniasis (kala-azar): spiking fevers, hepatosplenomegaly, pancytopenia	Sandfly	Macrophages containing amastigotes	Sodium stibogluconate
Plasmodium *P. vivax* *P. ovale* *P. malariae* *P. falciparum* Trophozoite ring form in RBC RBC schizont with merozoites	Malaria: cyclic fever, headache, anemia, splenomegaly Malaria—severe (cerebral) with *P. falciparum* *P. vivax* and *P. ovale* have dormant forms in liver (hypnozoites) → relapsing malaria	Mosquito (*Anopheles*)	Blood smear	Chloroquine (primaquine to prevent relapse caused by *P. vivax*, *P. ovale*), sulfadoxine + pyrimethamine, mefloquine, quinine

Medically important protozoa—single-celled organisms *(continued)*

Organism	Disease	Transmission	Diagnosis	Treatment
Babesia RBC Maltese cross and ring forms	Babesiosis: fever and hemolytic anemia; predominantly in northeastern United States	*Ixodes* tick	Blood smear, no RBC pigment, appears as "Maltese cross"	Quinine, clindamycin
Cryptosporidium Acid-fast cysts	Severe diarrhea in AIDS Mild disease (watery diarrhea) in non-immunocompromised	Cysts in water	Cysts on acid-fast stain	None
Toxoplasma gondii	Brain abscess in HIV, birth defects (ring-enhancing brain lesions)	Cysts in meat or cat feces; crosses placenta (pregnant women should avoid cats)	Serology, biopsy	Sulfadiazine + pyrimethamine
Entamoeba histolytica RBCs Trophozoite Cyst with 4 nuclei	Amebiasis: bloody diarrhea, (dysentery), liver abscess, RUQ pain	Cysts in water	Serology and/or trophozoites or cysts in stool; RBCs in cytoplasm of entamoeba	Metronidazole and iodoquinol
Naegleria fowleri	Rapidly fatal meningoencephalitis	Swimming in freshwater lakes (enter via cribriform plate)	Amoebas in spinal fluid	None

Medically important helminths Multicellular organisms. Life cycle involves stages in other organisms.

Organism	Transmission/disease	Treatment
Nematodes (roundworms)		
Enterobius vermicularis (pinworm)	Food contaminated with eggs; intestinal infection; causes anal pruritus (the Scotch tape test).	Mebendazole/pyrantel pamoate
Ascaris lumbricoides (giant roundworm)	Eggs are visible in feces; intestinal infection.	Mebendazole/pyrantel pamoate
Trichinella spiralis	Undercooked meat, usually pork; inflammation of muscle (larvae encyst in muscle), periorbital edema.	Thiabendazole
Strongyloides stercoralis	Larvae in soil penetrate the skin; intestinal infection; causes vomiting, diarrhea, and anemia.	Ivermectin/thiabendazole
Ancylostoma duodenale, *Necator americanus* (hookworms)	Larvae penetrate skin of feet; intestinal infection can cause anemia (sucks blood from intestinal walls).	Mebendazole/pyrantel pamoate (worms are **BEND**y; treat with me**BEND**azole)
Dracunculus medinensis	In drinking water; skin inflammation and ulceration.	Niridazole
Onchocerca volvulus	Transmitted by female blackflies; causes **river** blindness, with skin nodules and "lizard skin." Can have allergic reaction to microfilaria.	**Iver**mectin (**IVER**mectin for r**IVER** blindness)
Loa loa	Transmitted by deer fly, horse fly, and mango fly; causes swelling in skin (can see worm crawling in conjunctiva).	Diethylcarbamazine
Wuchereria bancrofti	Female mosquito; causes blockage of lymphatic vessels (elephantiasis).	Diethylcarbamazine
Toxocara canis	Food contaminated with eggs; causes granulomas (if in retina → blindness) and visceral larva migrans.	Diethylcarbamazine
Cestodes (tapeworms)		
Taenia solium	Ingestion of larvae encysted in undercooked pork leads to intestinal tapeworms. Ingestion of eggs causes cysticercosis and neurocysticercosis, mass lesions in brain ("swiss cheese" appearance).	Praziquantel for intestinal worms and cysticercosis; albendazole for neurocysticercosis
Echinococcus granulosus	Eggs in dog feces when ingested can cause cysts in liver; causes anaphylaxis if echinococcal antigens are released from cysts (see Image 112).	Albendazole
Trematodes (flukes)		
Schistosoma	Snails are host; cercariae penetrate skin of humans; causes granulomas, fibrosis, and inflammation of the spleen and liver.	Praziquantel
Clonorchis sinensis	Undercooked fish; causes inflammation of the biliary tract → pigmented gallstones. Also associated with cholangiocarcinoma.	Praziquantel
Paragonimus westermani	Undercooked crab meat; causes inflammation and 2° bacterial infection of the lung.	Praziquantel

▶ MICROBIOLOGY–PARASITOLOGY *(continued)*

Nematode routes of infection	Ingested—*Enterobius, Ascaris, Trichinella.* Cutaneous—*Strongyloides, Ancylostoma, Necator.*	You'll get sick if you **EAT** these! These get into your feet from the **SAN**d.
Parasite hints	**Findings** Brain cysts, seizures Liver cysts B_{12} deficiency Biliary tract disease Hemoptysis Portal hypertension Hematuria, bladder cancer Microcytic anemia Perianal pruritus	**Organism** *Taenia solium* (cysticercosis) *Echinococcus granulosus* *Diphyllobothrium latum* *Clonorchis sinensis* *Paragonimus westermani* *Schistosoma mansoni* *Schistosoma haematobium* *Ancylostoma, Necator* *Enterobius*
"Tricky T's"	Typhoid fever—caused by bacterium *Salmonella typhi.* Typhus—caused by bacteria *Rickettsia rickettsii* (endemic) and *Rickettsia prowazekii* (epidemic). *Chlamydia* ***trach****omatis*—bacteria, STD. ***Trep****onema*—spirochete; causes syphilis (*T. pallidum*) or yaws (*T. pertenue*). ***Trich****omonas vaginalis*—protozoan, STD. ***Tryp****anosoma*—protozoan, causes Chagas' disease (*T. cruzi*) or African sleeping sickness. *Toxoplasma*—protozoan, a TORCH infection. ***Trich****inella spiralis*—nematode in undercooked meat.	

▶ MICROBIOLOGY–VIROLOGY

DNA viral genomes	All DNA viruses except the Parvoviridae are dsDNA. All are linear except papilloma, polyoma, and hepadnaviruses (circular).	All are dsDNA (like our cells), except "**part-of-a-virus**" (**parvovirus**) is ssDNA.
RNA viral genomes	All RNA viruses except Reoviridae are ssRNA.	All are ssRNA (like our mRNA), except "**repeato**-virus" (**reo**virus) is dsRNA.
Naked viral genome infectivity	Purified nucleic acids of most dsDNA (except poxviruses and HBV) and (+) strand ssRNA (≈ mRNA) viruses are infectious. Naked nucleic acids of (–) strand ssRNA and dsRNA viruses are not infectious. They require enzymes contained in the complete virion.	

Viral envelopes	**Naked** (nonenveloped) viruses include **C**alicivirus, **P**icornavirus, **R**eovirus, **P**arvovirus, **A**denovirus, **P**apilloma, and **P**olyoma. Generally, enveloped viruses acquire their envelopes from plasma membrane when they exit from cell. Exceptions are herpesviruses, which acquire envelopes from nuclear membrane.	**Naked CPR** and **PAPP** smear.

Virus ploidy	All viruses are haploid (with 1 copy of DNA or RNA) except retroviruses, which have 2 identical ssRNA molecules (≈ diploid).

Viral replication	
DNA viruses	All replicate in the nucleus (except poxvirus).
RNA viruses	All replicate in the cytoplasm (except influenza virus and retroviruses).

Viral pathogens	
Structure	**Viruses**
DNA enveloped viruses	Herpesviruses (HSV types 1 and 2, VZV, CMV, EBV), HBV, smallpox virus
DNA nucleocapsid viruses	Adenovirus, papillomaviruses, parvovirus
RNA enveloped viruses	Influenza virus, parainfluenza virus, RSV, measles virus, mumps virus, rubella virus, rabies virus, HTLV, HIV
RNA nucleocapsid viruses	Enteroviruses (poliovirus, coxsackievirus, echovirus, HAV), rhinovirus, reovirus (rotavirus)

Viral structure—general features

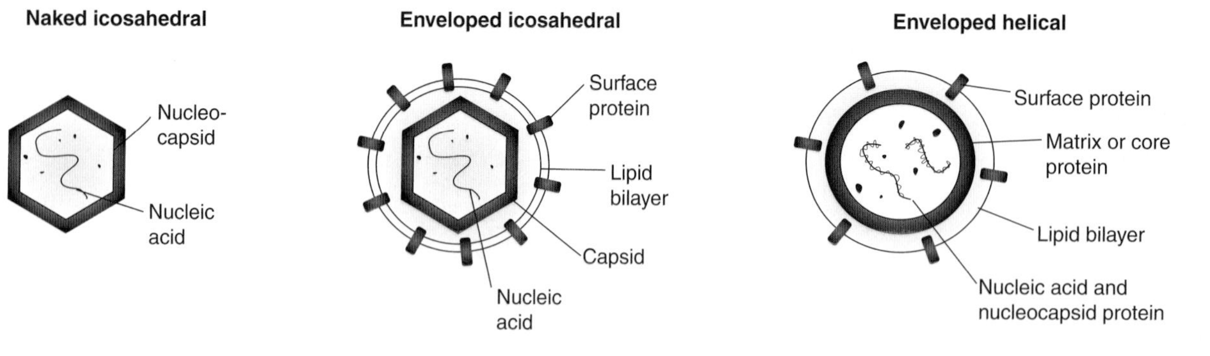

DNA virus characteristics

Some general rules—all DNA viruses:

1. Are **HHAPPPPy** viruses — **H**epadna, **H**erpes, **A**deno, **P**ox, **P**arvo, **P**apilloma, **P**olyoma.
2. Are double stranded — EXCEPT parvo (single stranded).
3. Are linear — EXCEPT papilloma and polyoma (circular, supercoiled) and hepadna (circular, incomplete).
4. Are icosahedral — EXCEPT pox (complex).
5. Replicate in the nucleus — EXCEPT pox (carries own DNA-dependent RNA polymerase).

DNA viruses

Viral Family	Envelope	DNA Structure	Medical Importance
Herpesviruses	Yes	DS – linear	HSV-1—oral (and some genital) lesions, keratoconjunctivitis HSV-2—genital (and some oral) lesions VZV—chickenpox, zoster, shingles EBV—mononucleosis, Burkitt's lymphoma CMV—infection in immunosuppressed patients, especially transplant recipients; congenital defects HHV-6—roseola (exanthem subitum) HHV-8—Kaposi's sarcoma–associated herpesvirus (KSHV)
Hepadnavirus	Yes	DS – partial circular	HBV Acute or chronic hepatitis Vaccine available—use has increased tremendously Not a retrovirus but has reverse transcriptase
Adenovirus	No	DS – linear	Febrile pharyngitis—sore throat Pneumonia Conjunctivitis—"pink eye"
Parvovirus	No	SS – linear (–) (smallest DNA virus)	B19 virus—aplastic crises in sickle cell disease, "slapped cheeks" rash—erythema infectiosum (fifth disease), hydrops fetalis
Papillomavirus*	No	DS – circular	HPV—warts, CIN, cervical cancer
Polyomavirus*	No	DS – circular	JC—progressive multifocal leukoencephalopathy (PML) in HIV
Poxvirus	Yes	DS – linear (largest DNA virus)	Smallpox, although eradicated, could be used in germ warfare Vaccinia—cowpox ("milkmaid's blisters") Molluscum contagiosum

*Papillomavirus and polyomavirus are two new classifications originally grouped as "papovavirus."

HIGH-YIELD PRINCIPLES

MICROBIOLOGY

RNA viruses

Viral Family	Envelope	RNA Structure	Capsid Symmetry	Medical Importance
Picornaviruses	No	SS + linear	Icosahedral	Poliovirus—polio-Salk/Sabin vaccines—IPV/OPV Echovirus—aseptic meningitis Rhinovirus—"common cold" Coxsackievirus—aseptic meningitis herpangina—febrile pharyngitis hand, foot, and mouth disease myocarditis HAV—acute viral hepatitis
Caliciviruses	No	SS + linear	Icosahedral	HEV Norwalk virus—viral gastroenteritis
Reoviruses	No	DS linear 10–12 segments	Icosahedral (double)	Reovirus—Colorado tick fever Rotavirus—#1 cause of fatal diarrhea in children
Flaviviruses	Yes	SS + linear	Icosahedral	HCV Yellow fever* Dengue* St. Louis encephalitis* West Nile virus*
Togaviruses	Yes	SS + linear	Icosahedral	Rubella (German measles) Eastern equine encephalitis* Western equine encephalitis*
Retroviruses	Yes	SS + linear	Icosahedral	Have reverse transcriptase HIV—AIDS HTLV—T-cell leukemia
Coronaviruses	Yes	SS + linear	Helical	Coronavirus—"common cold" and SARS
Orthomyxoviruses	Yes	SS – linear 8 segments	Helical	Influenza virus
Paramyxoviruses	Yes	SS – linear Nonsegmented	Helical	**P**a**R**a**M**yxovirus: **P**arainfluenza—croup **R**SV—bronchiolitis in babies; Rx—ribavirin Rubeola (**M**easles) **M**umps
Rhabdoviruses	Yes	SS – linear	Helical	Rabies
Filoviruses	Yes	SS – linear	Helical	Ebola/Marburg hemorrhagic fever—often fatal!
Arenaviruses	Yes	SS – circular	Helical	LCV—lymphocytic choriomeningitis Lassa fever encephalitis—spread by mice
Bunyaviruses	Yes	SS – circular 3 segments	Helical	California encephalitis* Sandfly/Rift Valley fevers Crimean-Congo hemorrhagic fever* Hantavirus—hemorrhagic fever, pneumonia
Deltavirus	Yes	SS – circular	Helical	HDV

SS, single-stranded; DS, double-stranded; +, + sense; –, – sense; * = arbovirus

(Adapted, with permission, from Levinson W, Jawetz E. *Medical Microbiology and Immunology: Examination and Board Review,* 6th ed. New York: McGraw-Hill, 2000: 182.)

Viral vaccines	Live attenuated vaccines induce humoral and cell-mediated immunity but have reverted to virulence on rare occasions. Killed vaccines induce only humoral immunity but are stable. Live attenuated—measles, mumps, rubella, Sabin polio, VZV, yellow fever, smallpox. Killed—**R**abies, **I**nfluenza, Salk **P**olio, and HAV vaccines. Recombinant—HBV (antigen = recombinant HBsAg).	Dangerous to give live vaccines to immunocompromised patients or their close contacts. MMR = measles, mumps, rubella. Sal**K** = **K**illed. **RIP** **A**lways.
Viral genetics		
Recombination	Exchange of genes between 2 chromosomes by crossing over within regions of significant base sequence homology.	
Reassortment	When viruses with segmented genomes (e.g., influenza virus) exchange segments. High-frequency recombination. Cause of worldwide influenza pandemics.	
Complementation	When 1 of 2 viruses that infect the cell has a mutation that results in a nonfunctional protein. The nonmutated virus "complements" the mutated one by making a functional protein that serves both viruses.	
Phenotypic mixing	Occurs with simultaneous infection of a cell with 2 viruses. Genome of virus A can be partially or completely coated (forming pseudovirion) with the surface proteins of virus B. Type B protein coat determines the infectivity of the phenotypically mixed virus. However, the progeny from this infection have a type A coat that is encoded by its type A genetic material.	
Negative-stranded viruses	Must transcribe negative strand to positive using RNA polymerase. They include **A**renaviruses, **B**unyaviruses, **P**aramyxoviruses, **O**rthomyxoviruses, **F**iloviruses, **R**habdoviruses, and **H**epatitis delta virus.	**A**lways **B**ring **P**olymerase **O**r **F**ail **R**eplication **H**orribly.
Segmented viruses	All are RNA viruses. They include **B**unyaviruses, **O**rthomyxoviruses (influenza viruses), **A**renaviruses, and **R**eoviruses. Influenza virus consists of 8 segments of negative-stranded RNA. These segments can undergo reassortment, causing antigenic shifts that lead to worldwide pandemics of the flu.	**BOAR**.

Herpesviruses

Virus	Diseases	Route of transmission	
HSV-1	Gingivostomatitis, keratoconjunctivitis, temporal lobe encephalitis, herpes labialis	Respiratory secretions, saliva	Get herpes in a **CHEV**rolet: CMV HSV EBV VZV
HSV-2	Herpes genitalis (see Color Image 11), neonatal herpes	Sexual contact, perinatal	
VZV	Varicella-zoster (shingles), encephalitis, pneumonia (see Color Image 15)	Respiratory secretions	
EBV	Infectious mononucleosis, Burkitt's lymphoma	Respiratory secretions, saliva	
CMV	Congenital infection, mononucleosis (negative Monospot), pneumonia. Infected cells have characteristic "owl's eye" appearance (see Color Image 6)	Congenital, transfusion, sexual contact, saliva, urine, transplant	
HHV-8	Kaposi's sarcoma (HIV patients)	Sexual contact	

HSV identification	Tzanck test—a smear of an opened skin vesicle to detect multinucleated giant cells. Used to assay for HSV-1, HSV-2, and VZV. Infected cells also have intranuclear Cowdry A inclusions.	**Tzanck** heavens I do not have herpes.
EBV	A herpesvirus. Can cause mononucleosis. Infects B cells. Characterized by fever, hepatosplenomegaly, pharyngitis, and lymphadenopathy (especially posterior auricular nodes). Peak incidence 15–20 years old. Positive heterophil antibody test. Abnormal circulating cytotoxic T cells (atypical lymphocytes). Also associated with development of Hodgkin's and endemic Burkitt's lymphomas.	Most common during peak kissing years ("kissing disease"). Monospot test—heterophil antibodies detected by agglutination of sheep RBCs.
Picornavirus	Includes **P**oliovirus, **E**chovirus, **R**hinovirus, **C**oxsackievirus, **H**AV. RNA is translated into 1 large polypeptide that is cleaved by proteases into functional viral proteins. Can cause aseptic (viral) meningitis (except rhinovirus and HAV).	Pico**RNA**virus = small **RNA** virus. **PERCH** on a **"peak"** (pico).
Rhinovirus	A picornavirus. Nonenveloped RNA virus. Cause of common cold; > 100 serologic types.	**Rhino** has a runny nose.
Yellow fever virus	A flavivirus (also an arbovirus) transmitted by *Aedes* mosquitos. Virus has a monkey or human reservoir. Symptoms: high fever, black vomitus, and jaundice. Councilman bodies (acidophilic inclusions) may be seen in liver.	*Flavi* = yellow.

Rubella virus	A togavirus. Causes German (3-day) measles. Fever, lymphadenopathy, arthralgias, fine truncal rash. Causes mild disease in children but serious congenital disease (a TORCH infection).	
Rotavirus 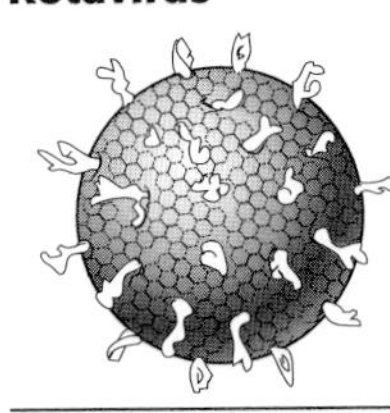	Rotavirus, the most important global cause of infantile gastroenteritis, is a segmented dsRNA virus (a reovirus). Major cause of acute diarrhea in the United States during winter. Villous destruction with atrophy leads to ↓ absorption of Na^+ and water.	**ROTA** = **R**ight **O**ut **T**he **A**nus.
Influenza viruses	Orthomyxoviruses. Enveloped, single-stranded RNA viruses with segmented genome. Contain hemagglutinin and neuraminidase antigens. Responsible for worldwide influenza epidemics; patients at risk for fatal bacterial superinfection. Rapid genetic changes.	Killed viral vaccine is major mode of protection; reformulated vaccine offered each fall to elderly, health-care workers, etc.
Genetic shift (pandemic)	Reassortment of viral genome (such as when human flu A virus recombines with swine flu A virus).	**S**udden **S**hift is more deadly than gra**D**ual **D**rift.
Genetic drift (epidemic)	Minor (antigenic drift) changes based on random mutation.	
Treatment	Amantadine and rimantadine useful for influenza A (especially prophylaxis). High level of resistance to these drugs; no longer used. Zanamivir and oseltamivir (neuraminidase inhibitors) useful for both influenza A and B.	
Paramyxoviruses	Paramyxoviruses cause disease in children. They include those that cause parainfluenza (croup), mumps, and measles as well as RSV, which causes respiratory tract infection (bronchiolitis, pneumonia) in infants.	
Rubeola (measles) virus	A paramyxovirus that causes measles. Koplik spots (red spots with blue-white center on buccal mucosa) are diagnostic. SSPE (years later), encephalitis (1:2000), and giant cell pneumonia (rarely, in immunosuppressed) are possible sequelae. Rash spreads from head to toe.	3 C's of measles: Cough Coryza Conjunctivitis Also look for **K**oplik spots.
Mumps virus	A paramyxovirus. Symptoms: **P**arotitis, **O**rchitis (inflammation of testes), and aseptic **M**eningitis. Can cause sterility (especially after puberty).	Mumps makes your parotid glands and testes as big as **POM**-poms.

Rabies virus 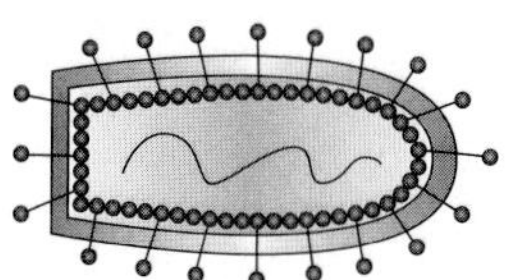	Negri bodies (see Image 113) are characteristic cytoplasmic inclusions in neurons infected by rabies virus. Has bullet-shaped capsid. Rabies has long incubation period (weeks to months). Causes fatal encephalitis with seizures, hydrophobia, hypersalivation, and pharyngeal spasm. More commonly from bat, raccoon, and skunk bites than from dog bites in the United States.	Travels to the CNS by migrating in a retrograde fashion up nerve axons.
Arboviruses	Transmitted by arthropods (mosquitoes, ticks). Classic examples are dengue fever (also known as break-bone fever) and yellow fever. A variant of dengue fever in Southeast Asia is hemorrhagic shock syndrome.	**ARBO**virus—**AR**thropod-**BO**rne virus, including some members of **F**lavivirus, **T**ogavirus, and **B**unyavirus. **F**ever **T**ransmitted by **B**ites.
"Lots of spots"		
Rubella	Togavirus; German 3-day measles.	
Rubeola	Paramyxovirus; measles.	
Varicella	Herpesvirus; chickenpox and zoster.	
Variola	Poxvirus; smallpox (no longer present outside of labs).	
Vaccinia	Poxvirus; strain used for smallpox vaccine.	
Hepatitis viruses	The hepatitis viruses belong to 5 different viral families.	
	HAV (RNA picornavirus) is transmitted primarily by fecal-oral route. Short incubation (3 weeks). No carriers.	Hep **A**: **A**symptomatic (usually), **A**cute, **A**lone (no carriers).
	HBV (DNA hepadnavirus) is transmitted primarily by parenteral, sexual, and maternal-fetal routes. Long incubation (3 months). Carriers. Cellular RNA polymerase transcribes RNA from DNA template. Reverse transcriptase transcribes DNA genome from RNA intermediate. However, the virion enzyme is a DNA-dependent DNA polymerase.	Hep **B**: **B**lood borne.
	HCV (RNA flavivirus) is transmitted primarily via blood and resembles HBV in its course and severity. Carriers. Common cause of hepatitis among IV drug users in the United States.	Hep **C**: **C**hronic, **C**irrhosis, **C**arcinoma, **C**arriers.
	HDV (delta agent) is a defective virus that requires HBsAg as its envelope. HDV can coinfect with HBV or superinfect; the latter has a worse prognosis. Carriers.	Hep **D**: **D**efective, **D**ependent on HBV.
	HEV (RNA calicivirus) is transmitted enterically and causes water-borne epidemics. Resembles HAV in course, severity, incubation. High mortality rate in pregnant women.	Hep **E**: **E**nteric, **E**xpectant mothers, **E**pidemics.
	Both HBV and HCV predispose a patient to chronic active hepatitis, cirrhosis, and hepatocellular carcinoma.	A and E by fecal-oral route: "The **vowels** hit your **bowels**."

Hepatitis serologic markers

IgG HAVAb	Indicates prior infection; protective against reinfection.
IgM HAVAb	IgM antibody to HAV; best test to detect active hepatitis A.
HBsAg	Antigen found on surface of HBV; continued presence indicates carrier state.
HBsAb	Antibody to HBsAg; **provides immunity** to hepatitis B.
HBcAg	Antigen associated with core of HBV.
HBcAb	Antibody to HBcAg; positive during **window period.** IgM HBcAb is an indicator of recent disease. IgG HBcAb signifies chronic disease.
H**Be**Ag	A second, different antigenic determinant in the HBV core. Important indicator of active viral replication and therefore transmissibility (**Be**ware!)
HBeAb	Antibody to e antigen; indicates low transmissibility.

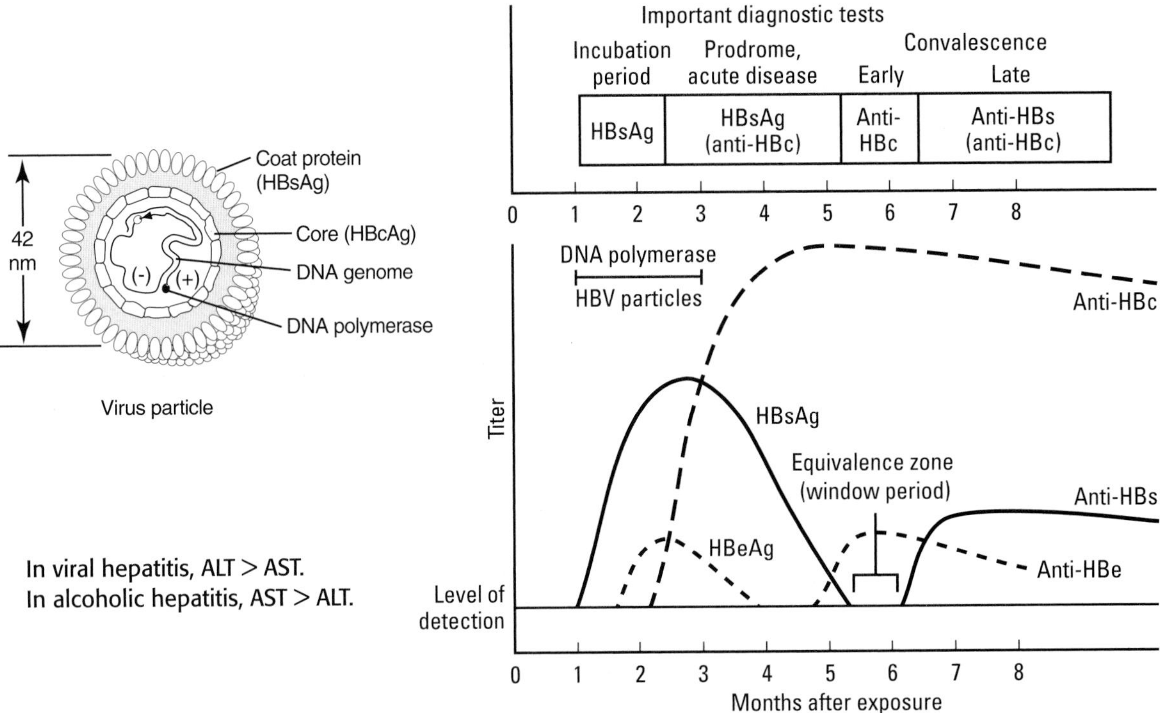

In viral hepatitis, ALT > AST.
In alcoholic hepatitis, AST > ALT.

Test	Acute Disease	Window Phase	Complete Recovery	Chronic Carrier	Immunized
HBsAg	+	–	–	+	–
HBsAb	–	–[b]	+	–	+
HBcAb	+[a]	+	+	+	–

[a]IgM in acute stage; IgG in chronic or recovered stage.

[b]Patient has surface antibody but available antibody is bound to HBsAg, so not detected in assay.

HIV

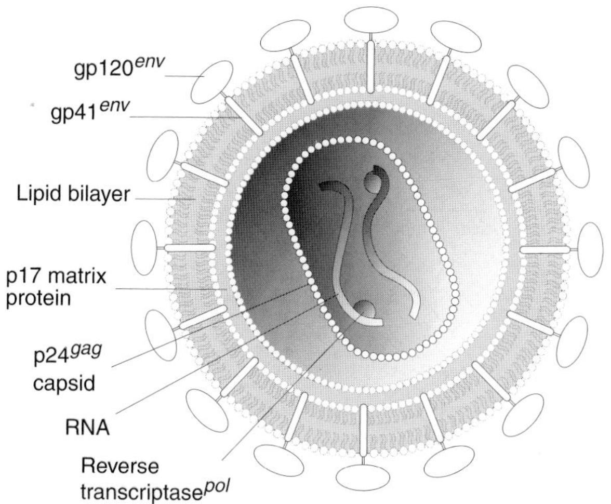

(Adapted, with permission, from Levinson W. *Medical Microbiology and Immunology: Examination and Board Review*, 8th ed. New York: McGraw-Hill, 2004: 314.)

Diploid genome (2 molecules of RNA).
p24 = rectangular capsid protein.
gp41 and gp120 = envelope proteins.

Reverse transcriptase synthesizes dsDNA from RNA; dsDNA integrates into host genome.

Virus binds CXCR4 and CD4 on T cells; binds CCR5 and CD4 on macrophages. Homozygous CCR5 mutation = immunity. Heterozygous CCR5 mutation = slower course.

HIV diagnosis	Presumptive diagnosis made with ELISA (sensitive, high false-positive rate and low threshold, RULE OUT test); positive results are then confirmed with Western blot assay (specific, high false-negative rate and high threshold, RULE IN test). HIV PCR/viral load tests are increasing in popularity: they allow physician to monitor the effect of drug therapy on viral load. AIDS diagnosis ≤ 200 CD4+, HIV positive with AIDS indicator condition (e.g., PCP), or CD4/CD8 ratio < 1.5.	ELISA/Western blot tests look for antibodies to viral proteins; these tests are often falsely negative in the first 1–2 months of HIV infection and falsely positive initially in babies born to infected mothers (anti-gp120 crosses placenta).

Time course of HIV infection

4 stages of infection:

1. **Flulike** (acute)
2. **Feeling fine** (latent)
3. **Falling count**
4. **Final crisis**

During latent phase, virus replicates in lymph nodes.

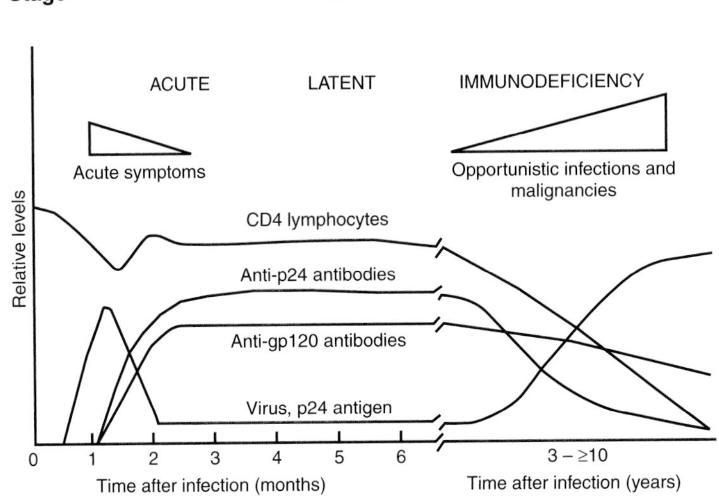

(Adapted, with permission, from Levinson W. *Medical Microbiology and Immunology: Examination and Board Review,* 8th ed. New York: McGraw-Hill, 2004: 318.)

Opportunistic infections and disease in AIDS

Organ system	Infection/disease
Brain	Cryptococcal meningitis, toxoplasmosis, CMV encephalopathy, AIDS dementia, PML (JC virus)
Eyes	CMV retinitis
Mouth and throat	Thrush (*Candida albicans*), HSV, CMV, oral hairy leukoplakia (EBV)
Lungs	*Pneumocystis jiroveci* pneumonia (PJP), TB, histoplasmosis
GI	Cryptosporidiosis, *Mycobacterium avium–intracellulare* complex, CMV colitis, non-Hodgkin's lymphoma (EBV), *Isospora belli*
Skin	Shingles (VZV), Kaposi's sarcoma (HHV-8)
Genitals	Genital herpes, warts, and cervical cancer (HPV)

HIV-associated infections and CD4 count

Risk increases at CD4 level of:	Infection
< 400	Oral thrush, tinea pedis, reactivation VZV, reactivation tuberculosis, other bacterial infections (e.g., *H. influenzae*, *S. pneumoniae*, *Salmonella*)
< 200	Reactivation HSV, cryptosporidiosis, *Isospora*, disseminated coccidioidomycosis, *Pneumocystis* pneumonia
< 100	Candidal esophagitis, toxoplasmosis, histoplasmosis
< 50	CMV retinitis and esophagitis, disseminated *M. avium–intracellulare*, cryptococcal meningoencephalitis

Neoplasms associated with HIV

Kaposi's sarcoma (HHV-8), invasive cervical carcinoma (HPV), 1° CNS lymphoma, non-Hodgkin's lymphoma.

HIV encephalitis

Occurs late in the course of HIV infection. Virus gains CNS access via infected macrophages. Microglial nodules with multinucleated giant cells.

Prions — Infectious agents that do not contain RNA or DNA (consist only of proteins); encoded by cellular genes. Diseases include Creutzfeldt-Jakob disease (CJD—rapid progressive dementia), kuru, scrapie (sheep), and "mad cow disease." Prions are associated with spongiform encephalopathy. Normal prions have α-helix conformation; pathologic prions (like CJD) are β-pleated sheets.

▶ MICROBIOLOGY—SYSTEMS

Normal flora: dominant

Skin—*Staphylococcus epidermidis.*
Nose—*S. Epidermidis;* colonized by *S. aureus.*
Oropharynx—Viridans group streptococci.
Dental plaque—*Streptococcus mutans.*
Colon—*Bacteroides fragilis* > *E. coli.*
Vagina—*Lactobacillus,* colonized by *E. coli* and group B strep.

Neonates delivered by cesarean section have no flora but are rapidly colonized after birth.

Common causes of pneumonia

Neonates (< 4 wk)	Children (4 wk–18 yr)	Adults (18–40 yr)	Adults (40–65 yr)	Elderly
Group B streptococci	Viruses (**R**SV)	*Mycoplasma*	*S. pneumoniae*	*S. pneumoniae*
E. coli	***M**ycoplasma*	*C. pneumoniae*	*H. influenzae*	Viruses
	Chlamydia pneumoniae	*S. pneumoniae*	Anaerobes	Anaerobes
	***S**treptococcus pneumoniae*		Viruses	*H. influenzae*
	Runts **M**ay **C**ough **S**putum		*Mycoplasma*	Gram-negative rods

Special groups:

Nosocomial (hospital acquired)	*Staphylococcus,* gram-negative rods
Immunocompromised	*Staphylococcus,* gram-negative rods, fungi, viruses, *Pneumocystis jiroveci*—with HIV
Aspiration	Anaerobes
Alcoholic/IV drug user	*S. pneumoniae, Klebsiella, Staphylococcus*
Postviral	*Staphylococcus, H. influenzae*
Atypical	*Mycoplasma, Legionella, Chlamydia*

Common causes of meningitis

Newborn (0–6 mos)	Children (6 mos–6 yrs)	6–60 yrs	60 yrs +
Group B streptococci	*Streptococcus pneumoniae*	*N. meningitidis*	*S. pneumoniae*
E. coli	*Neisseria meningitidis*	Enteroviruses	Gram-negative rods
Listeria	*Haemophilus influenzae* type B	*S. pneumoniae*	*Listeria*
	Enteroviruses	HSV	

Viral causes of meningitis—enteroviruses (esp. coxsackievirus), HSV, HIV, West Nile virus, VZV.

In HIV—*Cryptococcus*, CMV, toxoplasmosis (brain abscess), JC virus (PML).

Note: Incidence of *H. influenzae* meningitis has ↓ greatly with introduction of *H. influenzae* vaccine in last 10–15 years.

CSF findings in meningitis

	Pressure	Cell type	Protein	Sugar
Bacterial	↑	↑ PMNs	↑	↓
Fungal/TB	↑	↑ lymphocytes	↑	↓
Viral	Normal/↑	↑ lymphocytes	Normal	Normal

Osteomyelitis

Most people—*S. aureus*.

Sexually active—*Neisseria gonorrhoeae* (rare), septic arthritis more common.

Diabetics and drug addicts—*Pseudomonas aeruginosa*.

Sickle cell—*Salmonella*.

Prosthetic replacement—*S. aureus* and *S. epidermidis*.

Vertebral—*Mycobacterium tuberculosis* (Pott's disease).

Cat and dog bites or scratches—*Pasteurella multocida*.

Assume *S. aureus* if no other information.

Most osteomyelitis occurs in children.

Elevated CRP and ESR classic but nonspecific.

Urinary tract infections

Ambulatory—*E. coli* (50–80%), *Klebsiella* (8–10%).

Staphylococcus saprophyticus (10–30%) is the 2nd most common cause of UTI in young, sexually active, ambulatory women.

Hospital—*E. coli, Proteus, Klebsiella, Serratia, Pseudomonas*.

Epidemiology: women to men—10:1 (short urethra colonized by fecal flora).

Predisposing factors: flow obstruction, kidney surgery, catheterization, gynecologic abnormalities, diabetes, and pregnancy.

UTIs mostly caused by ascending infections. In males: babies with congenital defects; elderly with enlarged prostates.

UTI—dysuria, frequency, urgency, suprapubic pain.

Pyelonephritis—fever, chills, flank pain, and CVA tenderness.

UTI bugs

SSEEK PP.

Diagnostic markers:

Leukocyte esterase—positive = bacterial.

Nitrite test—positive = gram negative.

Species	Features of the organism
Serratia marcescens	Some strains produce a red pigment; often nosocomial and drug resistant.
Staphylococcus saprophyticus	2nd leading cause of community-acquired UTI in sexually active women.
Escherichia coli	Leading cause of UTI. Colonies show metallic sheen on EMB agar.
Enterobacter cloacae	Often nosocomial and drug resistant.
Klebsiella pneumoniae	Large mucoid capsule and viscous colonies.
Proteus mirabilis	Motility causes "swarming" on agar; produces urease; associated with struvite stones.
Pseudomonas aeruginosa	Blue-green pigment and fruity odor; usually nosocomial and drug resistant.

ToRCHeS infections

These important infections are transmitted in utero or during vaginal birth.

Major clinical manifestations

Toxoplasma gondii—"classic triad" of chorioretinitis, intracranial calcifications, and hydrocephalus. May be asymptomatic at birth.

Rubella—deafness, cataracts, heart defects (PDA, pulmonary artery stenosis), and mental retardation.

CMV—petechial rash, intracranial calcifications, mental retardation, hepatosplenomegaly, microcephaly, jaundice. 90% are asymptomatic at birth.

HIV—hepatosplenomegaly, neurologic abnormalities, frequent infections.

HSV type 2—encephalitis, conjunctivitis, vesicular skin lesions. Often asymptomatic at birth.

Syphilis—cutaneous lesions, hepatosplenomegaly, jaundice, saddle nose, saber shins, Hutchinson teeth, CN VIII deafness, rhinitis ("snuffles").

Other important congenital infections

Listeria, *E. coli*, and group B streptococci can be acquired placentally or from birth canal.

Sexually transmitted diseases

Disease	Clinical features	Organism
Gonorrhea	Urethritis, cervicitis, PID, prostatitis, epididymitis, arthritis, creamy purulent discharge	*Neisseria gonorrhoeae*
1° syphilis	Painless chancre	*Treponema pallidum*
2° syphilis	Fever, lymphadenopathy, skin rashes, condylomata lata	
3° syphilis	Gummas, tabes dorsalis, general paresis, aortitis, Argyll Robertson pupil	
Genital herpes	Painful penile, vulvar, or cervical ulcers; can cause systemic symptoms such as fever, headache, myalgia.	HSV-2
Chlamydia	Urethritis, cervicitis, conjunctivitis, Reiter's syndrome, PID	*Chlamydia trachomatis* (D–K)
Lymphogranuloma venereum	Ulcers, lymphadenopathy, rectal strictures	*C. trachomatis* (L1–L3)
Trichomoniasis	Vaginitis, strawberry-colored mucosa	*Trichomonas vaginalis*
AIDS	Opportunistic infections, Kaposi's sarcoma, lymphoma	HIV
Condylomata acuminata	Genital warts, koilocytes	HPV 6 and 11
Hepatitis B	Jaundice	HBV
Chancroid	Painful genital ulcer, inguinal adenopathy	*Haemophilus ducreyi*
Bacterial vaginosis	Noninflammatory, malodorous discharge (fishy smell); positive whiff test, clue cells	*Gardnerella vaginalis*

Pelvic inflammatory disease

Top bugs—*Chlamydia trachomatis* (subacute, often undiagnosed), *Neisseria gonorrhoeae* (acute, high fever). *C. trachomatis* is the most common STD in the United States (3–4 million cases per year). Cervical motion tenderness (chandelier sign), purulent cervical discharge. PID may include salpingitis, endometritis, hydrosalpinx, and tubo-ovarian abscess.

Salpingitis is a risk factor for ectopic pregnancy, infertility, chronic pelvic pain, and adhesions.

Other STDs include *Gardnerella* (clue cells) and *Trichomonas* (motile on wet prep).

Nosocomial infections

Pathogen	Risk factor
CMV, RSV	Newborn nursery
E. coli, Proteus mirabilis	Urinary catheterization
Pseudomonas aeruginosa	Respiratory therapy equipment
HBV	Work in renal dialysis unit
Candida albicans	Hyperalimentation
Legionella	Water aerosols

Notes

The 2 most common causes of nosocomial infections are *E. coli* (UTI) and *S. aureus* (wound infection).

Presume *Pseudomonas* ***AIR****uginosa* when **AIR** or burns are involved.

Legionella when water source is involved.

Bug hints (if all else fails)	Pus, empyema, abscess—*S. aureus.* Pediatric infection—*Haemophilus influenzae* (including epiglottitis). Pneumonia in cystic fibrosis, burn infection—*Pseudomonas aeruginosa.* Branching rods in oral infection—*Actinomyces israelii.* Traumatic open wound—*Clostridium perfringens.* Surgical wound—*S. aureus.* Dog or cat bite—*Pasteurella multocida.* Currant jelly sputum—*Klebsiella.* Sepsis/meningitis in newborn—group B strep.

▶ MICROBIOLOGY–ANTIMICROBIALS

Antimicrobial therapy

Mechanism of action	Drugs
1. Block cell wall synthesis by inhibition of peptidoglycan cross-linking	Penicillin, ampicillin, ticarcillin, piperacillin, imipenem, aztreonam, cephalosporins
2. Block peptidoglycan synthesis	Bacitracin, vancomycin
3. Disrupt bacterial cell membranes	Polymyxins
4. Block nucleotide synthesis	Sulfonamides, trimethoprim
5. Block DNA topoisomerases	Quinolones
6. Block mRNA synthesis	Rifampin
7. Block protein synthesis at 50S ribosomal subunit	Chloramphenicol, macrolides, clindamycin, streptogramins (quinupristin, dalfopristin), linezolid
8. Block protein synthesis at 30S ribosomal subunit	Aminoglycosides, tetracyclines

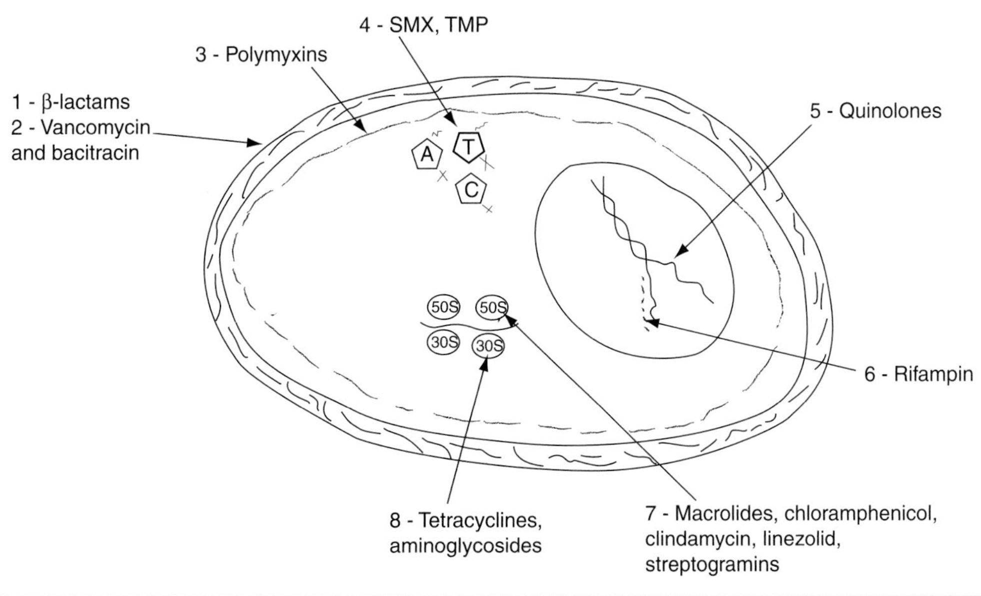

Bacteriostatic vs. bacteriocidal antibiotics

Bacteriostatic	**E**rythromycin, **C**lindamycin, **S**ulfamethoxazole, **T**rimethoprim, **T**etracyclines, **C**hloramphenicol.	"We're **ECSTaTiC** about bacteriostatics."
Bactericidal	**V**ancomycin, **F**luoroquinolones, **P**enicillin, **A**minoglycosides, **C**ephalosporins, **M**etronidazole.	"**V**ery **F**inely **P**roficient **A**t **C**ell **M**urder."

Penicillin

	Penicillin G (IV form), penicillin V (oral). Prototype β-lactam antibiotics.
Mechanism	1. Bind penicillin-binding proteins 2. Block transpeptidase cross-linking of cell wall 3. Activate autolytic enzymes
Clinical use	Bactericidal for gram-positive cocci, gram-positive rods, gram-negative cocci, and spirochetes. Not penicillinase resistant.
Toxicity	Hypersensitivity reactions, hemolytic anemia.

Methicillin, nafcillin, dicloxacillin (penicillinase-resistant penicillins)

Mechanism	Same as penicillin. Narrow spectrum; penicillinase resistant because of bulkier R group.	"Use **naf** (nafcillin) for **staph.**"
Clinical use	*S. aureus* (except MRSA; resistant because of altered penicillin-binding protein target site).	
Toxicity	Hypersensitivity reactions; methicillin—interstitial nephritis.	

Ampicillin, amoxicillin (aminopenicillins)

Mechanism	Same as penicillin. Wider spectrum; penicillinase sensitive. Also combine with clavulanic acid (penicillinase inhibitor) to enhance spectrum. AmOxicillin has greater **O**ral bioavailability than ampicillin.	
Clinical use	Extended-spectrum penicillin—certain gram-positive bacteria and gram-negative rods (***H**aemophilus influenzae*, ***E**. coli*, ***L**isteria monocytogenes*, ***P**roteus mirabilis*, ***S**almonella*, enterococci).	Coverage: ampicillin/amoxicillin **HELPS** kill enterococci.
Toxicity	Hypersensitivity reactions; ampicillin rash; pseudomembranous colitis.	

Ticarcillin, carbenicillin, piperacillin (antipseudomonals)

Mechanism	Same as penicillin. Extended spectrum.	**TCP**: Takes Care of *Pseudomonas*.
Clinical use	*Pseudomonas* spp. and gram-negative rods; susceptible to penicillinase; use with clavulanic acid.	
Toxicity	Hypersensitivity reactions.	

Cephalosporins

Mechanism	β-lactam drugs that inhibit cell wall synthesis but are less susceptible to penicillinases. Bactericidal.	
Clinical use	1st generation (cefazolin, cephalexin)—gram-positive cocci, ***Proteus mirabilis*, *E. coli*, *Klebsiella* ***pneumoniae*.	1st generation—**PEcK.**
	2nd generation (cefoxitin, cefaclor, cefuroxime)—gram-positive cocci, ***Haemophilus influenzae*, *Enterobacter aerogenes*, *Neisseria*** spp., ***Proteus mirabilis*, *E. coli*, *Klebsiella pneumoniae*, *Serratia*** *marcescens*.	2nd generation—**HEN PEcKS.**
	3rd generation (ceftriaxone, cefotaxime, ceftazidime)—serious gram-negative infections resistant to other β-lactams; meningitis (most penetrate the blood-brain barrier). Examples: ceftazidime for *Pseudomonas*; ceftriaxone for gonorrhea.	
	4th generation (cefepime)—↑ activity against *Pseudomonas* and gram-positive organisms.	
Toxicity	Hypersensitivity reactions. Cross-hypersensitivity with penicillins occurs in 5–10% of patients. ↑ nephrotoxicity of aminoglycosides; disulfiram-like reaction with ethanol (in cephalosporins with a methylthiotetrazole group, e.g., cefamandole).	

Penicillin

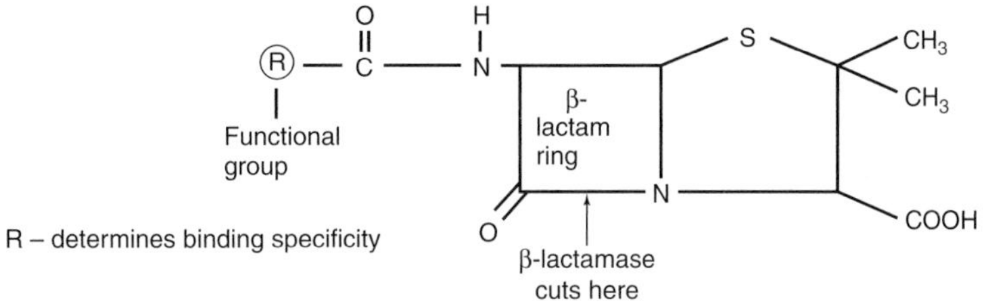

R – determines binding specificity
Functional group
β-lactam ring
β-lactamase cuts here
CH_3
CH_3
COOH

Cephalosporin

R_1 Functional group
β-lactam ring
β-lactamase cuts here
COO^{-}
R_2 Functional group

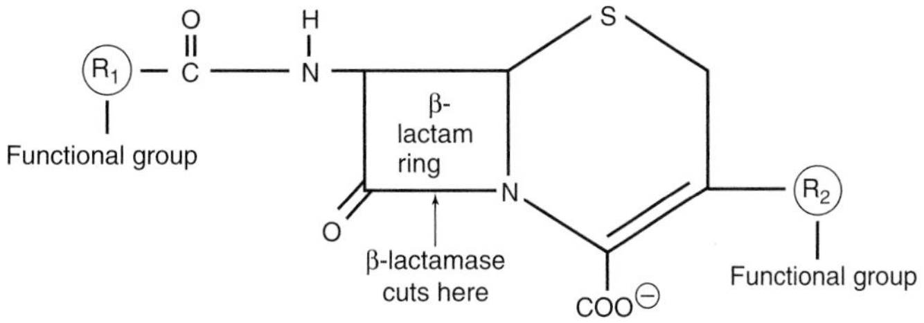

Aztreonam

Mechanism	A monobactam resistant to β-lactamases. Inhibits cell wall synthesis (binds to PBP3). Synergistic with aminoglycosides. No cross-allergenicity with penicillins.
Clinical use	Gram-negative rods—*Klebsiella* spp., *Pseudomonas* spp., *Serratia* spp. No activity against gram-positives or anaerobes. For penicillin-allergic patients and those with renal insufficiency who cannot tolerate aminoglycosides.
Toxicity	Usually nontoxic; occasional GI upset. No cross-sensitivity with penicillins or cephalosporins.

Imipenem/cilastatin, meropenem

Mechanism	Imipenem is a broad-spectrum, β-lactamase-resistant carbapenem. Always administered with cilastatin (inhibitor of renal dihydropeptidase I) to ↓ inactivation in renal tubules.	With imipenem, "the kill is **LASTIN'** with ci**LASTATIN**."
Clinical use	Gram-positive cocci, gram-negative rods, and anaerobes. Drug of choice for *Enterobacter*. The significant side effects limit use to life-threatening infections, or after other drugs have failed. Meropenem, however, has a reduced risk of seizures and is stable to dihydropeptidase I.	
Toxicity	GI distress, skin rash, and CNS toxicity (seizures) at high plasma levels.	

Vancomycin

Mechanism	Inhibits cell wall mucopeptide formation by binding D-ala D-ala portion of cell wall precursors. Bactericidal. Resistance occurs with amino acid change of D-ala D-ala to D-ala D-lac.
Clinical use	Used for serious, gram-positive multidrug-resistant organisms, including *S. aureus* and *Clostridium difficile* (pseudomembranous colitis).
Toxicity	**N**ephrotoxicity, **O**totoxicity, **T**hrombophlebitis, diffuse flushing—"red man syndrome" (can largely prevent by pretreatment with antihistamines and slow infusion rate). Well tolerated in general—does **NOT** have many problems.

Protein synthesis inhibitors

30S inhibitors:
A = **A**minoglycosides (streptomycin, gentamicin, tobramycin, amikacin) [bactericidal]
T = **T**etracyclines [bacteriostatic]

"Buy **AT 30, CCELL** (sell) at **50**."

50S inhibitors:
C = **C**hloramphenicol, **C**lindamycin [bacteriostatic]
E = **E**rythromycin [bacteriostatic]
L = **L**incomycin [bacteriostatic]
L = **L**inezolid [variable]

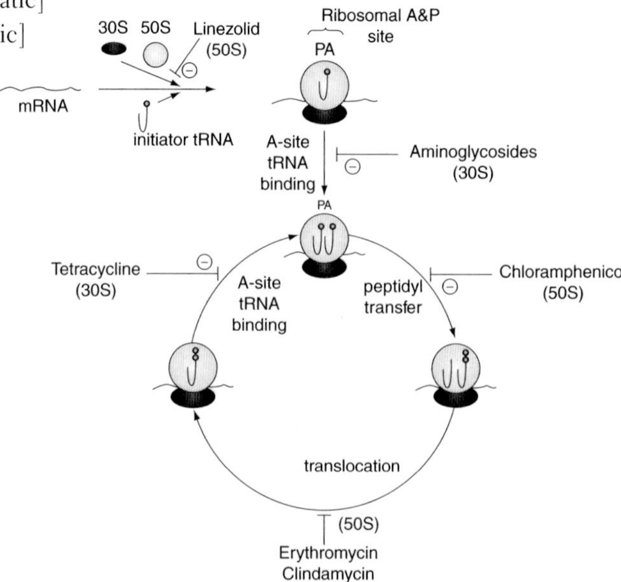

Aminoglycosides	**G**entamicin, **N**eomycin, **A**mikacin, **T**obramycin, **S**treptomycin.	**"Mean" GNATS** can**NOT** kill anaerobes.
Mechanism	Bactericidal; inhibit formation of initiation complex and cause misreading of mRNA. Require O_2 for uptake; therefore ineffective against anaerobes.	
Clinical use	Severe gram-negative rod infections. Synergistic with β-lactam antibiotics. Neomycin for bowel surgery.	
Toxicity	**N**ephrotoxicity (especially when used with cephalosporins), **O**totoxicity (especially when used with loop diuretics). **T**eratogen.	

Tetracyclines	Tetracycline, doxycycline, demeclocycline, minocycline.	Demeclocycline—ADH antagonist; acts as a **D**iuretic in SIADH.
Mechanism	Bacteriostatic; bind to 30S and prevent attachment of aminoacyl-tRNA; limited CNS penetration. Doxycycline is fecally eliminated and can be used in patients with renal failure. Must NOT take with milk, antacids, or iron-containing preparations because divalent cations inhibit its absorption in the gut.	
Clinical use	***V****ibrio cholerae*, **A**cne, ***C****hlamydia*, ***U****reaplasma* ***U****realyticum*, ***M****ycoplasma pneumoniae*, **T**ularemia, ***H****. pylori*, ***B****orrelia burgdorferi* (Lyme disease), ***R****ickettsia*.	**VACUUM THe BedRoom.**
Toxicity	GI distress, discoloration of teeth and inhibition of bone growth in children, photosensitivity. Contraindicated in pregnancy.	

Macrolides	Erythromycin, azithromycin, clarithromycin.
Mechanism	Inhibit protein synthesis by blocking translocation; bind to the 23S rRNA of the 50S ribosomal subunit. Bacteriostatic.
Clinical use	URIs, pneumonias, STDs—gram-positive cocci (streptococcal infections in patients allergic to penicillin), *Mycoplasma*, *Legionella*, *Chlamydia*, *Neisseria*.
Toxicity	GI discomfort (most common cause of noncompliance), acute cholestatic hepatitis, eosinophilia, skin rashes. Increases serum concentration of theophyllines, oral anticoagulants.

Chloramphenicol	
Mechanism	Inhibits 50S peptidyltransferase activity. Bacteriostatic.
Clinical use	Meningitis (*Haemophilus influenzae*, *Neisseria meningitidis*, *Streptococcus pneumoniae*). Conservative use owing to toxicities.
Toxicity	Anemia (dose dependent), aplastic anemia (dose independent), gray baby syndrome (in premature infants because they lack liver UDP-glucuronyl transferase).

Clindamycin

Mechanism	Blocks peptide bond formation at 50S ribosomal subunit. Bacteriostatic.	Treats anaerobes above the diaphragm.
Clinical use	Treat anaerobic infections (e.g., *Bacteroides fragilis, Clostridium perfringens*).	
Toxicity	Pseudomembranous colitis (*C. difficile* overgrowth), fever, diarrhea.	

Sulfonamides Sulfamethoxazole (SMX), sulfisoxazole, triple sulfas, sulfadiazine.

Mechanism	PABA antimetabolites inhibit dihydropteroate synthetase. Bacteriostatic.
Clinical use	Gram-positive, gram-negative, *Nocardia, Chlamydia.* Triple sulfas or SMX for simple UTI.
Toxicity	Hypersensitivity reactions, hemolysis if G6PD deficient, nephrotoxicity (tubulointerstitial nephritis), photosensitivity, kernicterus in infants, displace other drugs from albumin (e.g., warfarin).

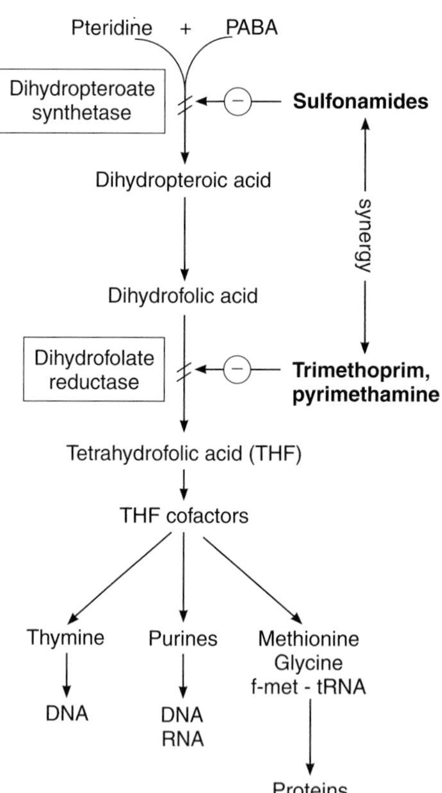

(Adapted, with permission, from Katzung BG. *Basic and Clinical Pharmacology,* 7th ed. Stamford, CT: Appleton & Lange, 1997: 762.)

Trimethoprim		
Mechanism	Inhibits bacterial dihydrofolate reductase. Bacteriostatic.	Trimethoprim = **TMP**: "**T**reats **M**arrow **P**oorly."
Clinical use	Used in combination with sulfonamides (trimethoprim-sulfamethoxazole [TMP-SMX]), causing sequential block of folate synthesis. Combination used for recurrent UTIs, *Shigella*, *Salmonella*, *Pneumocystis jiroveci* pneumonia.	
Toxicity	Megaloblastic anemia, leukopenia, granulocytopenia. (May alleviate with supplemental folinic acid.)	
Sulfa drug allergies	Patients who do not tolerate sulfa drugs should not be given sulfonamides or other sulfa drugs, such as sulfasalazine, sulfonylureas, thiazide diuretics, acetazolamide, or furosemide.	
Fluoroquinolones	Ciprofloxacin, norfloxacin, ofloxacin, sparfloxacin, moxifloxacin, gatifloxacin, enoxacin (fluoroquinolones), nalidixic acid (a quinolone).	
Mechanism	Inhibit DNA gyrase (topoisomerase II). Bactericidal. Must not be taken with antacids.	Fluoroquino**LONES** hurt attachments to your **BONES.**
Clinical use	Gram-negative rods of urinary and GI tracts (including *Pseudomonas*), *Neisseria*, some gram-positive organisms.	
Toxicity	GI upset, superinfections, skin rashes, headache, dizziness. Contraindicated in pregnant women and in children because animal studies show damage to cartilage. Tendonitis and tendon rupture in adults; leg cramps and myalgias in kids.	
Metronidazole		
Mechanism	Forms toxic metabolites in the bacterial cell that damage DNA. Bactericidal.	
Clinical use	Antiprotozoal. *Giardia*, *Entamoeba*, *Trichomonas*, *Gardnerella vaginalis*, Anaerobes (*Bacteroides*, *Clostridium*). Used with bismuth and amoxicillin (or tetracycline) for "triple therapy" against *H. Pylori*.	**GET GAP** on the **Metro!** Anaerobic infection below the diaphragm.
Toxicity	Disulfiram-like reaction with alcohol; headache, metallic taste.	
Polymyxins	Polymyxin B, polymyxin E.	'**MYXins MIX up** membranes.
Mechanism	Bind to cell membranes of bacteria and disrupt their osmotic properties. Polymyxins are cationic, basic proteins that act like detergents.	
Clinical use	Resistant gram-negative infections.	
Toxicity	Neurotoxicity, acute renal tubular necrosis.	

Antimycobacterial drugs

Bacterium	Prophylaxis	Treatment
M. tuberculosis	Isoniazid	Isoniazid, rifampin, ethambutol, pyrazinamide
M. avium–intracellulare	Azithromycin	Azithromycin, rifampin, ethambutol, streptomycin
M. leprae	N/A	Dapsone, rifampin, clofazimine

Anti-TB drugs

Streptomycin, **P**yrazinamide, **I**soniazid (INH), **R**ifampin, **E**thambutol.
Cycloserine (2nd-line therapy).
Important side effect of ethambutol is optic neuropathy (red-green color blindness). For other drugs, hepatotoxicity.

INH-SPIRE (inspire).

Isoniazid (INH)

Mechanism	↓ synthesis of mycolic acids.	**INH** **I**njures **N**eurons and **H**epatocytes.
Clinical use	*Mycobacterium tuberculosis*. The only agent used as solo prophylaxis against TB.	Different INH half-lives in fast vs. slow acetylators.
Toxicity	Hemolysis if G6PD deficient, neurotoxicity, hepatotoxicity, SLE-like syndrome. Pyridoxine (vitamin B_6) can prevent neurotoxicity.	

Rifampin

Mechanism	Inhibits DNA-dependent RNA polymerase.	Rifampin's **4 R's**:
Clinical use	*Mycobacterium tuberculosis*; delays resistance to dapsone when used for leprosy. Used for meningococcal prophylaxis and chemoprophylaxis in contacts of children with *Haemophilus influenzae* type B.	**R**NA polymerase inhibitor **R**evs up microsomal P-450 **R**ed/orange body fluids **R**apid resistance if used alone
Toxicity	Minor hepatotoxicity and drug interactions (↑ P-450); orange body fluids (nonhazardous side effect).	

Resistance mechanisms for various antibiotics

Drug	Most common mechanism
Penicillins/cephalosporins	β-lactamase cleavage of β-lactam ring, or altered PBP in case of MRSA
Aminoglycosides	Modification via acetylation, adenylation, or phosphorylation
Vancomycin	Terminal D-ala of cell wall component replaced with D-lac; ↓ affinity
Chloramphenicol	Modification via acetylation
Macrolides	Methylation of rRNA near erythromycin's ribosome-binding site
Tetracycline	↓ uptake or ↑ transport out of cell
Sulfonamides	Altered enzyme (bacterial dihydropteroate synthetase), ↓ uptake, or ↑ PABA synthesis
Quinolones	Altered gyrase or reduced uptake

Nonsurgical antimicrobial prophylaxis	
Meningococcal infection	Rifampin (drug of choice), minocycline.
Gonorrhea	Ceftriaxone.
Syphilis	Benzathine penicillin G.
History of recurrent UTIs	TMP-SMX.
Pneumocystis jiroveci pneumonia	TMP-SMX (drug of choice), aerosolized pentamidine.
Endocarditis with surgical or dental procedures	Penicillins.

Treatment of highly resistant bacteria	MRSA—vancomycin. VRE—linezolid and streptogramins (quinupristin/dalfopristin).

Antifungal therapy

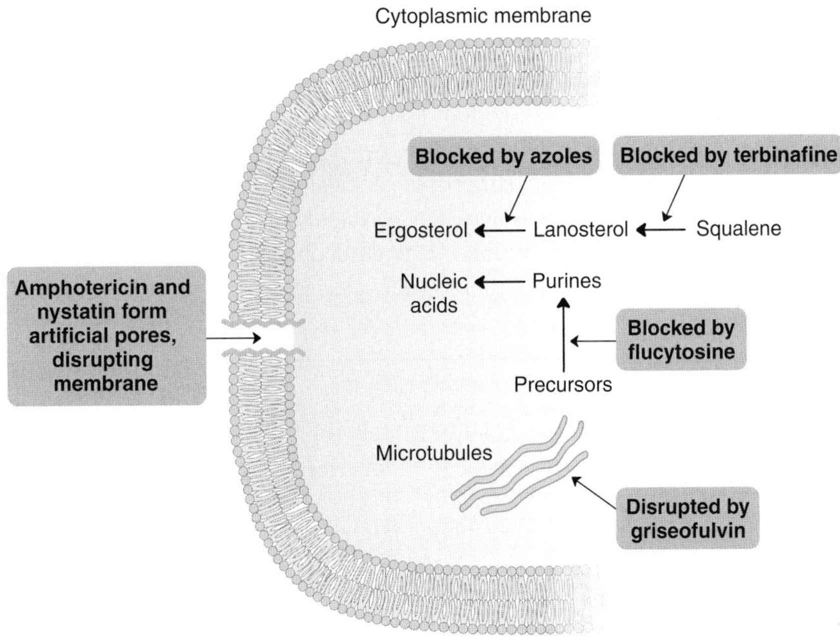

(Adapted, with permission, from Katzung BG, Trevor AJ. *USMLE Road Map: Pharmacology*, 1st ed. New York: McGraw-Hill, 2003: 120.)

Amphotericin B

Mechanism	Binds ergosterol (unique to fungi); forms membrane pores that allow leakage of electrolytes.	Amphotericin "tears" holes in the fungal membrane by forming pores.
Clinical use	Used for wide spectrum of systemic mycoses. *Cryptococcus, Blastomyces, Coccidioides, Aspergillus, Histoplasma, Candida, Mucor* (systemic mycoses). Intrathecally for fungal meningitis; does not cross blood-brain barrier.	
Toxicity	Fever/chills ("shake and bake"), hypotension, nephrotoxicity, arrhythmias, anemia, IV phlebitis ("amphoterrible"). Hydration reduces nephrotoxicity. Liposomal amphotericin reduces toxicity.	

Nystatin

Mechanism	Binds to ergosterol, disrupting fungal membranes. Too toxic for systemic use.
Clinical use	"Swish and swallow" for oral candidiasis (thrush); topical for diaper rash or vaginal candidiasis.

Azoles

	Fluconazole, ketoconazole, clotrimazole, miconazole, itraconazole, voriconazole.
Mechanism	Inhibit fungal steroid (ergosterol) synthesis.
Clinical use	Systemic mycoses. Fluconazole for cryptococcal meningitis in AIDS patients (because it can cross blood-brain barrier) and candidal infections of all types (i.e., yeast infections). Ketoconazole for *Blastomyces, Coccidioides, Histoplasma, Candida albicans;* hypercortisolism. Clotrimazole and miconazole for topical fungal infections.
Toxicity	Hormone synthesis inhibition (gynecomastia), liver dysfunction (inhibits cytochrome P-450), fever, chills.

Flucytosine

Mechanism	Inhibits DNA synthesis by conversion to fluorouracil, which competes with uracil.
Clinical use	Used in systemic fungal infections (e.g., *Candida, Cryptococcus*) in combination with amphotericin B.
Toxicity	Nausea, vomiting, diarrhea, bone marrow suppression.

Caspofungin

Mechanism	Inhibits cell wall synthesis.
Clinical use	Invasive aspergillosis.
Toxicity	GI upset, flushing.

Terbinafine

Mechanism	Inhibits the fungal enzyme squalene epoxidase.
Clinical use	Used to treat dermatophytoses (especially onychomycosis).

Griseofulvin

Mechanism	Interferes with microtubule function; disrupts mitosis. Deposits in keratin-containing tissues (e.g., nails).
Clinical use	Oral treatment of superficial infections; inhibits growth of dermatophytes (tinea, ringworm).
Toxicity	Teratogenic, carcinogenic, confusion, headaches, ↑ P-450 and warfarin metabolism.

Antiviral chemotherapy

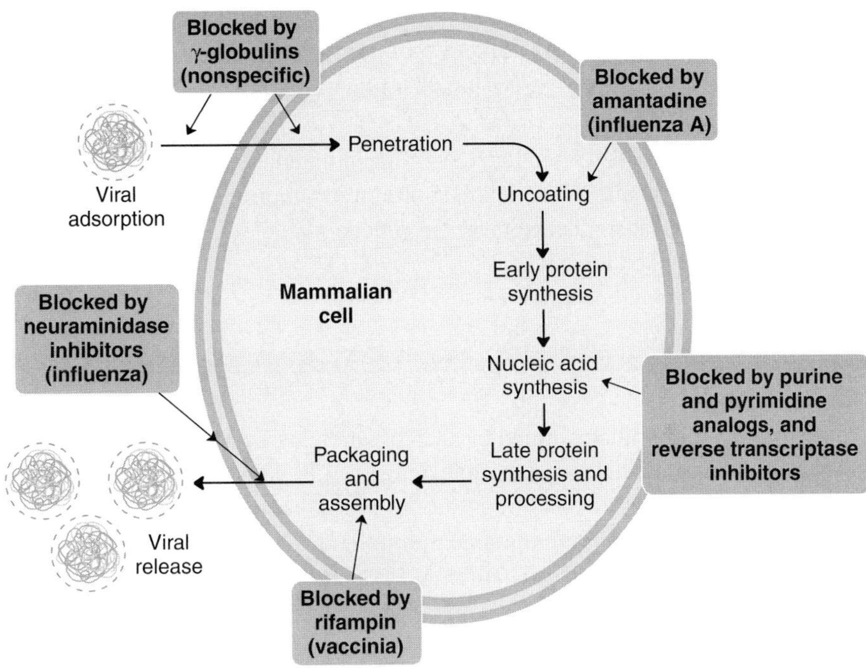

(Adapted, with permission, from Katzung BG, Trevor AJ. *USMLE Road Map: Pharmacology*, 1st ed. New York: McGraw-Hill, 2003: 120.)

Amantadine

Mechanism	Blocks viral penetration/un**coating** (M2 protein); may buffer pH of endosome. Also causes the release of dopamine from intact nerve terminals.	**"A man to dine"** takes off his **coat.**
Clinical use	Prophylaxis and treatment for influenza A; Parkinson's disease.	Amantadine blocks influenza **A** and rubell**A** and causes problems with the cerebell**A.**
Toxicity	Ataxia, dizziness, slurred speech.	
Mechanism of resistance	Mutated M2 protein. 90% of all influenza A strains are resistant to amantadine, so not used.	Rimantidine is a derivative with fewer CNS side effects. Does not cross the blood-brain barrier.

Zanamivir, oseltamivir

Mechanism	Inhibit influenza neuraminidase, decreasing the release of progeny virus.
Clinical use	Both influenza A and B.

Ribavirin

Mechanism	Inhibits synthesis of guanine nucleotides by competitively inhibiting IMP dehydrogenase.
Clinical use	RSV, chronic hepatitis C.
Toxicity	Hemolytic anemia. Severe teratogen.

Acyclovir

Mechanism	Monophosphorylated by HSV/VZV thymidine kinase. Triphosphate formed by cellular enzymes. Preferentially inhibits viral DNA polymerase by chain termination.
Clinical use	HSV, VZV, EBV. Used for HSV-induced mucocutaneous and genital lesions as well as for encephalitis. Prophylaxis in immunocompromised patients. For herpes zoster, use a related agent, famciclovir. No effect on latent forms of HSV and VZV.
Toxicity	Generally well tolerated.
Mechanism of resistance	Lack of thymidine kinase.

Ganciclovir

Mechanism	5'-monophosphate formed by a CMV viral kinase or HSV/VZV thymidine kinase. Triphosphate formed by cellular kinases. Preferentially inhibits viral DNA polymerase.
Clinical use	CMV, especially in immunocompromised patients.
Toxicity	Leukopenia, neutropenia, thrombocytopenia, renal toxicity. More toxic to host enzymes than acyclovir.
Mechanism of resistance	Mutated CMV DNA polymerase or lack of viral kinase.

Foscarnet

Mechanism	Viral DNA polymerase inhibitor that binds to the pyrophosphate-binding site of the enzyme. Does not require activation by viral kinase.	**FOS**carnet = pyro**FOS**phate analog.
Clinical use	CMV retinitis in immunocompromised patients when ganciclovir fails; acyclovir-resistant HSV.	
Toxicity	Nephrotoxicity.	
Mechanism of resistance	Mutated DNA polymerase.	

HIV therapy		
Protease inhibitors	Saquin**avir**, riton**avir**, indin**avir**, nelfin**avir**, ampren**avir**.	All protease inhibitors end in *-navir.*
Mechanism	Inhibit assembly of new virus by blocking protease in progeny virions.	**NAVIR** (never) **TEASE** a **proTEASE**.
Toxicity	GI intolerance (nausea, diarrhea), hyperglycemia, lipodystrophy, thrombocytopenia (indinavir).	
Reverse transcriptase inhibitors		
Nucleosides	Zidovudine (ZDV, formerly AZT), didanosine (ddI), zalcitabine (ddC), stavudine (d4T), lamivudine (3TC), abacavir.	
Non-nucleosides	**N**evirapine, **E**favirenz, **D**elavirdine.	**N**ever **E**ver **D**eliver nucleosides.
Mechanism	Preferentially inhibit reverse transcriptase of HIV; prevent incorporation of DNA copy of viral genome into host DNA.	
Toxicity	Bone marrow suppression (neutropenia, anemia), peripheral neuropathy, lactic acidosis (nucleosides), rash (non-nucleosides), megaloblastic anemia (ZDV).	GM-CSF and erythropoietin can be used to reduce bone marrow suppression.
Clinical use	Highly active antiretroviral therapy (HAART) generally entails combination therapy with protease inhibitors and reverse transcriptase inhibitors. Initiated when patients have low CD4 counts (< 500 cells/mm^3) or high viral load. ZDV is used for general prophylaxis and during pregnancy to reduce risk of fetal transmission.	
Fusion inhibitors	Enfuvirtide.	
Mechanism	Bind viral gp41 subunit; inhibit conformational change required for fusion with CD4 cells. Therefore block entry and subsequent replication.	
Toxicity	Hypersensitivity reactions, reactions at subcutaneous injection site, ↑ risk of bacterial pneumonia.	
Clinical use	In patients with persistent viral replication in spite of antiretroviral therapy. Used in combination with other drugs.	

Interferons	
Mechanism	Glycoproteins from human leukocytes that block various stages of viral RNA and DNA synthesis. Induce ribonuclease that degrades viral mRNA.
Clinical use	IFN-α—chronic hepatitis B and C, Kaposi's sarcoma. IFN-β—MS. IFN-γ—NADPH oxidase deficiency.
Toxicity	Neutropenia.

► MICROBIOLOGY–ANTIMICROBIALS *(continued)*

Antibiotics to avoid in pregnancy	**S**ulfonamides—kernicterus. **A**minoglycosides—ototoxicity. **F**luoroquinolones—cartilage damage. **E**rythromycin—acute cholestatic hepatitis in mom (and clarithromycin—embryotoxic). **M**etronidazole—mutagenesis. **T**etracyclines—discolored teeth, inhibition of bone growth. **R**ibavirin (antiviral)—teratogenic. **G**riseofulvin (antifungal)—teratogenic. **C**hloramphenicol—"gray baby."	**SAFE M**oms **T**ake **R**eally **G**ood **C**are.

HIGH-YIELD PRINCIPLES IN

Immunology

"I hate to disappoint you, but my rubber lips are immune to your charms."
—*Batman & Robin*

"No State shall abridge the privileges or immunities of its citizens."
—The United States Constitution

Immunology can be confusing and complicated, but luckily the USMLE tests only basic principles and facts in this area. Cell surface markers are important to know because they are clinically useful (for example, in identifying specific types of immune deficiency or cancer) and are functionally critical to the jobs immune cells carry out. By spending a little extra effort here, it is possible to turn a traditionally difficult subject into one that is high yield.

IMMUNOLOGY—HIGH-YIELD CLINICAL VIGNETTES

- Patient with *Mycoplasma pneumoniae* exhibits cryoagglutinins during recovery phase. — What types of immunoglobulins are reacting? — IgM.
- Young child presents with tetany and candidiasis. Hypocalcemia and immunosuppression are found. — What immune cell is deficient? — T cell (DiGeorge).
- Young child has recurrent lung infections and granulomatous lesions. — What enzyme is deficient in neutrophils? — NADPH oxidase (chronic granulomatous disease).
- Patient presents with recurrent *Neisseria* infections. — What complement proteins are deficient? — C6–C8.
- Woman complains of a malar rash and arthritis. — The presence of which antibodies are specific for SLE? — Anti-dsDNA and anti-Smith.
- Patient presents with dermatitis, enteritis, and hepatitis after bone marrow transplantation. — What disease process is occurring? — Graft-versus-host disease.

Lymph node A 2° lymphoid organ that has many afferents, 1 or more efferents. Encapsulated, with trabeculae. Functions are nonspecific filtration by macrophages, storage and activation of B and T cells, antibody production.

Follicle: Site of B-cell localization and proliferation. In outer cortex. 1° follicles are dense and dormant. 2° follicles have pale central germinal centers and are active.

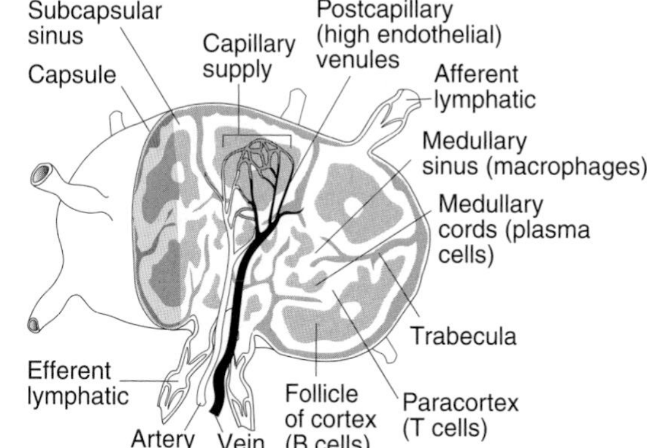

Medulla: Consists of medullary cords (closely packed lymphocytes and plasma cells) and medullary sinuses. Medullary sinuses communicate with efferent lymphatics and contain reticular cells and macrophages.

Paracortex: Houses T cells. Region of cortex between follicles and medulla. Contains high endothelial venules through which T and B cells enter from blood. In an extreme cellular immune response, paracortex becomes greatly enlarged. Not well developed in patients with DiGeorge syndrome.

Paracortex enlarges in an extreme cellular immune response (i.e., viral).

Lymph drainage

Area of body	1° lymph node drainage site
1. Upper limb, lateral breast	1. Axillary
2. Stomach	2. Celiac
3. Duodenum, jejunum	3. Superior mesenteric
4. Sigmoid colon	4. Colic → inferior mesenteric
5. Rectum (lower part), anal canal above pectinate line	5. Internal iliac
6. Anal canal below pectinate line	6. Superficial inguinal
7. Testes	7. Superficial and deep plexuses → para-aortic
8. Scrotum	8. Superficial inguinal
9. Thigh (superficial)	9. Superficial inguinal
10. Lateral side of dorsum of foot	10. Popliteal

Right lymphatic duct—drains right arm and right half of head.

Thoracic duct—drains everything else.

▶ IMMUNOLOGY–LYMPHOID STRUCTURES *(continued)*

Sinusoids of spleen	Long, vascular channels in red pulp with fenestrated "barrel hoop" basement membrane. Macrophages found nearby.	T cells are found in the periarterial lymphatic sheath (PALS) and in the red pulp of the spleen. B cells are found in follicles within the white pulp of the spleen. Macrophages in the spleen remove encapsulated bacteria.
Thymus	Site of T-cell differentiation and maturation. Encapsulated. From epithelium of 3rd branchial pouches. Lymphocytes of mesenchymal origin. Cortex is dense with immature T cells; medulla is pale with mature T cells and epithelial reticular cells and contains Hassall's corpuscles. Positive (MHC restriction) and negative selection (nonreactive to self) occur at the corticomedullary junction.	**T** cells = **T**hymus. **B** cells = **B**one marrow.

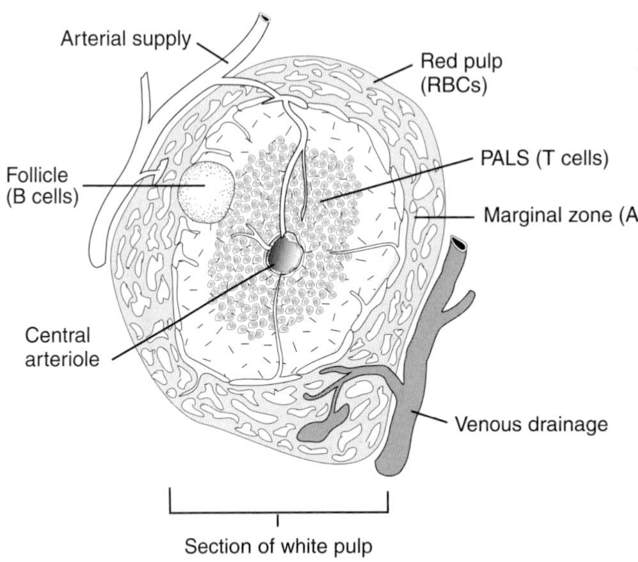

Innate vs. adaptive immunity

Innate—receptors that recognize pathogens are germline encoded. Response to pathogens is fast and nonspecific. No memory. Consists of neutrophils, macrophages, dendritic cells, and complement.

Adaptive—receptors that recognize pathogens undergo VDJ recombination during lymphocyte development. Response is slow on first exposure, but memory response is faster and more robust. Consists of T cells, B cells, and circulating antibody.

Differentiation of T cells

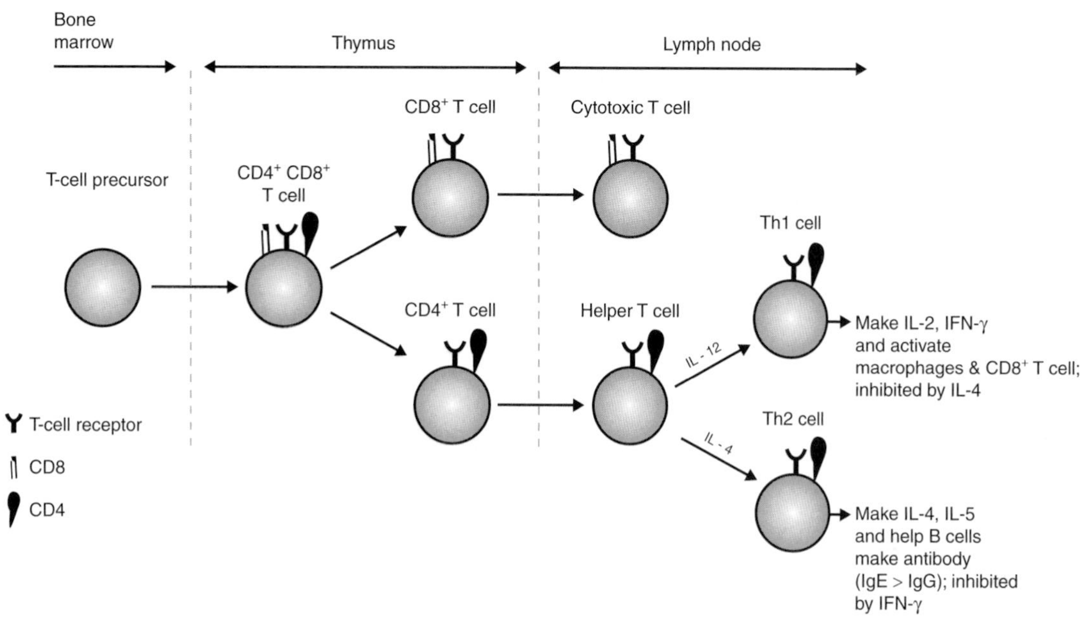

MHC I and II

MHC = major histocompatibility complex, encoded by **H**uman **L**eukocyte **A**ntigen (HLA) genes.

MHC I = HLA-A, HLA-B, HLA-C.
- Expressed on almost all nucleated cells.
- Antigen is loaded in RER of mostly intracellular peptides.
- Mediates viral immunity.
- Pairs with β_2-microglobulin.

MHC II = HLA-DR, HLA-DP, HLA-DQ.
- Expressed only on antigen-presenting cells (APCs).
- Antigen is loaded in an acidified endosome.

MHC I—HLA I letter (A, B, C).

MHC II—HLA II letters (DR, DP, DQ).

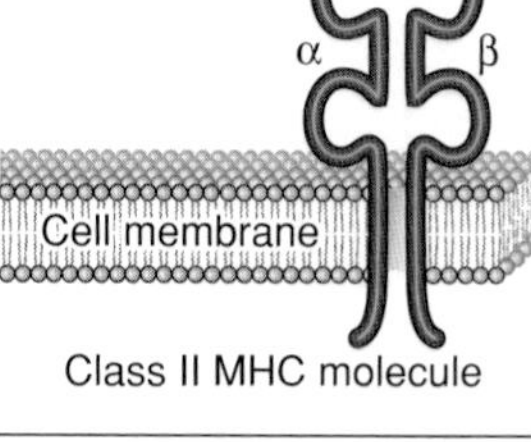

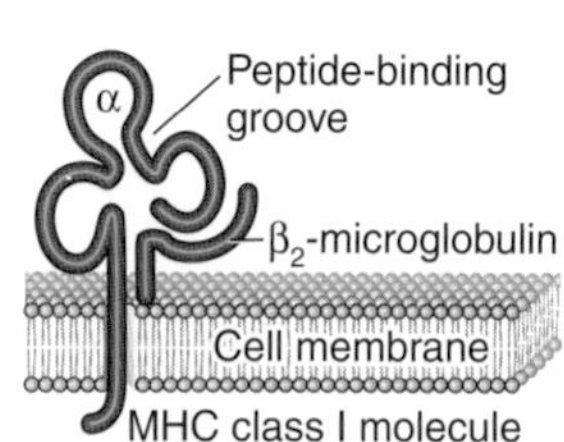

Major function of B and T cells

B cells	T cells
Make antibody	CD4+ T cells help B cells make antibody and produce γ-interferon, which activates macrophages
IgG antibodies opsonize bacteria, viruses	Kill virus-infected cells directly (CD8+ T cells)
Allergy (type I hypersensitivity): IgE	Delayed cell-mediated hypersensitivity (type IV)
Cytotoxic (type II) and immune complex (type III) hypersensitivity: IgG	
Antibodies cause organ rejection (hyperacute)	Organ (allograft) rejection (acute and chronic)

T-cell glycoproteins

Helper T cells have CD4, which binds to MHC II on APCs. Cytotoxic T cells have CD8, which binds to MHC I on virus-infected cells.

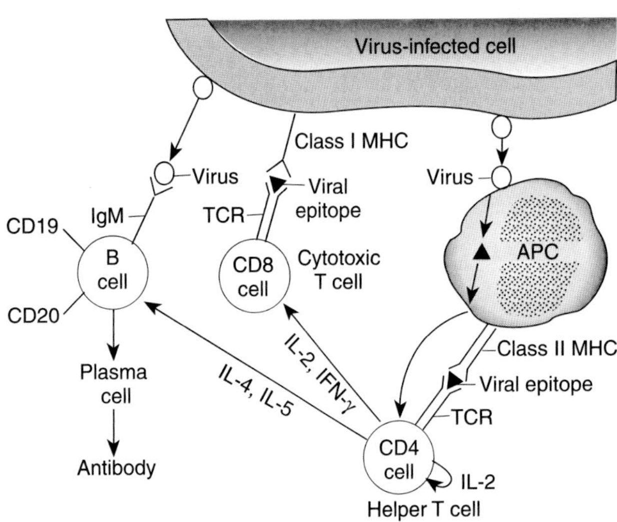

Product of CD and MHC = 8 (CD4 × MHC **II** = 8 = CD8 × MHC **I**).

CD3 complex—cluster of polypeptides associated with a T-cell receptor. Important in signal transduction.

APCs:

1. Macrophage
2. B cell
3. Dendritic cell

T-cell activation	2 signals are required for T-cell activation—signal 1 and signal 2. Th activation: 1. Foreign body is phagocytosed by APC 2. Foreign antigen is presented on MHC II and recognized by TCR on Th cell (signal 1) 3. "Costimulatory signal" is given by interaction of B7 and CD28 (signal 2) 4. Th cell activated to produce cytokines Tc activation: 1. Endogenously synthesized (viral or self) proteins are presented on MHC I and recognized by TCR on Tc cell (signal 1) 2. IL-2 from Th cell activates Tc cell to kill virus-infected cell (signal 2)

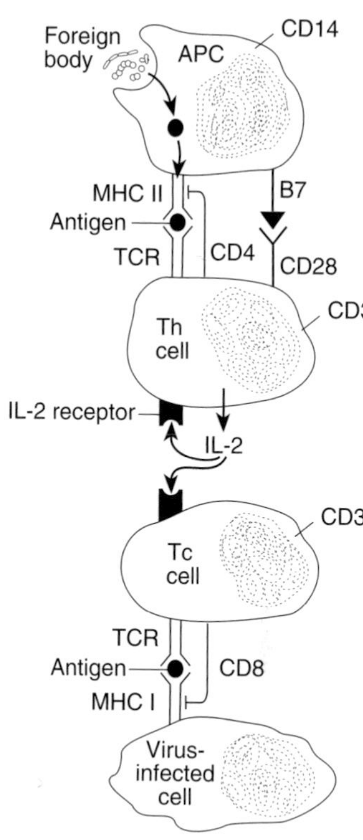

Antibody structure and function

Variable part of L and H chains recognizes antigens. Fc portion of IgM and IgG fixes complement. Heavy chain contributes to Fc and Fab fractions. Light chain contributes only to Fab fraction.

Fab: antigen-binding fragment

Fc:
- Constant
- Carboxy terminal
- Complement-binding (IgG + IgM only)
- Carbohydrate side chains

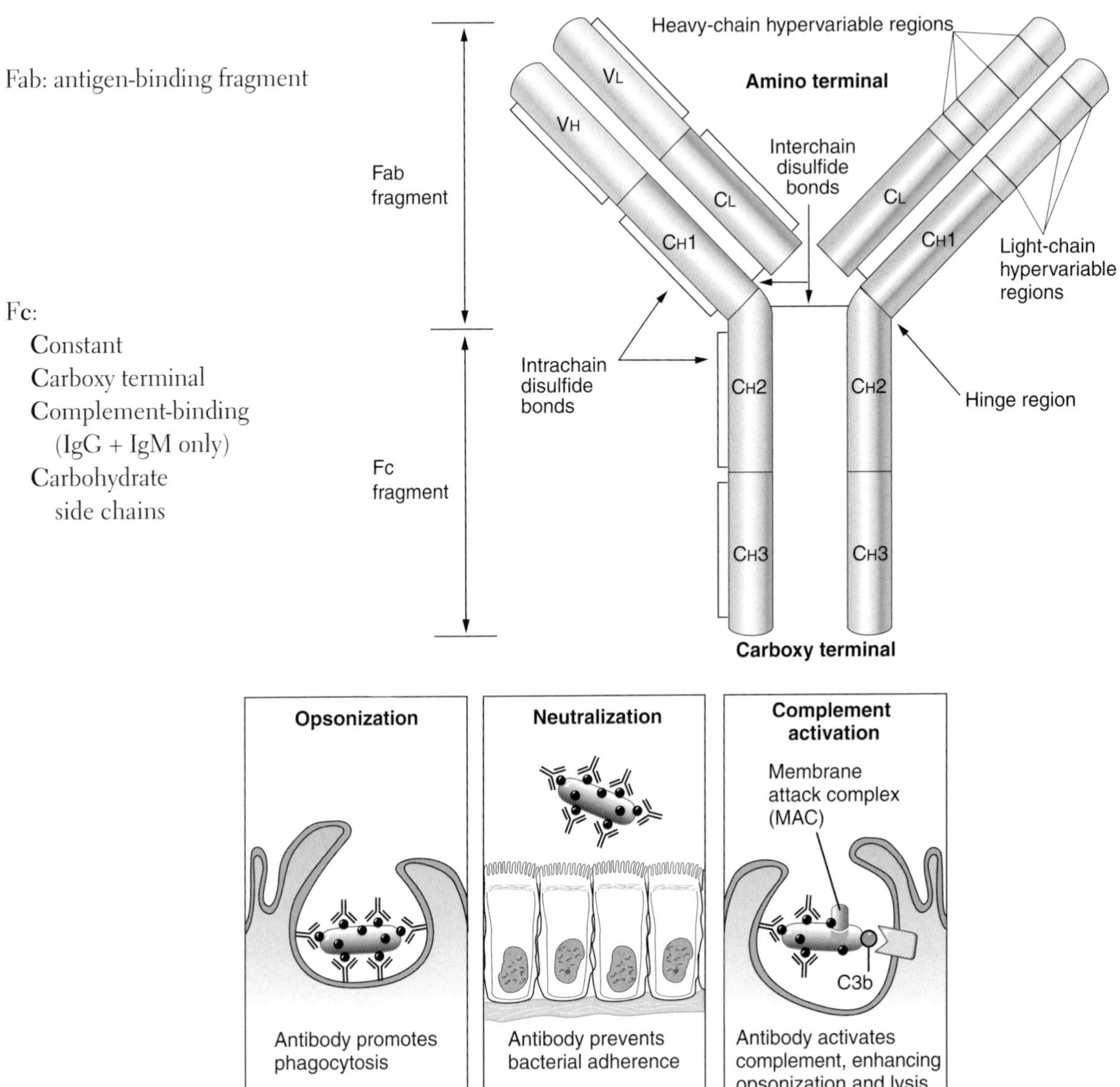

Antibody diversity is generated by:

1. Random "recombination" of VJ (light-chain) or VDJ (heavy-chain) genes
2. Random combination of heavy chains with light chains
3. Somatic hypermutation
4. Addition of nucleotides to DNA during "recombination" (see #1) by terminal deoxynucleotidyl transferase

Immunoglobulin isotypes	Mature B lymphocytes express IgM and IgD on their surfaces. They may differentiate by isotype switching (mediated by cytokines and CD40 ligand) into plasma cells that secrete IgA, IgE, or IgG.	
IgG	Main antibody in 2° response. Most abundant. Fixes complement, crosses the placenta, opsonizes bacteria, neutralizes bacterial toxins and viruses.	
IgA	Prevents attachment of bacteria and viruses to mucous membranes, does not fix complement. Monomer or dimer. Found in secretions. Picks up secretory component from epithelial cells before secretion.	
IgM	Produced in the 1° response to an antigen. Fixes complement but does not cross the placenta. Antigen receptor on the surface of B cells. Monomer on B cell or pentamer.	
IgD	Unclear function. Found on the surface of many B cells and in serum.	
IgE	Mediates immediate (type I) hypersensitivity by inducing the release of mediators from mast cells and basophils when exposed to allergen. Mediates immunity to worms by activating eosinophils. Lowest concentration in serum.	
Ig epitopes	**All**otype (polymorphism)—Ig epitope that differs among members of same species. Can be on light chain or heavy chain.	**ALL**otypes represent different **ALL**eles.
	Isotype (IgG, IgA, etc.)—Ig epitope common to a single class of Ig (5 classes, determined by heavy chain).	Isotype = *iso* (same). Common to same class.
	Idiotype (specific for a given antigen)—Ig epitope determined by antigen-binding site.	Idiotype = *idio* (unique). Hypervariable region is unique.

▶ IMMUNOLOGY–IMMUNE RESPONSES

Important cytokines

IL-1	Secreted by macrophages. Causes acute inflammation. Induces chemokine production to recruit leukocytes; activates endothelium to express adhesion molecules. An endogenous pyrogen.	IL-2: stimulates T cells. IL-3: stimulates bone marrow. IL-4: stimulates IgE production. IL-5: stimulates IgA production.
IL-2	Secreted by Th cells. Stimulates growth of helper and cytotoxic T cells.	
IL-3	Secreted by activated T cells. Supports the growth and differentiation of bone marrow stem cells. Has a function similar to GM-CSF.	
IL-4	Secreted by Th2 cells. Promotes growth of B cells. Enhances class switching to IgE and IgG.	
IL-5	Secreted by Th2 cells. Promotes differentiation of B cells. Enhances class switching to IgA. Stimulates production and activation of eosinophils.	
IL-6	Secreted by Th cells and macrophages. Stimulates production of acute-phase reactants and immunoglobulins.	
IL-8	Secreted by macrophages. Major chemotactic factor for neutrophils.	"Clean up on **aisle 8.**" Neutrophils are recruited by **IL**-8 to clear infections.
IL-10	Secreted by regulatory T cells. Inhibits actions of activated T cells.	
IL-12	Secreted by B cells and macrophages. Activates NK and Th1 cells.	
γ-interferon	Secreted by Th1 cells. Stimulates macrophages.	
TNF	Secreted by macrophages. Mediates septic shock. Causes leukocyte recruitment, vascular leak.	

Cell surface proteins

Helper T cells	CD4, TCR, CD3, CD28, CD40L.
Cytotoxic T cells	CD8, TCR, CD3.
B cells	IgM, B7, CD19, CD20, CD21, CD40, MHC II.
Macrophages	MHC II, B7, CD40, CD14. Receptors for Fc and C3b.
NK cells	Receptors for MHC I, CD16, CD56.
All cells except mature red cells	MHC I.

Complement

System of proteins that interact to play a role in humoral immunity and inflammation.

Membrane attack complex of complement defends against gram-negative bacteria. Activated by **IgG** or **IgM** in the **classic** pathway, and activated by molecules on the surface of microbes (especially endotoxin) in the **alternative** pathway.

C3b and IgG are the two 1° opsonins in bacterial defense.

Decay-accelerating factor (DAF) and C1 esterase inhibitor help prevent complement activation on self-cells.

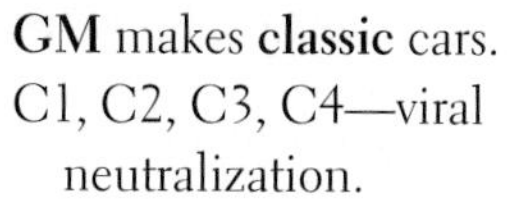

GM makes **classic** cars.
C1, C2, C3, C4—viral neutralization.
C3**b**—opsonization. **B**inds **B**acteria.
C3**a**, C5**a**—**A**naphylaxis.
C5a—neutrophil chemotaxis.
C5b-9—cytolysis by membrane attack complex (MAC).
Deficiency of C1 esterase inhibitor leads to hereditary angioedema.
Deficiency of C3 leads to severe, recurrent pyogenic sinus and respiratory tract infections.
Deficiency of C6–C8 leads to *Neisseria* bacteremia.
Deficiency of DAF leads to complement-mediated lysis of RBCs and paroxysmal nocturnal hemoglobinuria (PNH).

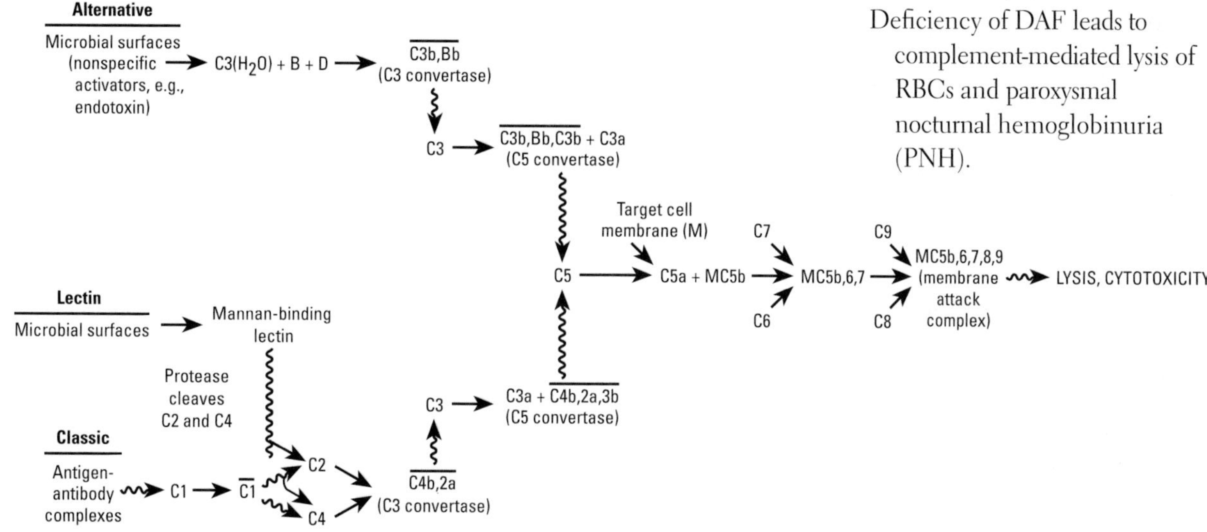

(Adapted, with permission, from Levinson W. *Medical Microbiology and Immunology: Examination and Board Review,* 8th ed. New York: McGraw-Hill, 2004: 432.)

Interferon mechanism

Interferons (α, β, γ) are proteins that place uninfected cells in an antiviral state. Interferons induce the production of a ribonuclease that inhibits viral protein synthesis by degrading viral mRNA (but not host mRNA).

Interferes with viruses:

1. α- and β-interferons inhibit viral protein synthesis
2. γ-interferons ↑ MHC I and II expression and antigen presentation in all cells
3. Activates NK cells to kill virus-infected cells

▶ IMMUNOLOGY–IMMUNE RESPONSES *(continued)*

Passive vs. active immunity		
Active	Induced after exposure to foreign antigens. Slow onset. Long-lasting protection (memory).	After exposure to **T**etanus toxin, **B**otulinum toxin, **H**BV, or **R**abies, patients are given preformed antibodies (passive)—**T**o **B**e **H**ealed **R**apidly.
Passive	Based on receiving preformed antibodies from another host. Rapid onset. Short life span of antibodies (half-life = 3 weeks).	
Antigen variation	Classic examples: Bacteria—*Salmonella* (2 flagellar variants), *Borrelia* (relapsing fever), *Neisseria gonorrhoeae* (pilus protein). Virus—influenza (major = shift, minor = drift). Parasites—trypanosomes (programmed rearrangement).	Some mechanisms for variation include DNA rearrangement and RNA segment reassortment (e.g., influenza major shift).
Anergy	Self-reactive T cells become nonreactive without costimulatory molecule. B cells also become anergic, but tolerance is less complete than in T cells.	

Hypersensitivity

Type I 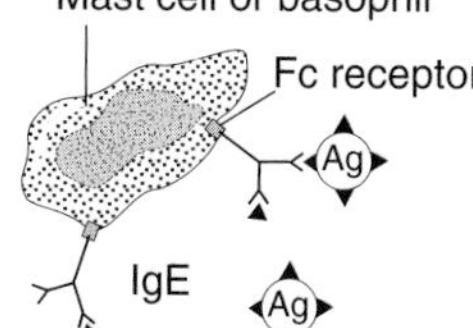	**Anaphylactic and atopic**—free antigen cross-links IgE on presensitized mast cells and basophils, triggering release of vasoactive amines (i.e., histamine). Reaction develops rapidly after antigen exposure due to preformed antibody.	**F**irst and **F**ast (anaphylaxis). Types I, II, and III are all antibody mediated.
Type II 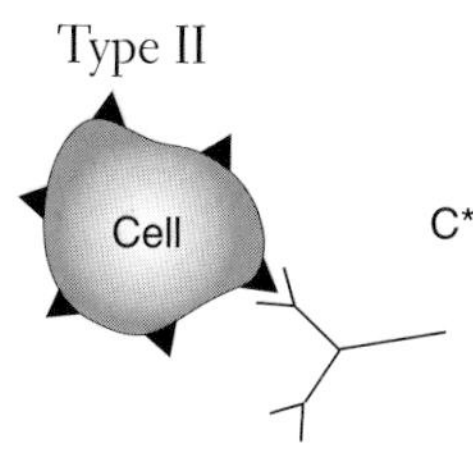	**Antibody mediated**—IgM, IgG bind to fixed antigen on "enemy" cell, leading to lysis (by complement) or phagocytosis.	Cy-2-toxic. Antibody and complement lead to membrane attack complex (MAC).
Type III 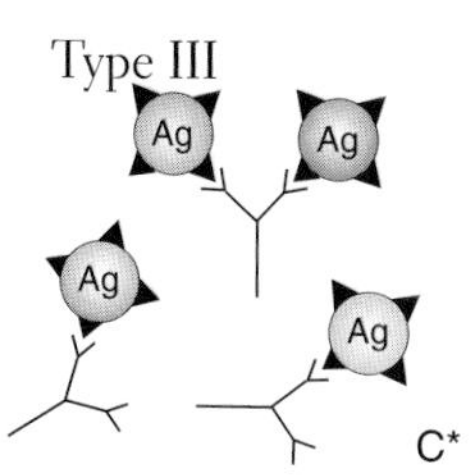	**Immune complex**—antigen-antibody complexes activate complement, which attracts neutrophils; neutrophils release lysosomal enzymes. **Serum sickness**—an immune complex disease (type III) in which antibodies to the foreign proteins are produced (takes 5 days). Immune complexes form and are deposited in membranes, where they fix complement (leads to tissue damage). More common than Arthus reaction. **Arthus reaction**—a local subacute antibody-mediated hypersensitivity (type III) reaction. Intradermal injection of antigen induces antibodies, which form antigen-antibody complexes in the skin. Characterized by edema, necrosis, and activation of complement.	Imagine an immune complex as **3** things stuck together: antigen-antibody-complement. Most serum sickness is now caused by drugs (not serum). Fever, urticaria, arthralgias, proteinuria, lymphadenopathy 5–10 days after antigen exposure. Antigen-antibody complexes cause the Arthus reaction.
Type IV	**Delayed (T-cell-mediated) type**—sensitized T lymphocytes encounter antigen and then release lymphokines (leads to macrophage activation).	**4th** and last—delayed. Cell mediated; therefore, it is not transferable by serum. **4 T's** = **T** lymphocytes, **T**ransplant rejections, **T**B skin tests, **T**ouching (contact dermatitis). **ACID**: **A**naphylactic and **A**topic (type I) **C**ytotoxic (antibody mediated) (type II) **I**mmune complex (type III) **D**elayed (cell mediated) (type IV)

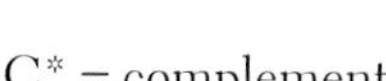

C* = complement

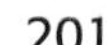

Diseases caused by hypersensitivity

Reaction	Disorder
Type I	Anaphylaxis
	Allergic rhinitis (hay fever)
Type II	Hemolytic anemia
	Idiopathic thrombocytopenic purpura
	Erythroblastosis fetalis
	Rheumatic fever
	Goodpasture's syndrome
	Bullous pemphigoid
	Graves' disease
	Myasthenia gravis
Type III	SLE
	Rheumatoid arthritis
	Polyarteritis nodosum
	Poststreptococcal glomerulonephritis
	Serum sickness
	Arthus reaction
	Hypersensitivity pneumonitis
Type IV	Type 1 diabetes mellitus
	Multiple sclerosis
	Guillain-Barré syndrome
	Hashimoto's thyroiditis
	Graft-versus-host disease
	PPD (test for *M. tuberculosis*)
	Contact dermatitis

Immune deficiencies

1. **↓ production of:**

B cells—**B**ruton's agammaglobulinemia	X-linked recessive defect in a tyrosine kinase gene associated with low levels of all classes of immunoglobulins. ↓ number of B cells. Associated with recurrent **B**acterial infections after 6 months of age, when levels of maternal IgG antibody decline. Occurs in **B**oys (X-linked).
T cells—Thymic aplasia (DiGeorge syndrome)	Thymus and parathyroids fail to develop owing to failure of development of the 3rd and 4th pharyngeal pouches. Presents with Tetany owing to hypocalcemia. Recurrent viral and fungal infections due to T-cell deficiency. Congenital defects of heart and great vessels. 22q11 deletion.
B and T cells—severe combined immunodeficiency (SCID)	Defect in early stem-cell differentiation. Presents with recurrent viral, bacterial, fungal, and protozoal infections. May have multiple causes (e.g., failure to synthesize MHC II antigens, defective IL-2 receptors, or adenosine deaminase deficiency).

2. **↓ activation of:**

T cells—IL-12 receptor deficiency	Presents with disseminated mycobacterial infections due to ↓ Th1 response.
B cells—hyper-IgM syndrome	Defect in CD40 ligand on CD4 T helper cells leads to inability to class switch. Presents early in life with severe pyogenic infections. High levels of IgM; very low levels of IgG, IgA, and IgE.
B cells—**W**iskott-Aldrich syndrome	X-linked defect in the ability to mount an IgM response to capsular polysaccharides of bacteria. Associated with elevated IgA levels (**A**ldrich = ↑ Ig**A**), normal IgE levels, and low IgM levels. Triad of symptoms includes recurrent pyogenic **I**nfections, thrombocytopenic **P**urpura, **E**czema (**WIPE**).
Macrophages—Job's syndrome	Failure of IFN-γ production by helper T cells. Neutrophils fail to respond to chemotactic stimuli. Presents with coarse **F**acies, cold (noninflamed) staphylococcal **A**bscesses, retained primary **T**eeth, ↑ IgE, and **D**ermatologic problems (eczema) **(FATED).**

3. **Phagocytic cell deficiency:**

Leukocyte adhesion deficiency syndrome (type 1)	Defect in LFA-1 integrin proteins on phagocytes. Presents early with recurrent bacterial infections, absent pus formation, and delayed separation of umbilicus.
Chédiak-Higashi disease	Autosomal recessive. Defect in microtubular function and lysosomal emptying of phagocytic cells. Presents with recurrent pyogenic infections by staphylococci and streptococci, partial albinism, and peripheral neuropathy.
Chronic granulomatous disease	Defect in phagocytosis of neutrophils owing to lack of NADPH oxidase activity or similar enzymes. Presents with marked susceptibility to opportunistic infections with bacteria, especially *S. aureus*, *E. coli*, and *Aspergillus*. Diagnosis confirmed with negative nitroblue tetrazolium dye reduction test.

4. **Idiopathic dysfunction of:**

T cells—chronic mucocutaneous candidiasis	T-cell dysfunction specifically against *Candida albicans*. Presents with skin and mucous membrane *Candida* infections.
B cells—selective immunoglobulin deficiency	Deficiency in a specific class of immunoglobulins—possibly due to a defect in isotype switching. Selective IgA deficiency is the most common selective immunoglobulin deficiency. Presents with sinus and lung infections; milk allergies and diarrhea are common.
B cells—ataxia-telangiectasia	Defect in DNA repair enzymes with associated IgA deficiency. Presents with cerebellar problems (ataxia) and spider angiomas (telangiectasia).
B cells—common variable immunodeficiency	Normal numbers of circulating B cells, ↓ plasma cells (defect in B-cell maturation), ↓ Ig, can be acquired in 20s–30s.

▶ IMMUNOLOGY–IMMUNE RESPONSES *(continued)*

Autoantibodies

Autoantibody	Associated disorder
Antinuclear antibodies (ANA)	SLE
Anti-dsDNA, anti-Smith	Specific for SLE
Antihistone	Drug-induced lupus
Anti-IgG (rheumatoid factor)	Rheumatoid arthritis
Anticentromere	Scleroderma (CREST)
Anti-Scl-70	Scleroderma (diffuse)
Antimitochondrial	1° biliary cirrhosis
Antigliadin	Celiac disease
Anti–basement membrane	Goodpasture's syndrome
Anti–epithelial cell	Pemphigus vulgaris
Antimicrosomal, antithyroglobulin	Hashimoto's thyroiditis
Anti-Jo-1	Polymyositis, dermatomyositis
Anti-SS-A (anti-Ro)	Sjögren's syndrome
Anti-SS-B (anti-La)	Sjögren's syndrome
Anti-U1 RNP (ribonucleoprotein)	Mixed connective tissue disease
Anti–smooth muscle	Autoimmune hepatitis
Anti–glutamate decarboxylase	Type 1 diabetes mellitus
c-ANCA	Wegener's granulomatosis
p-ANCA	Other vasculitides

HLA subtypes

B27	**P**soriasis, **A**nkylosing spondylitis, **I**nflammatory bowel disease, **R**eiter's syndrome.	**PAIR.**
B8	Graves' disease, celiac sprue.	
DR2	Multiple sclerosis, hay fever, SLE, Goodpasture's.	
DR3	Diabetes mellitus type 1.	
DR4	Rheumatoid arthritis, diabetes mellitus type 1.	
DR5	Pernicious anemia → B_{12} deficiency, Hashimoto's thyroiditis.	
DR7	Steroid-responsive nephrotic syndrome.	

Grafts

Autograft	From self.
Syngeneic graft	From identical twin or clone.
Allograft	From nonidentical individual of same species.
Xenograft	From different species.

▶ IMMUNOLOGY–IMMUNOSUPPRESSANTS

Cyclosporine

Mechanism	Binds to cyclophilins. Complex blocks the differentiation and activation of T cells by inhibiting calcineurin, thus preventing the production of IL-2 and its receptor.
Clinical use	Suppresses organ rejection after transplantation; selected autoimmune disorders.
Toxicity	Predisposes patients to viral infections and lymphoma; nephrotoxic (preventable with mannitol diuresis).

Tacrolimus (FK506)

Mechanism	Similar to cyclosporine; binds to FK-binding protein, inhibiting secretion of IL-2 and other cytokines.
Clinical use	Potent immunosuppressive used in organ transplant recipients.
Toxicity	Significant—nephrotoxicity, peripheral neuropathy, hypertension, pleural effusion, hyperglycemia.

Azathioprine

Mechanism	Antimetabolite precursor of 6-mercaptopurine that interferes with the metabolism and synthesis of nucleic acids. Toxic to proliferating lymphocytes.
Clinical use	Kidney transplantation, autoimmune disorders (including glomerulonephritis and hemolytic anemia).
Toxicity	Bone marrow suppression. Active metabolite mercaptopurine is metabolized by xanthine oxidase; thus, toxic effects may be ↑ by allopurinol.

Muromonab-CD3 (OKT3)

Mechanism	Monoclonal antibody that binds to CD3 (epsilon chain) on the surface of T cells. Blocks cellular interaction with CD3 protein responsible for T-cell signal transduction.
Clinical use	Immunosuppression after kidney transplantation.
Toxicity	Cytokine release syndrome, hypersensitivity reaction.

Sirolimus (rapamycin)

Mechanism	Binds to mTOR. Inhibits T-cell proliferation in response to IL-2.
Clinical use	Immunosuppression after kidney transplantation in combination with cyclosporine and corticosteroids.
Toxicity	Hyperlipidemia, thrombocytopenia, leukopenia.

Mycophenolate mofetil

Mechanism	Inhibits de novo guanine synthesis and blocks lymphocyte production.

Daclizumab

Mechanism	Monoclonal antibody with high affinity for the IL-2 receptor on activated T cells.

Recombinant cytokines and clinical uses

Agent	Clinical uses
Aldesleukin (interleukin-2)	Renal cell carcinoma, metastatic melanoma
Erythropoietin (epoetin)	Anemias (especially in renal failure)
Filgrastim (granulocyte colony-stimulating factor)	Recovery of bone marrow
Sargramostim (granulocyte-macrophage colony-stimulating factor)	Recovery of bone marrow
α-interferon	Hepatitis B and C, Kaposi's sarcoma, leukemias, malignant melanoma
β-interferon	Multiple sclerosis
γ-interferon	Chronic granulomatous disease
Oprelvekin (interleukin-11)	Thrombocytopenia
Thrombopoietin	Thrombocytopenia

▶ IMMUNOLOGY–IMMUNOSUPPRESSANTS *(continued)*

Transplant rejection

Hyperacute rejection	Antibody mediated due to the presence of preformed antidonor antibodies in the transplant recipient. Occurs within minutes after transplantation.
Acute rejection	Cell mediated due to cytotoxic T lymphocytes reacting against foreign MHCs. Occurs weeks after transplantation. Reversible with immunosuppressants such as cyclosporine and OKT3.
Chronic rejection	Antibody-mediated vascular damage (fibrinoid necrosis); occurs months to years after transplantation. Irreversible.
Graft-versus-host disease	Grafted immunocompetent T cells proliferate in the irradiated immunocompromised host and reject cells with "foreign" proteins, resulting in severe organ dysfunction. Major symptoms include a maculopapular rash, jaundice, hepatosplenomegaly, and diarrhea.

HIGH-YIELD PRINCIPLES IN

Pathology

- High-Yield Clinical Vignettes
- Inflammation
- Amyloidosis
- Neoplasia

"Digressions, objections, delight in mockery, carefree mistrust are signs of health; everything unconditional belongs in pathology."

—Friedrich Nietzsche

The fundamental principles of pathology are key to understanding diseases in all organ systems. Major topics such as inflammation and neoplasia appear frequently in questions aimed at many different organ systems and are definitely high yield. For example, the concepts of cell injury and inflammation are key to knowing the inflammatory response that follows myocardial infarction, a very common subject of boards questions. Likewise, a familiarity with the early cellular changes that culminate in the development of neoplasias—for example, esophageal or colon cancer—is critical. Finally, make sure you recognize the major tumor-associated genes and are comfortable with key cancer concepts such as tumor staging and metastasis.

▶ PATHOLOGY—HIGH-YIELD CLINICAL VIGNETTES

Vignette	Question	Answer
Prostate biopsy shows neoplastic proliferation of well-differentiated glands with evidence of tumor spread to regional lymph nodes.	What is the Gleason score and stage of the prostate cancer?	Low Gleason score (low "grade") and high stage.
Boy presents with mental retardation, facial angiofibromas, and seizures.	What type of cancers are most often associated with his disease?	Cardiac rhabdomyomas and astrocytomas (in tuberous sclerosis).
Patient with marked leukocytosis and presence of myeloid blast cells in the peripheral blood is found to have lymphadenopathy and splenomegaly.	What oncogene most likely became translocated in the myeloid stem cells?	*abl* (to form the fusion protein *bcr-abl*).
Mother notices that her daughter has a white pupil, which is later confirmed to be inherited retinoblastoma.	Her daughter has an ↑ risk of what other type of cancer?	Osteosarcoma (*Rb* tumor suppressor gene mutation).
Woman's Pap smear shows dysplastic changes.	What HPV types are most often associated with cervical carcinoma?	Types 16 and 18.
Man complains of joint pain following chemotherapy for AML.	What is the side effect of his cancer treatment?	↑ nucleic acid turnover from dying cancer cells leads to hyperuricemia (tumor lysis syndrome).
Elderly woman on chronic hemodialysis treatment has a biopsy of her joint spaces that shows amyloid deposits.	From what protein is the amyloid derived?	β_2-microglobulin.

Apoptosis

Programmed cell death; ATP required. Mediated by caspases.

Characterized by cell shrinkage, chromatin condensation (pyknosis), membrane blebbing, DNA fragmentation (karyorrhexis), nuclear fragmentation (karyolysis), and formation of apoptotic bodies, which are then phagocytosed. No significant inflammation.

Occurs during embryogenesis, hormone induction (menstruation), immune cell–mediated death, injurious stimuli (e.g., radiation, hypoxia), atrophy (e.g., endometrial lining during menopause).

Necrosis

Enzymatic degradation of a cell resulting from exogenous injury.

Characterized by enzymatic digestion and protein denaturation, with release of intracellular components.

Inflammatory.

Morphologically occurs as coagulative (heart, liver, kidney), liquefactive (brain), caseous (tuberculosis), fat (pancreas), fibrinoid (blood vessels), or gangrenous (limbs, GI tract).

Cell injury

Reversible	Irreversible
Cellular swelling	Plasma membrane damage
Nuclear chromatin clumping	Lysosomal rupture
↓ ATP synthesis	Ca^{2+} influx → oxidative phosphorylation
Ribosomal detachment	Nuclear pyknosis, karyolysis, karyorrhexis
Glycogen depletion	Mitochondrial permeability
Fatty change	

Inflammation

Characterized by *rubor* (redness), *dolor* (pain), *calor* (heat), *tumor* (swelling), and *functio laesa* (loss of function).

Fluid exudation	↑ vascular permeability, vasodilation, endothelial injury.	
Leukocyte activation	Emigration (rolling, tight binding, diapedesis); chemotaxis (bacterial products, complement, chemokines); phagocytosis and killing.	
Fibrosis	Fibroblast emigration and proliferation; deposition of ECM.	
Acute	Neutrophil, eosinophil, and antibody mediated.	
Chronic	Mononuclear cell mediated: Characterized by persistent destruction and repair. Granuloma—nodular collections of epithelioid macrophages and giant cells.	Granulomatous diseases: TB (caseating), syphilis, leprosy, *Bartonella*, some fungal pneumonias, sarcoidosis, Crohn's disease.
Resolution	Restoration of normal structure. Granulation tissue—highly vascularized, fibrotic. Abscess—fibrosis surrounding pus. Fistula—abnormal communication. Scarring—collagen deposition resulting in altered structure and function.	

	Transudate	Exudate
Transudate vs. exudate	Hypocellular	Cellular
	Protein poor	Protein rich
	Specific gravity < 1.012	Specific gravity > 1.020
	Due to:	Due to:
	↑ hydrostatic pressure	Lymphatic obstruction
	↑ oncotic pressure	Inflammation
	Na^+ retention	

Leukocyte extravasation

Neutrophils exit from blood vessels at sites of tissue injury and inflammation in 4 steps:

1. Rolling—mediated by E-selectin and P-selectin on vascular endothelium binding to sialyl Lewis^X on the leukocyte
2. Tight binding—mediated by **I**CAM-1 on vascular endothelium binding to LFA-1 (**I**ntegrin) on the leukocyte
3. Diapedesis—leukocyte travels between endothelial cells and exits blood vessel
4. Migration—leukocyte travels through the interstitium to the site of injury or infection guided by chemotactic signals (e.g., cytokines)

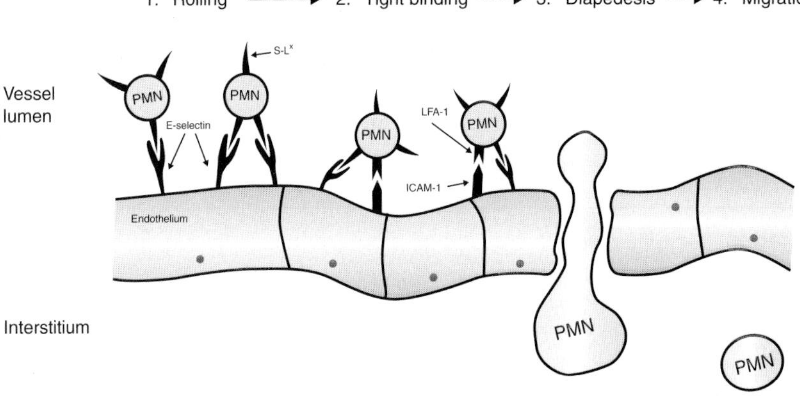

Free radical injury

Initiated via radiation exposure, metabolism of drugs (phase I), redox reaction, nitric oxide, transition metals, leukocyte oxidative burst.

Induces cell injury through membrane lipid peroxidation, protein modification, DNA breakage.

Free radical degradation produced through enzymes (catalase, superoxide dismutase, glutathione peroxidase), spontaneous decay, antioxidants (vitamins E and A).

Reperfusion after anoxia induces free radical production (e.g., superoxide) and is a major cause of injury after thrombolytic therapy.

▶ PATHOLOGY—AMYLOIDOSIS

Structure β-pleated sheet demonstrable by apple-green birefringence of Congo red stain under polarized light; affected tissue has waxy appearance.

Types	Protein	Derived from	
Primary	AL	Ig light chains (multiple myeloma)	**AL** = **L**ight chain.
Secondary	AA	Serum amyloid-associated (SAA) protein (chronic inflammatory disease)	**AA** = **A**cute-phase reactant.
Senile cardiac	Transthyretin	AF	**AF** = old **F**ogies.
Diabetes mellitus type 2	Amylin	AE	**AE** = **E**ndocrine.
Medullary carcinoma of the thyroid	A-CAL	Calcitonin	**A-CAL** = **CAL**citonin.
Alzheimer's disease	Amyloid precursor protein (APP)	β-amyloid	
Dialysis-associated	β_2-microglobulin	MHC class I proteins	

▶ PATHOLOGY–NEOPLASIA

Neoplastic progression

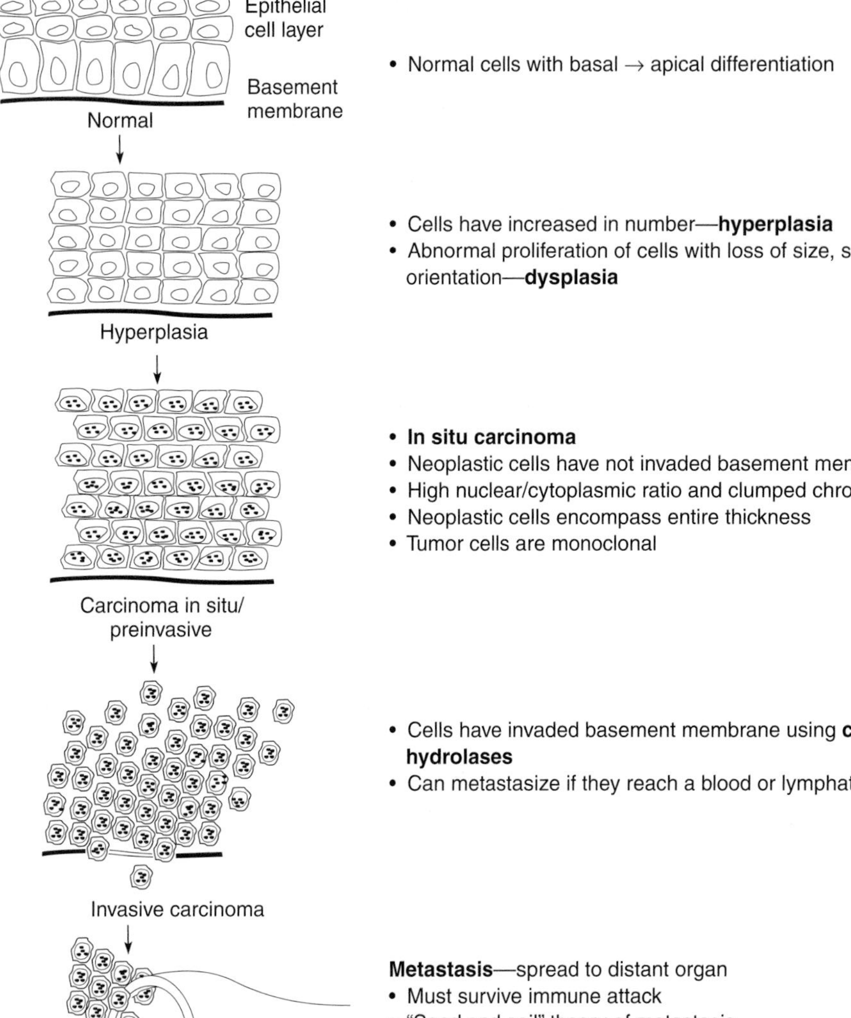

- Normal cells with basal → apical differentiation

- Cells have increased in number—**hyperplasia**
- Abnormal proliferation of cells with loss of size, shape, and orientation—**dysplasia**

- **In situ carcinoma**
- Neoplastic cells have not invaded basement membrane
- High nuclear/cytoplasmic ratio and clumped chromatin
- Neoplastic cells encompass entire thickness
- Tumor cells are monoclonal

- Cells have invaded basement membrane using **collagenases** and **hydrolases**
- Can metastasize if they reach a blood or lymphatic vessel

Metastasis—spread to distant organ
- Must survive immune attack
- "Seed and soil" theory of metastasis
  - Seed = tumor embolus
  - Soil = target organ—liver, lungs, bone, brain. . .
  - Angiogenesis allows for tumor survival

(Adapted, with permission, from McPhee S et al. *Pathophysiology of Disease: An Introduction to Clinical Medicine,* 3rd ed. New York: McGraw-Hill, 2000: 84.)

-plasia definitions

Reversible	Hyperplasia—↑ in number of cells.
	Metaplasia—1 adult cell type is replaced by another. Often 2° to irritation and/or environmental exposure (e.g., squamous metaplasia in trachea and bronchi of smokers).
	Dysplasia—abnormal growth with loss of cellular orientation, shape, and size in comparison to normal tissue maturation; commonly preneoplastic.
Irreversible	Anaplasia—abnormal cells lacking differentiation; like primitive cells of same tissue, often equated with undifferentiated malignant neoplasms.
	Neoplasia—a clonal proliferation of cells that is uncontrolled and excessive.
	Desmoplasia—fibrous tissue formation in response to neoplasm.

Tumor grade vs. stage

Grade	Degree of cellular differentiation based on histologic appearance of tumor. Usually graded I–IV based on degree of differentiation and number of mitoses per high-power field; character of tumor itself.	Stage usually has more prognostic value than grade. Stage = Spread. TNM staging system: **T** = size of **T**umor **N** = **N**ode involvement **M** = **M**etastases
Stage	Degree of localization/spread based on site and size of 1° lesion, spread to regional lymph nodes, presence of metastases; spread of tumor in a specific patient.	

Tumor nomenclature

Cell type	**Benign**	**Malignant**[a]
Epithelium	Adenoma, papilloma	Adenocarcinoma, papillary carcinoma
Mesenchyme		
Blood cells		Leukemia, lymphoma
Blood vessels	Hemangioma	Angiosarcoma
Smooth muscle	Leiomyoma	Leiomyosarcoma
Skeletal muscle	Rhabdomyoma	Rhabdomyosarcoma
Bone	Osteoma	Osteosarcoma
Fat	Lipoma	Liposarcoma
> 1 cell type	Mature teratoma (women)	Immature teratoma and mature teratoma (men)

[a]The term **carcinoma** implies epithelial origin, whereas **sarcoma** denotes mesenchymal origin. Both terms imply malignancy.

Tumor differences

Benign	Usually well differentiated, slow growing, well demarcated, no metastasis.
Malignant	May be poorly differentiated, erratic growth, locally invasive/diffuse, may metastasize.

Disease associations with neoplasms

Condition	Neoplasm
1. **Down** syndrome	1. **ALL** (we **ALL** fall **Down**), AML
2. Xeroderma pigmentosum, albinism	2. Melanoma, basal cell carcinoma, and especially squamous cell carcinomas of skin
3. Chronic atrophic gastritis, pernicious anemia, postsurgical gastric remnants	3. Gastric adenocarcinoma
4. Tuberous sclerosis (facial angiofibroma, seizures, mental retardation)	4. Astrocytoma, angiomyolipoma, and cardiac rhabdomyoma
5. Actinic keratosis	5. Squamous cell carcinoma of skin
6. Barrett's esophagus (chronic GI reflux)	6. Esophageal adenocarcinoma
7. Plummer-Vinson syndrome (atrophic glossitis, esophageal webs, anemia; all due to iron deficiency)	7. Squamous cell carcinoma of esophagus
8. Cirrhosis (alcoholic, hepatitis B or C)	8. Hepatocellular carcinoma
9. Ulcerative colitis	9. Colonic adenocarcinoma
10. Paget's disease of bone	10. 2° osteosarcoma and fibrosarcoma
11. Immunodeficiency states	11. Malignant lymphomas
12. AIDS	12. Aggressive malignant lymphomas (non-Hodgkin's) and Kaposi's sarcoma
13. Autoimmune diseases (e.g., Hashimoto's thyroiditis, myasthenia gravis)	13. Benign and malignant lymphomas
14. Acanthosis nigricans (hyperpigmentation and epidermal thickening)	14. Visceral malignancy (stomach, lung, breast, uterus)
15. Dysplastic nevus	15. Malignant melanoma
16. Radiation exposure	16. Sarcoma

Oncogenes

Gain of function → cancer. Need damage to only 1 allele.

Gene	Associated tumor
abl	CML
c-*myc*	Burkitt's lymphoma
bcl-2	Follicular and undifferentiated lymphomas (inhibits apoptosis)
erb-B2	Breast, ovarian, and gastric carcinomas
ras	Colon carcinoma
L-*myc*	**L**ung tumor
N-*myc*	**N**euroblastoma
ret	Multiple endocrine neoplasia (MEN) types II and III
c-*kit*	Gastrointestinal stromal tumor (GIST)

Tumor suppressor genes

Loss of function → cancer; both alleles must be lost for expression of disease.

Gene	Chromosome	Associated tumor	
Rb	13q	Retinoblastoma, osteosarcoma	
BRCA1	17q	Breast and ovarian cancer	
BRCA2	13q	Breast cancer	
p53	17p	Most human cancers, Li-Fraumeni syndrome	
p16	9p	Melanoma	
APC	5q	Colorectal cancer	
WT1	11p	Wilms' tumor	
NF1	17q	Neurofibromatosis type 1	
NF2	22q	Neurofibromatosis type 2	
DPC	18q	Pancreatic cancer	DPC—Deleted in Pancreatic Cancer.
DCC	18q	Colon cancer	DCC—Deleted in Colon Cancer.

Tumor markers

Tumor markers should not be used as the 1° tool for cancer diagnosis. They may be used to confirm diagnosis, to monitor for tumor recurrence, and to monitor response to therapy.

PSA	Prostate-specific antigen. Used to screen for prostate carcinoma.
Prostatic acid phosphatase	Prostate carcinoma.
CEA	Carcinoembryonic antigen. Very nonspecific but produced by ~ 70% of colorectal and pancreatic cancers; also produced by gastric and breast carcinomas.
α-fetoprotein	Normally made by fetus. Hepatocellular carcinomas. Nonseminomatous germ cell tumors of the testis (e.g., yolk sac tumor).
β-hCG	**H**ydatidiform moles, **C**horiocarcinomas, and **G**estational trophoblastic tumors.
CA-125	Ovarian, malignant epithelial tumors.
S-100	Melanoma, neural tumors, astrocytomas.
Alkaline phosphatase	Metastases to bone, obstructive biliary disease, Paget's disease of bone.
Bombesin	Neuroblastoma, lung and gastric cancer.
TRAP	Tartrate-resistant acid phosphatase. Hairy cell leukemia—a B-cell neoplasm.
CA-19-9	Pancreatic adenocarcinoma.

Oncogenic viruses

Virus	Associated cancer
HTLV-1	Adult T-cell leukemia
HBV, HCV	Hepatocellular carcinoma
EBV	Burkitt's lymphoma, nasopharyngeal carcinoma
HPV	Cervical carcinoma (16, 18), penile/anal carcinoma
HHV-8 (Kaposi's sarcoma–associated herpesvirus)	Kaposi's sarcoma, body cavity fluid B-cell lymphoma

Chemical carcinogens

Toxin	Affected organ
Aflatoxins	Liver (hepatocellular carcinoma)
Vinyl chloride	Liver (angiosarcoma)
CCl_4	Liver (centrilobular necrosis, fatty change)
Nitrosamines (e.g., in smoked foods)	Esophagus, stomach
Cigarette smoke	Larynx, lung, renal cell carcinoma, transitional cell carcinoma
Asbestos	Lung (mesothelioma and bronchogenic carcinoma)
Arsenic	Skin (squamous cell carcinoma)
Naphthalene (aniline) dyes	Bladder (transitional cell carcinoma)
Alkylating agents	Blood (leukemia)

Paraneoplastic effects of tumors

Neoplasm	Causes	Effect
Small cell lung carcinoma	ACTH or ACTH-like peptide	Cushing's syndrome
Small cell lung carcinoma and intracranial neoplasms	ADH	SIADH
Squamous cell lung carcinoma, renal cell carcinoma, and breast carcinoma	PTH-related peptide, TGF-β, TNF, IL-1	Hypercalcemia
Renal cell carcinoma, hemangioblastoma	Erythropoietin	Polycythemia
Thymoma, small cell lung carcinoma	Antibodies against presynaptic Ca^{2+} channels at neuromuscular junction	Lambert-Eaton syndrome (muscle weakness)
Leukemias and lymphomas	Hyperuricemia due to excess nucleic acid turnover (i.e., cytotoxic therapy)	Gout, urate nephropathy

Psammoma bodies

Laminated, concentric, calcific spherules seen in:

1. Papillary adenocarcinoma of thyroid
2. Serous papillary cystadenocarcinoma of ovary
3. Meningioma
4. Malignant mesothelioma

PSaMMoma:
Papillary (thyroid)
Serous (ovary)
Meningioma
Mesothelioma

Metastasis to brain

1° tumors that metastasize to brain—**L**ung, **B**reast, **S**kin (melanoma), **K**idney (renal cell carcinoma), **G**I. Overall, approximately 50% of brain tumors are from metastases.

Lots of **B**ad **S**tuff **K**ills **G**lia.
Typically multiple well-circumscribed tumors at gray-white border.

Metastasis to liver

The liver and lung are the most common sites of metastasis after the regional lymph nodes. 1° tumors that metastasize to the liver—**C**olon > **S**tomach > **P**ancreas > **B**reast > **L**ung.

Metastases >> 1° liver tumors.
Cancer **S**ometimes **P**enetrates **B**enign **L**iver.

Metastasis to bone	These 1° tumors metastasize to bone—**P**rostate, **T**hyroid, **T**estes, **B**reast, **L**ung, **K**idney. Metastases from breast and prostate are most common. Metastatic bone tumors are far more common than 1° bone tumors.	**P. T. B**arnum **L**oves **K**ids. **L**ung = **L**ytic. Prostate = blastic. **B**reast = **B**oth lytic and blastic.

Cancer epidemiology

	Male	Female	
Incidence	Prostate (32%) Lung (16%) Colon and rectum (12%)	Breast (32%) Lung (13%) Colon and rectum (13%)	Deaths from lung cancer have plateaued in males but continue to ↑ in females. Cancer is the 2nd leading cause of death in the United States (heart disease is 1st).
Mortality	Lung (33%) Prostate (13%)	Lung (23%) Breast (18%)	

NOTES

HIGH-YIELD PRINCIPLES IN

Pharmacology

"Take me, I am the drug; take me, I am hallucinogenic."
—Salvador Dali

"I was under medication when I made the decision not to burn the tapes."
—Richard Nixon

Preparation for questions on pharmacology is straightforward. Memorizing all the key drugs and their characteristics (e.g., mechanisms, clinical use, and important side effects) is high yield. Focus on understanding the prototype drugs in each class. Avoid memorizing obscure derivatives. Learn the "classic" and distinguishing toxicities of the major drugs. Do not bother with drug dosages or trade names. Reviewing associated biochemistry, physiology, and microbiology can be useful while studying pharmacology. There is a strong emphasis on ANS, CNS, antimicrobial, and cardiovascular agents as well as on NSAIDs. Much of the material is clinically relevant. Newer drugs on the market are also fair game.

PHARMACOLOGY—HIGH-YIELD CLINICAL VIGNETTES

Vignette	Question	Answer
28-year-old chemist presents with MPTP exposure.	What neurotransmitter is depleted?	Dopamine.
Woman taking tetracycline exhibits photosensitivity.	What are the clinical manifestations?	Rash on sun-exposed regions of the body.
African-American man who goes to Africa develops a hemolytic anemia after taking malaria prophylaxis.	What is the enzyme deficiency?	Glucose-6-phosphate dehydrogenase.
Farmer presents with dyspnea, salivation, miosis, diarrhea, cramping, and blurry vision.	What caused this, and what is the mechanism of action?	Insecticide poisoning; inhibition of acetylcholinesterase.
27-year-old woman with a history of psychiatric illness now has urinary retention due to a neuroleptic.	What do you treat it with?	Bethanechol.
Recent kidney transplant patient who is on cyclosporine for immunosuppression requires an antifungal agent for candidiasis.	What antifungal drug would result in cyclosporine toxicity?	Ketoconazole.
Patient is on carbamazepine.	What routine workup should always be done?	LFTs.
23-year-old woman who is on rifampin for TB prophylaxis and on birth control (estrogen) gets pregnant.	Why?	Rifampin augments estrogen metabolism in the liver, rendering it less effective.

Enzyme kinetics

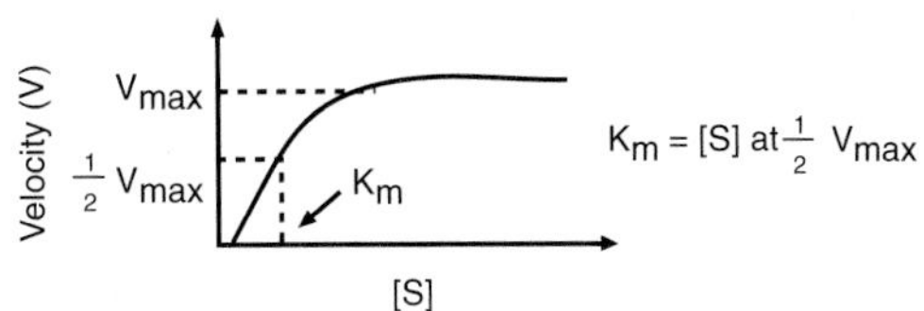

K_m reflects the affinity of the enzyme for its substrate.

V_{max} is directly proportional to the enzyme concentration.

The lower the K_m, the higher the affinity.

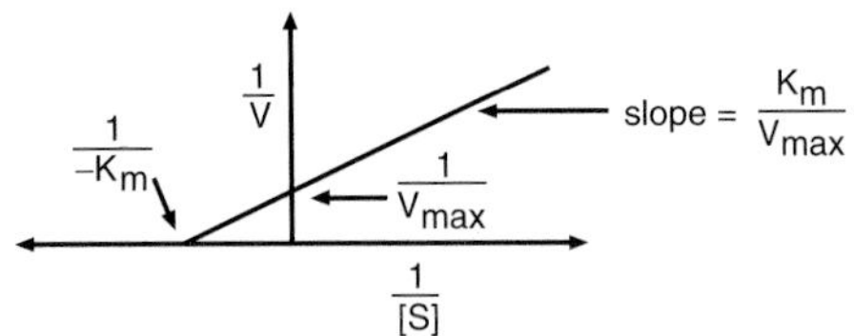

The higher the y-intercept, the lower the V_{max}.

The further to the right the x-intercept, the greater the K_m.

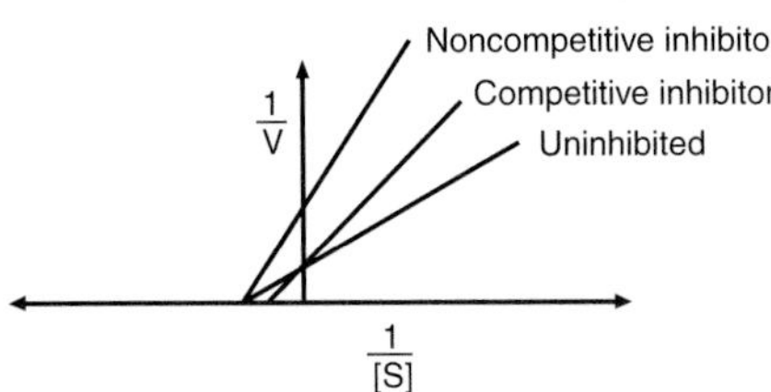

HINT: Competitive inhibitors cross each other competitively, while noncompetitive inhibitors do not.

	Competitive inhibitors	Noncompetitive inhibitors
Resemble substrate	Yes	No
Overcome by ↑ [S]	Yes	No
Bind active site	Yes	No
Effect on V_{max}	Unchanged	↓
Effect on K_m	↑	Unchanged

Pharmacokinetics

Volume of distribution (V_d)

Relates the amount of drug in the body to the plasma concentration. V_d of plasma protein–bound drugs can be altered by liver and kidney disease.

$$V_d = \frac{\text{amount of drug in the body}}{\text{plasma drug concentration}}$$

Drugs with:

- Low V_d (4–8 L) distribute in blood.
- Medium V_d distribute in extracellular space or body water.
- High V_d (> body weight) distribute in tissues.

Clearance (CL)

Relates the rate of elimination to the plasma concentration.

$$CL = \frac{\text{rate of elimination of drug}}{\text{plasma drug concentration}} = V_d \times K_e \text{ (elimination constant)}$$

Half-life ($t_{1/2}$)

The time required to change the amount of drug in the body by ½ during elimination (or during a constant infusion). A drug infused at a constant rate reaches about 94% of steady state after 4 $t_{1/2}$.

$$t_{1/2} = \frac{0.7 \times V_d}{CL}$$

# of half-lives	1	2	3	4
Concentration	50%	75%	87.5%	93.75%

Dosage calculations	Loading dose = $C_p \times V_d/F$. Maintenance dose = $C_p \times CL/F$ where C_p = target plasma concentration and F = bioavailability = 1 when drug is given IV. In patients with impaired renal or hepatic function, the loading dose remains unchanged, although the maintenance dose is ↓.	
Elimination of drugs		
Zero-order elimination	Rate of elimination is constant regardless of C (i.e., constant **amount** of drug eliminated per unit time). C_p ↓ linearly with time. Examples of drugs—**P**henytoin, **E**thanol, and **A**spirin (at high or toxic concentrations).	**PEA.**
First-order elimination	Rate of elimination is proportional to the drug concentration (i.e., constant **fraction** of drug eliminated per unit time). C_p ↓ exponentially with time.	

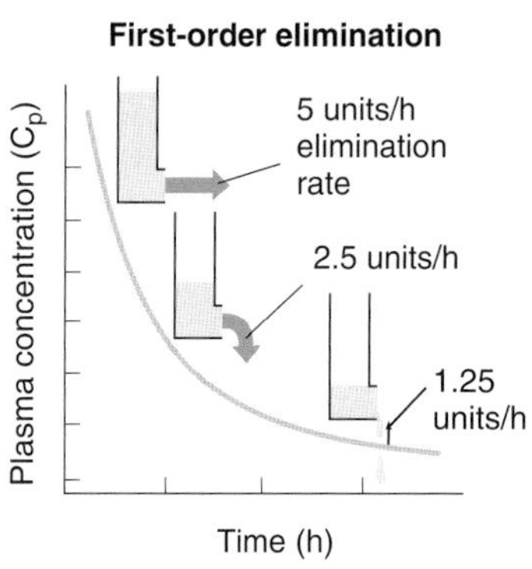

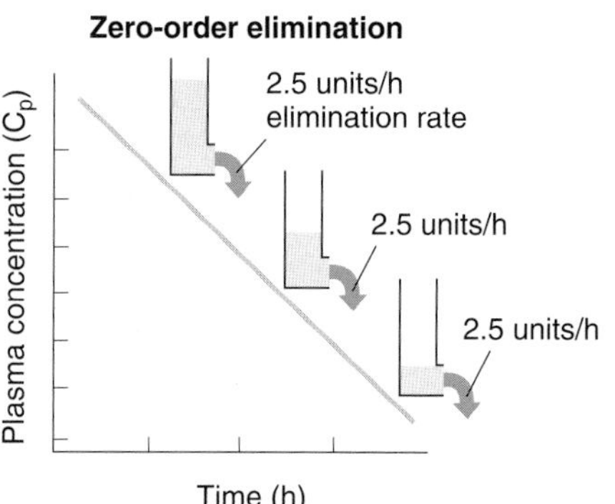

(Adapted, with permission, from Katzung BG, Trevor AJ. *Pharmacology: Examination & Board Review,* 5th ed. Stamford, CT: Appleton & Lange, 1998: 5.)

Urine pH and drug elimination	Ionized species get trapped.	
Weak acids	Trapped in basic environments. Treat overdose with bicarbonate.	
Weak bases	Trapped in acidic environments. Treat overdose with ammonium chloride.	
Phase I vs. phase II metabolism	Phase I (reduction, oxidation, hydrolysis) usually yields slightly polar, water-soluble metabolites (often still active). Phase II (acetylation, glucuronidation, sulfation) usually yields very polar, inactive metabolites (renally excreted).	Phase I—cytochrome P-450. Phase II—conjugation. Geriatric patients lose phase I first.

Pharmacodynamics

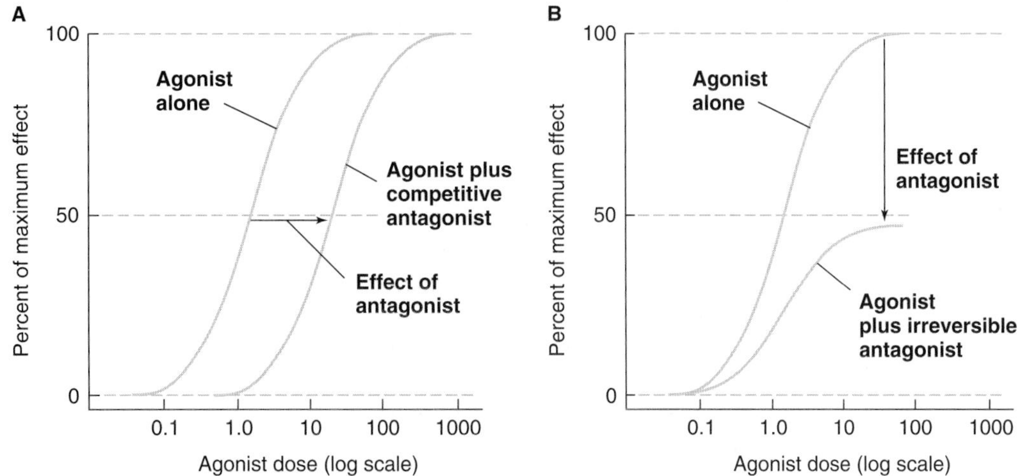

(Adapted, with permission, from Katzung BG, Trevor AJ. *Pharmacology: Examination & Board Review,* 5th ed. Stamford, CT: Appleton & Lange, 1998: 13–14.)

A. A competitive antagonist shifts curve to the right, decreasing potency and increasing EC_{50}. **B.** A noncompetitive antagonist shifts the agonist curve downward, decreasing efficacy.

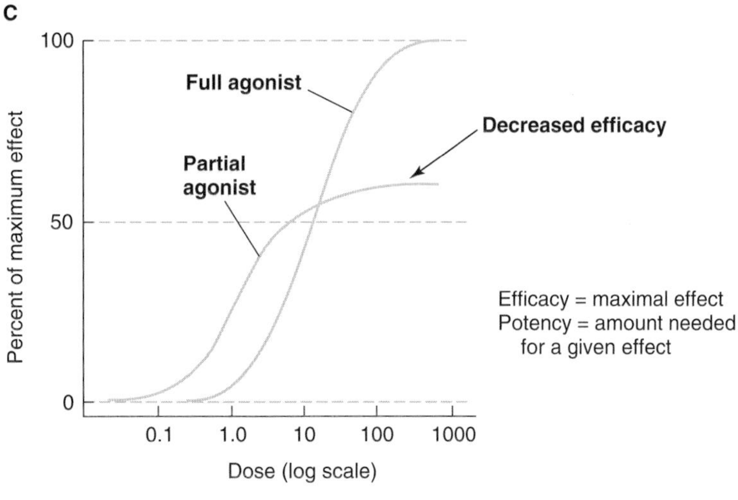

(Adapted, with permission, from Katzung BG. *Basic and Clinical Pharmacology,* 7th ed. Stamford, CT: Appleton & Lange, 1997: 13.)

C. Comparison of dose-response curves for a full agonist and a partial agonist. The **partial agonist** acts on the same receptor system as the full agonist but has a **lower maximal efficacy** regardless of the dose. A partial agonist may be more potent (as in the figure), less potent, or equally potent; **potency is an independent factor.**

Therapeutic index	$\frac{LD_{50}}{ED_{50}} = \frac{\text{median toxic dose}}{\text{median effective dose}}$	TILE: **TI** = LD_{50} / ED_{50}. Safer drugs have higher TI values.

Central and peripheral nervous system

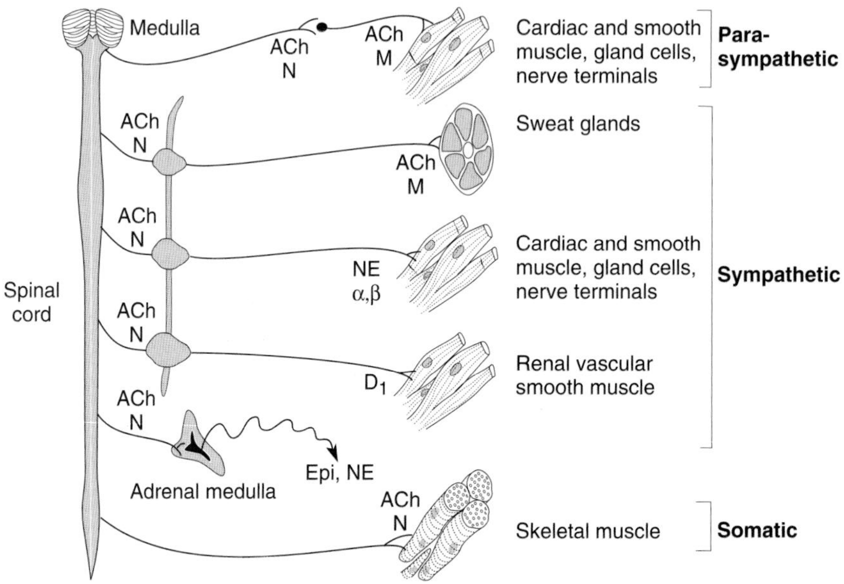

(Adapted, with permission, from Katzung BG. *Basic and Clinical Pharmacology,* 7th ed. Stamford, CT: Appleton & Lange, 1997: 74.)

ACh receptors	Nicotinic ACh receptors are ligand-gated Na^+/K^+ channels. Muscarinic ACh receptors are G-protein-coupled receptors that act through 2nd messengers.

G-protein-linked 2nd messengers

Receptor	G-protein class	Major functions
α_1	q	↑ vascular smooth muscle contraction
α_2	i	↓ sympathetic outflow, ↓ insulin release
β_1	s	↑ heart rate, ↑ contractility, ↑ renin release, ↑ lipolysis, maintains aqueous humor formation
β_2	s	Vasodilation, bronchodilation, ↑ heart rate, ↑ contractility, ↑ lipolysis, ↑ glucagon release
M_1	q	CNS, enteric nervous system
M_2	i	↓ heart rate and contractility
M_3	q	↑ exocrine gland secretions, ↑ gut peristalsis, ↑ bladder contraction
D_1	s	Relaxes renal vascular smooth muscle
D_2	i	Modulates transmitter release, especially in brain
H_1	q	↑ nasal and bronchial mucus production, contraction of bronchioles, pruritus, and pain
H_2	s	↑ gastric acid secretion
V_1	q	↑ vascular smooth muscle contraction
V_2	s	↑ H_2O permeability and reabsorption in the collecting tubules of the kidney

"**Qiss** (kiss) and **qiq** (kick) till you're **siq** (sick) of **sqs** (sex)."

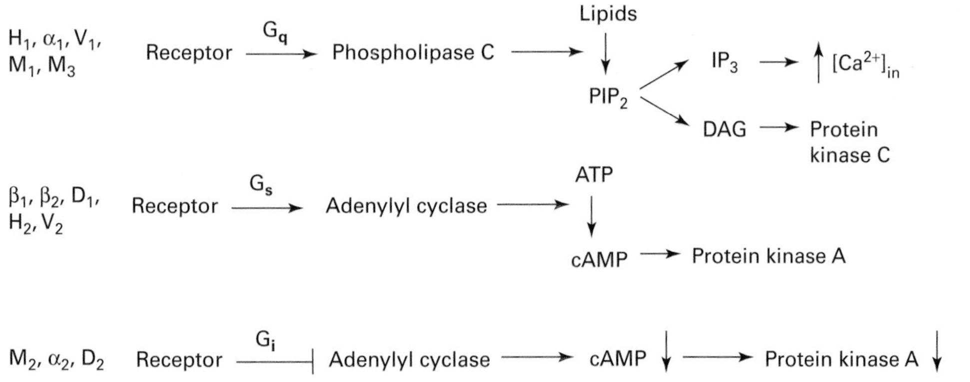

H_1, α_1, V_1, M_1, M_3 — Receptor —G_q→ Phospholipase C → Lipids ↓ PIP_2 → IP_3 → ↑ $[Ca^{2+}]_{in}$; PIP_2 → DAG → Protein kinase C

HAVe 1 M&M.

β_1, β_2, D_1, H_2, V_2 — Receptor —G_s→ Adenylyl cyclase → ATP ↓ cAMP → Protein kinase A

M_2, α_2, D_2 — Receptor —G_i⊣ Adenylyl cyclase → cAMP ↓ → Protein kinase A ↓

MAD 2's.

Autonomic drugs

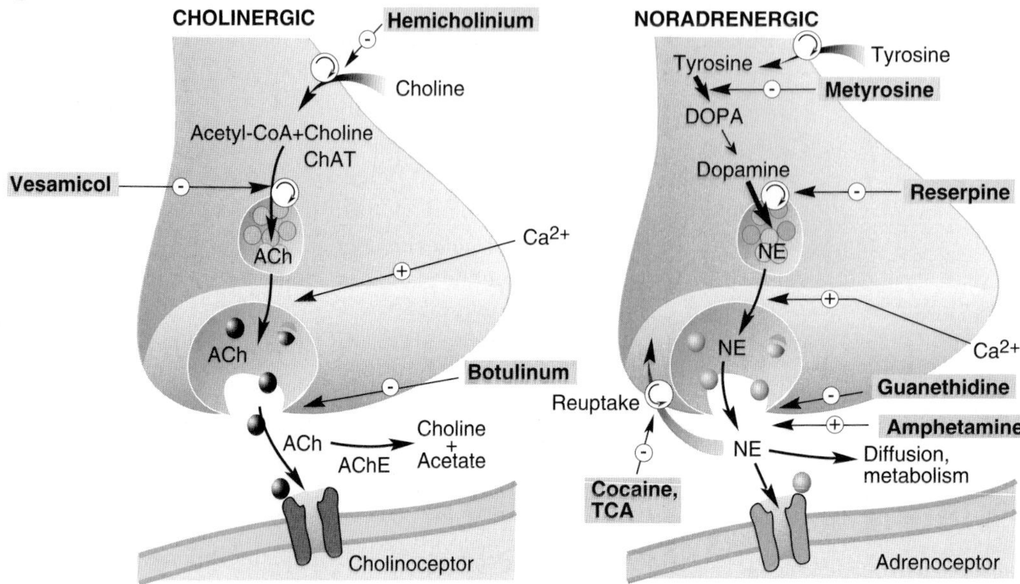

(Adapted, with permission, from Katzung BG, Trevor AJ. *Pharmacology: Examination & Board Review,* 5th ed. Stamford, CT: Appleton & Lange, 1998: 42.)

Circles with rotating arrows represent transporters; ChAT, choline acetyltransferase; ACh, acetylcholine; AChE, acetylcholinesterase; NE, norepinephrine.

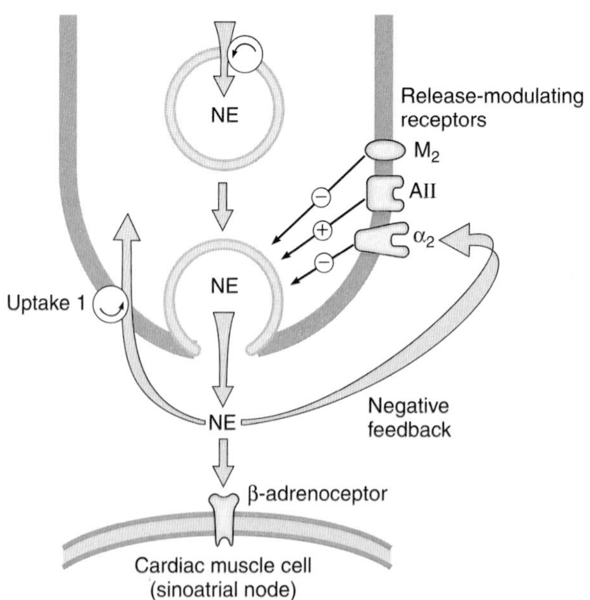

(Adapted, with permission, from Katzung BG, Trevor AJ. *Pharmacology: Examination & Board Review,* 5th ed. Stamford, CT: Appleton & Lange, 1998: 42.)

Release of NE from a sympathetic nerve ending is modulated by NE itself, acting on presynaptic α_2 autoreceptors, and by ACh, angiotensin II, and other substances.

Cholinergic agents		
Drug	Clinical applications	Action
Direct agonists		
Bethanechol	Postoperative and neurogenic ileus and urinary retention	Activates **B**owel and **B**ladder smooth muscle; resistant to AChE. **Beth Anne, call (bethanechol)** me if you want to activate your **B**owels and **B**ladder.
Carbachol	Glaucoma, pupillary contraction, and release of intraocular pressure	
Pilocarpine	Potent stimulator of sweat, tears, saliva	Contracts ciliary muscle of eye (open angle), pupillary sphincter (narrow angle); resistant to AChE. **PILE** on the sweat and tears.
Methacholine	Challenge test for diagnosis of asthma	Stimulates muscarinic receptors in airway when inhaled.
Indirect agonists (anticholinesterases)		
Neostigmine	Postoperative and neurogenic ileus and urinary retention, myasthenia gravis, reversal of neuromuscular junction blockade (postoperative)	↑ endogenous ACh; no CNS penetration. **NEO** CNS = **NO** CNS penetration.
Pyridostigmine	Myasthenia gravis (long acting); does not penetrate CNS	↑ endogenous ACh; ↑ strength.
Edrophonium	Diagnosis of myasthenia gravis (extremely short acting)	↑ endogenous ACh.
Physostigmine	Glaucoma (crosses blood-brain barrier → CNS) and atropine overdose	↑ endogenous ACh. **PHYS** is for **EYES.**
Echothiophate	Glaucoma	↑ endogenous ACh.

Cholinesterase inhibitor poisoning	Symptoms include **D**iarrhea, **U**rination, **M**iosis, **B**ronchospasm, **B**radycardia, **E**xcitation of skeletal muscle and CNS, **L**acrimation, **S**weating, and **S**alivation (also abdominal cramping). Antidote—atropine (muscarinic antagonist) plus pralidoxime (chemical antagonist used to regenerate active cholinesterase).	**DUMBBELSS.** Parathion and other organophosphates. Irreversible inhibitors.

Muscarinic antagonists

Drug	Organ system	Application
Atropine, homatropine, tropicamide	Eye	Produce mydriasis and cycloplegia
Benztropine	CNS	**PARK**inson's disease—**PARK** my **BENZ**
Scopolamine	CNS	Motion sickness
Ipratropium	Respiratory	Asthma, COPD
Methscopolamine, oxybutynin, glycopyrrolate	Genitourinary	Reduce urgency in mild cystitis and reduce bladder spasms
Pirenzepine, propantheline	Gastrointestinal	Peptic ulcer treatment

Glaucoma drugs

α_1 stimulation → mydriasis (pupillary dilator muscle); M3 stimulation → miosis (pupillary constrictor muscle) and ciliary muscle contraction.

Drug	Mechanism	Side effects
α-agonists		
Epinephrine	↓ aqueous humor synthesis due to vasoconstriction	Mydriasis, stinging; do not use in closed-angle glaucoma
Brimonidine	↓ aqueous humor synthesis	No pupillary or vision changes
β-blockers		
Timolol, betaxolol, carteolol	↓ aqueous humor secretion	No pupillary or vision changes
Diuretics		
Acetazolamide	↓ aqueous humor secretion due to ↓ HCO_3^- (via inhibition of carbonic anhydrase)	No pupillary or vision changes
Cholinomimetics		
Pilocarpine, carbachol, physostigmine, echothiophate	↑ outflow of aqueous humor; contract ciliary muscle and open trabecular meshwork; use pilocarpine in emergencies; very effective at opening canal of Schlemm	Miosis, cyclospasm
Prostaglandin		
Latanoprost ($PGF_{2\alpha}$)	↑ outflow of aqueous humor	Darkens color of iris (browning)

Atropine	Muscarinic antagonist.	
Organ system		
Eye	↑ pupil dilation, cycloplegia.	Blocks **DUMBBELSS.**
Airway	↓ secretions.	
Stomach	↓ acid secretion.	
Gut	↓ motility.	
Bladder	↓ urgency in cystitis.	
Toxicity	↑ body temperature; rapid pulse; dry mouth; dry, flushed skin; cycloplegia; constipation; disorientation. Can cause acute angle-closure glaucoma in elderly, urinary retention in men with prostatic hypertrophy, and hyperthermia in infants.	**Side effects:** Hot as a hare Dry as a bone Red as a beet Blind as a bat Mad as a hatter

Hexamethonium	Nicotinic antagonist.
Clinical use	Ganglionic blocker. Used in experimental models to prevent vagal reflex responses to changes in blood pressure—e.g., prevents reflex bradycardia caused by NE.
Toxicity	Severe orthostatic hypotension, blurred vision, constipation, sexual dysfunction.

Sympathomimetics

Drug	Mechanism/selectivity	Applications
Direct sympathomimetics		
Epinephrine	α_1, α_2, β_1, β_2, low doses selective for β_1	Anaphylaxis, glaucoma (open angle), asthma, hypotension
NE	α_1, $\alpha_2 > \beta_1$	Hypotension (but ↓ renal perfusion)
Isoproterenol	$\beta_1 = \beta_2$	AV block (rare)
Dopamine	$D_1 = D_2 > \beta > \alpha$, inotropic and chronotropic	Shock (↑ renal perfusion), heart failure
Dobutamine	$\beta_1 > \beta_2$, inotropic but not chronotropic	Shock, heart failure, cardiac stress testing
Phenylephrine	$\alpha_1 > \alpha_2$	Pupillary dilation, vasoconstriction, nasal decongestion
Albuterol, terbutaline	$\beta_2 > \beta_1$	Albuterol for acute asthma; terbutaline reduces premature uterine contractions
Ritodrine	β_2	Reduces premature uterine contractions
Indirect sympathomimetics		
Amphetamine	Indirect general agonist, releases stored catecholamines	Narcolepsy, obesity, attention deficit disorder
Ephedrine	Indirect general agonist, releases stored catecholamines	Nasal decongestion, urinary incontinence, hypotension
Cocaine	Indirect general agonist, uptake inhibitor	Causes vasoconstriction and local anesthesia
Sympathoplegics		
Clonidine, α-methyldopa	Centrally acting α_2-agonist, ↓ central adrenergic outflow	Hypertension, especially with renal disease (no ↓ in blood flow to kidney)

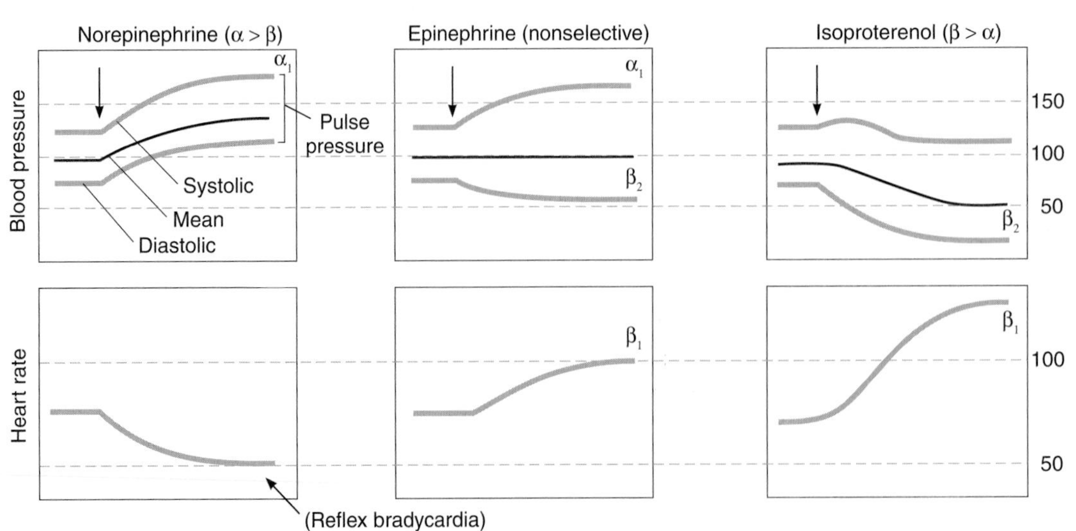

(Adapted, with permission, from Katzung BG, Trevor AJ. *Pharmacology: Examination & Board Review,* 5th ed. Stamford, CT: Appleton & Lange, 1998: 72.)

Selective β_2-agonists	Metaproterenol, Albuterol, Salmeterol, Terbutaline.	MAST.

α-blockers

Drug	Application	Toxicity
Nonselective		
Phenoxybenzamine (irreversible) and phentolamine (reversible)	Pheochromocytoma (use phenoxybenzamine before removing tumor, since high levels of released catecholamines will not be able to overcome blockage)	Orthostatic hypotension, reflex tachycardia
α_1 selective		
Prazosin, terazosin, doxazosin	Hypertension, urinary retention in BPH	1st-dose orthostatic hypotension, dizziness, headache
α_2 selective		
Mirtazapine	Depression	Sedation, ↑ serum cholesterol, ↑ appetite

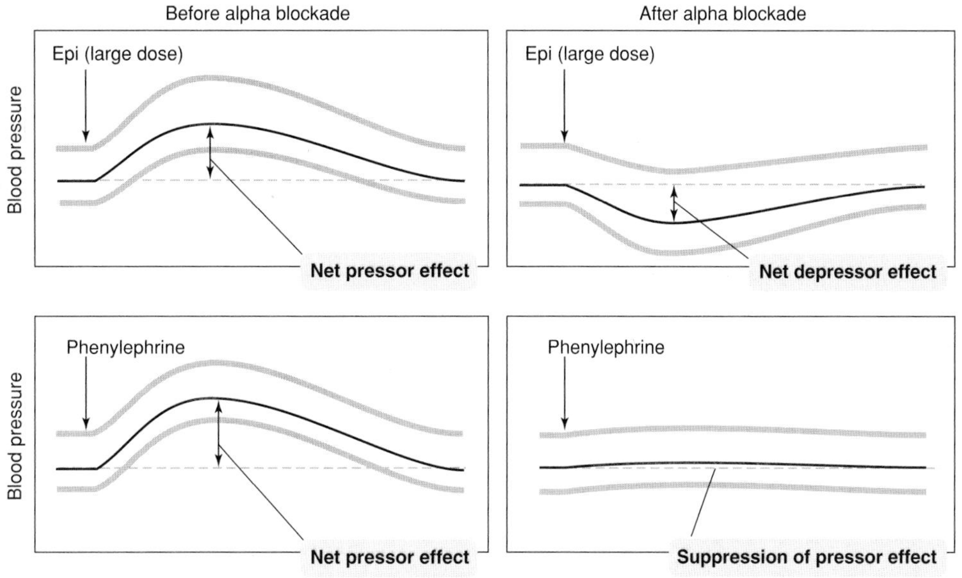

(Adapted, with permission, from Katzung BG, Trevor AJ. *Pharmacology: Examination & Board Review,* 5th ed. Stamford, CT: Appleton & Lange, 1998: 80.)

Shown above are the effects of an α-blocker (e.g., phentolamine) on blood pressure responses to epinephrine and phenylephrine. The epinephrine response exhibits reversal of the mean blood pressure change, from a net increase (the α response) to a net decrease (the β_2 response). The response to phenylephrine is suppressed but not reversed because phenylephrine is a "pure" α-agonist without β action.

β-blockers	Propranolol, metoprolol, atenolol, nadolol, timolol, pindolol, esmolol, labetalol.	
Application	**Effect**	
Hypertension	↓ cardiac output, ↓ renin secretion	
Angina pectoris	↓ heart rate and contractility, resulting in ↓ O_2 consumption	
MI	β-blockers ↓ mortality	
SVT (propranolol, esmolol)	↓ AV conduction velocity (class II antiarrhythmic)	
CHF	Slows progression of chronic failure	
Glaucoma (timolol)	↓ secretion of aqueous humor	
Toxicity	Impotence, exacerbation of asthma, cardiovascular adverse effects (bradycardia, AV block, CHF), CNS adverse effects (sedation, sleep alterations); use with caution in diabetics	
Selectivity	Nonselective antagonists ($\beta_1 = \beta_2$)—propranolol, timolol, nadolol, pindolol, and labetalol	
	β_1-selective antagonists ($\beta_1 > \beta_2$)—**A**cebutolol (partial agonist), **B**etaxolol, **E**smolol (short acting), **A**tenolol, **M**etoprolol	**A BEAM** of β_1-blockers.
	Nonselective α- and β-antagonists—carvedilol, labetalol	
	Partial β-agonists—acebutolol, pindolol	

Specific antidotes

Toxin	Antidote/treatment
1. Acetaminophen	1. N-acetylcysteine
2. Salicylates	2. $NaHCO_3$ (alkalinize urine), dialysis
3. Amphetamines (basic)	3. NH_4Cl (acidify urine)
4. Anticholinesterases, organophosphates	4. Atropine, pralidoxime
5. Antimuscarinic, anticholinergic agents	5. Physostigmine salicylate
6. β-blockers	6. Glucagon
7. Digitalis	7. Stop dig, normalize K^+, lidocaine, anti-dig Fab fragments, Mg^{2+}
8. Iron	8. Deferoxamine
9. Lead	9. CaEDTA, dimercaprol, succimer, penicillamine
10. Arsenic, mercury, gold	10. Dimercaprol (BAL), succimer
11. Copper, arsenic, gold	11. Penicillamine
12. Cyanide	12. Nitrite, hydroxocobalamin, thiosulfate
13. Methemoglobin	13. Methylene blue
14. Carbon monoxide	14. 100% O_2, hyperbaric O_2
15. Methanol, ethylene glycol (antifreeze)	15. Ethanol, dialysis, fomepizole
16. Opioids	16. Naloxone/naltrexone
17. Benzodiazepines	17. Flumazenil
18. TCAs	18. $NaHCO_3$ (serum alkalinization)
19. Heparin	19. Protamine
20. Warfarin	20. Vitamin K, fresh frozen plasma
21. tPA, streptokinase	21. Aminocaproic acid

Lead poisoning

Lead Lines on gingivae and on epiphyses of long bones on x-ray.
Encephalopathy and Erythrocyte basophilic stippling.
Abdominal colic and sideroblastic Anemia.
Drops—wrist and foot drop. Dimercaprol and EDTA 1st line of treatment. **Succ**imer for kids.

LEAD.
High risk in houses with chipped paint.

It "**sucks**" to be a kid who eats lead.

Iron poisoning

Iron overdose is one of the leading causes of fatality from toxicologic agents in children.

Mechanism: Cell death due to peroxidation of membrane lipids.

Symptoms: Acute—gastric bleeding.
Chronic—metabolic acidosis, scarring leading to GI obstruction.

Drug reactions

Drug reaction by system	Causal agent
Cardiovascular	
Atropine-like side effects	Tricyclics
Coronary vasospasm	Cocaine, sumatriptan
Cutaneous flushing	Niacin, Ca^{2+} channel blockers, adenosine, vancomycin
Dilated cardiomyopathy	Doxorubicin (Adriamycin), daunorubicin
Torsades des pointes	Class III (sotalol), class IA (quinidine) antiarrhythmics, cisapride
Hematologic	
Agranulocytosis	Clozapine, carbamazepine, colchicine, propylthiouracil, methimazole
Aplastic anemia	Chloramphenicol, benzene, NSAIDs, propylthiouracil, methimazole
Direct Coombs-positive hemolytic anemia	Methyldopa
Gray baby syndrome	Chloramphenicol
Hemolysis in G6PD-deficient patients	**I**soniazid (INH), **S**ulfonamides, **P**rimaquine, **A**spirin, **I**buprofen, **N**itrofurantoin (hemolysis **IS PAIN**)
Thrombotic complications	OCPs (e.g., estrogens and progestins)
Respiratory	
Cough	ACE inhibitors (note: ARBs like losartan—no cough)
Pulmonary fibrosis	Bleomycin, busulfan, amiodarone
GI	
Acute cholestatic hepatitis	Macrolides
Focal to massive hepatic necrosis	Halothane, valproic acid, acetaminophen, *Amanita phalloides*
Hepatitis	INH
Pseudomembranous colitis	Clindamycin, ampicillin
Reproductive/endocrine	
Adrenocortical insufficiency	Glucocorticoid withdrawal (HPA suppression)
Gynecomastia	**S**pironolactone, **D**igitalis, **C**imetidine, chronic **A**lcohol use, estrogens, **K**etoconazole (**S**ome **D**rugs **C**reate **A**wesome **K**nockers)
Hot flashes	Tamoxifen, clomiphene
Musculoskeletal/connective tissue	
Gingival hyperplasia	Phenytoin
Gout	Furosemide, thiazides
Osteoporosis	Corticosteroids, heparin
Photosensitivity	**S**ulfonamides, **A**miodarone, **T**etracycline (**SAT** for a **photo**)
SLE-like syndrome	**H**ydralazine, **I**NH, **P**rocainamide, **P**henytoin (it's not **HIPP** to have lupus)
Tendonitis, tendon rupture, and cartilage damage (kids)	Fluoroquinolones

Drug reactions *(continued)*

Renal	
Fanconi's syndrome	Expired tetracycline
Interstitial nephritis	Methicillin, NSAIDs
Hemorrhagic cystitis	Cyclophosphamide, ifosfamide (prevent by coadministrating with mesna)
Neurologic	
Cinchonism	Quinidine, quinine
Diabetes insipidus	Lithium, demeclocycline
Seizures	Bupropion, imipenem/cilastatin
Tardive dyskinesia	Antipsychotics
Multiorgan	
Disulfiram-like reaction	Metronidazole, certain cephalosporins, procarbazine, 1st-generation sulfonylureas
Nephrotoxicity/ neurotoxicity	Polymyxins
Nephrotoxicity/ ototoxicity	Aminoglycosides, loop diuretics, cisplatin

P-450 interactions

Inducers	Inhibitors
Quinidine*	Isoniazid
Barbiturates	Sulfonamides
Phenytoin	Cimetidine
Rifampin	Ketoconazole
Griseofulvin	Erythromycin
Carbamazepine	Grapefruit juice
St. John's wort	

Inducers:
Queen **Barb** takes **Phen**-phen and **R**efuses **G**reasy **Carb** **S**hakes.

Inhibitors:
Inhibitors **S**top **Cy**ber-**K**ids from **E**ating **G**rapefruit.

*Quinidine can both induce and inhibit different isoforms of P-450. Induction is the more important effect.

Alcohol toxicity

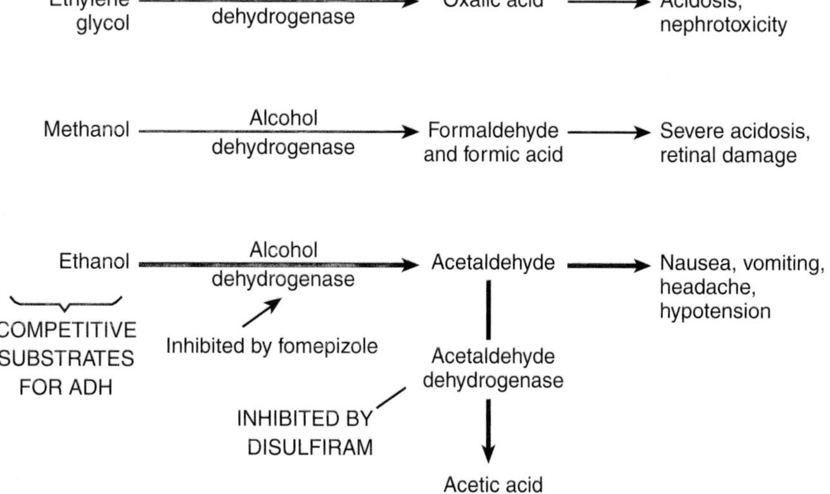

(Adapted, with permission, from Katzung BG, Trevor AJ. *Pharmacology: Examination & Board Review*, 5th ed. Appleton & Lange, 1998: 181.)

▶ PHARMACOLOGY–TOXICITIES AND SIDE EFFECTS *(continued)*

Sulfa drugs Drugs that can lead to allergies in sulfa-allergic patients—celecoxib, furosemide, thiazides, TMP-SMX, sulfonyureas, sulfasalazine.

▶ PHARMACOLOGY–MISCELLANEOUS

Herbal agents

Agent	Clinical uses	Toxicities
Echinacea	Common cold	GI distress, dizziness, and headache
Ephedra	As for ephedrine	CNS and cardiovascular stimulation; arrhythmias, stroke, and seizures at high doses
Feverfew	Migraine	GI distress, mouth ulcers, antiplatelet actions
Ginkgo	Intermittent claudication	GI distress, anxiety, insomnia, headache, antiplatelet actions
Kava	Chronic anxiety	GI distress, sedation, ataxia, hepatotoxicity, phototoxicity, dermatotoxicity
Milk thistle	Viral hepatitis	Loose stools
Saw palmetto	Benign prostatic hyperplasia	GI distress, ↓ libido, hypertension
St. John's wort	Mild to moderate depression	GI distress and phototoxicity; serotonin syndrome with SSRIs; induces P-450 system
Dehydroepi-androsterone	Symptomatic improvement in females with SLE or AIDS	Androgenization (premenopausal women), estrogenic effects (postmenopausal), feminization (young men)
Melatonin	Jet lag, insomnia	Sedation, suppresses midcycle LH, hypoprolactinemia

(Adapted, with permission, from Katzung BG, Trevor AJ. *USMLE Road Map: Pharmacology*, 1st ed. New York: McGraw-Hill, 2003.)

Drug name

Ending	Category	Example
-afil	Erectile dysfunction	Sildenafil
-ane	Inhalational general anesthetic	Halothane
-azepam	Benzodiazepine	Diazepam
-azine	Phenothiazine (neuroleptic, antiemetic)	Chlorpromazine
-azole	Antifungal	Ketoconazole
-barbital	Barbiturate	Phenobarbital
-caine	Local anesthetic	Lidocaine
-cillin	Penicillin	Methicillin
-cycline	Antibiotic, protein synthesis inhibitor	Tetracycline
-ipramine	TCA	Imipramine
-navir	Protease inhibitor	Saquinavir
-olol	β-antagonist	Propranolol
-operidol	Butyrophenone (neuroleptic)	Haloperidol
-oxin	Cardiac glycoside (inotropic agent)	Digoxin
-phylline	Methylxanthine	Theophylline
-pril	ACE inhibitor	Captopril
-terol	β_2 agonist	Albuterol
-tidine	H_2 antagonist	Cimetidine
-triptyline	TCA	Amitriptyline
-tropin	Pituitary hormone	Somatotropin
-zosin	α_1 antagonist	Prazosin

SECTION III

High-Yield Organ Systems

- Approaching the Organ Systems
- Cardiovascular
- Endocrine
- Gastrointestinal
- Hematology and Oncology
- Musculoskeletal and Connective Tissue
- Neurology
- Psychiatry
- Renal
- Reproductive
- Respiratory

In this section, we have divided the High-Yield Facts into the major **Organ Systems.** Within each Organ System are several subsections, including **Anatomy, Physiology, Pathology,** and **Pharmacology.** As you progress through each Organ System, refer back to information in the previous subsections to organize these basic science subsections into a "vertical" framework for learning. Below is some general advice for studying the organ systems by these subsections.

Anatomy

Several topics fall under this heading, including embryology, gross anatomy, histology, and neuroanatomy. Do not memorize all the small details; however, do not ignore anatomy altogether. Review what you have already learned and what you wish you had learned. Many questions require two steps. The first step is to identify a structure on anatomic cross section, electron micrograph, or photomicrograph. The second step may require an understanding of the clinical significance of the structure.

When studying, stress clinically important material. For example, be familiar with gross anatomy related to specific diseases (e.g., Pancoast's tumor, Horner's syndrome), traumatic injuries (e.g., fractures, sensory and motor nerve deficits), procedures (e.g., lumbar puncture), and common surgeries (e.g., cholecystectomy). There are also many questions on the exam involving x-rays, CT scans, and neuro MRI scans. Many students suggest browsing through a general radiology atlas, pathology atlas, and histology atlas. Focus on learning basic anatomy at key levels in the body (e.g., sagittal brain MRI; axial CT of the midthorax, abdomen, and pelvis). Basic neuroanatomy (especially pathways, blood supply, and functional anatomy) also has good yield. Use this as an opportunity to learn associated neuropathology and neurophysiology. Basic embryology (especially congenital malformations) is worth reviewing as well.

Physiology

The portion of the examination dealing with physiology is broad and concept oriented and thus does not lend itself as well to fact-based review. Diagrams are often the best study aids, especially given the increasing number of questions requiring the interpretation of diagrams. Learn to apply basic physiologic relationships in a variety of ways (e.g., the Fick equation, clearance equations). You are seldom asked to perform complex calculations. Hormones are the focus of many questions, so learn their sites of production and action as well as their regulatory mechanisms.

A large portion of the physiology tested on the USMLE Step 1 is now clinically relevant and involves understanding physiologic changes associated with pathologic processes (e.g., changes in pulmonary function with COPD). Thus, it is worthwhile to review the physiologic changes that are found with common pathologies of the major organ systems (e.g., heart, lungs, kidneys, GI tract) and endocrine glands.

Pathology

Questions dealing with this discipline are difficult to prepare for because of the sheer volume of material involved. Review the basic principles and hallmark characteristics of the key diseases. Given the increasingly clinical orientation of Step 1, it is no longer sufficient to know only the "trigger word" associations of certain diseases (e.g., café-au-lait macules and neurofibromatosis); you must also know the clinical descriptions of these findings.

Given the clinical slant of the USMLE Step 1, it is also important to review the classic presenting signs and symptoms of diseases as well as their associated laboratory findings. Delve into the signs, symptoms, and pathophysiology of major diseases that have a high prevalence in the United States (e.g., alcoholism, diabetes, hypertension, heart failure, ischemic heart disease, infectious disease). Be prepared to think one step beyond the simple diagnosis to treatment or complications.

The examination includes a number of color photomicrographs and photographs of gross specimens that are presented in the setting of a brief clinical history. However, read the question and the choices carefully before looking at the illustration, because the history will help you identify the pathologic process. Flip through an illustrated pathology textbook, color atlases, and appropriate Web sites in order to look at the pictures in the days before the exam. Pay attention to potential clues such as age, sex, ethnicity, occupation, recent activities and exposures, and specialized lab tests.

Pharmacology

Preparation for questions on pharmacology is straightforward. Memorizing all the key drugs and their characteristics (e.g., mechanisms, clinical use, and important side effects) is high yield. Focus on understanding the prototype drugs in each class. Avoid memorizing obscure derivatives. Learn the "classic" and distinguishing toxicities of the major drugs. Do not bother with drug dosages or trade names. Reviewing associated biochemistry, physiology, and microbiology can be useful while studying pharmacology. There is a strong emphasis on ANS, CNS, antimicrobial, and cardiovascular agents as well as on NSAIDs. Much of the material is clinically relevant. Newer drugs on the market are also fair game.

HIGH-YIELD SYSTEMS

Cardiovascular

"As for me, except for an occasional heart attack, I feel as young as I ever did."
—Robert Benchley

"Hearts will never be practical until they are made unbreakable."
—*The Wizard of Oz*

"As the arteries grow hard, the heart grows soft."
—H. L. Mencken

"Nobody has ever measured, not even poets, how much the heart can hold."
—Zelda Fitzgerald

Vignette	Question	Answer
Pregnant woman in 3rd trimester has normal blood pressure when standing and sitting. When supine, blood pressure drops to 90/50.	What is the diagnosis?	Compression of the IVC.
35-year-old man has high blood pressure in his arms and low pressure in his legs.	What is the diagnosis?	Coarctation of the aorta.
5-year-old boy presents with a systolic murmur and wide, fixed split S2.	What is the diagnosis?	ASD.
During a game, a young football player collapses and dies immediately.	What is the most likely type of cardiac disease?	Hypertrophic cardiomyopathy.
Patient has a stroke after incurring multiple long bone fractures in trauma stemming from a motor vehicle accident.	What caused the infarct?	Fat emboli.
Elderly woman presents with a headache and jaw pain. Labs show elevated ESR.	What is the diagnosis?	Temporal arteritis.
80-year-old man presents with a systolic crescendo-decrescendo murmur.	What is the most likely cause?	Aortic stenosis.
Man starts a medication for hyperlipidemia. He then develops a rash, pruritus, and GI upset.	What drug is it?	Niacin.
Patient develops a cough and must discontinue captopril.	What is a good replacement drug, and why doesn't it have the same side effects?	Losartan, an angiotensin II receptor antagonist, does not ↑ bradykinin as captopril does.
Patient presents with ringing in the ears, dizziness, headaches, and GI distress.	What drug is it?	Quinidine.
Patient with a history of hypertension presents with sudden sharp, tearing pain radiating to the back.	What is the CXR finding?	Mediastinal widening.
On auscultation, a pansystolic murmur at the apex with radiation to the axilla is noted.	What is the likely cause?	Mitral insufficiency.

Carotid sheath	3 structures inside: 1. Internal jugular **V**ein (lateral) 2. Common carotid **A**rtery (medial) 3. Vagus **N**erve (posterior)	VAN.
Coronary artery anatomy	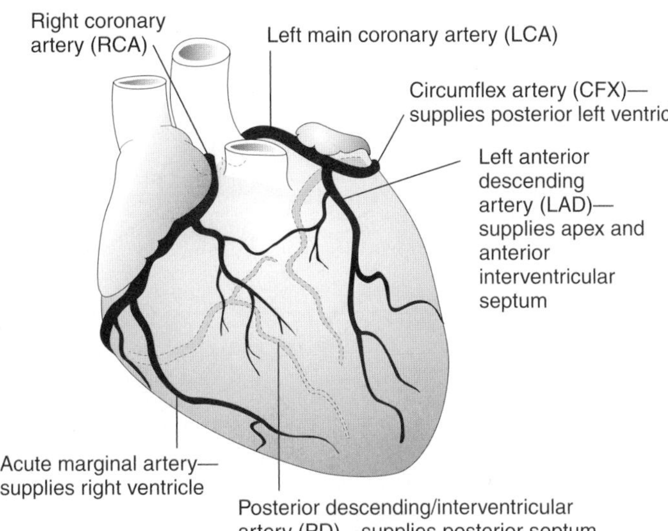 (Adapted, with permission, from Ganong WF. *Review of Medical Physiology,* 19th ed. Stamford, CT: Appleton & Lange, 1999: 592.)	In the majority of cases, the SA and AV nodes are supplied by the RCA. 80% of the time, the RCA supplies the inferior portion of the left ventricle via the PD artery (= right dominant). 20% of the time, the PD arises from the CFX. Coronary artery occlusion most commonly occurs in the LAD, which supplies the anterior interventricular septum. Coronary arteries fill during diastole. The most posterior part of the heart is the left atrium; enlargement can cause dysphagia or hoarseness.

HIGH-YIELD SYSTEMS

CARDIOVASCULAR

Auscultation of the heart

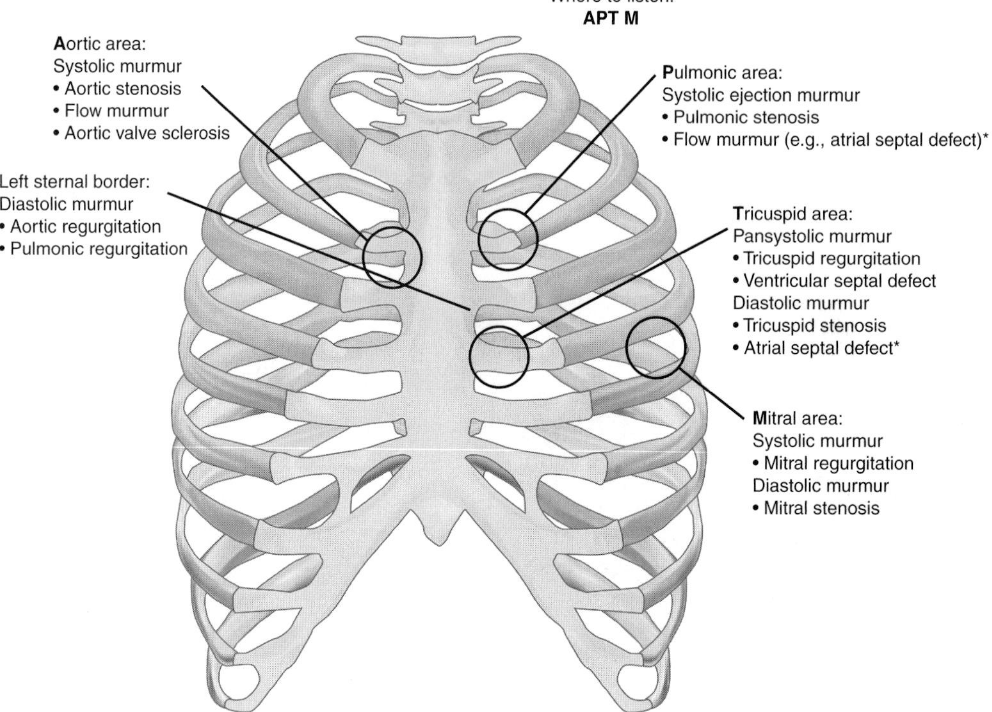

*ASD commonly presents with a pulmonary flow murmur (↑ flow through pulmonary valve) and a diastolic rumble (↑ flow across tricuspid). The murmur later progresses to a louder diastolic murmur of pulmonic regurgitation from dilatation of the pulmonary artery.

Cardiac output (CO)

Cardiac output (CO) = (stroke volume) × (heart rate).
Fick principle:

$$CO = \frac{\text{rate of } O_2 \text{ consumption}}{\text{arterial } O_2 \text{ content} - \text{venous } O_2 \text{ content}}$$

$$\text{Mean arterial pressure} = \begin{pmatrix}\text{cardiac}\\ \text{output}\end{pmatrix} \times \begin{pmatrix}\text{total peripheral}\\ \text{resistance}\end{pmatrix}$$

MAP = ⅔ diastolic pressure + ⅓ systolic pressure.
Pulse pressure = systolic pressure – diastolic pressure.
Pulse pressure is proportion to stroke volume.

$$SV = \frac{CO}{HR} = EDV - ESV$$

During exercise, CO ↑ initially as a result of an ↑ in SV. After prolonged exercise, CO ↑ as a result of an ↑ in HR.
If HR is too high, diastolic filling is incomplete and CO ↓ (e.g., ventricular tachycardia).

Cardiac output variables	**S**troke **V**olume affected by **C**ontractility, **A**fterload, and **P**reload. ↑ SV when ↑ preload, ↓ afterload, or ↑ contractility. Contractility (and SV) ↑ with: 1. Catecholamines (↑ activity of Ca^{2+} pump in sarcoplasmic reticulum) 2. ↑ intracellular calcium 3. ↓ extracellular sodium 4. Digitalis (↑ intracellular Na^+, resulting in ↑ Ca^{2+}) Contractility (and SV) ↓ with: 1. β_1 blockade 2. Heart failure 3. Acidosis 4. Hypoxia/hypercapnea 5. Non-dihydropyridine Ca^{2+} channel blockers	**SV CAP.** SV ↑ in anxiety, exercise, and pregnancy. A failing heart has ↓ SV. Myocardial O_2 demand is ↑ by: 1. ↑ afterload (∝ arterial pressure) 2. ↑ contractility 3. ↑ heart rate 4. ↑ heart size (↑ wall tension)
Preload and afterload	Preload = ventricular EDV. Afterload = mean arterial pressure (proportional to peripheral resistance). Venodilators (e.g., nitroglycerin) ↓ preload. Vasodilators (e.g., hydralazine) ↓ afterload.	Preload ↑ with exercise (slightly), ↑ blood volume (overtransfusion), and excitement (sympathetics). Preload pumps up the heart.
Starling curve	Force of contraction is proportional to initial length of cardiac muscle fiber (preload).	

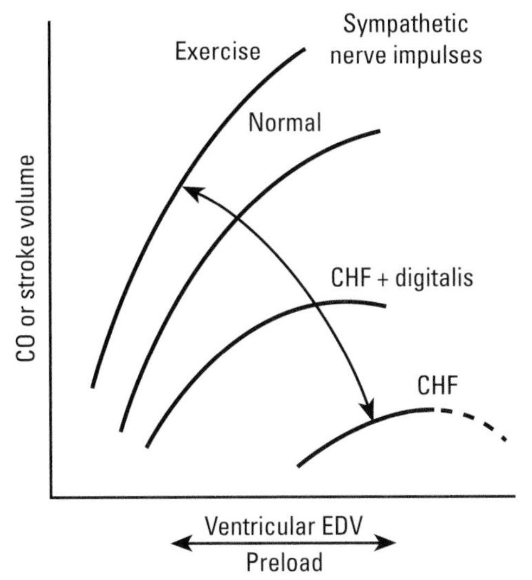

CONTRACTILE STATE OF MYOCARDIUM

⊕	⊖
Circulating catecholamines	Pharmacologic depressants
Digitalis	Loss of myocardium (MI)
Sympathetic stimulation	

Ejection fraction (EF)

$$EF = \frac{SV}{EDV} = \frac{EDV - ESV}{EDV}$$

EF is an index of ventricular contractility.
EF is normally ≥ 55%.

Resistance, pressure, flow

$\Delta P = Q \times R$

Similar to Ohm's law: $\Delta V = IR$.

$$\text{Resistance} = \frac{\text{driving pressure } (\Delta P)}{\text{flow } (Q)} = \frac{8\eta \text{ (viscosity)} \times \text{length}}{\pi r^4}$$

Viscosity depends mostly on hematocrit.

Viscosity ↑ in:

1. Polycythemia
2. Hyperproteinemic states (e.g., multiple myeloma)
3. Hereditary spherocytosis

Resistance is directly proportional to viscosity and inversely proportional to the radius to the 4th power.

Arterioles account for most of total peripheral resistance → regulate capillary flow.

Cardiac and vascular function curves

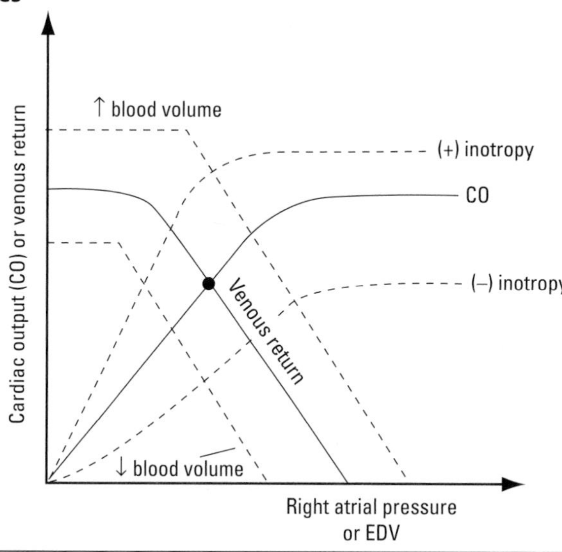

Cardiac cycle

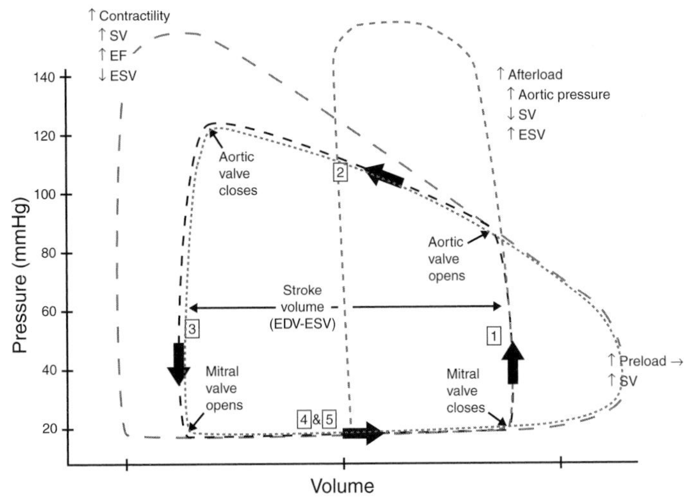

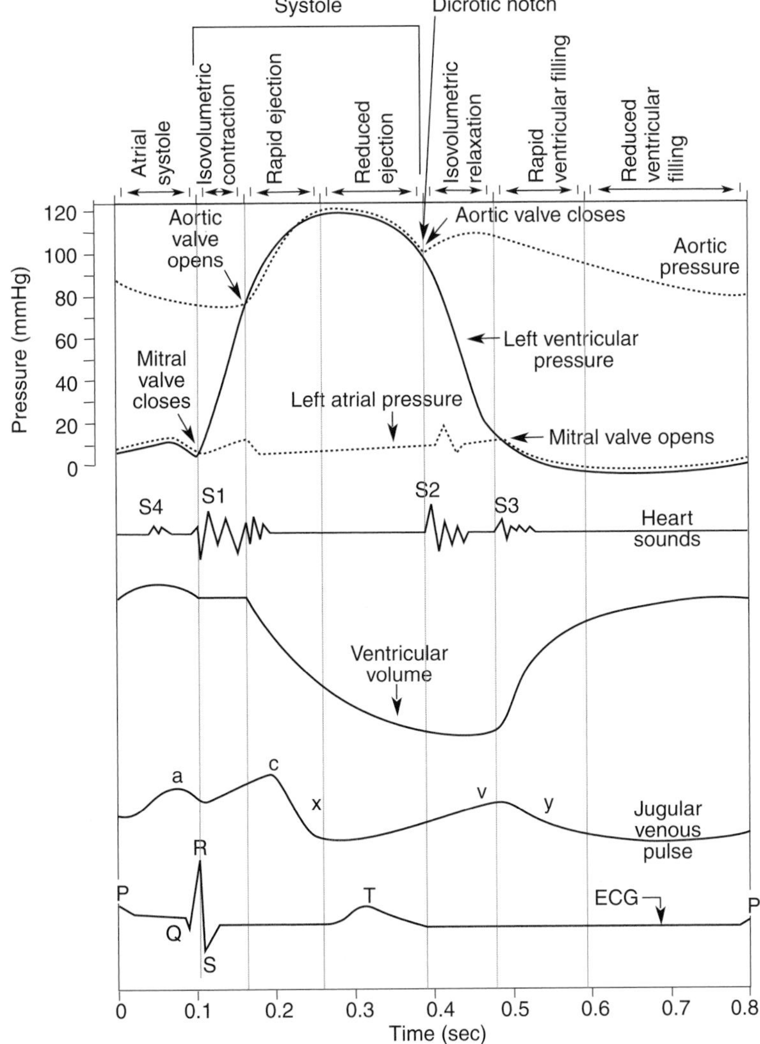

(Adapted, with permission, from Ganong WF. *Review of Medical Physiology,* 22nd ed. New York: McGraw-Hill, 2005.)

Phases—left ventricle:

1. Isovolumetric contraction—period between mitral valve closure and aortic valve opening; period of highest O_2 consumption
2. Systolic ejection—period between aortic valve opening and closing
3. Isovolumetric relaxation—period between aortic valve closing and mitral valve opening
4. Rapid filling—period just after mitral valve opening
5. Reduced filling—period just before mitral valve closure

Sounds:

S1—mitral and tricuspid valve closure. Loudest at mitral area.

S2—aortic and pulmonary valve closure. Loudest at left sternal border.

S3—in early diastole during rapid ventricular filling phase. Associated with ↑ filling pressures and more common in dilated ventricles (but normal in children).

S4 ("atrial kick")—high atrial pressure. Associated with ventricular hypertrophy.

a wave—**a**trial contraction.

c wave—RV **c**ontraction (tricuspid valve bulging into atrium).

v wave—↑ atrial pressure due to filling against closed tricuspid **v**alve.

S2 splitting: aortic valve closes before pulmonic; inspiration ↑ this difference.

Normal:
Expiration | || (S_1 A_2 P_2)
Inspiration | | |

Wide splitting (associated with pulmonic stenosis):
Expiration | | | (S_1 A_2 P_2)
Inspiration | | |

Fixed splitting (associated with ASD):
Expiration | | | (S_1 A_2 P_2)
Inspiration | | |

Paradoxical splitting (associated with aortic stenosis):
Expiration | | | (S_1 P_2 A_2)
Inspiration | ||

Heart murmurs

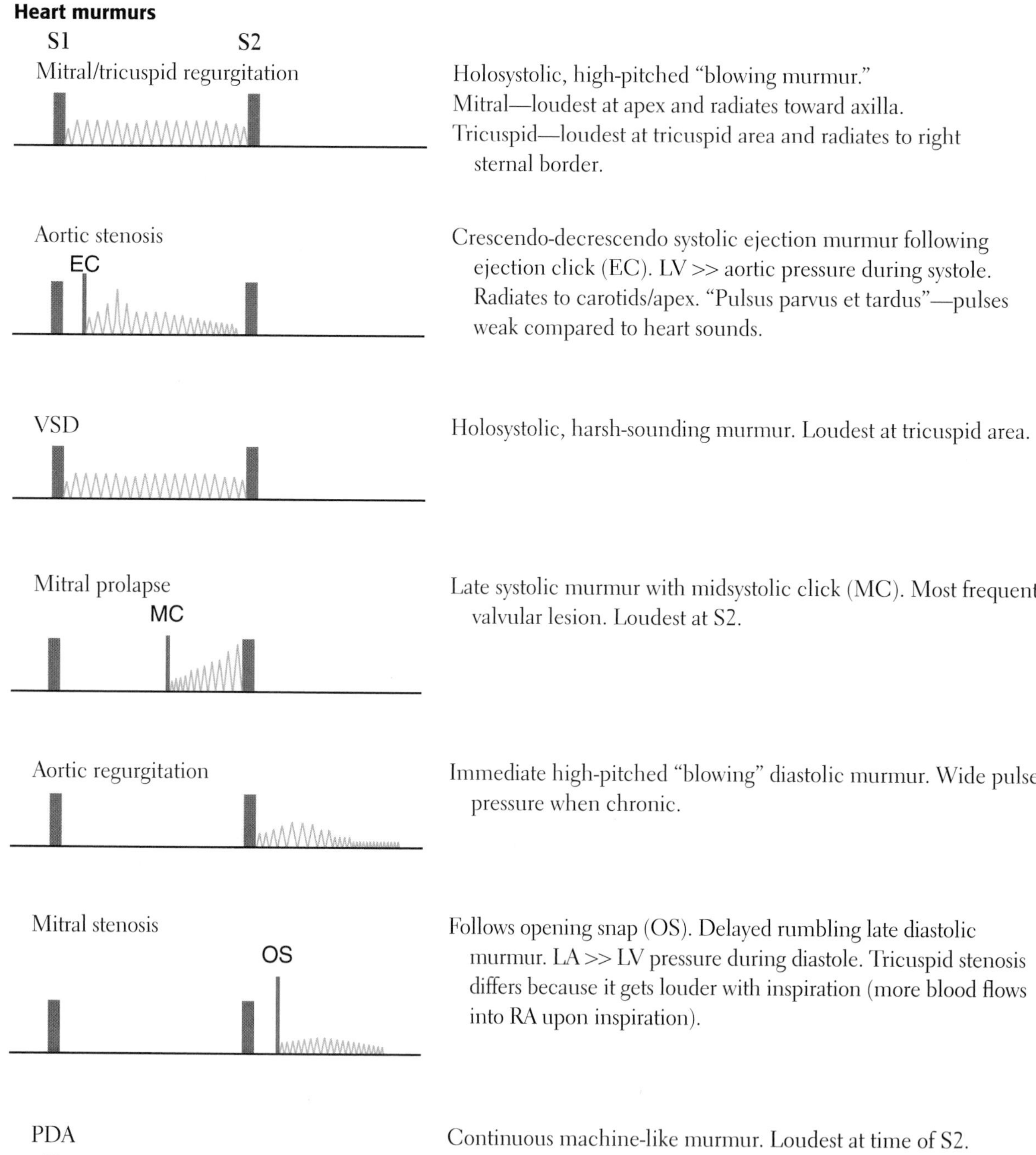

Murmur	Description
Mitral/tricuspid regurgitation	Holosystolic, high-pitched "blowing murmur." Mitral—loudest at apex and radiates toward axilla. Tricuspid—loudest at tricuspid area and radiates to right sternal border.
Aortic stenosis	Crescendo-decrescendo systolic ejection murmur following ejection click (EC). LV >> aortic pressure during systole. Radiates to carotids/apex. "Pulsus parvus et tardus"—pulses weak compared to heart sounds.
VSD	Holosystolic, harsh-sounding murmur. Loudest at tricuspid area.
Mitral prolapse	Late systolic murmur with midsystolic click (MC). Most frequent valvular lesion. Loudest at S2.
Aortic regurgitation	Immediate high-pitched "blowing" diastolic murmur. Wide pulse pressure when chronic.
Mitral stenosis	Follows opening snap (OS). Delayed rumbling late diastolic murmur. LA >> LV pressure during diastole. Tricuspid stenosis differs because it gets louder with inspiration (more blood flows into RA upon inspiration).
PDA	Continuous machine-like murmur. Loudest at time of S2.

Cardiac myocyte physiology

Cardiac muscle contraction is dependent on extracellular calcium, which enters the cells during plateau of action potential and stimulates calcium release from the cardiac muscle sarcoplasmic reticulum (calcium-induced calcium release).

In contrast to skeletal muscle:

1. Cardiac muscle action potential has a plateau, which is due to Ca^{2+} influx
2. Cardiac nodal cells spontaneously depolarize, resulting in automaticity
3. Cardiac myocytes are electrically coupled to each other by gap junctions

Ventricular action potential

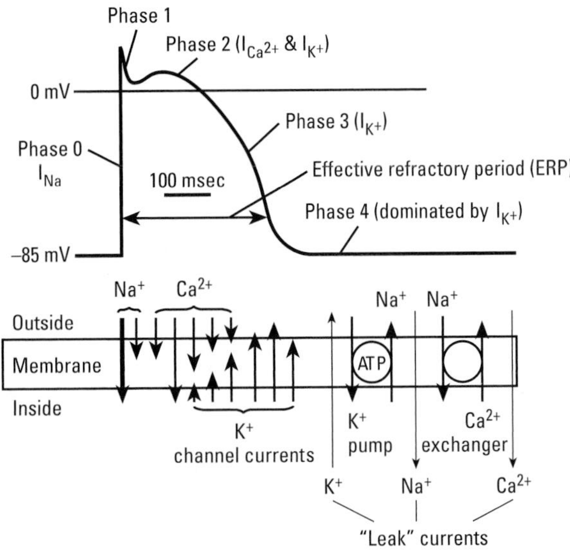

Occurs in atrial and ventricular myocytes and Purkinje fibers.

Phase 0 = rapid upstroke—voltage-gated Na^+ channels open.

Phase 1 = initial repolarization—inactivation of voltage-gated Na^+ channels. Voltage-gated K^+ channels begin to open.

Phase 2 = plateau—Ca^{2+} influx through voltage-gated Ca^{2+} channels balances K^+ efflux. Ca^{2+} influx triggers Ca^{2+} release from sarcoplasmic reticulum and myocyte contraction.

Phase 3 = rapid repolarization—massive K^+ efflux due to opening of voltage-gated slow K^+ channels and closure of voltage-gated Ca^{2+} channels.

Phase 4 = resting potential—high K^+ permeability through K^+ channels.

Pacemaker action potential

Occurs in the SA and AV nodes. Key differences from the ventricular action potential include:

Phase 0 = upstroke—opening of voltage-gated Ca^{2+} channels. These cells lack fast voltage-gated Na^+ channels. Results in a slow conduction velocity that is used by the AV node to prolong transmission from the atria to ventricles.

Phase 2 = plateau is absent.

Phase 3 = inactivation of the Ca^{2+} channels and ↑ activation of K^+ channels → ↑ K^+ efflux.

Phase 4 = slow diastolic depolarization—membrane potential spontaneously depolarizes as Na^+ conductance ↑ (I_f different from I_{Na} above). Accounts for automaticity of SA and AV nodes. The slope of phase 4 in the SA node determines heart rate. ACh ↓ the rate of diastolic depolarization and ↓ heart rate, while catecholamines ↑ depolarization and ↑ heart rate.

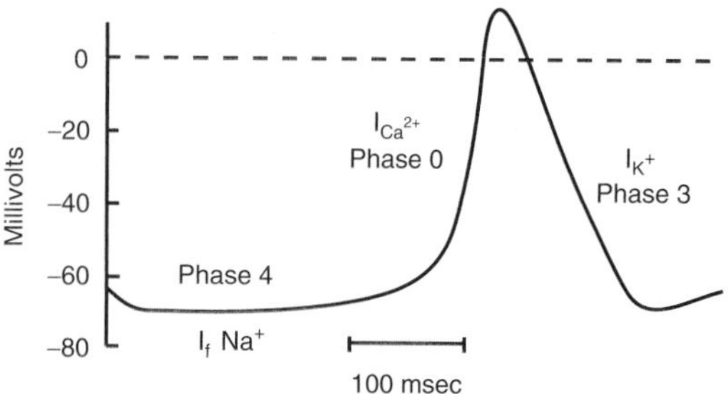

(Adapted, with permission, from Ganong WF. *Review of Medical Physiology,* 22nd ed. New York: McGraw-Hill, 2005.)

Electrocardiogram

P wave—atrial depolarization.
PR interval—conduction delay through AV node (normally < 200 msec).
QRS complex—ventricular depolarization (normally < 120 msec).
QT interval—mechanical contraction of the ventricles.
T wave—ventricular repolarization.
Atrial repolarization is masked by QRS complex.
ST segment—isoelectric, ventricles depolarized.
U wave—caused by hypokalemia, bradycardia.

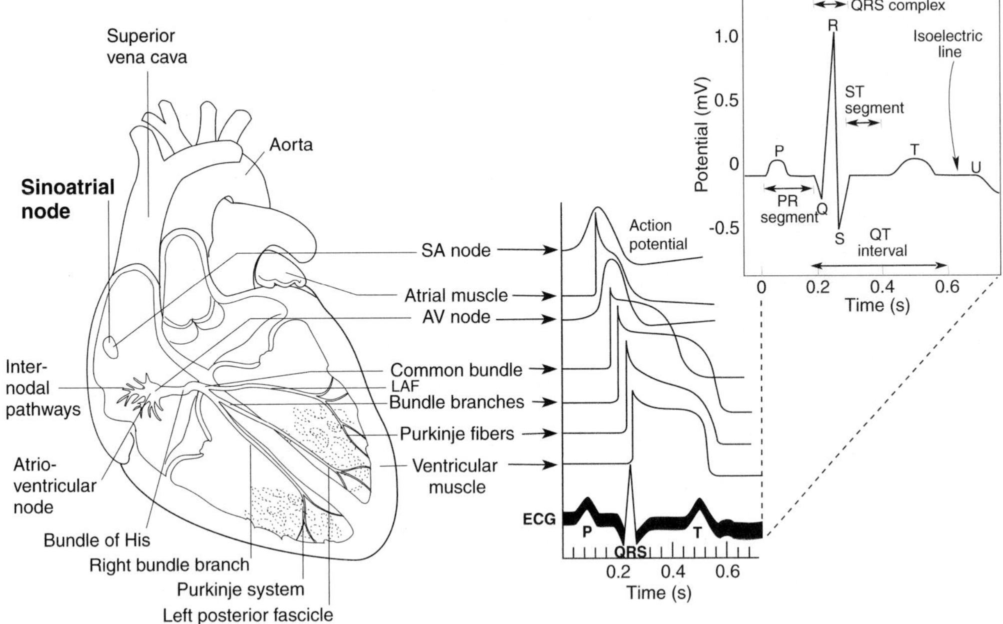

SA node "pacemaker" inherent dominance with slow phase of upstroke
AV node - 100-msec delay - atrioventricular delay

(Adapted, with permission, from Ganong WF. *Review of Medical Physiology,* 22nd ed. New York: McGraw-Hill, 2005: 548, 550.)

Torsades des pointes

Ventricular tachycardia characterized by shifting sinusoidal waveforms on ECG. Can progress to V-fib. Anything that prolongs the QT interval can predispose to torsades des pointes.

Wolff-Parkinson-White syndrome

δ wave

Accessory conduction pathway from atria to ventricle (bundle of Kent), bypassing AV node. As a result, ventricles begin to partially depolarize earlier, giving rise to characteristic delta wave on ECG. May result in reentry current leading to supraventricular tachycardia.

ECG tracings

Atrial fibrillation Chaotic and erratic baseline (irregularly irregular) with no discrete P waves in between irregularly spaced QRS complexes.

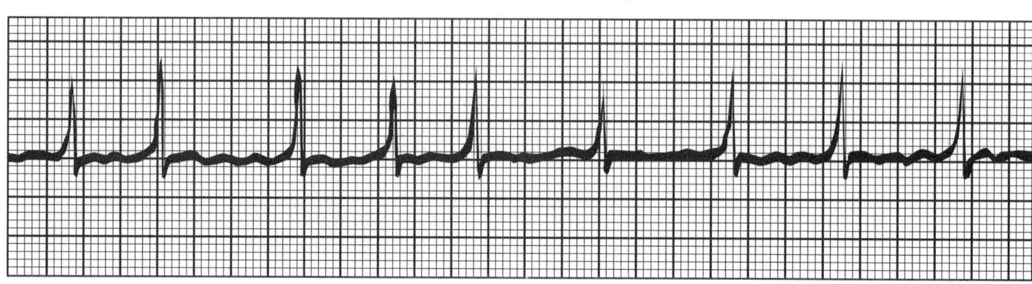

Atrial flutter A rapid succession of identical, back-to-back atrial depolarization waves. The identical appearance accounts for the "sawtooth" appearance of the flutter waves.

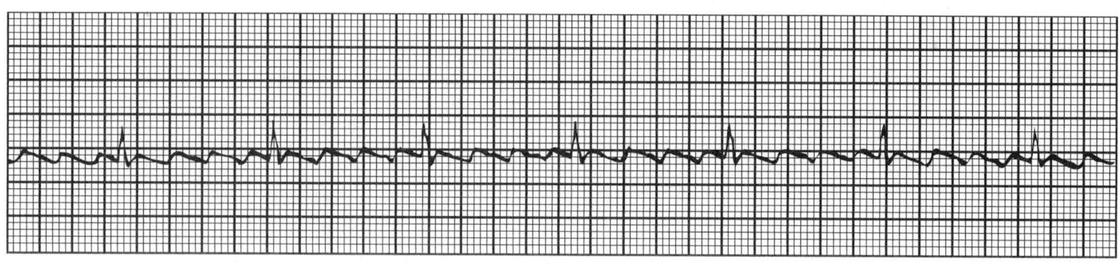

AV block

1st degree The PR interval is prolonged (> 200 msec). Asymptomatic.

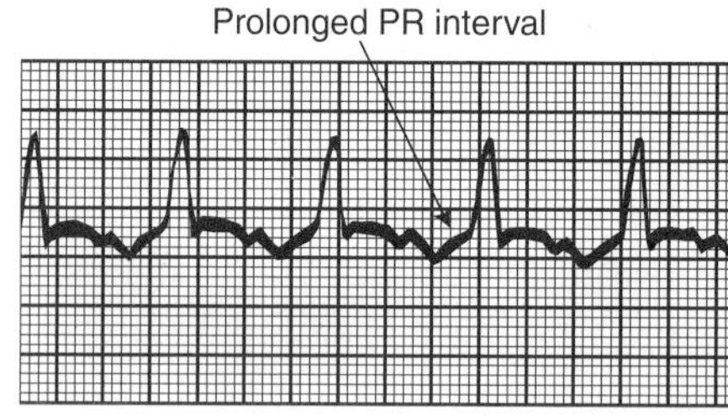

2nd degree

Mobitz type I (Wenckebach) Progressive lengthening of the PR interval until a beat is "dropped" (a P wave not followed by a QRS complex). Usually asymptomatic.

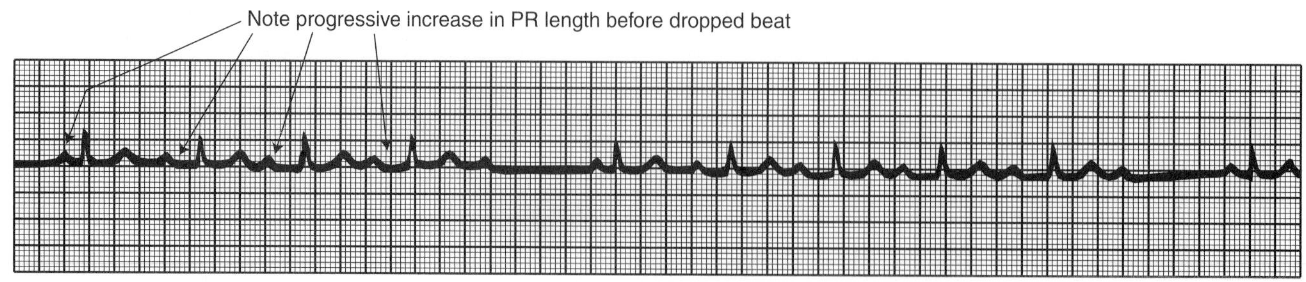

ECG tracings *(continued)*

Mobitz type II — Dropped beats that are not preceded by a change in the length of the PR interval (as in type I). These abrupt, nonconducted P waves result in a pathologic condition. It is often found as 2:1 block, where there are 2 P waves to 1 QRS response. May progress to 3rd-degree block.

No QRS following P wave, normal PR intervals

3rd degree (complete) — The atria and ventricles beat independently of each other. Both P waves and QRS complexes are present, although the P waves bear no relation to the QRS complexes. The atrial rate is faster than the ventricular rate. Usually treat with pacemaker.

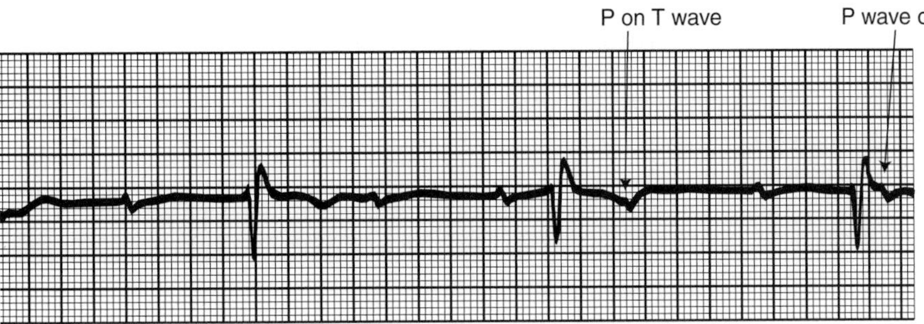

Ventricular fibrillation — A completely erratic rhythm with no identifiable waves. Fatal arrhythmia without immediate CPR and defibrillation.

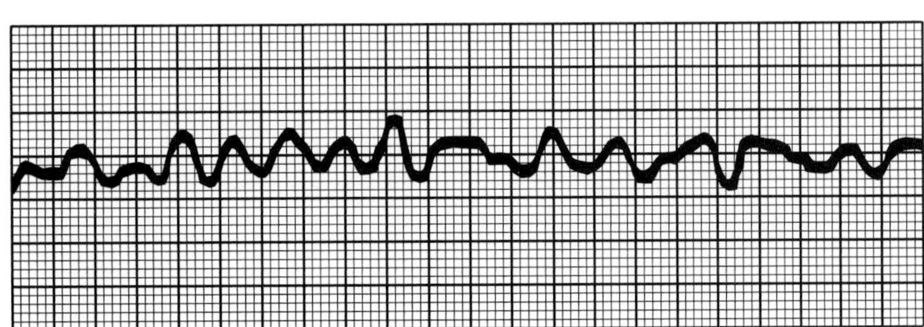

(Adapted, with permission, from Hurst JW. *Introduction to Electrocardiography.* New York: McGraw-Hill, 2001.)

Control of mean arterial pressure

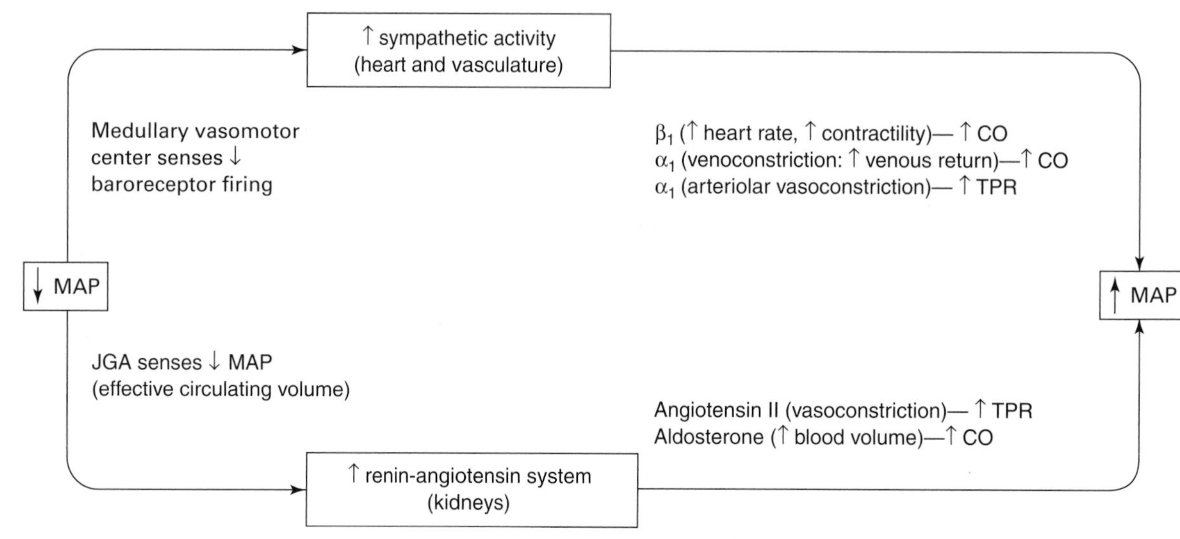

Baroreceptors and chemoreceptors

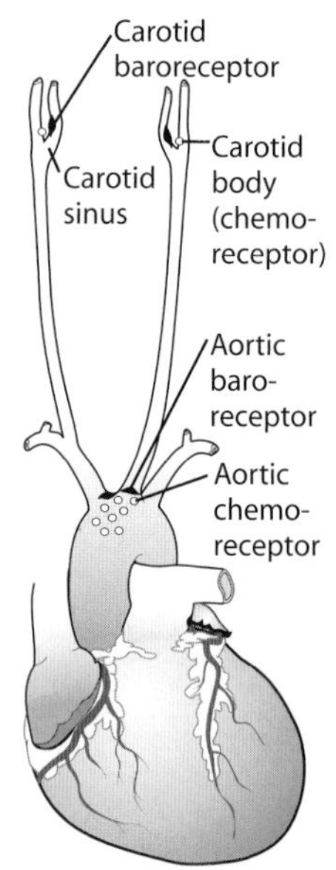

Receptors:

1. Aortic arch transmits via vagus nerve to medulla (responds only to ↑ BP)
2. Carotid sinus transmits via glossopharyngeal nerve to medulla (responds to ↓ and ↑ in BP).

Baroreceptors:

1. Hypotension—↓ arterial pressure → ↓ stretch → ↓ afferent baroreceptor firing → ↑ efferent sympathetic firing and ↓ efferent parasympathetic stimulation → vasoconstriction, ↑ HR, ↑ contractility, ↑ BP. Important in the response to severe hemorrhage.
2. Carotid massage—↑ pressure on carotid artery → ↑ stretch → ↑ afferent baroreceptor firing → ↓ HR.

Chemoreceptors:

1. Peripheral—carotid and aortic bodies respond to ↓ P_{O_2} (< 60 mmHg), ↑ P_{CO_2}, and ↓ pH of blood.
2. Central—respond to changes in pH and P_{CO_2} of brain interstitial fluid, which in turn are influenced by arterial CO_2. Do not directly respond to P_{O_2}. Responsible for Cushing reaction— ↑ intracranial pressure constricts arterioles → cerebral ischemia → hypertension (sympathetic response) and reflex bradycardia. Note: Cushing triad = hypertension, bradycardia, respiratory depression.

Circulation through organs

Liver	Largest share of systemic cardiac output.
Kidney	Highest blood flow per gram of tissue.
Heart	Large arteriovenous O_2 difference. ↑ O_2 demand is met by ↑ coronary blood flow, not by ↑ extraction of O_2.

Normal pressures

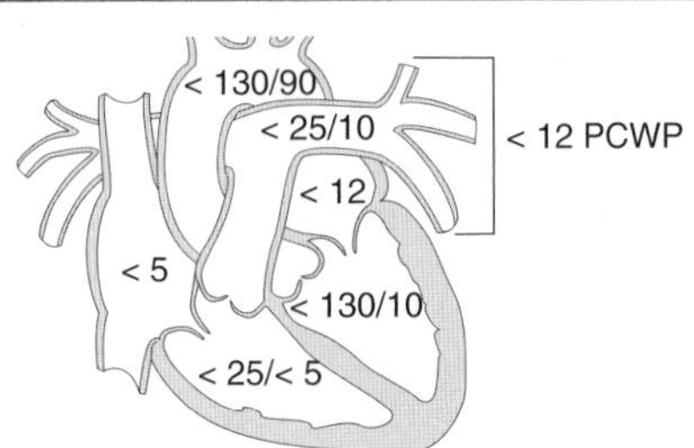

PCWP—pulmonary capillary wedge pressure (in mmHg) is a good approximation of left atrial pressure.
Measured with Swan-Ganz catheter.

Autoregulation

Organ	Factors determining autoregulation
Heart	Local metabolites—O_2, adenosine, NO
Brain	Local metabolites—CO_2 (pH)
Kidneys	Myogenic and tubuloglomerular feedback
Lungs	Hypoxia causes vasoconstriction
Skeletal muscle	Local metabolites—lactate, adenosine, K^+
Skin	Sympathetic stimulation most important mechanism—temperature control

Note: the pulmonary vasculature is unique in that hypoxia causes vasoconstriction. In other organs, hypoxia causes vasodilation.

Capillary fluid exchange

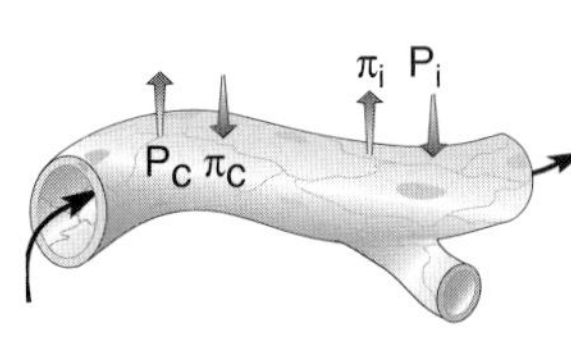

Starling forces determine fluid movement through capillary membranes:

1. P_c = capillary pressure—pushes fluid out of capillary
2. P_i = interstitial fluid pressure—pushes fluid into capillary
3. π_c = plasma colloid osmotic pressure—pulls fluid into capillary
4. π_i = interstitial fluid colloid osmotic pressure—pulls fluid out of capillary

Thus, net filtration pressure = $P_{net} = [(P_c - P_i) - (\pi_c - \pi_i)]$.
K_f = filtration constant (capillary permeability).
Net fluid flow = $(P_{net})(K_f)$.
Edema—excess fluid outflow into interstitium commonly caused by:

1. ↑ capillary pressure (↑ P_c; heart failure)
2. ↓ plasma proteins (↓ π_c; nephrotic syndrome, liver failure)
3. ↑ capillary permeability (↑ K_f; toxins, infections, burns)
4. ↑ interstitial fluid colloid osmotic pressure (↑ π_i; lymphatic blockage)

▶ CARDIOVASCULAR–PATHOLOGY

Congenital heart disease

Right-to-left shunts (early cyanosis)—"blue babies"

1. Tetralogy of Fallot (most common cause of early cyanosis)
2. Transposition of great vessels
3. Truncus arteriosus
4. Tricuspid atresia
5. Total anomalous pulmonary venous return (TAPVR)

The **5 T**'s:
Tetralogy
Transposition
Truncus
Tricuspid
TAPVR
Children may squat to ↑ systemic vascular resistance.

Left-to-right shunts (late cyanosis)—"blue kids"

1. VSD (most common congenital cardiac anomaly)
2. ASD (loud S1; wide, fixed split S2)
3. PDA (close with indomethacin)

Frequency—VSD > ASD > PDA.
↑ pulmonary resistance due to arteriolar thickening.
→ progressive pulmonary hypertension; right-to-left shunt (Eisenmenger's).

Eisenmenger's syndrome

Uncorrected VSD, ASD, or PDA leads to progressive pulmonary hypertension. As pulmonary resistance ↑, the shunt reverses from L → R to R → L, which causes late cyanosis (clubbing and polycythemia).

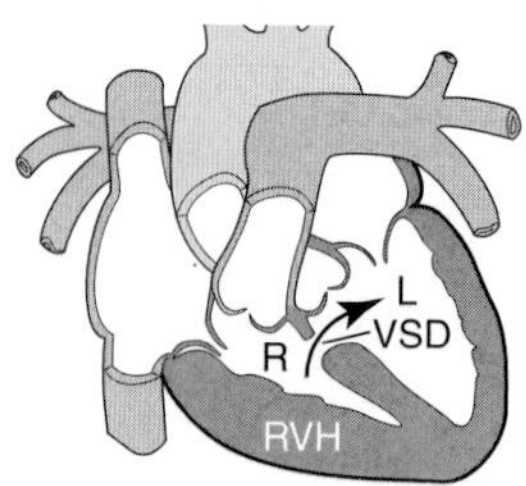

Tetralogy of Fallot

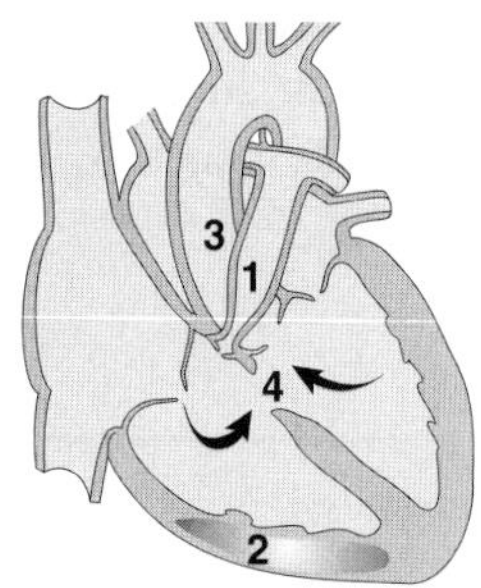

1. **P**ulmonary stenosis (most important determinant for prognosis)
2. **RV**H
3. **O**verriding aorta (overrides the VSD)
4. **V**SD

Early cyanosis is caused by a right-to-left shunt across the VSD. On x-ray, boot-shaped heart due to RVH. Patients suffer "cyanotic spells."

Tetralogy of Fallot is caused by anterosuperior displacement of the infundibular septum.

PROVe.

Patient learns to squat to improve symptoms: compression of femoral arteries ↑ pressure, thereby ↓ the right-to-left shunt and directing more blood from the RV to the lungs.

Transposition of great vessels

Aorta leaves RV (anterior) and pulmonary trunk leaves LV (posterior) → separation of systemic and pulmonary circulations. Not compatible with life unless a shunt is present to allow adequate mixing of blood (e.g., VSD, PDA, or patent foramen ovale).

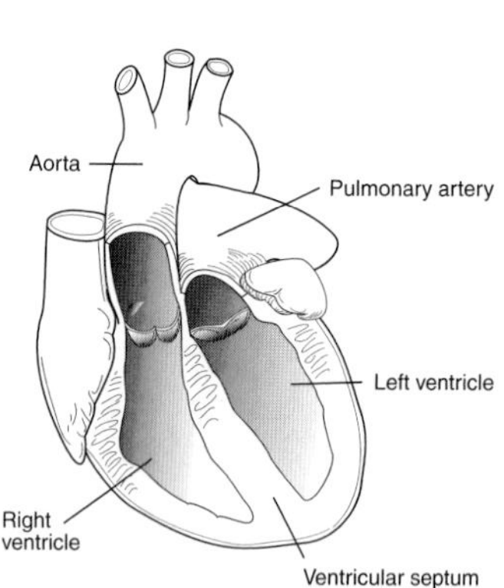

Due to failure of the aorticopulmonary septum to spiral.

Without surgical correction, most infants die within the first few months of life.

Coarctation of the aorta

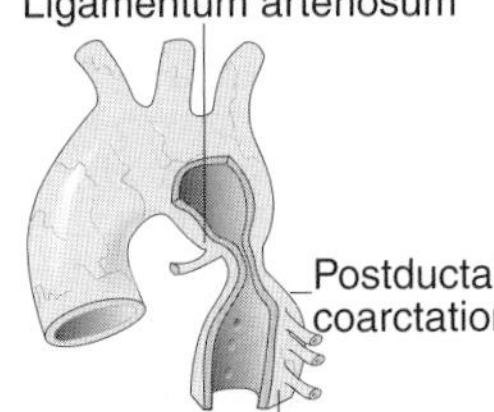

Infantile type—aortic stenosis proximal to insertion of ductus arteriosus (preductal).

Adult type—stenosis is distal to ductus arteriosus (postductal). Associated with notching of the ribs (due to collateral circulation), hypertension in upper extremities, weak pulses in lower extremities.

Associated with Turner's syndrome.

Male-to-female ratio 3:1.

Check femoral pulses on physical exam.

INfantile: **IN** close to the heart.

ADult: **D**istal to **D**uctus.

Patent ductus arteriosus

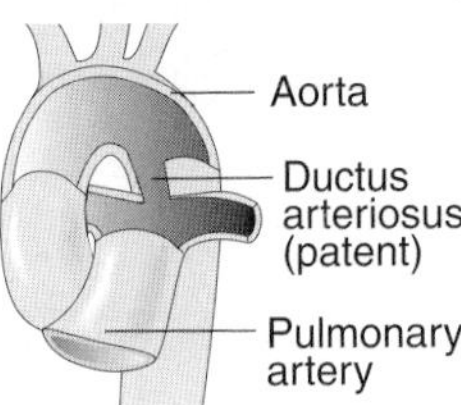

In fetal period, shunt is right to left (normal). In neonatal period, lung resistance ↓ and shunt becomes left to right with subsequent RVH and failure (abnormal). Associated with a continuous, "machine-like" murmur. Patency is maintained by PGE synthesis and low O_2 tension.

Indomethacin is used to close a PDA. PGE is used to keep a PDA open, which may be necessary to sustain life in conditions such as transposition of the great vessels.

PDA is normal in utero and normally closes only after birth.

Congenital cardiac defect associations

Disorder	Defect
22q11 syndromes	Truncus arteriosus, tetralogy of Fallot
Down syndrome	ASD, VSD, AV septal defect (endocardial cushion defect)
Congenital rubella	Septal defects, PDA, pulmonary artery stenosis
Turner's syndrome	Coarctation of aorta
Marfan's syndrome	Aortic insufficiency (late complication)
Offspring of diabetic mother	Transposition of great vessels

Hypertension

Defined as BP ≥ 140/90.

Risk factors	↑ age, obesity, diabetes, smoking, genetics, black > white > Asian.
Features	90% of hypertension is 1° (essential) and related to ↑ CO or ↑ TPR; remaining 10% mostly 2° to renal disease. Malignant hypertension is severe and rapidly progressing.
Predisposes to	Atherosclerosis, stroke, CHF, renal failure, retinopathy, and aortic dissection.

Hyperlipidemia signs

Atheromas	Plaques in blood vessel walls.
Xanthomas	Plaques or nodules composed of lipid-laden histiocytes in the skin, especially the eyelids.
Tendinous xanthoma	Lipid deposit in tendon, especially Achilles.
Corneal arcus	Lipid deposit in cornea, nonspecific (arcus senilis).

Arteriosclerosis

Mönckeberg	Calcification in the media of the arteries, especially radial or ulnar. Usually benign; "pipestem" arteries.
Arteriolosclerosis	Hyaline thickening of small arteries in essential hypertension. Hyperplastic "onion skinning" in malignant hypertension.
Atherosclerosis	Fibrous plaques and atheromas form in intima of arteries.

Aortic dissection — Longitudinal intraluminal tear forming a false lumen. Associated with hypertension or cystic medial necrosis (component of Marfan's syndrome). Presents with tearing chest pain radiating to the back. CXR shows mediastinal widening. Can result in aortic rupture and death.

Atherosclerosis — Disease of elastic arteries and large and medium-sized muscular arteries (see Color Image 79).

- Risk factors: Smoking, hypertension, diabetes mellitus, hyperlipidemia, family history.
- Progression: Endothelial cell dysfunction → macrophage and LDL accumulation → foam cell formation → fatty streaks → smooth muscle migration → fibrous plaque → complex atheromas.
- Complications: Aneurysms, ischemia, infarcts, peripheral vascular disease, thrombus, emboli.
- Location: Abdominal aorta > coronary artery > popliteal artery > carotid artery.
- Symptoms: Angina, claudication, but can be asymptomatic.

Ischemic heart disease — Possible manifestations:

1. **Angina** (CAD narrowing > 75%):
   a. Stable—mostly 2° to atherosclerosis (retrosternal chest pain with exertion)
   b. Prinzmetal's variant—occurs at rest 2° to coronary artery spasm
   c. Unstable/crescendo—thrombosis but no necrosis (worsening chest pain)
2. **Myocardial infarction**—most often acute thrombosis due to coronary artery atherosclerosis; results in myocyte necrosis
3. **Sudden cardiac death**—death from cardiac causes within 1 hour of onset of symptoms, most commonly due to a lethal arrhythmia
4. **Chronic ischemic heart disease**—progressive onset of CHF over many years due to chronic ischemic myocardial damage

Infarcts: red vs. pale — Red (hemorrhagic) infarcts occur in loose tissues with collaterals, such as liver, lungs, intestine, or liver, or following reperfusion.

Pale infarcts occur in solid tissues with single blood supply, such as heart, kidney, and spleen.

REd = **RE**perfusion.

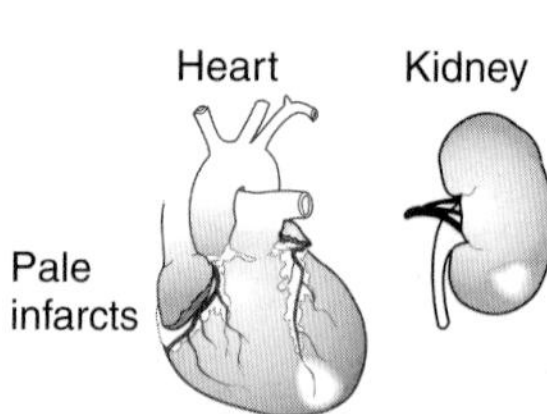

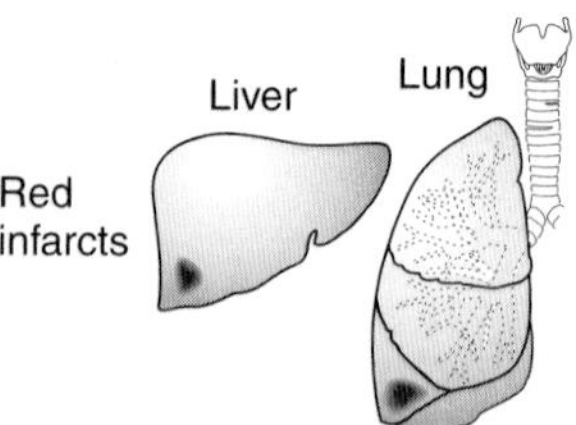

Evolution of MI

Coronary artery occlusion: LAD > RCA > circumflex.

Symptoms: diaphoresis, nausea, vomiting, severe retrosternal pain, pain in left arm and/or jaw, shortness of breath, fatigue, adrenergic symptoms (see Color Image 80).

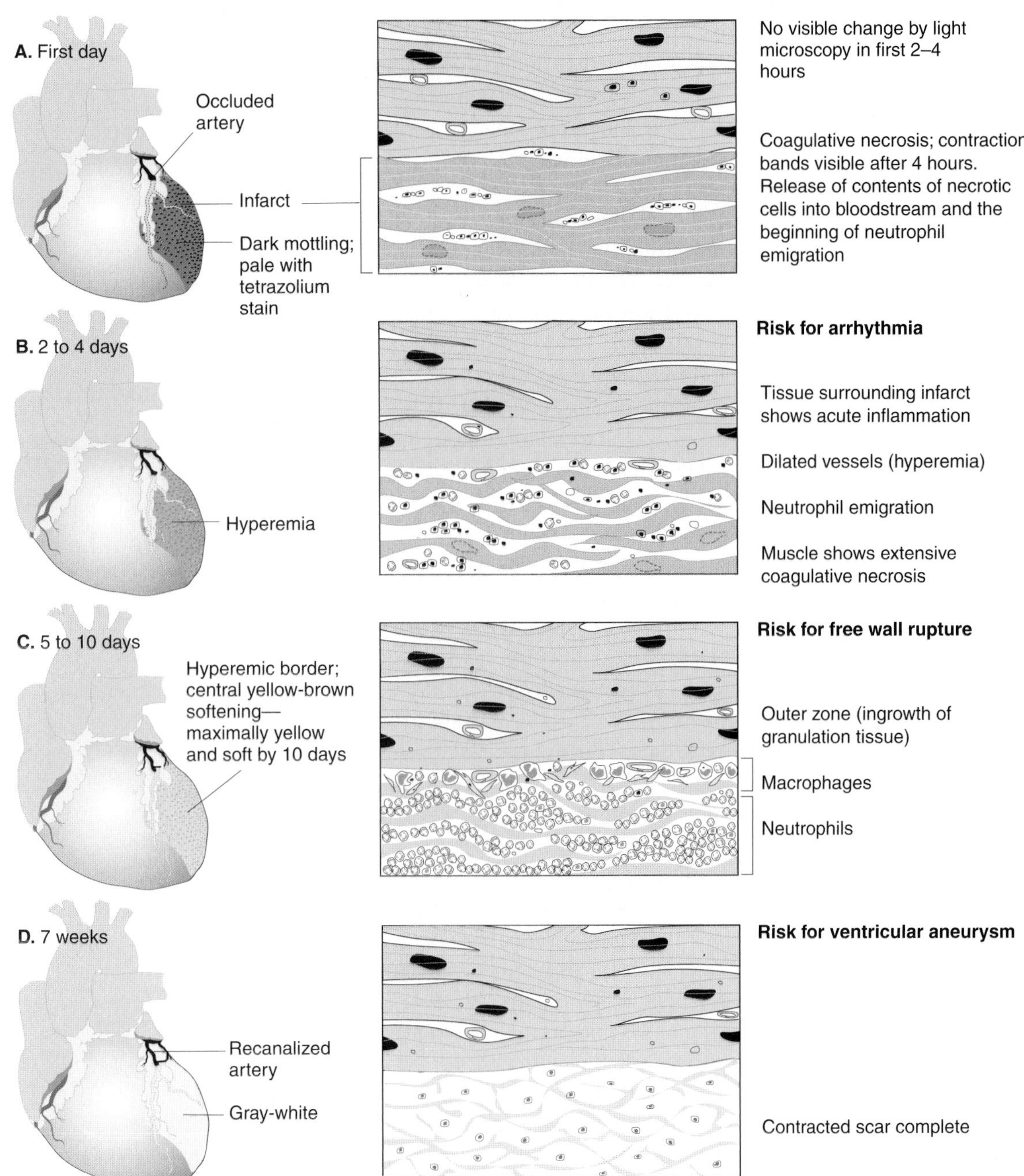

(Adapted, with permission, from Chandrasoma P. *Pathology Notes.* Stamford, CT: Appleton & Lange, 1991: 244.)

Diagnosis of MI

In the first 6 hours, ECG is the gold standard.

Cardiac troponin I rises after 4 hours and is elevated for 7–10 days; more specific than other protein markers.

CK-MB is predominantly found in myocardium but can also be released from skeletal muscle.

AST is nonspecific and can be found in cardiac, liver, and skeletal muscle cells.

ECG changes can include ST elevation (transmural infarct), ST depression (subendocardial infarct), and pathological Q waves (transmural infarct).

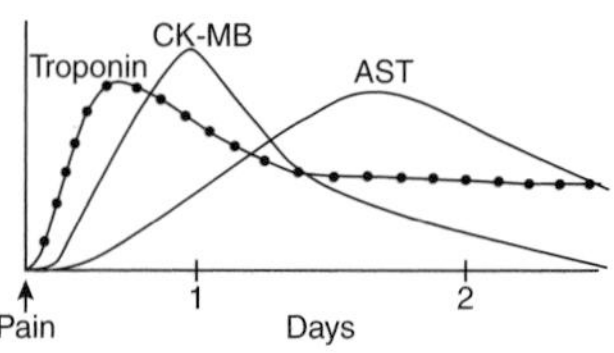

MI complications

1. Cardiac arrhythmia—important cause of death before reaching hospital; common in first few days
2. LV failure and pulmonary edema
3. Cardiogenic shock (large infarct—high risk of mortality)
4. Ventricular free wall rupture → cardiac tamponade; papillary muscle → severe mitral regurgitation; and interventricular septal rupture → VSD
5. Aneurysm formation—↓ CO, risk of arrhythmia, embolus from mural thrombus
6. Fibrinous pericarditis—friction rub (3–5 days post-MI)
7. Dressler's syndrome—autoimmune phenomenon resulting in fibrinous pericarditis (several weeks post-MI)

Cardiomyopathies

Dilated (congestive) cardiomyopathy	Most common cardiomyopathy (90% of cases). Etiologies include chronic **A**lcohol abuse, **B**eriberi, **C**oxsackie B virus myocarditis, chronic **C**ocaine use, **C**hagas' disease, **D**oxorubicin toxicity, and peripartum cardiomyopathy. Heart dilates and looks like a balloon on chest x-ray.	Systolic dysfunction ensues.
Hypertrophic cardiomyopathy	Hypertrophy often asymmetric and involving the interventricular septum. Normal heart size. 50% of cases are familial, autosomal dominant. Cause of sudden death in young athletes. Findings: loud S4, apical impulses, systolic murmur. Treat with β-blocker or non-dihydropyridine calcium channel blocker (e.g., verapamil).	Diastolic dysfunction ensues.
Restrictive/obliterative cardiomyopathy	Major causes include sarcoidosis, amyloidosis, postradiation fibrosis, endocardial fibroelastosis (thick fibroelastic tissue in endocardium of young children), Löffler's syndrome (endomyocardial fibrosis with a prominent eosinophilic infiltrate), and hemochromatosis (dilated cardiomyopathy can also occur).	Diastolic dysfunction ensues.

CHF

Abnormality	Cause
Dyspnea on exertion	Failure of LV output to ↑ during exercise.
Cardiac dilation	Greater ventricular end-diastolic volume.
Pulmonary edema, paroxysmal nocturnal dyspnea	LV failure → ↑ pulmonary venous pressure → pulmonary venous distention and transudation of fluid. Presence of hemosiderin-laden macrophages ("heart failure" cells) in the lungs.
Orthopnea (shortness of breath when supine)	↑ venous return in supine position exacerbates pulmonary vascular congestion.
Hepatomegaly (nutmeg liver)	↑ central venous pressure → ↑ resistance to portal flow. Rarely, leads to "cardiac cirrhosis."
Ankle, sacral edema	RV failure → ↑ venous pressure → fluid transudation.
Jugular venous distention	Right heart failure → ↑ venous pressure.

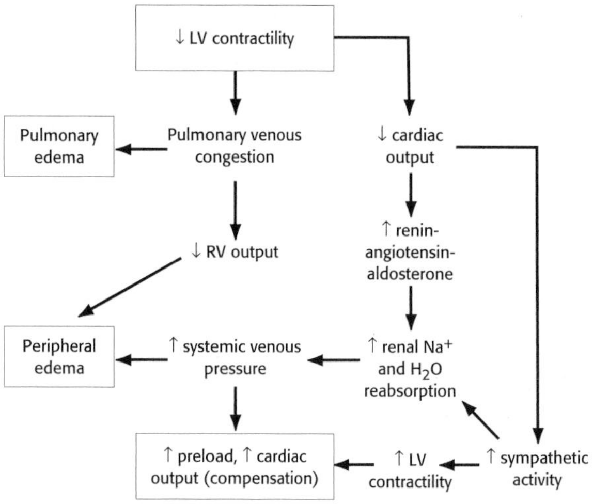

Right heart failure most often results from left heart failure. Isolated right heart failure is usually due to cor pulmonale.

Embolus types	**F**at, **A**ir, **T**hrombus, **B**acteria, **A**mniotic fluid, **T**umor. Fat emboli are associated with long bone fractures and liposuction. Amniotic fluid emboli can lead to DIC, especially postpartum. Pulmonary embolus—chest pain, tachypnea, dyspnea.	An embolus moves like a **FAT BAT.** Approximately 95% of pulmonary emboli arise from deep leg veins.
Deep venous thrombosis	Predisposed by Virchow's triad: 1. Stasis 2. Hypercoagulability 3. Endothelial damage	Can lead to pulmonary embolism.

Bacterial endocarditis	**Fever,** Roth's spots (round white spots on retina surrounded by hemorrhage), Osler's nodes (tender raised lesions on finger or toe pads), new **murmur, Janeway lesions** (small erythematous lesions on palm or sole), anemia, **splinter hemorrhages** on nail bed. Valvular damage may cause new murmur. Multiple blood cultures necessary for diagnosis (see Color Image 82). 1. Acute—*S. aureus* (high virulence). Large vegetations on previously normal valves. Rapid onset. 2. Subacute—viridans streptococcus (low virulence). Smaller vegetations on congenitally abnormal or diseased valves. Sequela of dental procedures. More insidious onset. Endocarditis may also be nonbacterial 2° to malignancy or hypercoagulable state (marantic/thrombotic endocarditis).	Mitral valve is most frequently involved. **Tri**cuspid valve endocarditis is associated with IV **drug** abuse (don't **tri drugs**). Complications: chordae rupture, glomerulonephritis, suppurative pericarditis, emboli. Bacteria **FROM JANE:** **F**ever **R**oth's spots **O**sler's nodes **M**urmur **J**aneway lesions **A**nemia **N**ail-bed hemorrhage **E**mboli
Libman-Sacks endocarditis	Verrucous vegetations occur on both sides of the valve (can be associated with mitral regurgitation and, less commonly, mitral stenosis). Seen in lupus.	**SLE** causes **LSE.**
Rheumatic heart disease	Rheumatic fever is a consequence of pharyngeal infection with group A β-hemolytic streptococci. Early deaths due to myocarditis. Late sequelae include rheumatic heart disease, which affects heart valves—mitral > aortic >> tricuspid (high-pressure valves affected most). Associated with Aschoff bodies (granuloma with giant cells), Anitschkow's cells (activated histiocytes), migratory polyarthritis, erythema marginatum, elevated ASO titers. Immune mediated (type II hypersensitivity); not direct effect of bacteria (see Color Image 85).	**FEVERSS:** **F**ever **E**rythema marginatum **V**alvular damage (vegetation and fibrosis) **E**SR ↑ **R**ed-hot joints (polyarthritis) **S**ubcutaneous nodules (Aschoff bodies) **S**t. Vitus' dance (chorea)
Cardiac tamponade	Compression of heart by fluid (e.g., blood, effusions) in pericardium, leading to ↓ CO. Equilibration of diastolic pressures in all 4 chambers. Findings: hypotension, ↑ venous pressure (JVD), distant heart sounds, ↑ HR, pulsus paradoxus; ECG shows electrical alternans (beat-to-beat alternations of QRS complex height). **Pulsus paradoxus** (Kussmaul's pulse)—↓ in amplitude of pulse during inspiration. Seen in severe cardiac tamponade, asthma, obstructive sleep apnea, pericarditis, and croup.	

Pericarditis		
Serous	Caused by SLE, rheumatoid arthritis, viral infection, uremia.	
Fibrinous	Uremia, MI (Dressler's syndrome), rheumatic fever.	
Hemorrhagic	TB, malignancy (e.g., melanoma). Findings: pericardial pain, friction rub, pulsus paradoxus, distant heart sounds. Findings include ECG changes with diffuse ST-segment elevation. Can resolve without scarring or lead to chronic adhesive or chronic constrictive pericarditis.	
Syphilitic heart disease	3° syphilis disrupts the vasa vasorum of the aorta with consequent dilation of the aorta and valve ring. May see calcification of the aortic root and ascending aortic arch. Leads to "tree bark" appearance of the aorta.	Can result in aneurysm of the ascending aorta or aortic arch and aortic valve incompetence.
Cardiac tumors	Myxomas are the most common 1° cardiac tumor in adults (see Color Image 88). 90% occur in the atria (mostly LA). Myxomas are usually described as a "ball-valve" obstruction in the LA (associated with multiple syncopal episodes). Rhabdomyomas are the most frequent 1° cardiac tumor in children (associated with tuberous sclerosis). Metastases most common heart tumor (melanoma, lymphoma). Kussmaul's sign: ↑ in jugular venous pressure on inspiration.	
Telangiectasia	Arteriovenous malformation in small vessels. Looks like dilated capillary. Hereditary hemorrhagic telangiectasia (Osler-Weber-Rendu syndrome)—autosomal-dominant inheritance. Presents with nosebleeds and skin discolorations.	Affects small vessels.
Raynaud's disease	↓ blood flow to the skin due to arteriolar vasospasm in response to cold temperature or emotional stress. Most often in the fingers and toes (see Color Image 106). Called Raynaud's phenomenon when 2° to a mixed connective tissue disease, SLE, or CREST syndrome.	Affects small vessels.
Wegener's granulomatosis	Characterized by triad of focal necrotizing vasculitis, necrotizing granulomas in the **lung and upper airway,** and necrotizing glomerulonephritis.	Affects small vessels.
Symptoms	Perforation of nasal septum, chronic sinusitis, otitis media, mastoiditis, cough, dyspnea, hemoptysis, hematuria.	
Findings	**c-ANCA** is a strong marker of disease; chest x-ray may reveal large nodular densities; hematuria and red cell casts.	
Treatment	Cyclophosphamide and corticosteroids.	

Other ANCA-positive vasculitides		
Microscopic polyangiitis	Like Wegener's but lacks granulomas. **p-ANCA.**	All affect small vessels.
1° pauci-immune crescentic glomerulonephritis	Vasculitis limited to kidney. **Pauci**-immune = **paucit**y of antibodies.	
Churg-Strauss syndrome	Granulomatous vasculitis with eosinophilia. Involves lung, heart, skin, kidneys, nerves. Often seen in atopic patients. **p-ANCA.**	
Sturge-Weber disease	Congenital vascular disorder that affects capillary-sized blood vessels. Manifests with port-wine stain on face and leptomeningeal angiomatosis (intracerebral AVM).	Affects small vessels.
Henoch-Schönlein purpura	Most common form of childhood systemic vasculitis. Skin rash (palpable purpura), arthralgia, intestinal hemorrhage, abdominal pain, and melena. Follows URIs. Multiple lesions of the same age.	Affects small vessels. Common triad: 1. Skin 2. Joints 3. GI
Buerger's disease	Also known as thromboangiitis obliterans; idiopathic, segmental, thrombosing vasculitis of small and medium peripheral arteries and veins. Seen in **heavy smokers.**	Affects small and medium vessels.
Symptoms	Intermittent claudication, superficial nodular phlebitis, cold sensitivity (Raynaud's phenomenon), severe pain in affected part. May lead to gangrene.	
Treatment	Smoking cessation.	
Kawasaki disease	Acute, self-limiting disease of infants/kids. Acute necrotizing vasculitis of small/medium-sized vessels. Fever, congested conjunctiva, changes in lips/oral mucosa ("strawberry tongue"), lymphadenitis. May develop **coronary aneurysms.**	Affects small and medium vessels.
Polyarteritis nodosa	Characterized by necrotizing immune complex inflammation of medium-sized muscular arteries.	Affects medium arteries. Typically involves renal and visceral vessels. Lesions are of different ages.
Symptoms	Fever, weight loss, malaise, abdominal pain, melena, headache, myalgia, hypertension, neurologic dysfunction, cutaneous eruptions.	
Findings	Hepatitis B seropositivity in 30% of patients. Multiple aneurysms and constrictions on arteriogram. Typically not associated with ANCA.	
Treatment	Corticosteroids, cyclophosphamide.	

Takayasu's arteritis	Known as "pulseless disease"—granulomatous thickening of aortic arch and/or proximal great vessels. Associated with an ↑ ESR. Primarily affects Asian females < 40 years old. **F**ever, **A**rthritis, **N**ight sweats, **MY**algia, **SKIN** nodules, **O**cular disturbances, **W**eak pulses in upper extremities.	Affects medium and large arteries. **FAN MY SKIN On Wednesday.**
Temporal arteritis (giant cell arteritis)	Most common vasculitis that affects medium and large arteries, usually branches of carotid artery. Focal, granulomatous inflammation. Affects elderly females.	Affects medium and large arteries. **TEM**poral arteritis has signs near **TEM**ples.
Symptoms	Unilateral headache, jaw claudication, impaired vision (occlusion of ophthalmic artery).	
Findings	Associated with an ↑ ESR. Half of patients have systemic involvement and polymyalgia rheumatica.	
Treatment	High-dose steroids.	

▶ CARDIOVASCULAR–PHARMACOLOGY

Cardiovascular therapy

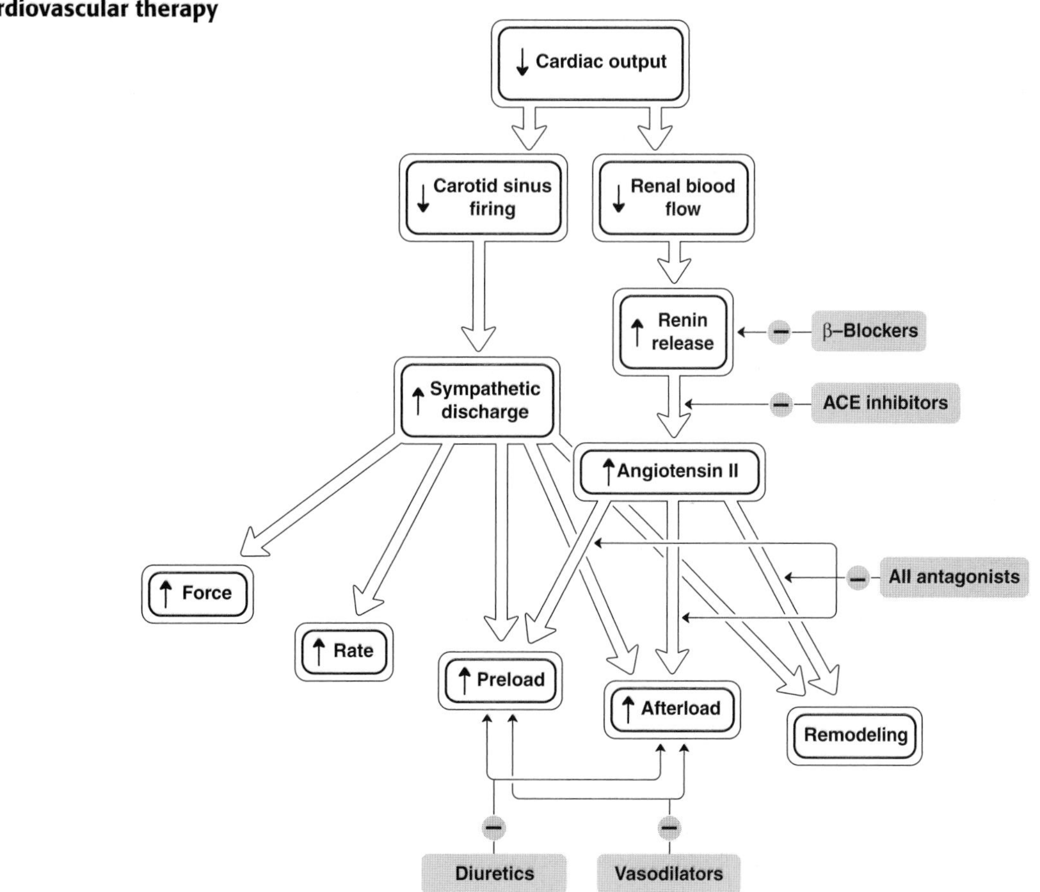

(Adapted, with permission, from Katzung BG, Trevor AJ. *USMLE Road Map: Pharmacology*, 1st ed. New York: McGraw-Hill, 2003: 39.)

Antihypertensive drugs

Drug	Adverse effects
Diuretics	
Hydrochlorothiazide	Hypokalemia, mild hyperlipidemia, hyperuricemia, lassitude, hypercalcemia, hyperglycemia
Loop diuretics	Potassium wasting, metabolic alkalosis, hypotension, ototoxicity
Sympathoplegics	
Clonidine	Dry mouth, sedation, severe rebound hypertension
Methyldopa	Sedation, positive Coombs' test
Hexamethonium	Severe orthostatic hypotension, blurred vision, constipation, sexual dysfunction
Reserpine	Sedation, depression, nasal stuffiness, diarrhea
Guanethidine	Orthostatic and exercise hypotension, sexual dysfunction, diarrhea
Prazosin	1st-dose orthostatic hypotension, dizziness, headache
β-blockers	Impotence, asthma, cardiovascular effects (bradycardia, CHF, AV block), CNS effects (sedation, sleep alterations)
Vasodilators	
Hydralazine*	Nausea, headache, lupus-like syndrome, reflex tachycardia, angina, salt retention
Minoxidil*	Hypertrichosis, pericardial effusion, reflex tachycardia, angina, salt retention
Nifedipine, verapamil	Dizziness, flushing, constipation (verapamil), AV block (verapamil), nausea
Nitroprusside	Cyanide toxicity (releases CN)
Diazoxide	Hypoglycemia (reduces insulin release, hypotension)
ACE inhibitors	
Captopril Enalapril Fosinopril	Hyperkalemia, cough, angioedema, taste changes, hypotension, pregnancy problems (fetal renal damage), rash, ↑ renin
Angiotensin II receptor inhibitors	
Losartan	Fetal renal toxicity, hyperkalemia

*Use with β-blockers to prevent reflex tachycardia, diuretic to block salt retention.

Hydralazine

Mechanism	↑ cGMP → smooth muscle relaxation. Vasodilates arterioles > veins; afterload reduction.
Clinical use	Severe hypertension, CHF. First-line therapy for hypertension in pregnancy, with methyldopa.
Toxicity	Compensatory tachycardia (contraindicated in angina/CAD), fluid retention. Lupus-like syndrome.

Minoxidil

Mechanism	K^+ channel opener—hyperpolarizes and relaxes vascular smooth muscle.
Clinical use	Severe hypertension.
Toxicity	Hypertrichosis, pericardial effusion.

Calcium channel blockers	Nifedipine, verapamil, diltiazem.
Mechanism	Block voltage-dependent L-type calcium channels of cardiac and smooth muscle and thereby reduce muscle contractility. Vascular smooth muscle—nifedipine > diltiazem > verapamil. Heart—verapamil > diltiazem > nifedipine.
Clinical use	Hypertension, angina, arrhythmias (not nifedipine), Prinzmetal's angina, Raynaud's.
Toxicity	Cardiac depression, peripheral edema, flushing, dizziness, and constipation.

Nitroglycerin, isosorbide dinitrate

Mechanism	Vasodilate by releasing nitric oxide in smooth muscle, causing ↑ in cGMP and smooth muscle relaxation. Dilate veins >> arteries. ↓ preload.
Clinical use	Angina, pulmonary edema. Also used as an aphrodisiac and erection enhancer.
Toxicity	Tachycardia, hypotension, flushing, headache, "Monday disease" in industrial exposure, development of tolerance for the vasodilating action during the work week and loss of tolerance over the weekend, resulting in tachycardia, dizziness, and headache on reexposure.

Malignant hypertension treatment

Nitroprusside	Short acting; ↑ cGMP via direct release of NO.
Fenoldopam	Dopamine D_1 receptor agonist—relaxes renal vascular smooth muscle.
Diazoxide	K^+ channel opener—hyperpolarizes and relaxes vascular smooth muscle.

Antianginal therapy

Goal—reduction of myocardial O_2 consumption (MVO_2) by decreasing 1 or more of the determinants of MVO_2: end diastolic volume, blood pressure, heart rate, contractility, ejection time.

Component	Nitrates (affect preload)	β-blockers (affect afterload)	Nitrates + β-blockers
End diastolic volume	↓	↑	No effect or ↓
Blood pressure	↓	↓	↓
Contractility	↑ (reflex response)	↓	Little/no effect
Heart rate	↑ (reflex response)	↓	↓
Ejection time	↓	↑	Little/no effect
MVO_2	↓	↓	↓↓

Calcium channel blockers—**N**ifedipine is similar to **N**itrates in effect; verapamil is similar to β-blockers in effect.

Note: Labetalol, pindolol, and acebutolol are partial agonists—contraindicated in angina.

Lipid-lowering agents

Drug	Effect on LDL "bad cholesterol"	Effect on HDL "good cholesterol"	Effect on triglycerides	Mechanisms of action	Side effects/problems
HMG-CoA reductase inhibitors (lovastatin, pravastatin, simvastatin, atorvastatin)	↓↓↓	↑	↓	Inhibit cholesterol precursor, mevalonate	Expensive, reversible ↑ LFTs, myositis
Niacin	↓↓	↑↑	↓	Inhibits lipolysis in adipose tissue; reduces hepatic VLDL secretion into circulation	Red, flushed face, which is ↓ by aspirin or long-term use
Bile acid resins (cholestyramine, colestipol)	↓↓	Slightly ↑	Slightly ↑	Prevent intestinal reabsorption of bile acids; liver must use cholesterol to make more	Patients hate it—tastes bad and causes GI discomfort, ↓ absorption of fat-soluble vitamins
Cholesterol absorption blockers (ezetimibe)	↓↓	—	—	Prevent cholesterol reabsorption at small intestine brush border	Rare ↑ LFTs
"Fibrates" (gemfibrozil, clofibrate, bezafibrate, fenofibrate)	↓	↑	↓↓↓	Upregulate LPL → ↑ TG clearance	Myositis, ↑ LFTs

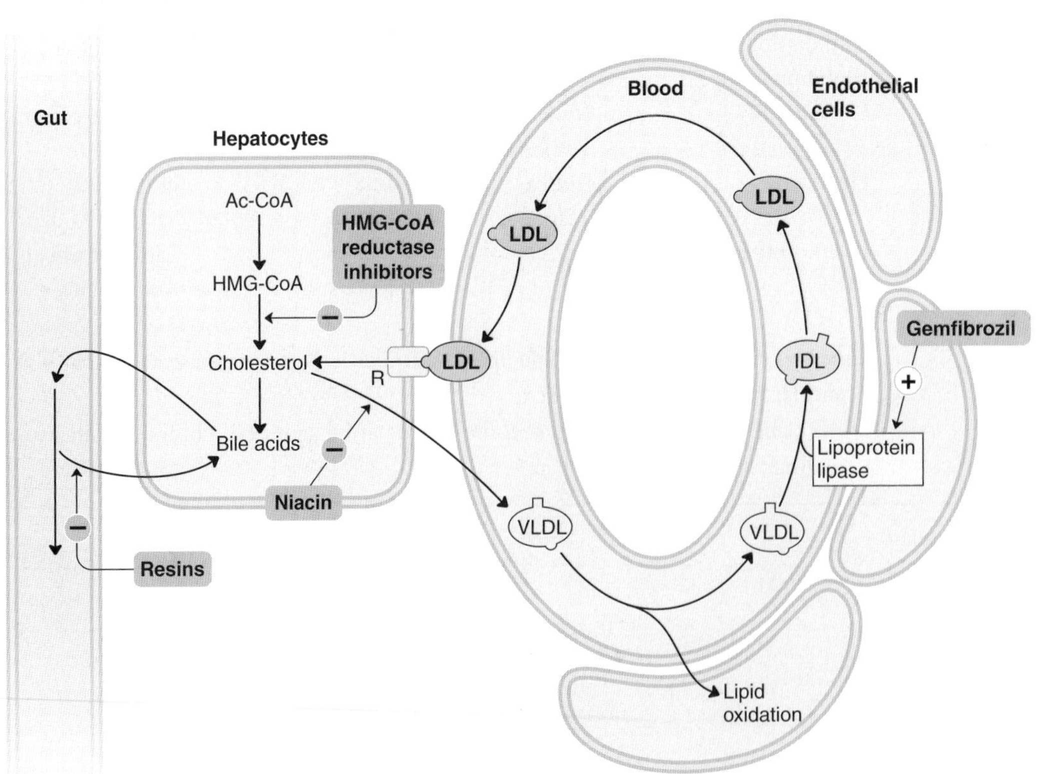

(Adapted, with permission, from Katzung BG, Trevor AJ. *USMLE Road Map: Pharmacology*, 1st ed. New York: McGraw-Hill, 2003: 56.)

Cardiac drugs: sites of action

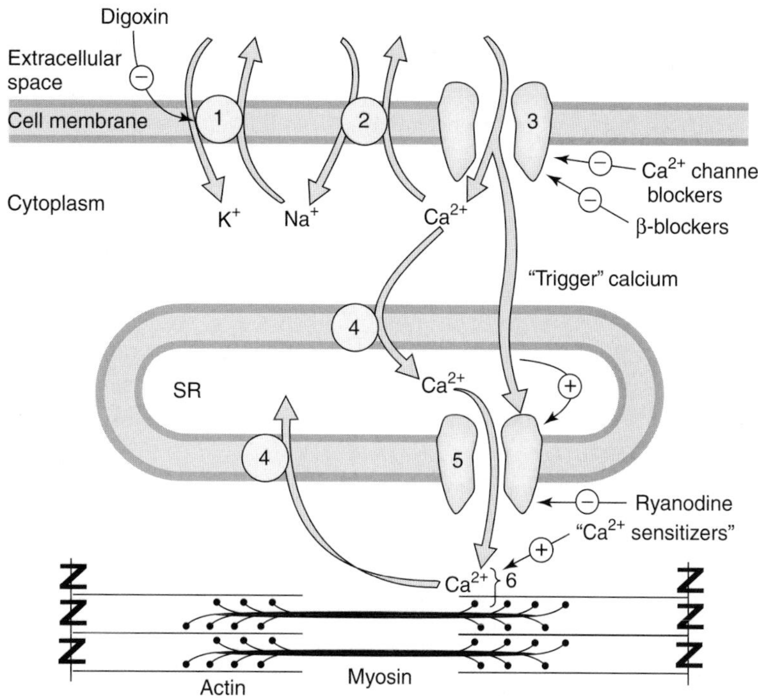

(Adapted, with permission, from Katzung BG. *Basic and Clinical Pharmacology,* 7th ed. Stamford, CT: Appleton & Lange, 1997: 198.)

Cardiac sarcomere is shown above with the cellular components involved in excitation-contraction coupling. Factors involved in excitation-contraction coupling are numbered. (1) Na^+/K^+ ATPase; (2) Na^+-Ca^{2+} exchanger; (3) voltage-gated calcium channel; (4) calcium pump in the wall of the sarcoplasmic reticulum (SR); (5) calcium release channel in the SR; (6) site of calcium interaction with troponin-tropomyosin system.

Cardiac glycosides	Digoxin—75% bioavailability, 20–40% protein bound, $t_{1/2}$ = 40 hours, urinary excretion.
Mechanism	Direct inhibition of Na^+/K^+ ATPase leads to indirect inhibition of Na^+/Ca^{2+} exchanger/antiport. ↑ $[Ca^{2+}]_i$ → positive inotropy.
Clinical use	CHF (↑ contractility); atrial fibrillation (↓ conduction at AV node and depression of SA node).
Toxicity	May cause ↑ PR, ↓ QT, scooping of ST segment, T-wave inversion of ECG. Also ↑ parasympathetic activity: nausea, vomiting, diarrhea, blurry yellow vision (think Van Gogh). Arrhythmia. Toxicities of digoxin are ↑ by renal failure (↓ excretion), hypokalemia (potentiates drug's effects), and quinidine (↓ digoxin clearance; displaces digoxin from tissue-binding sites).
Antidote	Slowly normalize K^+, lidocaine, cardiac pacer, anti-dig Fab fragments, Mg^{2+}.

Antiarrhythmics—Na^+ channel blockers (class I)

Local anesthetics. Slow or block (↓) conduction (especially in depolarized cells). ↓ slope of phase 4 depolarization and ↑ threshold for firing in abnormal pacemaker cells. Are state dependent (selectively depress tissue that is frequently depolarized, e.g., fast tachycardia).

Class IA	**Q**uinidine, **A**miodarone, **P**rocainamide, **Disopyramide**. ↑ AP duration, ↑ effective refractory period (ERP), ↑ QT interval. Affect both atrial and ventricular arrhythmias, especially reentrant and ectopic supraventricular and ventricular tachycardia. Toxicity: quinidine (cinchonism—headache, tinnitus; thrombocytopenia; torsades de pointes due to ↑ QT interval); procainamide (reversible SLE-like syndrome).	"**Q**ueen **A**my **P**roclaims Diso's **pyramid**."
Class **IB**	**Lid**ocaine, **Mexil**etine, **T**ocainide. ↓ AP duration. Affect ischemic or depolarized Purkinje and ventricular tissue. Useful in acute ventricular arrhythmias (especially post-MI) and in digitalis-induced arrhythmias. Toxicity: local anesthetic. CNS stimulation/depression, cardiovascular depression.	"I'd **B**uy **Lid**y's **Mex**ican **T**acos." Phenytoin can also fall into the IB category.
Class IC	Flecainide, encainide, propafenone. No effect on AP duration. Useful in V-tachs that progress to VF and in intractable SVT. Usually used only as last resort in refractory tachyarrhythmias. Toxicity: proarrhythmic, especially post-MI (contraindicated). Significantly prolongs refractory period in AV node.	

Hyperkalemia ↑ toxicity for all class I drugs.

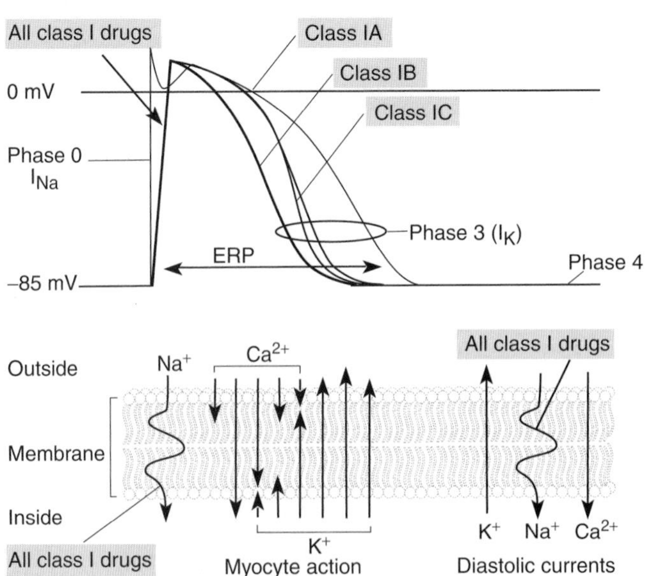

(Adapted, with permission, from Katzung BG, Trevor AJ. *Pharmacology: Examination & Board Review,* 5th ed. Stamford, CT: Appleton & Lange, 1998: 118.)

Antiarrhythmics—β-blockers (class II)	Propranolol, esmolol, metoprolol, atenolol, timolol.
Mechanism	↓ cAMP, ↓ Ca^{2+} currents. Suppress abnormal pacemakers by ↓ slope of phase 4. AV node particularly sensitive—↑ PR interval. Esmolol very short acting.
Clinical use	V-tach, SVT, slowing ventricular rate during atrial fibrillation and atrial flutter.
Toxicity	Impotence, exacerbation of asthma, cardiovascular effects (bradycardia, AV block, CHF), CNS effects (sedation, sleep alterations). May mask the signs of hypoglycemia. Metoprolol can cause dyslipidemia.

Antiarrhythmics—K^+ channel blockers (class III)	Sotalol, ibutilide, bretylium, amiodarone.	
Mechanism	↑ AP duration, ↑ ERP. Used when other antiarrhythmics fail. ↑ QT interval.	
Toxicity	Sotalol—torsades de pointes, excessive β block; ibutilide—torsades; bretylium—new arrhythmias, hypotension; amiodarone—**pulmonary fibrosis,** corneal deposits, **hepatotoxicity,** skin deposits resulting in photodermatitis, neurologic effects, constipation, cardiovascular effects (bradycardia, heart block, CHF), **hypothyroidism/ hyperthyroidism.**	Remember to check **PFT**s, **LFT**s, and **TFT**s when using amiodarone. Amiodarone is safe to use in Wolff-Parkinson-White syndrome.

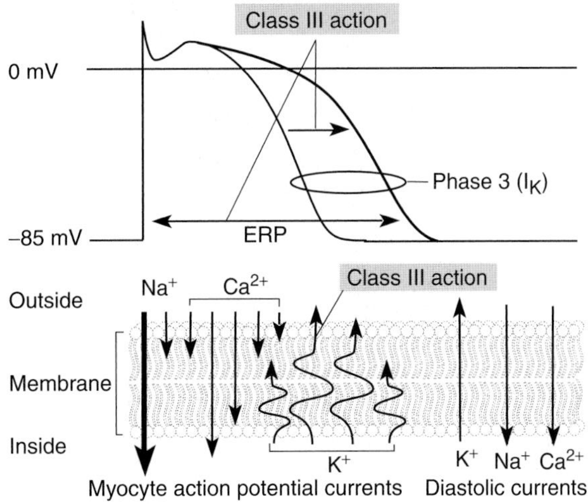

(Adapted, with permission, from Katzung BG, Trevor AJ. *Pharmacology: Examination & Board Review,* 5th ed. Stamford, CT: Appleton & Lange, 1998: 120.)

Antiarrhythmics—Ca^{2+} channel blockers (class IV) Verapamil, diltiazem.

Mechanism — Primarily affect AV nodal cells. ↓ conduction velocity, ↑ ERP, ↑ PR interval. Used in prevention of nodal arrhythmias (e.g., SVT).

Toxicity — Constipation, flushing, edema, CV effects (CHF, AV block, sinus node depression); torsades de pointes (bepridil).

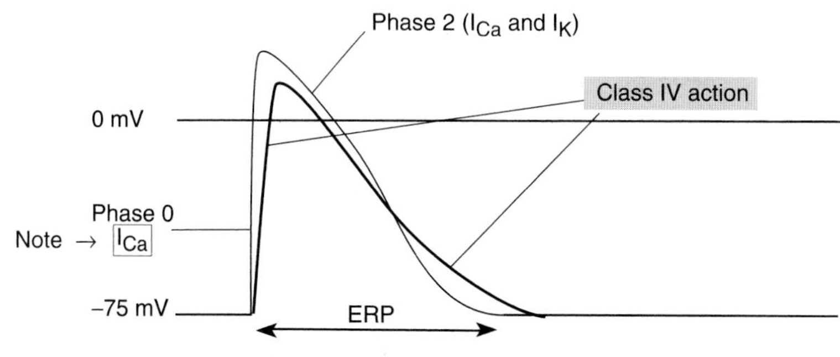

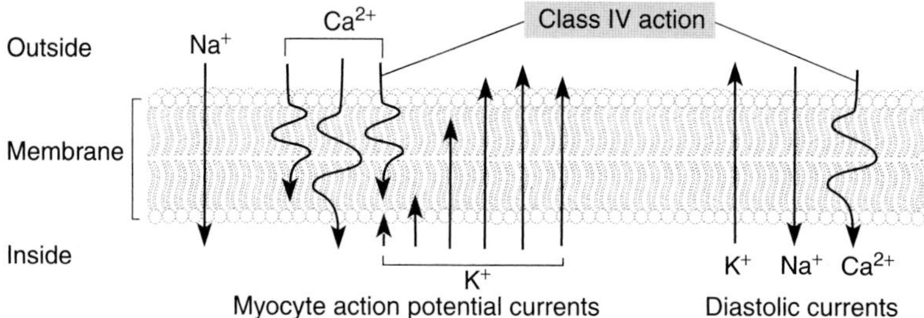

(Adapted, with permission, from Katzung BG, Trevor AJ. *Pharmacology: Examination & Board Review,* 5th ed. Stamford, CT: Appleton & Lange, 1998: 121.)

Other antiarrhythmics

Adenosine — ↑ K^+ out of cells → hyperpolarizing the cell. Drug of choice in diagnosing/abolishing AV nodal arrhythmias. Very short acting (~ 15 sec). Toxicity includes flushing, hypotension, chest pain.

K^+ — Depresses ectopic pacemakers in hypokalemia (e.g., digoxin toxicity).

Mg^{2+} — Effective in torsades de pointes and digoxin toxicity.

HIGH-YIELD SYSTEMS

Endocrine

"Chocolate causes certain endocrine glands to secrete hormones that affect your feelings and behavior by making you happy."

—Elaine Sherman, *Book of Divine Indulgences*

Woman presents with diffuse goiter and hyperthyroidism.	What are the expected values of TSH and thyroid hormones?	Low TSH and high thyroid hormones.
48-year-old woman presents with progressive lethargy and extreme sensitivity to cold temperatures.	What is the diagnosis?	Hypothyroidism.
Patient with elevated serum cortisol levels undergoes a dexamethasone suppression test. 1 mg of dexamethasone does not ↓ cortisol levels, but 8 mg does.	What is the diagnosis?	Pituitary tumor.
50-year-old man complains of diarrhea. On physical exam, his face is plethoric and a heart murmur is detected.	What is the diagnosis?	Carcinoid syndrome.
Woman of short stature presents with shortened 4th and 5th metacarpals.	What endocrine disorder comes to mind?	Albright's hereditary osteodystrophy, or pseudohypoparathyroidism.
Nondiabetic patient presents with hypoglycemia but low levels of C-peptide.	What is the diagnosis?	Surreptitious insulin injection.
Patient's MRI shows filling of sella turcica with cerebrospinal fluid.	What is the most likely clinical presentation?	Normal. Residual pituitary tissue is functional and can compensate (empty sella syndrome).
Patient complains of double vision, gynecomastia, and headaches.	What is the most likely diagnosis?	Prolactinoma.
Patient presents with hypotension and bronzed skin.	What is the most likely diagnosis?	1° adrenocortical deficiency (Addison's disease).

Adrenal cortex and medulla

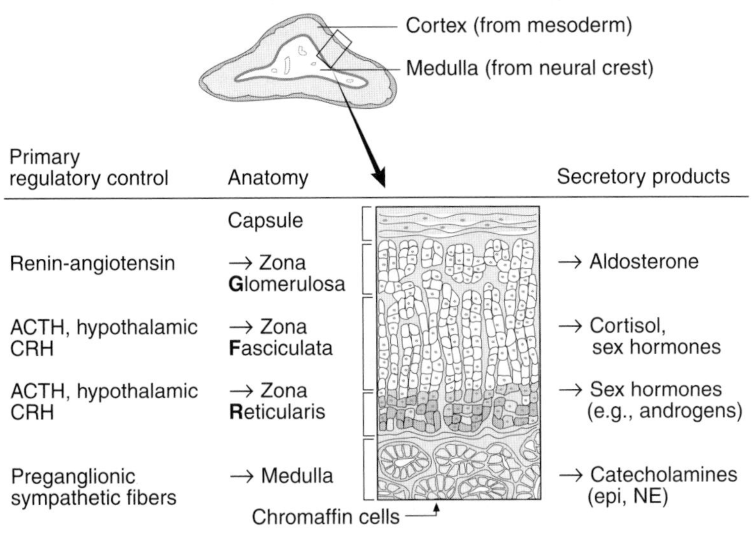

Cortex (from mesoderm)

Medulla (from neural crest)

Primary regulatory control	Anatomy	Secretory products
	Capsule	
Renin-angiotensin	→ Zona **G**lomerulosa	→ Aldosterone
ACTH, hypothalamic CRH	→ Zona **F**asciculata	→ Cortisol, sex hormones
ACTH, hypothalamic CRH	→ Zona **R**eticularis	→ Sex hormones (e.g., androgens)
Preganglionic sympathetic fibers	→ Medulla	→ Catecholamines (epi, NE)

Chromaffin cells

GFR corresponds with **S**alt (Na^+), **S**ugar (glucocorticoids), and **S**ex (androgens).

"The deeper you go, the sweeter it gets."

Pheochromocytoma—most common tumor of the adrenal medulla in adults.

Neuroblastoma—most common in children.

Pheochromocytoma causes episodic hypertension; neuroblastoma does not.

Adrenal gland drainage

Left adrenal → left adrenal vein → left renal vein → IVC.

Right adrenal → right adrenal vein → IVC.

Same as left and right gonadal vein.

Pituitary gland

Posterior pituitary (neurohypophysis) → vasopressin and oxytocin, made in the hypothalamus and shipped to pituitary. Derived from neuroectoderm.

Anterior pituitary (adenohypophysis) → FSH, LH, ACTH, GH, TSH, melanotropin (MSH), prolactin. Derived from oral ectoderm.

α subunit—common subunit to TSH, LH, FSH, and hCG.

β subunit—determines hormone specificity.

Acidophils—GH, prolactin.

B-Flat: **B**asophils—**F**SH, **L**H, **A**CTH, **T**SH.

FLAT PiG:
FSH
LH
ACTH
TSH
Prolactin
GH

Endocrine pancreas cell types

Islets of Langerhans are collections of α, β, and δ endocrine cells (most numerous in tail of pancreas). Islets arise from pancreatic buds. α = glucagon (peripheral); β = insulin (central); δ = somatostatin (interspersed).

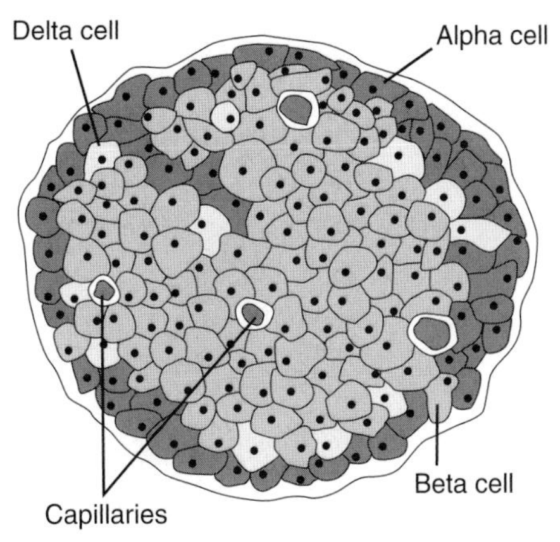

Prolactin regulation

Prolactin ↑ dopamine synthesis and secretion from the hypothalamus. Dopamine subsequently **inhibits** prolactin secretion. Dopamine agonists (e.g., bromocriptine) therefore **inhibit** prolactin secretion, whereas dopamine antagonists (e.g., most antipsychotics) stimulate prolactin secretion. In females, prolactin inhibits GnRH synthesis and release, which inhibits ovulation. Amenorrhea is commonly seen in prolactinomas.

Prolactin regulation

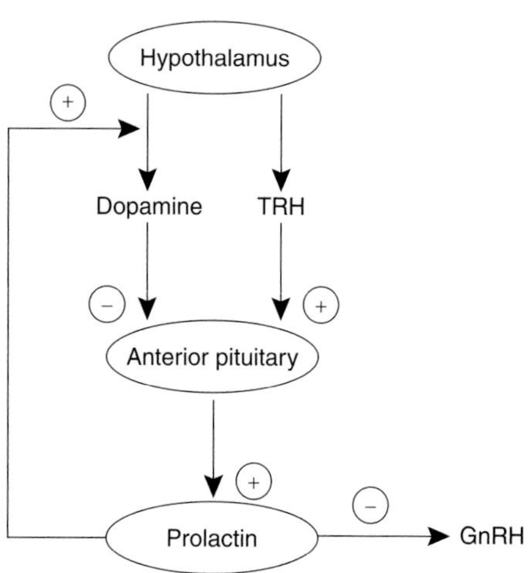

Hypothalamic-pituitary hormone regulation

TRH—⊕→ TSH, prolactin.
Dopamine—⊖→ prolactin.
CRH—⊕→ ACTH.
GHRH—⊕→ GH.
Somatostatin—⊖→ GH, TSH.
GnRH—⊕→ FSH, LH.

Adrenal steroids

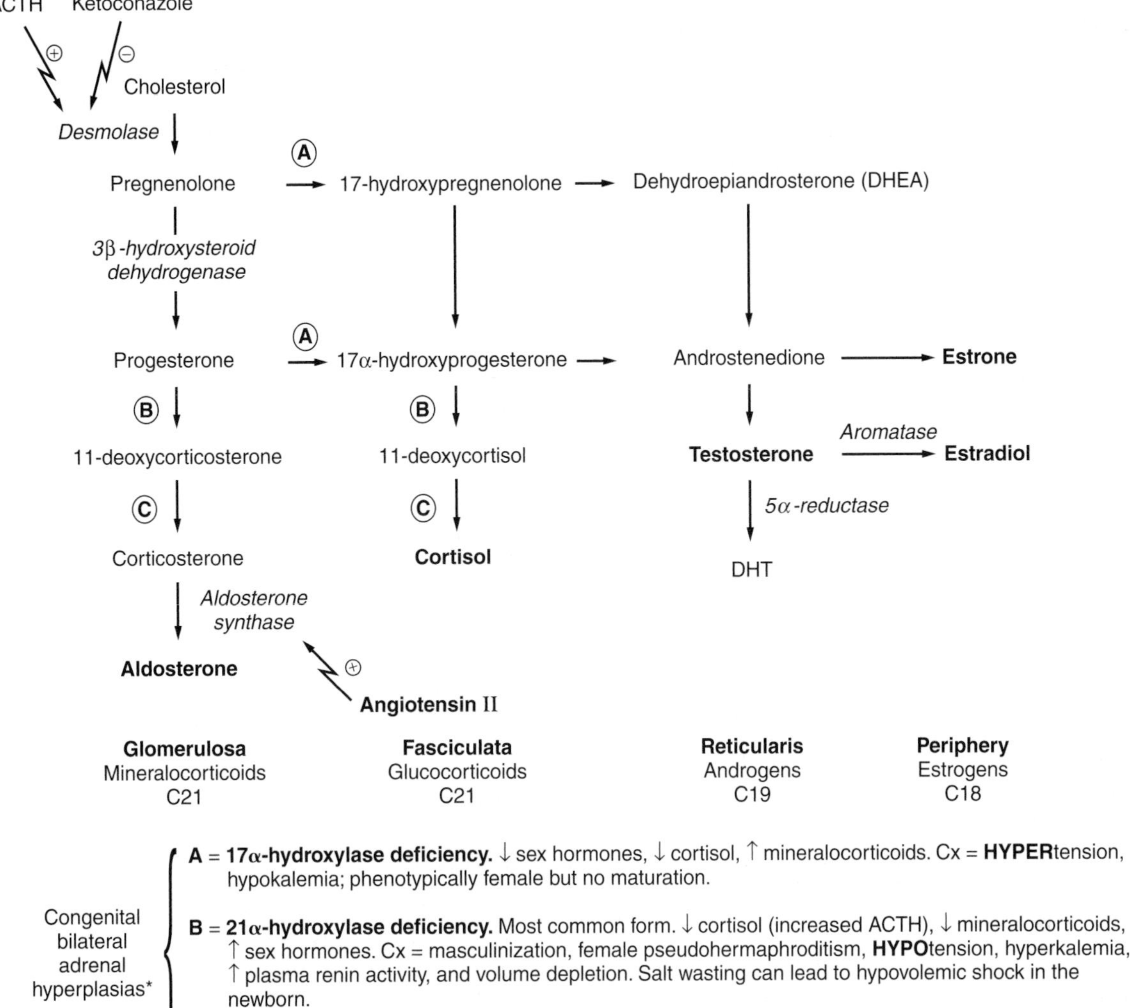

Congenital bilateral adrenal hyperplasias*

A = **17α-hydroxylase deficiency.** ↓ sex hormones, ↓ cortisol, ↑ mineralocorticoids. Cx = **HYPER**tension, hypokalemia; phenotypically female but no maturation.

B = **21α-hydroxylase deficiency.** Most common form. ↓ cortisol (increased ACTH), ↓ mineralocorticoids, ↑ sex hormones. Cx = masculinization, female pseudohermaphroditism, **HYPO**tension, hyperkalemia, ↑ plasma renin activity, and volume depletion. Salt wasting can lead to hypovolemic shock in the newborn.

C = **11β-hydroxylase deficiency.** ↓ cortisol, ↓ aldosterone and corticosterone, ↑ sex hormones. Cx = masculinization, **HYPER**tension (11-deoxycorticosterone is a mineralocorticoid and is secreted in excess).

*All congenital adrenal enzyme deficiencies are characterized by an enlargement of the adrenal glands due to an ↑ in ACTH stimulation because of the ↓ levels of cortisol.

PTH

Source	Chief cells of parathyroid.	
Function	1. ↑ bone resorption of calcium and phosphate 2. ↑ kidney reabsorption of calcium in distal convoluted tubule 3. ↓ kidney reabsorption of phosphate 4. ↑ 1,25-$(OH)_2$ vitamin D (calcitrol) production by stimulating kidney 1α-hydroxylase	PTH ↑ serum Ca^{2+}, ↓ serum $(PO_4)^{3-}$, ↑ urine $(PO_4)^{3-}$. PTH stimulates both osteoclasts and osteoblasts. **PTH** = **P**hosphate **T**rashing **H**ormone.
Regulation	↓ in free serum Ca^{2+} ↑ PTH secretion.	

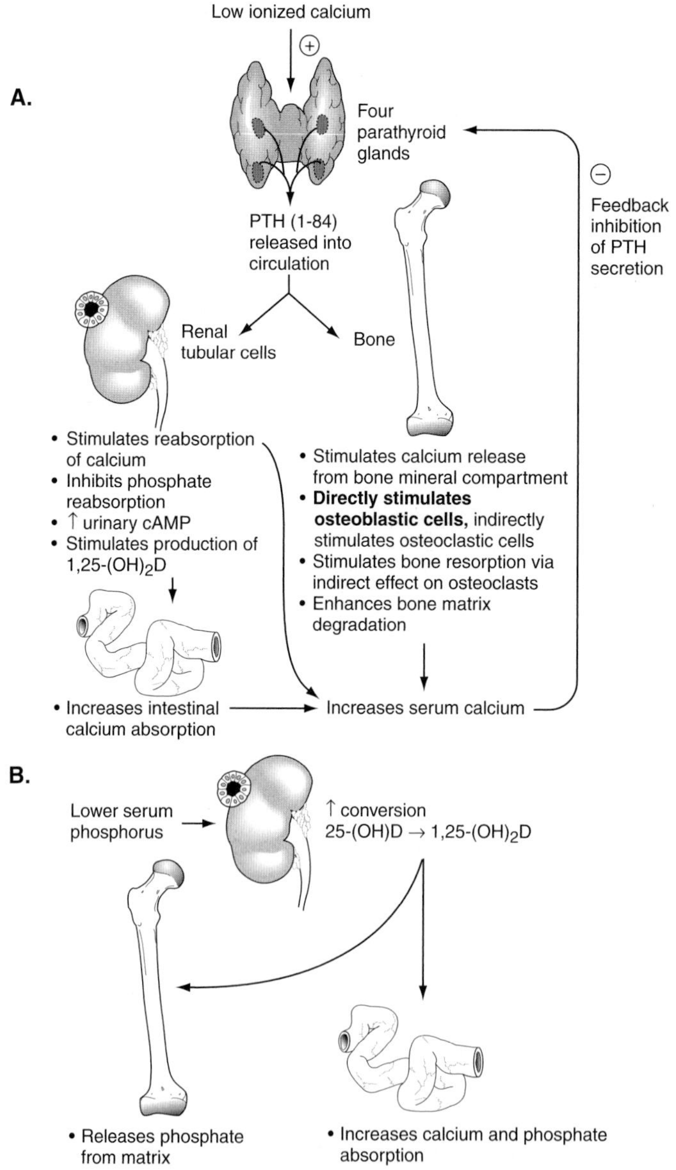

A.

Low ionized calcium

⊕

Four parathyroid glands

PTH (1-84) released into circulation

Renal tubular cells

Bone

⊖

Feedback inhibition of PTH secretion

- Stimulates reabsorption of calcium
- Inhibits phosphate reabsorption
- ↑ urinary cAMP
- Stimulates production of 1,25-$(OH)_2$D

- Stimulates calcium release from bone mineral compartment
- **Directly stimulates osteoblastic cells,** indirectly stimulates osteoclastic cells
- Stimulates bone resorption via indirect effect on osteoclasts
- Enhances bone matrix degradation

- Increases intestinal calcium absorption

Increases serum calcium

B.

Lower serum phosphorus

↑ conversion 25-(OH)D → 1,25-$(OH)_2$D

- Releases phosphate from matrix

- Increases calcium and phosphate absorption

(Adapted, with permission, from Chandrasoma P et al. *Concise Pathology,* 3rd ed. Stamford, CT: Appleton & Lange, 1998.)

Shown above are the main actions of PTH and 1,25-$(OH)_2$D in the maintenance of calcium (**A**) and phosphate (**B**) homeostasis.

Vitamin D

Source	Vitamin D_3 from sun exposure in skin. D_2 ingested from plants. Both converted to 25-OH vitamin D in liver and to 1,25-$(OH)_2$ vitamin D (active form) in kidney.	If you do not get vitamin D, you get rickets (kids) or osteomalacia (adults). 24,25-$(OH)_2$ vitamin D is an inactive form of vitamin D.
Function	1. ↑ absorption of dietary calcium 2. ↑ absorption of dietary phosphate 3. ↑ bone resorption of Ca^{2+} and $(PO_4)^{3-}$	
Regulation	↑ PTH causes ↑ 1,25-$(OH)_2$ vitamin D production. ↓ $[Ca^{2+}]$ ↑ 1,25-$(OH)_2$ vitamin D production. ↓ phosphate causes ↑ 1,25-$(OH)_2$ vitamin D production. 1,25-$(OH)_2$ vitamin D feedback inhibits its own production.	

Calcium, phosphate, and alkaline phosphatase levels

	Ca^{2+}	Phosphate	Alkaline phosphatase	PTH
Hyperparathyroidism	↑	↓	↑	↑
Paget's disease of bone	N/↑	N	↑↑↑	N
Vitamin D intoxication	↑	↑	N/↑	↓
Osteomalacia	↓	↓	↑	↑
Osteoporosis	N	N	N	N
Renal insufficiency	↓	↑	N	↑

N = no change.

Calcitonin

Source	Parafollicular cells (C cells) of thyroid.	Calcitonin opposes actions of PTH. It is probably not important in normal calcium homeostasis.
Function	↓ bone resorption of calcium.	
Regulation	↑ serum Ca^{2+} causes calcitonin secretion.	

Steroid/thyroid hormone mechanism

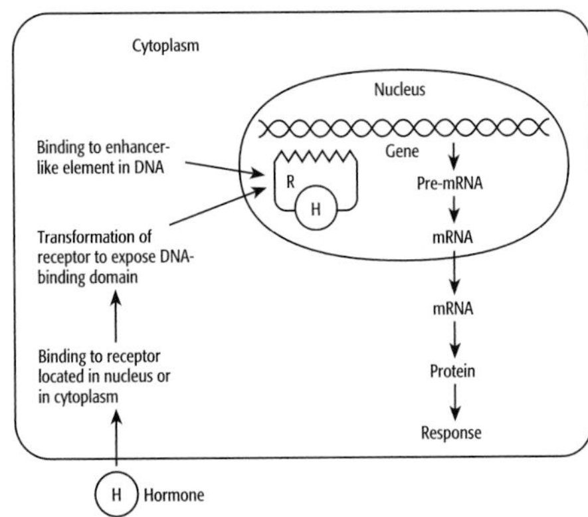

(Adapted, with permission, from Ganong WF. *Review of Medical Physiology,* 22th ed. New York: McGraw-Hill, 2005.)

The need for gene transcription and protein synthesis delays the onset of action of these hormones.

Steroid/thyroid hormones—**PET CAT:**

Progesterone
Estrogen
Testosterone
Cortisol
Aldosterone
Thyroxine and T_3

Steroid hormones are lipophilic and relatively insoluble in plasma; therefore, they must circulate bound to specific binding globulins, which ↑ solubility and allows for ↑ delivery of steroid to the target organ. ↑ levels of sex hormone–binding globulin (SHBG) lower free testosterone → gynecomastia. ↓ SHBG raises free testosterone → hirsutism.

Thyroid hormones (T_3/T_4)

Iodine-containing hormones that control the body's metabolic rate.

Source

Follicles of thyroid. Most T_3 formed in blood.

Function

1. Bone growth (synergism with GH)
2. CNS maturation
3. β-adrenergic effects (↑ CO, HR, SV, contractility)
4. ↑ basal metabolic rate via ↑ Na^+/K^+-ATPase activity = ↑ O_2 consumption, RR, ↑ body temperature
5. ↑ glycogenolysis, gluconeogenesis, lipolysis

Regulation

TRH (hypothalamus) stimulates TSH (pituitary), which stimulates follicular cells. Negative feedback by free T_3 to anterior pituitary ↓ sensitivity to TRH. TSI, like TSH, stimulates follicular cells (Graves' disease).

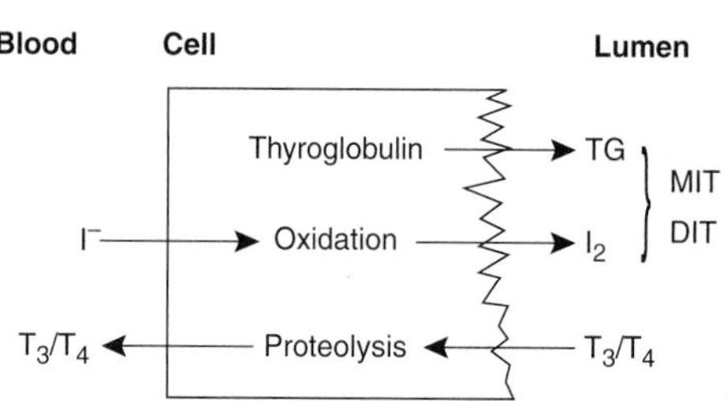

T_3 functions—4 **B**'s:
Brain maturation
Bone growth
Beta-adrenergic effects
BMR ↑

Thyroxine-binding globulin (TBG) binds most T_3/T_4 in blood; only free hormone is active. ↓ TBG in hepatic failure; ↑ TBG in pregnancy (estrogen ↑ TBG).

T_4 is major product.

T_4 is converted to T_3 by peripheral tissue. T_3 binds receptors with greater affinity than T_4.

Insulin-dependent organs

Skeletal muscle and adipose tissue depend on insulin for ↑ glucose uptake (GLUT-4). Brain and RBCs take up glucose independent of insulin levels (GLUT-1). Brain depends on glucose for metabolism under normal circumstances and uses ketone bodies in starvation. RBCs always depend on glucose.

Cortisol

Source

Adrenal fasciculata.

Function

1. Anti-inflammatory
2. ↑ gluconeogenesis, lipolysis, proteolysis
3. ↓ immune function
4. Maintains blood pressure
5. ↓ bone formation

Regulation

CRH (hypothalamus) stimulates ACTH release (pituitary), causing cortisol production in adrenal fasciculata.

Bound to corticosteroid-binding globulin (CBG).

Chronic stress induces prolonged secretion.

Signaling pathways of endocrine hormones

cAMP	cGMP	IP_3	Steroid receptor	Tyrosine kinase
ACTH	ANP	GnRH	Glucocorticoid	Insulin
LH	EDRF	TRH	Estrogen	IGF-1
FSH	NO	GHRH	Progesterone	FGF
TSH		ADH (V1)	Testosterone	
ADH (V2)		Oxytocin	Aldosterone	
hCG			Vitamin D	
MSH			T_3/T_4	
CRH				
PTH				
Calcitonin				
Glucagon				

▶ ENDOCRINE–PATHOLOGY

Cushing's syndrome

↑ cortisol due to a variety of causes.
Etiologies include:
1. Cushing's disease (1° pituitary adenoma); ↑ ACTH
2. 1° adrenal (hyperplasia/neoplasia); ↓ ACTH (see Color Image 68)
3. Ectopic ACTH production (e.g., small cell lung cancer); ↑ ACTH
4. Iatrogenic (e.g., chronic steroids); ↓ ACTH

The clinical picture includes hypertension, weight gain, moon facies, truncal obesity, buffalo hump, hyperglycemia (insulin resistance), skin changes (thinning, striae), osteoporosis, amenorrhea, and immune suppression (see Color Image 70).

Dexamethasone suppression test:
- Healthy—↓ cortisol after low dose.
- ACTH-producing pituitary tumor—↑ cortisol after low dose; ↓ cortisol after high dose.
- Ectopic ACTH-producing tumor (e.g., small cell carcinoma)—↑ cortisol after low dose; ↑ cortisol after high dose.
- Cortisol-producing tumor—↑ cortisol after low and high dose.

Hyperaldosteronism

Primary (Conn's syndrome): Caused by an aldosterone-secreting tumor, resulting in hypertension, hypokalemia, metabolic alkalosis, and **low** plasma renin.

Secondary: Due to renal artery stenosis, chronic renal failure, CHF, cirrhosis, or nephrotic syndrome. Kidney perception of low intravascular volume results in an overactive renin-angiotensin system. Therefore, it is associated with **high** plasma renin.

Treatment includes spironolactone, a K^+-sparing diuretic that works by acting as an aldosterone antagonist.

Addison's disease

1° deficiency of aldosterone and cortisol due to adrenal atrophy or destruction by disease, causing hypotension (hyponatremic volume contraction) and skin hyperpigmentation (due to MSH, a by-product of ↑ ACTH production from POMC). Characterized by **A**drenal **A**trophy and **A**bsence of hormone production; involves **A**ll 3 cortical divisions. Distinguish from 2° insufficiency, which has no skin hyperpigmentation (↓ pituitary ACTH production).

Waterhouse-Friderichsen syndrome	Acute adrenocortical insufficiency; adrenal hemorrhage syndrome associated with meningococcal septicemia.	
Tumors of the adrenal medulla		
Pheochromocytoma	The most common tumor of the adrenal medulla in adults. Derived from chromaffin cells (arise from neural crest) (see Color Image 69). VMA in urine.	Pheochromocytomas may be associated with neurofibromatosis, MEN types II and III.
Neuroblastoma	The most common tumor of the adrenal medulla in children, but it can occur anywhere along the sympathetic chain. HVA in urine. Less likely to develop hypertension. N-*myc* oncogene.	
Sheehan's syndrome	Postpartum hypopituitarism. Caused by infarction of the pituitary gland following severe bleeding and hypoperfusion during delivery. May cause fatigue, anorexia, poor lactation, and loss of pubic and axillary hair.	
Pheochromocytoma	Most of these tumors secrete epinephrine, NE, and dopamine. Urinary VMA levels and plasma catecholamines are elevated. Associated with MEN types II and III. Treated with α-antagonists, especially **phenoxybenzamine,** a nonselective, **irreversible** α-blocker. Episodic hyperadrenergic symptoms (**5 P's**): **P**ressure (elevated blood pressure) **P**ain (headache) **P**erspiration **P**alpitations (tachycardia) **P**allor	**Rule of 10's:** 10% malignant 10% bilateral 10% extra-adrenal 10% calcify 10% kids 10% familial Symptoms occur in "spells"—relapse and remit.
Multiple endocrine neoplasias (MEN)	MEN type I (Wermer's syndrome)—pancreas (e.g., Zollinger-Ellison syndrome, insulinomas, VIPomas), parathyroid, and pituitary tumors (prolactinoma). Presents with kidney stones and stomach ulcers. MEN type II (Sipple's syndrome)—medullary carcinoma of the thyroid, pheochromocytoma, parathyroid tumor. MEN type III (formerly MEN IIb)—medullary carcinoma of the thyroid, pheochromocytoma, and oral and intestinal ganglioneuromatosis (mucosal neuromas).	MEN I = **3 P's** (**P**ancreas, **P**ituitary, and **P**arathyroid). MEN II = **2 P's** (**P**heochromocytoma and **P**arathyroid). MEN III = **1 P** (**P**heochromocytoma). All MEN syndromes have autosomal-dominant inheritance. Associated with *ret* gene in MEN types II and III.

Hypothyroidism and hyperthyroidism		
Hypothyroidism	Cold intolerance, hypoactivity, weight gain, fatigue, lethargy, ↓ appetite, constipation, weakness, ↓ reflexes, myxedema (facial/periorbital), dry, cool skin, and coarse, brittle hair.	↑ TSH (sensitive test for 1° hypothyroidism), ↓ total T_4, ↓ free T_4, ↓ T_3 uptake. **Riedel's thyroiditis**—thyroid replaced by fibrous tissue (hypothyroid).
Hyperthyroidism	Heat intolerance, hyperactivity, weight loss, chest pain/palpitations, arrhythmias, diarrhea, ↑ reflexes, warm, moist skin, and fine hair.	↓ TSH (if 1°), ↑ total T_4, ↑ free T_4, ↑ T_3 uptake.
Graves' disease	An autoimmune hyperthyroidism with thyroid-stimulating/TSH receptor antibodies. Ophthalmopathy (proptosis, EOM swelling), pretibial myxedema, diffuse goiter (see Image 120). Often presents during stress (e.g., childbirth) (see Color Image 71).	Graves' is a type II hypersensitivity.
Thyroid storm	Underlying Graves' disease with a stress-induced catecholamine surge leading to death by arrhythmia.	
Hashimoto's thyroiditis	Autoimmune disorder resulting in hypothyroidism (can have thyrotoxicosis during follicular rupture). Slow course; moderately enlarged, nontender thyroid. Lymphocytic infiltrate with germinal centers. Antimicrosomal and antithyroglobulin antibodies. Associated with Hürthle cells on histology.	
Subacute thyroiditis (de Quervain's)	Self-limited hypothyroidism often following a flulike illness. Elevated ESR, jaw pain, early inflammation, and very tender thyroid gland. Histology shows granulomatous inflammation.	May be hyperthyroid early in course. Lymphocytic subacute thyroiditis is painless.
Toxic multinodular goiter	Iodine deprivation followed by iodine restoration. Causes release of T_3 and T_4. Nodules are not malignant. Jod-Basedow phenomenon—thyrotoxicosis if a patient with endemic goiter moves to iodine-replete area.	
Thyroid cancer	1. Papillary carcinoma—most common, excellent prognosis, "ground-glass" nuclei (Orphan Annie), psammoma bodies. ↑ risk with childhood irradiation. 2. Follicular carcinoma—good prognosis, uniform follicles. 3. Medullary carcinoma—from parafollicular "C cells"; produces calcitonin, sheets of cells in amyloid stroma. MEN types II and III. 4. Undifferentiated/anaplastic—older patients; very poor prognosis. 5. Lymphoma—associated with Hashimoto's thyroiditis.	
Cretinism	Endemic cretinism occurs wherever endemic goiter is prevalent (lack of dietary iodine); sporadic cretinism is caused by defect in T_4 formation or developmental failure in thyroid formation. Findings: pot-bellied, pale, puffy-faced child with protruding umbilicus and protuberant tongue.	Cretin means Christlike (French *chrétien*). Those affected were considered so mentally retarded as to be incapable of sinning. Still common in China.

Acromegaly	Excess GH in adults. Findings: large tongue with deep furrows, deep voice, large hands and feet, coarse facial features, impaired glucose tolerance (insulin resistance). ↑ GH in children → gigantism. Treat medically with octreotide.	↑ GH is normal in stress, exercise, and hypoglycemia. Test with oral glucose tolerance test.
Hyperparathyroidism		
Primary	Usually an adenoma. Hypercalcemia, hypercalciuria (**renal stones**), hypophosphatemia, ↑ PTH, ↑ alkaline phosphatase, ↑ cAMP in urine. Often asymptomatic, or may present with weakness and constipation ("**groans**").	"**Stones, bones, and groans.**" **Osteitis fibrosa cystica** (von Recklinghausen's syndrome)—cystic bone spaces filled with brown fibrous tissue (**bone pain**).
Secondary	2° hyperplasia due to ↓ serum Ca^{2+}, most often in chronic renal disease. Hypocalcemia, hyperphosphatemia, ↑ alkaline phosphatase, ↑ PTH.	**Renal osteodystrophy**—bone lesions due to 2° hyperparathyroidism due in turn to renal disease.
Hypoparathy-roidism	Hypocalcemia, tetany. Due to accidental surgical excision (thyroid surgery), autoimmune destruction or DiGeorge syndrome. Chvostek's sign—tap facial nerve → contraction of facial muscles. Trousseau's sign—occlusion of brachial artery with BP cuff → carpal spasm.	**Pseudohypoparathyroidism**—autosomal-dominant kidney unresponsiveness to PTH. Hypocalcemia, shortened 4th/5th digits, short stature.
Hypercalcemia	Caused by **C**alcium ingestion (milk-alkali syndrome), **H**yperparathyroid, **H**yperthyroid, **I**atrogenic (thiazides), **M**ultiple myeloma, **P**aget's disease, **A**ddison's disease, **N**eoplasms, **Z**ollinger-Ellison syndrome, **E**xcess vitamin D, **E**xcess vitamin A, **S**arcoidosis.	CHIMPANZEES.
Pituitary adenoma	Most commonly prolactinoma—amenorrhea, galactorrhea, low libido, infertility. Bromocriptine (dopamine agonist) causes shrinkage. Can impinge on optic chiasm → bitemporal hemianopia.	

Diabetes mellitus

Acute manifestations	Polydipsia, polyuria, polyphagia, weight loss, DKA (type 1), hyperosmolar coma (type 2), unopposed secretion of GH and epinephrine (exacerbating hyperglycemia).

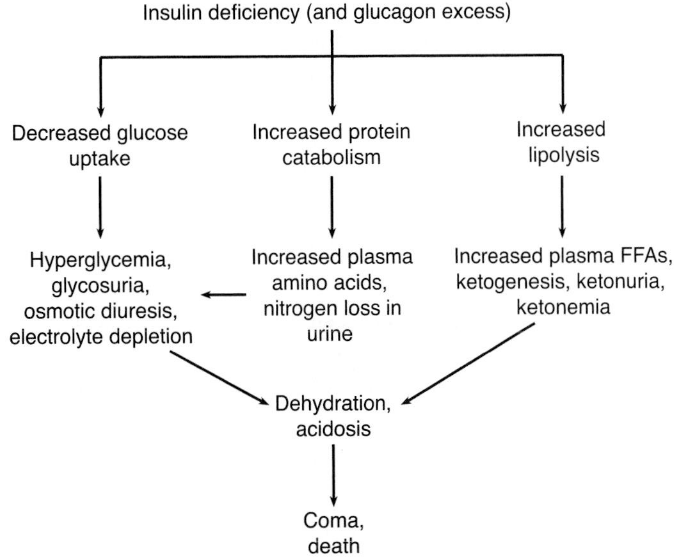

Chronic manifestations

Nonenzymatic glycosylation:

1. Small vessel disease (diffuse thickening of basement membrane) → retinopathy (hemorrhage, exudates, microaneurysms, vessel proliferation), glaucoma, nephropathy (nodular sclerosis, progressive proteinuria, chronic renal failure, arteriosclerosis leading to hypertension, Kimmelstiel-Wilson nodules)
2. Large vessel atherosclerosis, CAD, peripheral vascular occlusive disease and gangrene, cerebrovascular disease

Osmotic damage:

1. Neuropathy (motor, sensory, and autonomic degeneration)
2. Cataracts (sorbitol accumulation)

Tests

Fasting serum glucose, glucose tolerance test, HbA_{1c} (measures long-term diabetic control).

Type 1 vs. type 2 diabetes mellitus

Variable	Type 1—juvenile onset (IDDM)	Type 2—adult onset (NIDDM)
1° defect	Viral or immune destruction of β cells (see Color Image 67)	↑ resistance to insulin
Insulin necessary in treatment	Always	Sometimes
Age (exceptions commonly occur)	< 30	> 40
Association with obesity	No	Yes
Genetic predisposition	Weak, polygenic	Strong, polygenic
Association with HLA system	Yes (HLA-DR3 and 4)	No
Glucose intolerance	Severe	Mild to moderate
Ketoacidosis	Common	Rare
β-cell numbers in the islets	↓	Variable
Serum insulin level	↓	Variable
Classic symptoms of polyuria, polydipsia, thirst, weight loss	Common	Sometimes

Diabetic ketoacidosis	One of the most important complications of type 1 diabetes. Usually due to an ↑ in insulin requirements from an ↑ in stress (e.g., infection). Excess fat breakdown and ↑ ketogenesis from the ↑ in free fatty acids, which are then made into ketone bodies (β-hydroxybutyrate > acetoacetate).
Signs/symptoms	Kussmaul respirations (rapid/deep breathing), nausea/vomiting, abdominal pain, psychosis/delirium, dehydration. Fruity breath odor (due to exhaled acetone).
Labs	Hyperglycemia, ↑ H^+, ↓ HCO_3^- (anion gap metabolic acidosis), ↑ blood ketone levels, leukocytosis. Hyperkalemia, but depleted intracellular K^+ due to transcellular shift from ↓ insulin.
Complications	Life-threatening mucormycosis, *Rhizopus* infection, cerebral edema, cardiac arrhythmias, heart failure.
Treatment	Fluids, insulin, and potassium (to replete intracellular stores); glucose if necessary to prevent hypoglycemia.

Diabetes insipidus	Characterized by intense thirst and polyuria together with an inability to concentrate urine owing to lack of ADH (central DI—pituitary tumor, trauma, surgery, histiocytosis X) or to a lack of renal response to ADH (nephrogenic DI—hereditary or 2° to hypercalcemia, lithium, demeclocycline).
Diagnosis	Water deprivation test—urine osmolality doesn't ↑. Response to desmopressin distinguishes between central and nephrogenic.
Findings	Urine specific gravity < 1.006; serum osmolality > 290 mOsm/L.
Treatment	Adequate fluid intake. For central DI—intranasal desmopressin (ADH analog). For nephrogenic DI—hydrochlorothiazide, indomethacin, or amiloride.

SIADH	Syndrome of inappropriate antidiuretic hormone secretion: 1. Excessive water retention 2. Hyponatremia 3. Urine osmolarity > serum osmolarity Very low serum sodium levels can lead to seizures (correct slowly). Treat with demeclocycline or H_2O restriction.	Causes include: 1. Ectopic ADH (small cell lung cancer) 2. CNS disorders/head trauma 3. Pulmonary disease 4. Drugs (e.g., cyclophosphamide)
Carcinoid syndrome	Rare syndrome caused by carcinoid tumors (neuroendocrine cells), especially metastatic small bowel tumors, which secrete high levels of serotonin (5-HT). Not seen if tumor is limited to GI tract (5-HT undergoes first-pass metabolism in liver). Results in recurrent **diarrhea, cutaneous flushing, asthmatic wheezing,** and **right-sided valvular disease.** Most common tumor of appendix. ↑ 5-HIAA in urine.	**Rule of 1/3s:** 1/3 metastasize 1/3 present with 2nd malignancy 1/3 multiple Derived from neuroendocrine cells of GI tract. Treat with octreotide.

Zollinger-Ellison syndrome	Gastrin-secreting tumor of pancreas or duodenum. Causes recurrent ulcers. May be associated with MEN type I.

Diabetes drugs

Treatment strategy for type 1 DM—low-sugar diet, insulin replacement.

Treatment strategy for type 2 DM—dietary modification and exercise for weight loss; oral hypoglycemics.

Drug Classes	Action	Clinical Use	Toxicities
Insulin: Lispro (short-acting) Aspart (short-acting) NPH (intermediate) Lente (long-acting) Ultralente (long-acting)	**Bind insulin receptor** (tyrosine kinase activity). Liver: ↑ glucose stored as glycogen. Muscle: ↑ glycogen and protein synthesis, K^+ uptake. Fat: aids TG storage.	Type 1 DM. Also life-threatening hyperkalemia and stress-induced hyperglycemia.	Hypoglycemia, hypersensitivity reaction (very rare).
Sulfonylureas: First generation: Tolbutamide Chlorpropamide Second generation: Glyburide Glimepiride Glipizide	Close K^+ channel in β-cell membrane, so cell depolarizes → **triggering of insulin release** via ↑ Ca^{2+} influx.	Stimulate release of endogenous insulin in type 2 DM. Require some islet function, so useless in type 1 DM.	First generation: disulfiram-like effects. Second generation: hypoglycemia.
Biguanides: Metformin	Exact mechanism is unknown. Possibly ↓ **gluconeogenesis,** ↑ glycolysis, ↓ serum glucose levels.	Used as oral hypoglycemic. Can be used in patients without islet function.	Most grave adverse effect is lactic acidosis.
Glitazones: Pioglitazone Rosiglitazone	↑ target cell response to insulin.	Used as monotherapy in type 2 DM or combined with above agents.	Weight gain, edema. Hepatotoxicity, CV toxicity.
α-glucosidase inhibitors: Acarbose Miglitol	**Inhibit intestinal brush-border α-glucosidases.** Delayed sugar hydrolysis and glucose absorption lead to ↓ postprandial hyperglycemia.	Used as monotherapy in type 2 DM or in combination with above agents.	GI disturbances.

Orlistat

Mechanism	Alters fat metabolism by inhibiting pancreatic lipases.
Clinical use	Long-term obesity management (in conjunction with modified diet).
Toxicity	Steatorrhea, GI discomfort, reduced absorption of fat-soluble vitamins, headache.

Sibutramine

Mechanism	Sympathomimetic serotonin and norepinephrine reuptake inhibitor.
Clinical use	Short-term and long-term obesity management.
Toxicity	Hypertension and tachycardia.

Propylthiouracil, methimazole

Mechanism	Inhibit organification and coupling of thyroid hormone synthesis. Propylthiouracil also ↓ peripheral conversion of T_4 to T_3.
Clinical use	Hyperthyroidism.
Toxicity	Skin rash, agranulocytosis (rare), aplastic anemia.

Hypothalamic/pituitary drugs

Drug	Clinical use
GH	GH deficiency, Turner's syndrome
Somatostatin (octreotide)	Acromegaly, carcinoid, gastrinoma, glucagonoma
Oxytocin	Stimulates labor, uterine contractions, milk let-down; controls uterine hemorrhage
ADH (desmopressin)	Pituitary (central, not nephrogenic) DI

Levothyroxine, triiodothyronine

Mechanism	Thyroxine replacement.
Clinical use	Hypothyroidism, myxedema.
Toxicity	Tachycardia, heat intolerance, tremors, arrhythmias.

Glucocorticoids	Hydrocortisone, prednisone, triamcinolone, dexamethasone, beclomethasone.
Mechanism	↓ the production of leukotrienes and prostaglandins by inhibiting phospholipase A_2 and expression of COX-2.
Clinical use	Addison's disease, inflammation, immune suppression, asthma.
Toxicity	Iatrogenic Cushing's syndrome—buffalo hump, moon facies, truncal obesity, muscle wasting, thin skin, easy bruisability, osteoporosis, adrenocortical atrophy, peptic ulcers, diabetes (if chronic).

HIGH-YIELD SYSTEMS

Gastrointestinal

"A good set of bowels is worth more to a man than any quantity of brains."
—Josh Billings

"Man should strive to have his intestines relaxed all the days of his life."
—Moses Maimonides

"The colon is the playing field for all human emotions."
—Cyrus Kapadia, MD

Vignette	Question	Answer
Baby vomits milk when fed and has a gastric air bubble.	What kind of fistula is present?	Blind esophagus with lower segment of esophagus attached to the trachea.
After a stressful life event, 30-year-old man has diarrhea and blood per rectum; intestinal biopsy shows transmural inflammation.	What is the diagnosis?	Crohn's disease.
Young man presents with mental deterioration and tremors. He has brown pigmentation in a ring around the periphery of his cornea and altered LFTs.	What treatment should he receive?	Penicillamine for Wilson's disease.
20-year-old man presents with idiopathic hyperbilirubinemia.	What is the most common cause?	Gilbert's syndrome.
55-year-old man with chronic GERD presents with esophageal cancer.	What is the most likely histologic subtype?	Adenocarcinoma.
Woman presents with alternating bouts of painful diarrhea and constipation. Colonoscopy is normal.	What is the most likely diagnosis?	Irritable bowel syndrome.

Abdominal layers

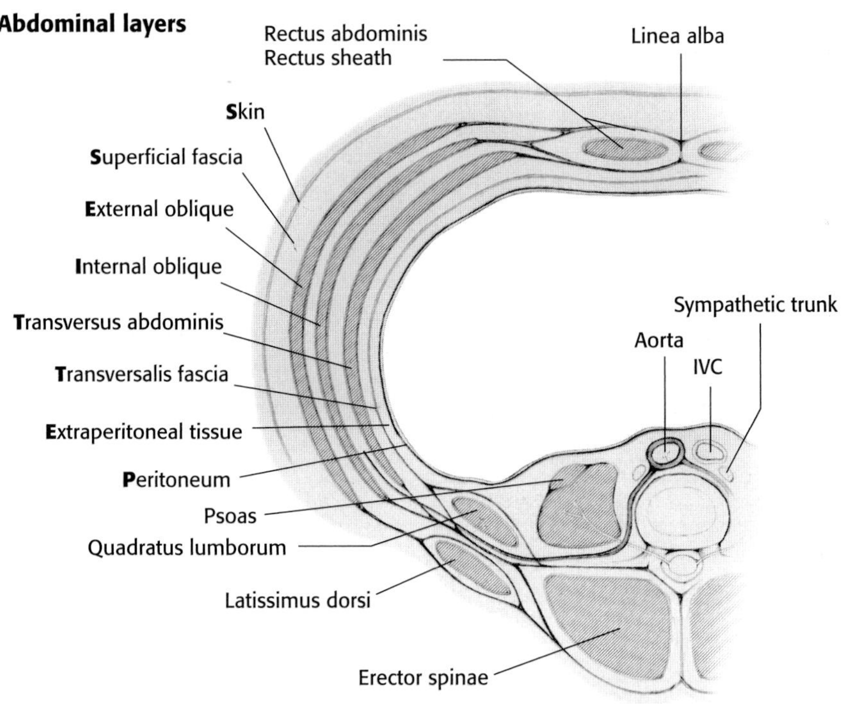

Sally Struthers Eats Indian Toddlers To Enlarge Peritoneum.

(Reproduced, with permission, from White JS. *USMLE Road Map: Gross Anatomy,* 1st ed. New York: McGraw-Hill, 2003: 67.)

Retroperitoneal structures

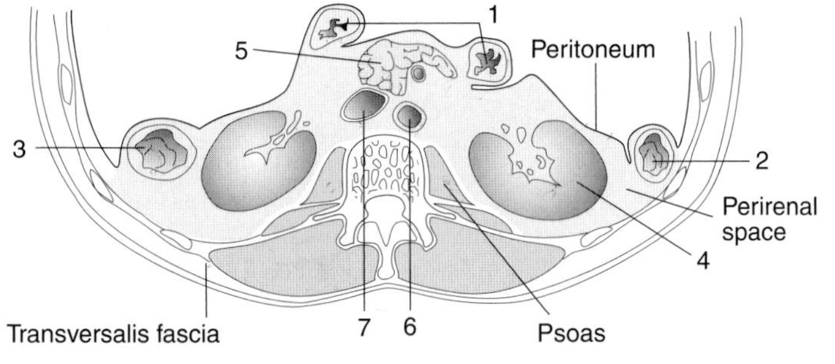

1. Duodenum (2nd, 3rd, 4th parts)
2. Descending colon
3. Ascending colon
4. Kidney and ureters
5. Pancreas (except tail)
6. Aorta
7. IVC

Adrenal glands and rectum (not shown in diagram)

GI blood supply and innervation

Embryonic gut region	Artery	Parasympathetic innervation	Vertebral level	Structures supplied
Foregut	Celiac	Vagus	T12/L1	Stomach to proximal duodenum; liver, gallbladder, pancreas
Midgut	SMA	Vagus	L1	Distal duodenum to proximal $^2/_3$ of transverse colon
Hindgut	IMA	Pelvic	L3	Distal $^1/_3$ of transverse colon to upper portion of rectum; splenic flexure is a watershed region

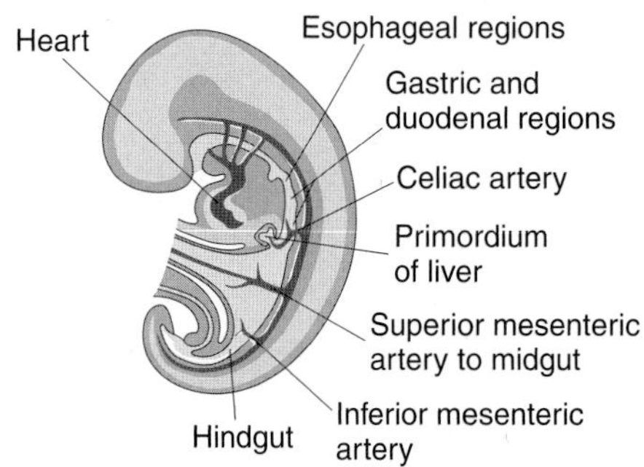

Celiac trunk

Branches of celiac trunk: common hepatic, splenic, left gastric. These comprise the main blood supply of the stomach.

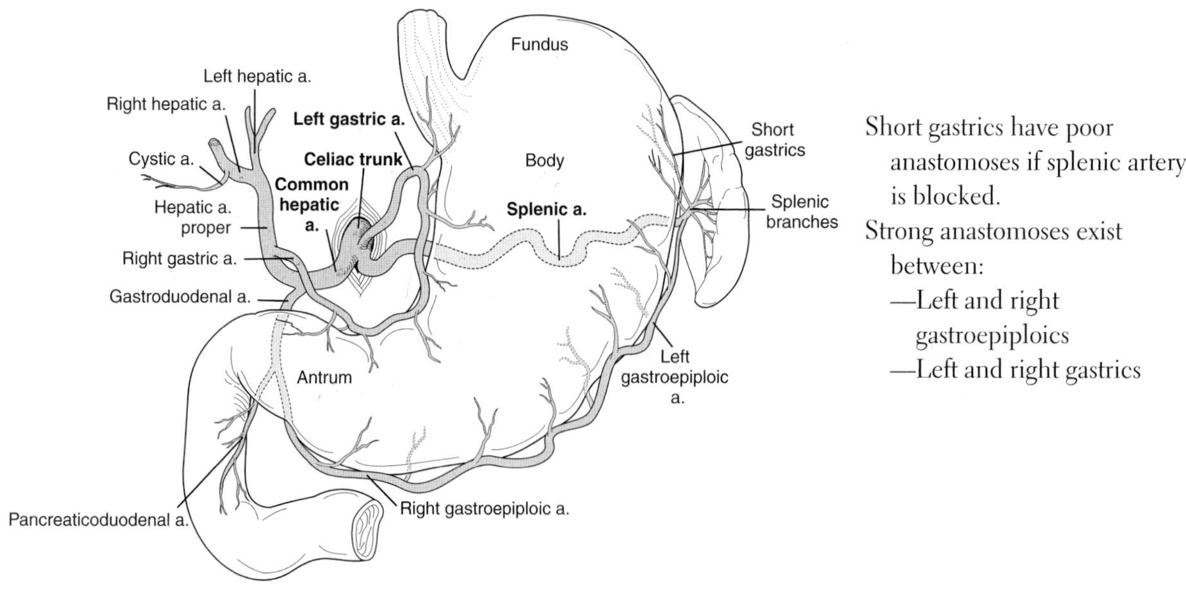

Short gastrics have poor anastomoses if splenic artery is blocked.

Strong anastomoses exist between:
—Left and right gastroepiploics
—Left and right gastrics

Collateral circulation

If the abdominal aorta is blocked, these arterial anastomoses (with origin) compensate:

1. Internal thoracic/mammary (subclavian) ↔ superior epigastric (internal thoracic) ↔ inferior epigastric (external iliac)
2. Superior pancreaticoduodenal (celiac trunk) ↔ inferior pancreaticoduodenal (SMA)
3. Middle colic (SMA) ↔ left colic (IMA)
4. Superior rectal (IMA) ↔ middle rectal (internal iliac)

Portosystemic anastomoses

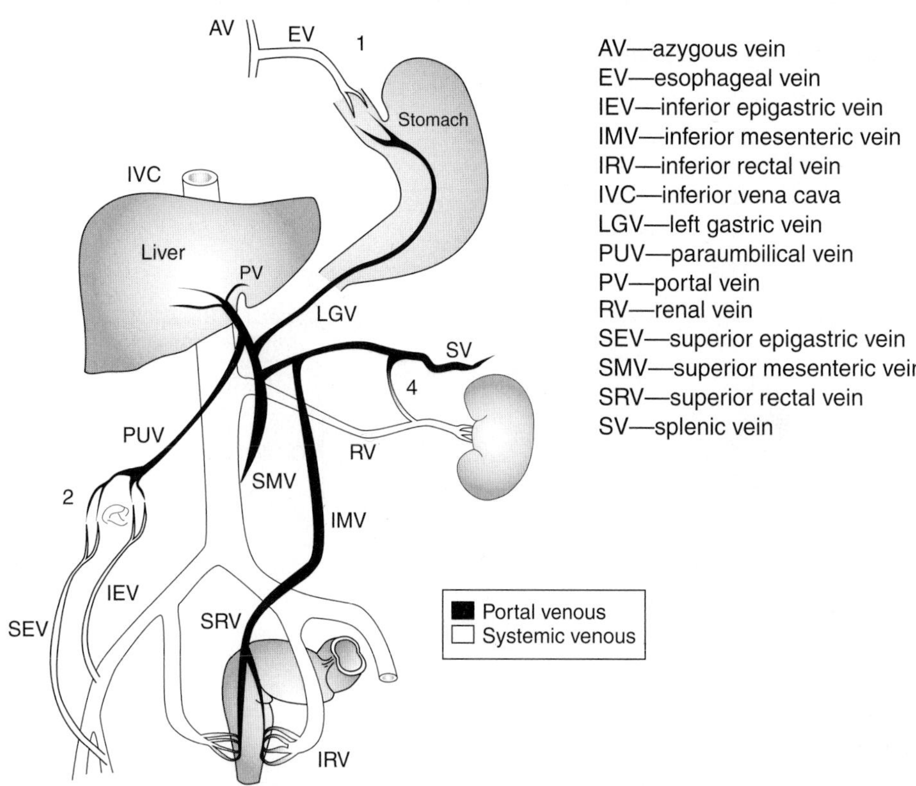

Site of anastomosis	Clinical sign	Portal ↔ systemic
1. Esophagus	Esophageal varices	Left gastric ↔ esophageal
2. Umbilicus	Caput medusae	Paraumbilical ↔ superficial and inferior epigastric
3. Rectum	Hemorrhoids	Superior rectal ↔ middle and inferior rectal

Varices of **gut, butt,** and **caput** are commonly seen with portal hypertension.

Inserting a portocaval shunt (4) between the splenic and left renal veins relieves portal hypertension by shunting blood to the systemic circulation.

Liver anatomy

Apical surface of hepatocytes faces bile canaliculi. Basolateral surface faces sinusoids.

Zone I: periportal zone:
—Affected 1st by viral hepatitis

Zone II: intermediate zone.

Zone III: pericentral vein (centrilobular) zone:
—Contains P-450 system
—Affected 1st by ischemia
—Most sensitive to toxic injury
—Alcoholic hepatitis

Sinusoids draining to central vein
Liver cell plates
Bile canaliculus
Kupffer cell
Bile ductule
Space of Disse (lymphatic drainage)
Central vein
Branch of portal vein
Branch of hepatic artery
Blood flow
Bile flow
Zone I
Zone II
Zone III

Sinusoids of liver

Irregular "capillaries" with fenestrated endothelium (pores 100–200 nm in diameter). No basement membrane. Allow macromolecules of plasma full access to basal surface of hepatocytes through perisinusoidal space (space of Disse).

Biliary structures

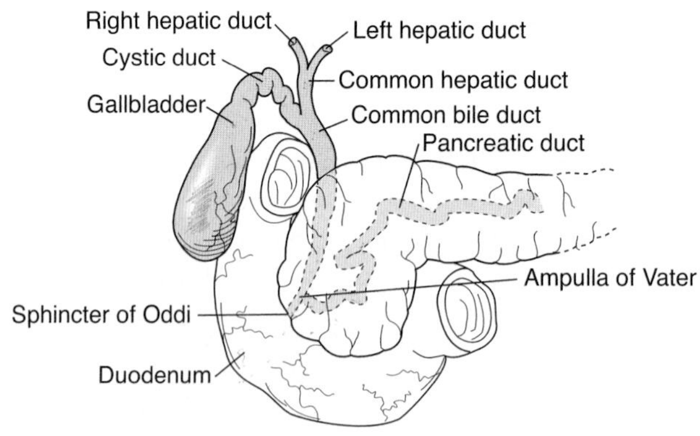

Important GI ligaments

Ligament	Connects	Structures contained	Notes
Falciform	Liver to anterior abdominal wall	Ligamentum teres	Derivative of fetal umbilical vein
Hepatoduodenal	Liver to duodenum	Portal triad: hepatic artery, portal vein, common bile duct	May be compressed between thumb and index finger placed in epiploic foramen (of Winslow) to control bleeding Connects greater and lesser sacs
Gastrohepatic	Liver to lesser curvature of stomach	Gastric arteries	Separates right greater and lesser sacs May be cut during surgery to access lesser sac
Gastrocolic	Greater curvature and transverse colon	Gastroepiploic arteries	Part of greater omentum
Gastrosplenic	Greater curvature and spleen	Short gastrics	Separates left greater and lesser sacs
Splenorenal	Spleen to posterior abdominal wall	Splenic artery and vein	

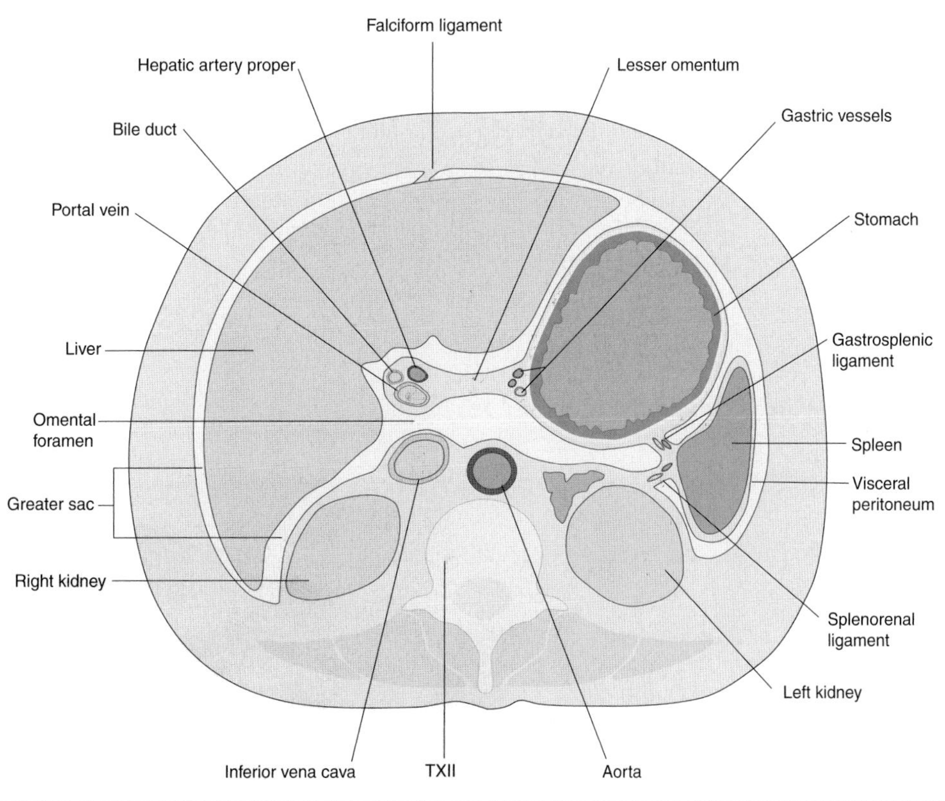

HIGH-YIELD SYSTEMS GASTROINTESTINAL

Esophageal anatomy

Upper ⅓	Striated muscle.
Middle ⅓	Striated and smooth muscle.
Lower ⅓	Smooth muscle.

Digestive tract anatomy

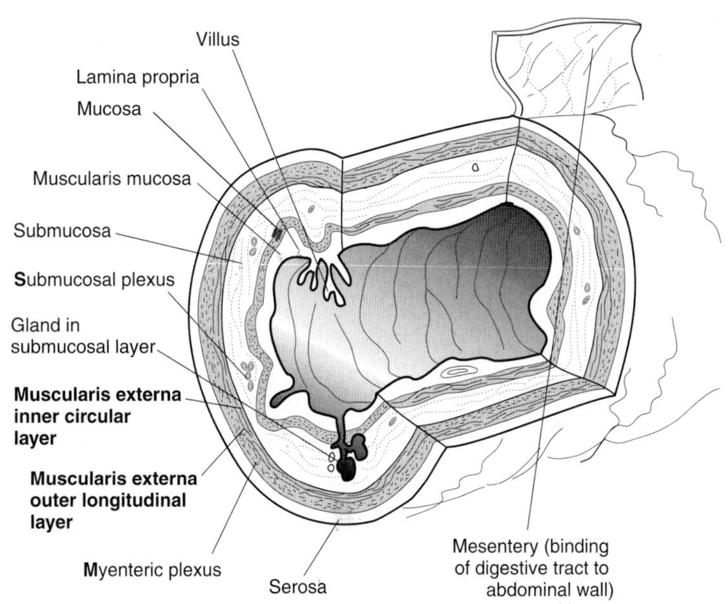

(Adapted, with permission, from McPhee S et al. *Pathophysiology of Disease: An Introduction to Clinical Medicine,* 3rd ed. New York: McGraw-Hill, 2000: 296.)

Layers of gut wall (inside to outside):

1. **Mucosa**—epithelium (absorption), lamina propria (support), muscularis mucosa (motility)
2. **Submucosa**—includes **S**ubmucosal nerve plexus (Meissner's)
3. **Muscularis externa**—includes **M**yenteric nerve plexus (Auerbach's)
4. **Serosa/adventitia**

Frequencies of basal electric rhythm (slow waves):
Stomach—3 waves/min
Duodenum—12 waves/min
Ileum—8–9 waves/min

Enteric nerve plexuses

Myenteric (Auerbach's)	Coordinates **M**otility along entire gut wall. Contains cell bodies of some parasympathetic terminal effector neurons. Located between inner (circular) and outer (longitudinal) layers of smooth muscle in GI tract wall.
Submucosal (Meissner's)	Regulates local **S**ecretions, blood flow, and absorption. Contains cell bodies of some parasympathetic terminal effector neurons. Located between mucosa and inner layer of smooth muscle in GI tract wall.

Pectinate line 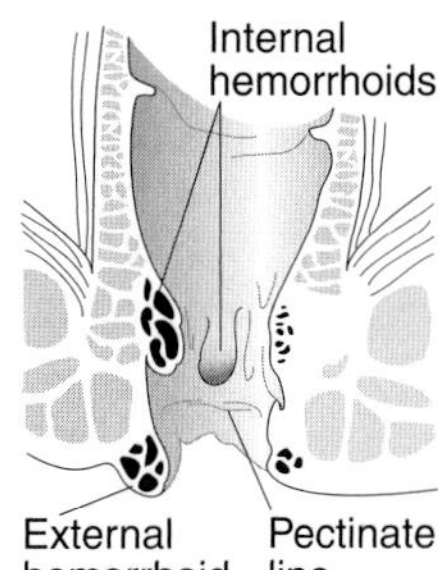 	Formed where hindgut meets ectoderm. **Above pectinate line**—internal hemorrhoids, adenocarcinoma. Arterial supply from superior rectal artery (branch of IMA). Venous drainage is to superior rectal vein → inferior mesenteric vein → portal system. **Below pectinate line**—external hemorrhoids (painful), squamous cell carcinoma. Somatic innervation. Arterial supply from inferior rectal artery (branch of internal pudendal artery). Venous drainage to inferior rectal vein → internal pudendal vein → internal iliac vein → IVC.	Internal hemorrhoids receive visceral innervation and are therefore NOT painful. External hemorrhoids receive somatic innervation and are therefore painful. Innervated by inferior rectal nerve—branch of pudendal nerve.

Femoral region

Organization	Lateral to medial: **N**erve-**A**rtery-**V**ein-**E**mpty space-**L**ymphatics.	**NAVEL.**
Femoral triangle	Contains femoral vein, artery, nerve.	
Femoral sheath	Fascial tube 3–4 cm below inguinal ligament. Contains femoral vein, artery, and canal (deep inguinal lymph nodes) but **not** femoral nerve.	

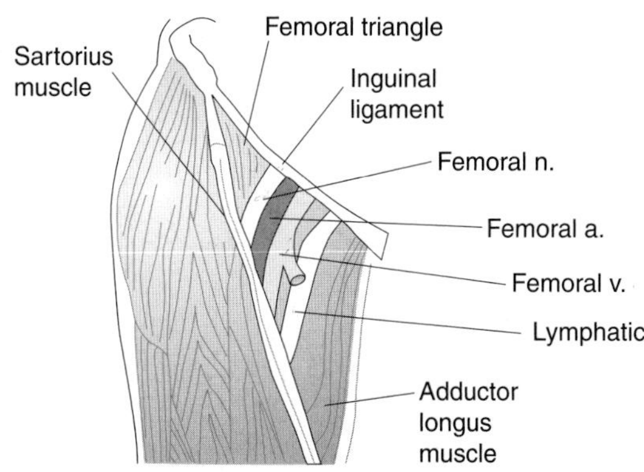

Inguinal canal

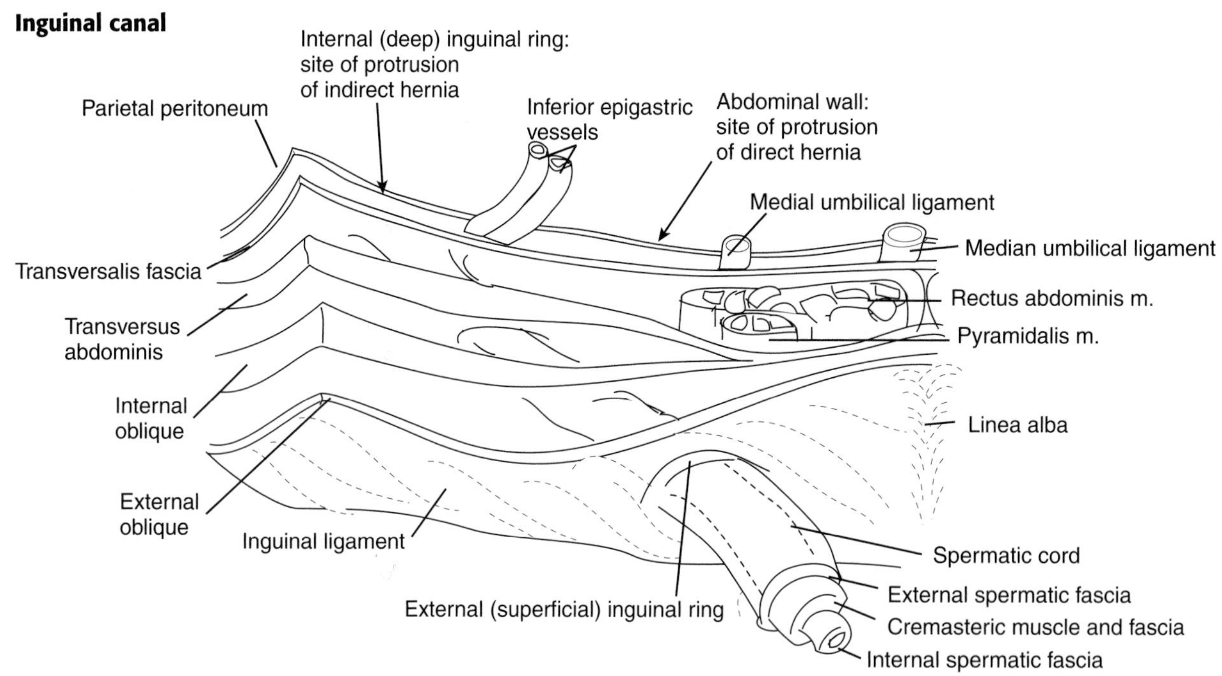

(Adapted, with permission, from White JS. *USMLE Road Map: Gross Anatomy,* 1st ed. New York: McGraw-Hill, 2003: 69.)

Hernias	A hernia is a protrusion of peritoneum through an opening, usually sites of weakness.	
Diaphragmatic hernia	Abdominal structures enter the thorax; may occur in infants as a result of defective development of pleuroperitoneal membrane. Most commonly a **hiatal hernia**, in which stomach herniates upward through the esophageal hiatus of the diaphragm.	**Hiatal hernias—sliding** (most common): GE junction is displaced **Paraesophageal:** GE junction is normal. Cardia moves into the thorax.
Indirect inguinal hernia	Goes through the **IN**ternal (deep) inguinal ring, external (superficial) inguinal ring, and **IN**to the scrotum. Enters internal inguinal ring lateral to inferior epigastric artery. Occur in **IN**fants owing to failure of processus vaginalis to close. Much more common in males.	Follows the path of the descent of the testes. Covered by all 3 layers of spermatic fascia.
Direct inguinal hernia	Protrudes through the inguinal (Hesselbach's) triangle. Bulges directly through abdominal wall medial to inferior epigastric artery. Goes through the external (superficial) inguinal ring only. Covered by transversalis fascia. Usually in older men.	**MD**s don't **LI**e: **M**edial to inferior epigastric artery = **D**irect hernia. **L**ateral to inferior epigastric artery = **I**ndirect hernia.
Femoral hernia	Protrudes below inguinal ligament through femoral canal below and lateral to pubic tubercle. More common in women.	Leading cause of bowel incarceration.

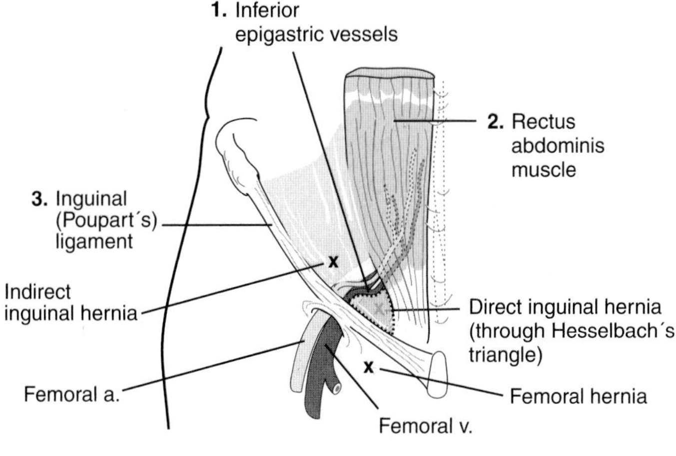

Hesselbach's triangle:
- Inferior epigastric artery
- Lateral border of rectus abdominis
- Inguinal ligament

HIGH-YIELD SYSTEMS GASTROINTESTINAL

Peyer's patches	Unencapsulated lymphoid tissue found in lamina propria and submucosa of small intestine. Contain specialized M cells that take up antigen. Stimulated B cells leave Peyer's patch and travel through lymph and blood to lamina propria of intestine, and differentiate into IgA-secreting plasma cells in mesenteric lymph nodes. IgA receives protective secretory component and is then transported across epithelium to gut to deal with intraluminal antigen.	Think of **IgA**, the **I**ntra-**g**ut **A**ntibody. And always say "secretory IgA."
Salivary secretion		
Source	Parotid (most serous), submandibular, submaxillary, and sublingual (most mucinous) glands.	**S**erous on the **S**ides (parotids); **M**ucinous in the **M**iddle (sublingual).
Function	1. α-amylase (ptyalin) begins starch digestion; inactivated by low pH on reaching stomach 2. Bicarbonate neutralizes oral bacterial acids, maintains dental health 3. Mucins (glycoproteins) lubricate food	Salivary secretion is stimulated by both sympathetic (T1–T3 superior cervical ganglion) and parasympathetic (facial, glossopharyngeal nerve) activity. Low flow rate → hypotonic. High flow rate → closer to isotonic. CN VII runs through parotid gland. Can be damaged during surgery.
Brunner's glands	Secrete alkaline mucus to neutralize acid contents entering the duodenum from the stomach. Located in **duodenal submucosa** (the only GI submucosal glands). Hypertrophy of Brunner's glands is seen in peptic ulcer disease.	

GI secretory products

Product	Source	Action	Regulation	Notes
Intrinsic factor	Parietal cells Stomach	Vitamin B_{12} binding protein (required for B_{12} uptake in terminal ileum)		Autoimmune destruction of parietal cells → chronic gastritis and pernicious anemia.
Gastric acid	Parietal cells Stomach	↓ stomach pH	↑ by histamine, ACh, gastrin ↓ by somatostatin, GIP, prostaglandin, secretin	**Gastrinoma:** gastrin-secreting tumor that causes continuous high levels of acid secretion and ulcers.
Pepsin	Chief cells Stomach	Protein digestion	↑ by vagal stimulation, local acid	Inactive pepsinogen → pepsin by H^+.
HCO_3^-	Mucosal cells Stomach Duodenum	Neutralizes acid Prevents autodigestion	↑ by secretin	HCO_3^- is trapped in mucus that covers the gastric epithelium.

GI hormones

Hormone	Source	Action	Regulation	Notes
Gastrin	G cells Antrum of stomach	↑ gastric H^+ secretion ↑ growth of gastric mucosa ↑ gastric motility	↑ by stomach distention, amino acids, peptides, vagal stimulation ↓ by stomach pH < 1.5	↑↑ in Zollinger-Ellison syndrome. Phenylalanine and tryptophan are potent stimulators.
Cholecystokinin	I cells Duodenum Jejunum	↑ pancreatic secretion ↑ gallbladder contraction ↓ gastric emptying	↑ by fatty acids, amino acids	In cholelithiasis, pain worsens after fatty food ingestion due to ↑ CCK.
Secretin	S cells Duodenum	↑ pancreatic HCO_3^- secretion ↓ gastric acid secretion ↑ bile secretion	↑ by acid, fatty acids in lumen of duodenum	↑ HCO_3^- neutralizes gastric acid in duodenum, allowing pancreatic enzymes to function.
Somatostatin	D cells Pancreatic islets GI mucosa	↓ gastric acid and pepsinogen secretion ↓ pancreatic and small intestine fluid secretion ↓ gallbladder contraction ↓ insulin and glucagon release	↑ by acid ↓ by vagal stimulation	Inhibitory hormone. Antigrowth hormone effects (digestion and absorption of substances needed for growth). Used to treat VIPoma and carcinoid tumors.
Gastric inhibitory peptide (GIP)	K cells Duodenum Jejunum	Exocrine: ↓ gastric H^+ secretion Endocrine: ↑ insulin release	↑ by fatty acids, amino acids, oral glucose	An oral glucose load is used more rapidly than the equivalent given by IV.
Vasoactive intestinal polypeptide (VIP)	Parasympathetic ganglia in sphincters, gallbladder, small intestine	↑ intestinal water and electrolyte secretion ↑ relaxation of intestinal smooth muscle and sphincters	↑ by distention and vagal stimulation ↓ by adrenergic input	**VIPoma**—non-α, non-β islet cell pancreatic tumor that secretes VIP. Copious diarrhea.
Nitric oxide		↑ smooth muscle relaxation, including lower esophageal sphincter		Loss of NO secretion is implicated in ↑ lower esophageal tone of achalasia.
Motilin	Small intestine	Produces migrating motor complexes (MMCs)	↑ in fasting state	

Regulation of gastric acid secretion

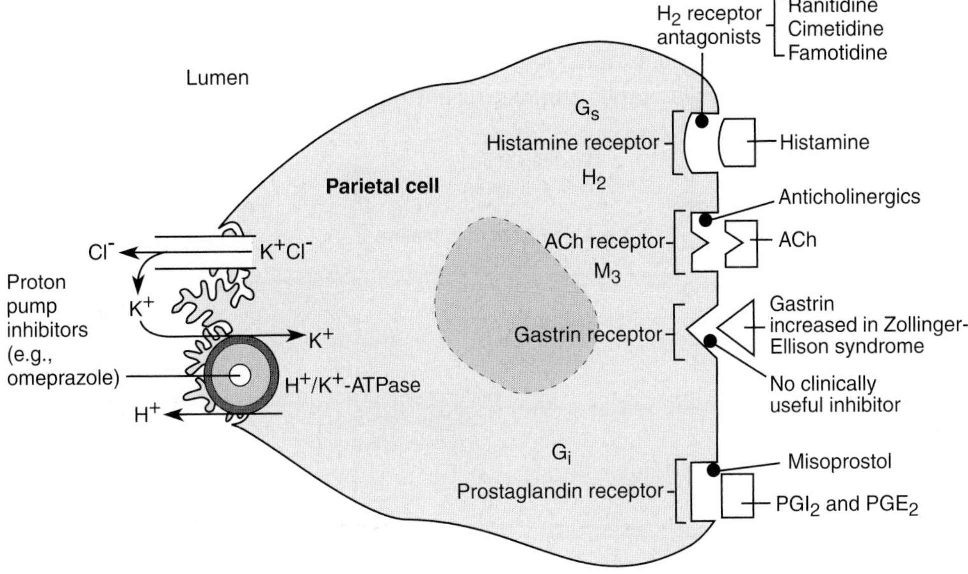

Pancreatic enzymes	α-amylase—starch digestion, secreted in active form. Lipase, phospholipase A, colipase—fat digestion. Proteases (trypsin, chymotrypsin, elastase, carboxypeptidases)—protein digestion, secreted as proenzymes also known as "zymogens." Trypsinogen is converted to active enzyme trypsin by **enterokinase/enteropeptidase,** an enzyme secreted from duodenal mucosa. Trypsin activates other proenzymes and more trypsinogen (positive feedback loop).
Carbohydrate digestion	
Salivary amylase	Starts digestion, hydrolyzes α-1,4 linkages to yield disaccharides (maltose, maltotriose, and α-limit dextrans).
Pancreatic amylase	Highest concentration in duodenal lumen, hydrolyzes starch to oligosaccharides and disaccharides.
Oligosaccharide hydrolases	At brush border of intestine, the rate-limiting step in carbohydrate digestion, produce monosaccharides from oligo- and disaccharides.
Carbohydrate absorption	Only monosaccharides (glucose, galactose, fructose) are absorbed by enterocytes. Glucose and galactose are taken up by SGLT1 (Na^+ dependent). Fructose is taken up by facilitated diffusion by GLUT-5. All are transported to blood by GLUT-2.
Bile	Composed of bile salts (bile acids conjugated to glycine or taurine, making them water soluble), phospholipids, cholesterol, bilirubin, water, and ions. The only significant mechanism for cholesterol excretion.

Bilirubin

Product of heme metabolism; actively taken up by hepatocytes. Direct bilirubin—conjugated with glucuronic acid; water soluble. Indirect bilirubin—unconjugated; water insoluble. Jaundice (yellow skin, sclerae) results from elevated bilirubin levels.

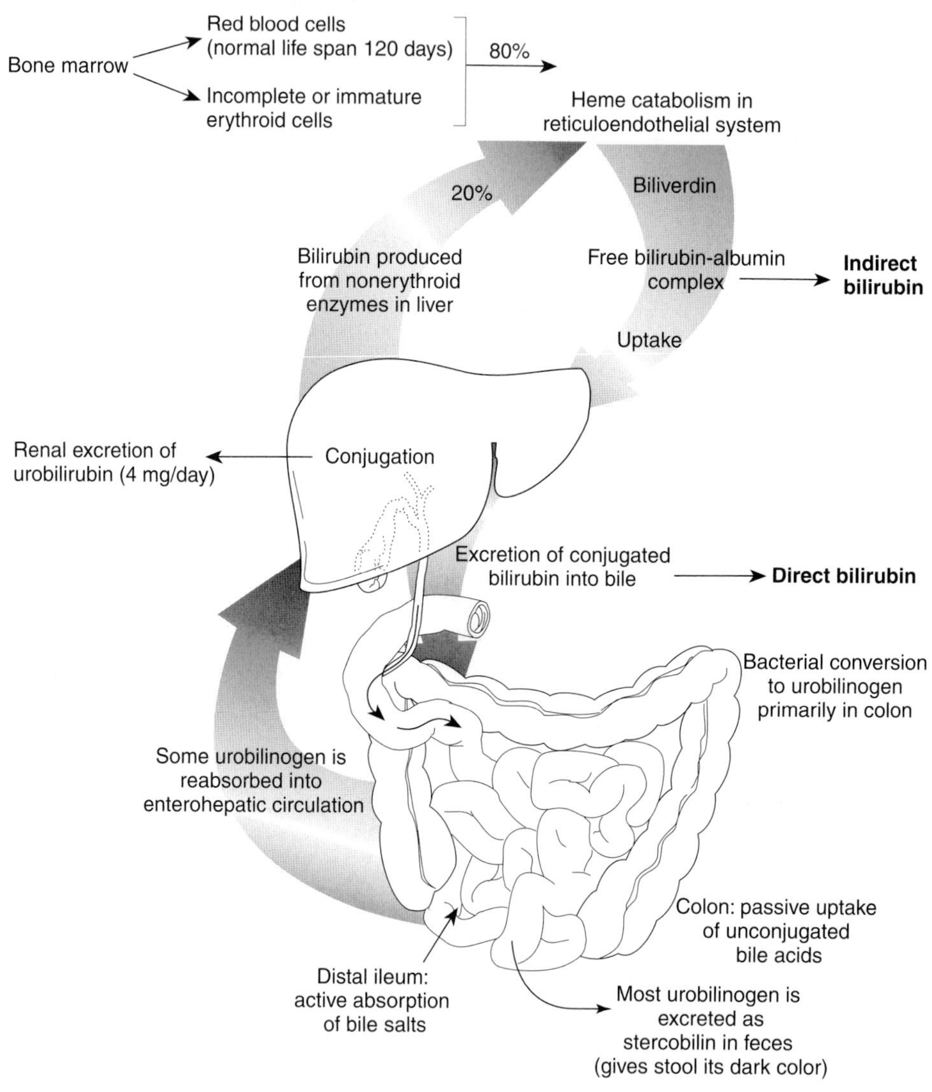

Achalasia

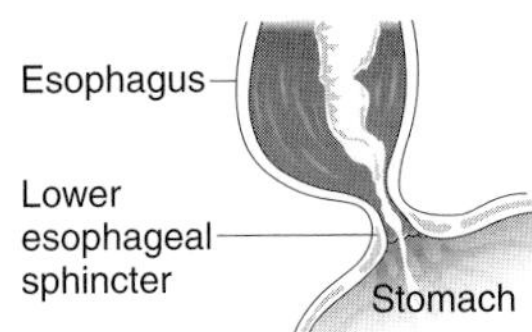

Failure of relaxation of lower esophageal sphincter (LES) due to loss of **myenteric (Auerbach's) plexus.** High LES opening pressure and uncoordinated peristalsis lead to progressive dysphagia. Barium swallow shows dilated esophagus with an area of distal stenosis. Associated with an ↑ risk of esophageal carcinoma.

A-*chalasia* = absence of relaxation.
"Bird's beak" on barium swallow.
2° achalasia may arise from Chagas' disease.
Scleroderma (CREST syndrome) is associated with esophageal dysmotility involving low pressure proximal to LES.

Esophageal pathologies

Gastroesophageal reflux disease (GERD)	Commonly presents as heartburn and regurgitation upon lying down.
Esophageal varices	**Painless** bleeding of submucosal veins in lower ⅓ of esophagus (see Color Image 33).
Mallory-Weiss syndrome	**Painful** mucosal lacerations at the gastroesophageal junction due to severe vomiting. Leads to hematemesis. Usually found in alcoholics and bulimics.
Boerhaave syndrome	Transmural esophageal rupture due to violent retching.
Esophageal strictures	Associated with lye ingestion.
Esophagitis	Associated with reflux, infection (HSV-1, CMV, *Candida*), or chemical ingestion.
Plummer-Vinson syndrome	Triad of: 1. Dysphagia (due to esophageal webs) 2. Glossitis 3. Iron deficiency anemia

Barrett's esophagus

Glandular metaplasia—replacement of nonkeratinized (stratified) squamous epithelium with intestinal (columnar) epithelium in the distal esophagus. Due to chronic acid reflux (GERD).

BARRett's = **B**ecomes **A**denocarcinoma, **R**esults from **R**eflux.

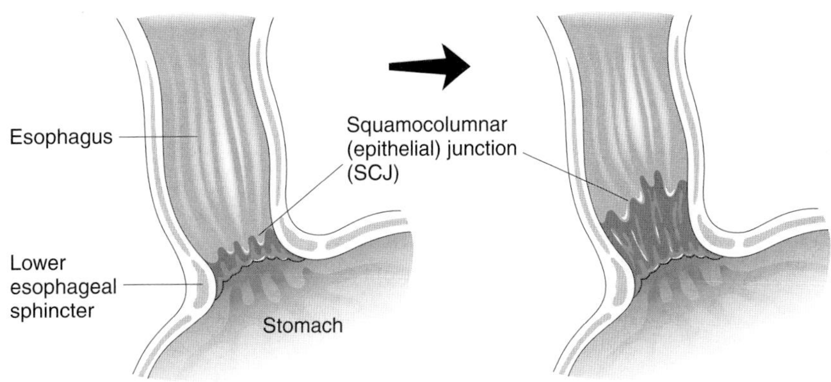

Esophageal cancer	Risk factors for esophageal cancer are: **A**lcohol/**A**chalasia **B**arrett's esophagus **C**igarettes **D**iverticuli (e.g., Zenker's diverticulum) **E**sophageal web (e.g., Plummer-Vinson)/ **E**sophagitis **F**amilial	ABCDEF. Worldwide, squamous cell is most common. In the United States, squamous and adenocarcinoma are equal in incidence. Squamous cell—upper and middle ⅓. Adenocarcinoma—lower ⅓.

Tracheoesophageal fistula

Abnormal connection between esophagus and trachea.

Most common subtype is blind upper esophagus with lower esophagus connected to trachea. Results in cyanosis, choking and vomiting with feeding, air bubble on CXR, and polyhydramnios.

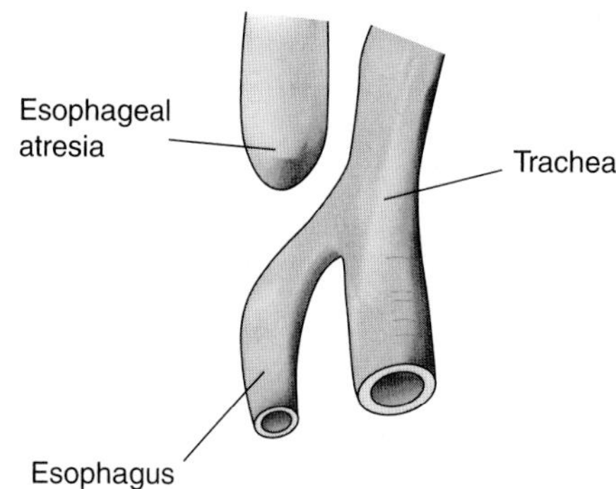

Congenital pyloric stenosis

Hypertrophy of the pylorus causes obstruction. Palpable "olive" mass in epigastric region and nonbilious projectile vomiting at ≈ 2 weeks of age. Treatment is surgical incision. Occurs in 1/600 live births, often in 1st-born males.

Malabsorption syndromes	Can cause diarrhea, steatorrhea, weight loss, weakness.
Celiac sprue	Autoantibodies to gluten (gliadin) in wheat and other grains. Proximal small bowel primarily.
Tropical sprue	Probably infectious; responds to antibiotics. Similar to celiac sprue, but can affect entire small bowel.
Whipple's disease	Infection with *Tropheryma whippelii* (gram positive); PAS-positive macrophages in intestinal lamina propria, mesenteric nodes. Arthralgias, cardiac and neurologic symptoms are common. Most often occurs in older men.
Disaccharidase deficiency	Most common is lactase deficiency → milk intolerance. Normal-appearing villi. Osmotic diarrhea.
Pancreatic insufficiency	Due to cystic fibrosis, obstructing cancer, and chronic pancreatitis. Causes malabsorption of protein, fat, vitamins A, D, E, K.

Celiac sprue	Autoimmune-mediated intolerance of gliadin (wheat) leading to steatorrhea. Associated with people of northern European descent. Findings include blunting of villi (see Color Image 32) and lymphocytes in the lamina propria. ↓ mucosal absorption that primarily affects jejunum. Serum levels of tissue transglutaminase are used for screening. Associated with dermatitis herpetiformis. Moderately ↑ risk of malignancy (most often T-cell lymphoma).	
Gastritis		
Acute gastritis (erosive)	Disruption of mucosal barrier → inflammation. Can be caused by stress, NSAIDs, alcohol, uricemia, burns (Curling's ulcer), and brain injury (Cushing's ulcer).	
Chronic gastritis (nonerosive)		
Type A (fundus/body)	Autoimmune disorder characterized by **A**utoantibodies to parietal cells, pernicious **A**nemia, and **A**chlorhydria.	**AB pairing**—pernicious **A**nemia affects gastric **B**ody.
Type B (antrum)	Caused by *H. pylori* infection. ↑ risk of MALT lymphoma.	*H. pylori* **B**acterium affects **A**ntrum.
Ménétrier's disease	Gastric hypertrophy with protein loss, parietal cell atrophy, and ↑ mucous cells. Precancerous.	
Stomach cancer	Almost always adenocarcinoma. Early aggressive local spread and node/liver mets. Associated with dietary nitrosamines (smoked foods), achlorhydria, chronic gastritis, type A blood. Termed linitis plastica when diffusely infiltrative (thickened, rigid appearance, "leather bottle"), signet ring cells (see Image 115), acanthosis nigricans.	Virchow's node—involvement of left supraclavicular node by mets from stomach. Krukenberg's tumor—bilateral mets to ovaries. Abundant mucus, signet ring cells.
Peptic ulcer disease		
Gastric ulcer	Pain can be greater with meals—weight loss. Often occurs in older patients. *H. pylori* infection in 70%; chronic NSAID use also implicated. Due to ↓ mucosal protection against gastric acid.	
Duodenal ulcer	Pain **D**ecreases with meals—weight gain. Almost 100% have *H. pylori* infection. Due to ↑ gastric acid secretion (e.g., Zollinger-Ellison syndrome) or ↓ mucosal protection. Hypertrophy of Brunner's glands. Tend to have clean, "punched-out" margins unlike the raised/irregular margins of carcinoma. Potential complications include bleeding, penetration into pancreas, perforation, and obstruction (not intrinsically precancerous) (see Image 114).	

Inflammatory bowel disease

	Crohn's disease	Ulcerative colitis
Possible etiology	Postinfectious.	Autoimmune.
Location	Any portion of the GI tract, usually the terminal ileum and colon. **Skip** lesions, **rec**tal sparing.	*Colitis* = colon inflammation. Continuous colonic lesions, always with rectal involvement.
Gross morphology	Transmural inflammation. **Cobblestone** mucosa, creeping **fat,** bowel wall thickening ("string sign" on barium swallow x-ray), linear ulcers, fissures, fistulas.	Mucosal and submucosal inflammation only. Friable mucosal pseudopolyps with freely hanging mesentery. "Lead pipe" appearance on imaging.
Microscopic morphology	Noncaseating **gran**ulomas and lymphoid aggregates.	Crypt abscesses and ulcers, bleeding, no granulomas.
Complications	Strictures, fistulas, perianal disease, malabsorption, nutritional depletion.	Severe stenosis, toxic megacolon, **colorectal carcinoma.**
Intestinal manifestation	Diarrhea that may or may not be bloody.	Bloody diarrhea.
Extraintestinal manifestations	Migratory polyarthritis, erythema nodosum, ankylosing spondylitis, uveitis, immunologic disorders.	Pyoderma gangrenosum, 1° sclerosing cholangitis.
Treatment	Corticosteroids.	Sulfasalazine.

For **Crohn's,** think of a **fat gran**ny and an old **crone skipping** down a **cobblestone** road away from the **wreck** (rectal sparing) (see Images 118, 119).

Appendicitis

All age groups; most common indication for emergent abdominal surgery in children.
Initial diffuse periumbilical pain → localized pain at McBurney's point. Nausea, fever; may perforate → peritonitis.
Differential: diverticulitis (elderly), ectopic pregnancy (use β-hCG to rule out).

Diverticular disease		
Diverticulum	Blind pouch leading off the alimentary tract that communicates with the lumen of the gut. Most diverticula (esophagus, stomach, duodenum, colon) are acquired and are termed "false" in that they lack or have an attenuated muscularis externa. Most often in sigmoid colon.	"**True**" diverticulum—all 3 gut wall layers outpouch. "**False**" diverticulum or pseudodiverticulum—only mucosa and submucosa outpouch. Occur especially where vasa recta perforate muscularis externa.
Diverticulosis	Many diverticula. Common (in ~50% of people > 60 years). Caused by ↑ intraluminal pressure and focal weakness in colonic wall. Associated with low-fiber diets. Most often in sigmoid colon.	Often asymptomatic or associated with vague discomfort and/or rectal bleeding.
Diverticulitis	Inflammation of diverticula classically causing LLQ pain, fever, leukocytosis. May perforate → peritonitis, abscess formation, or bowel stenosis (see Color Image 31). Give antibiotics.	May cause bright red rectal bleeding.

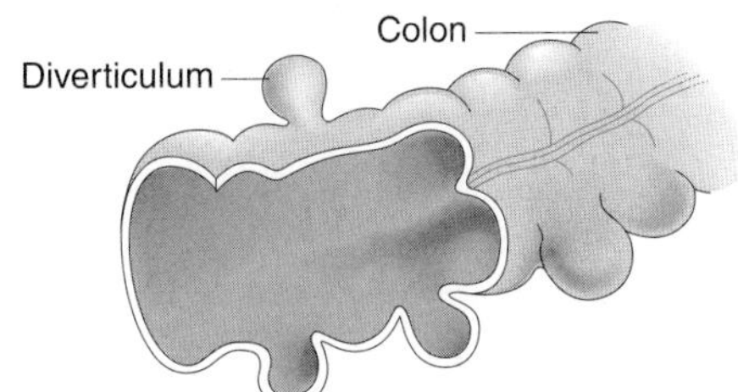

Zenker's diverticulum	False diverticulum. Herniation of mucosal tissue at junction of pharynx and esophagus. Presenting symptoms: halitosis, dysphagia, obstruction.	
Meckel's diverticulum 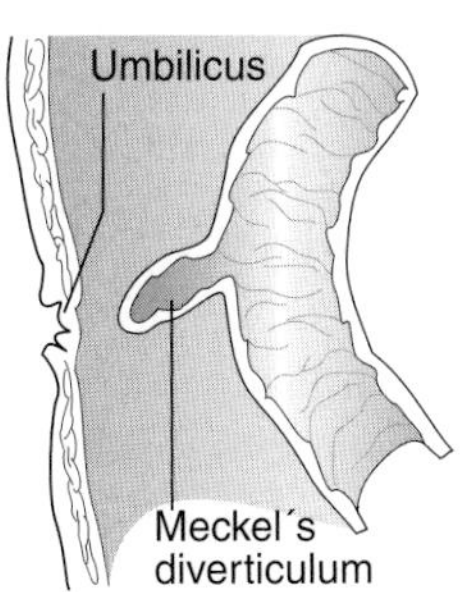	Persistence of the vitelline duct or yolk stalk. May contain ectopic acid–secreting gastric mucosa and/or pancreatic tissue. **Most common congenital anomaly of the GI tract.** Can cause bleeding, intussusception, volvulus, or obstruction near the terminal ileum. Contrast with omphalomesenteric cyst = cystic dilatation of vitelline duct.	The five 2's: 2 inches long. 2 feet from the ileocecal valve. 2% of population. Commonly presents in first 2 years of life. May have 2 types of epithelia (gastric/ pancreatic).

Intussusception and volvulus

Intussusception—"telescoping" of 1 bowel segment into distal segment; can compromise blood supply (see Color Image 34). Often due to intraluminal mass. Usually in infants.

Volvulus—twisting of portion of bowel around its mesentery; can lead to obstruction and infarction. May occur at sigmoid colon, where there is redundant mesentery. Usually in elderly.

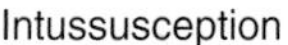

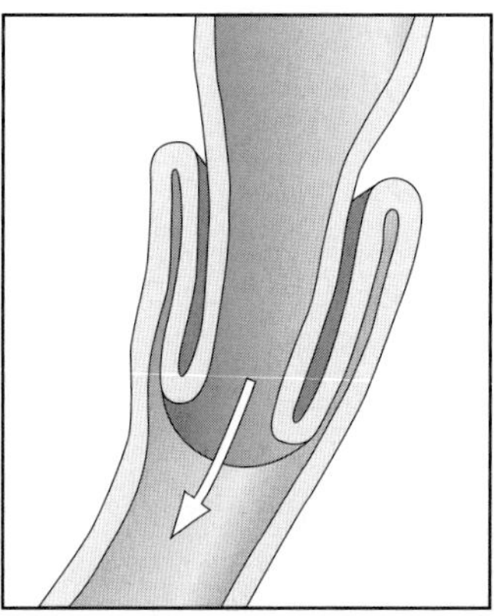

Volvulus

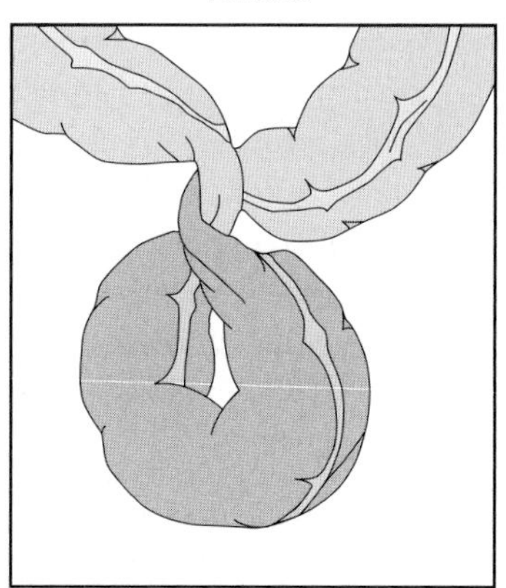

(Reproduced, with permission, from Kumar V et al. *Robbins & Cotran Pathologic Basis of Disease,* 7th ed. Atlanta: Elsevier, 2004: 856.)

Hirschsprung's disease

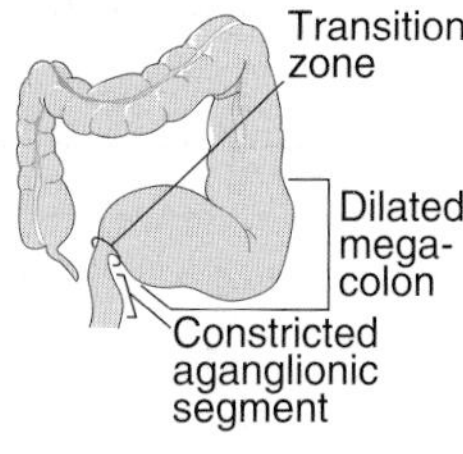

Congenital megacolon characterized by lack of ganglion cells/enteric nervous plexuses (Auerbach's and Meissner's plexuses) in segment on intestinal biopsy. Due to **failure of neural crest cell migration.**

Presents as chronic constipation early in life. Dilated portion of the colon proximal to the aganglionic segment, resulting in a "transition zone." Involves rectum. Usually failure to pass meconium.

Think of a giant spring that has **sprung** in the colon.
Risk ↑ with Down syndrome.

Other intestinal disorders

Duodenal atresia	Causes early bilious vomiting with proximal stomach distention ("double bubble") due to failure of recanalization of small bowel. Associated with Down syndrome.
Meconium ileus	In cystic fibrosis, meconium plug obstructs intestine, preventing stool passage.
Necrotizing enterocolitis	Necrosis of intestinal mucosa and possible perforation. Colon is usually involved, but can involve entire GI tract. In neonates, more common in preemies (↓ immunity).
Ischemic colitis	Reduction in intestinal blood causes ischemia. Typically affects elderly. Consequences include sepsis, bowel infarction, and death.
Adhesion	Acute bowel obstruction, commonly from a recent surgery. Can have well-demarcated necrotic zones.
Angiodysplasia	Tortuous dilation of vessels → bleeding. Most often found in cecum and ascending colon. More common in older patients. Confirmed by angiography.

Colonic polyps	90% are benign hyperplastic hamartomas, not neoplasms. Often rectosigmoid. Sawtooth appearance. The more villous the polyp, the more likely it is to be malignant (see Color Image 30).

Colorectal cancer	
Colorectal cancer (CRC)	3rd most common cancer. Most are sporadic, due to chromosomal instability (85%) or microsatellite instability (15%) (see Color Image 107). Risk factors: colorectal villous adenomas, chronic IBD (especially ulcerative colitis, ↑ age), FAP, HNPCC, past medical or family history; screen patients > 50 years of age with stool occult blood test and colonoscopy. "Apple core" lesion seen on barium enema x-ray. CEA tumor marker.
Familial adenomatous polyposis (FAP)	Autosomal-dominant mutation of *APC* gene on chromosome 5q. Two-hit hypothesis. Thousands of polyps; pancolonic; always involving the rectum. **Gardner's syndrome**—FAP with osseous and soft tissue tumors, retinal hyperplasia. **Turcot's syndrome**—FAP with possible brain involvement (glioblastoma).
HNPCC or Lynch syndrome	Mutations of DNA mismatch repair genes. ~80% progress to CRC. Proximal colon always involved.
Peutz-Jeghers syndrome	Benign polyposis syndrome. Associated with ↑ risk of CRC and other visceral malignancies (pancreas, breast, stomach, ovary). Findings: hamartomatous polyps of colon and small intestine; hyperpigmented mouth, lips, hands, genitalia.

Carcinoid tumor	Tumor of endocrine cells. Comprise 50% of small bowel tumors. Most common site is in small intestine. "Dense core bodies" seen on EM. Often produce 5-HT (depending on location → **carcinoid syndrome**). Classic symptoms: wheezing, right-sided heart murmurs, diarrhea, flushing.

Cirrhosis and portal hypertension

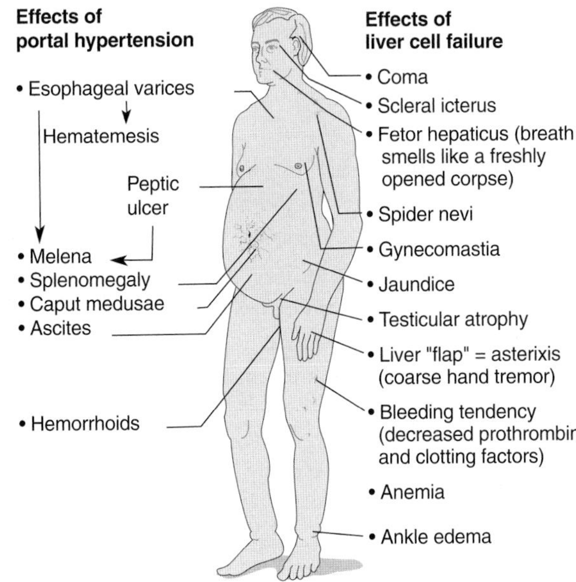

(Adapted, with permission, from Chandrasoma P, Taylor CE. *Concise Pathology,* 3rd ed. Stamford, CT: Appleton & Lange, 1998: 654.)

Cirrho (Greek) = tawny yellow.
Diffuse fibrosis of liver, destroys normal architecture.
Nodular regeneration.
Micronodular—nodules < 3 mm, uniform size. Due to metabolic insult (e.g., alcohol, hemochromatosis, Wilson's disease).
Macronodular—nodules > 3 mm, varied size. Usually due to significant liver injury leading to hepatic necrosis (e.g., postinfectious or drug-induced hepatitis). ↑ risk of hepatocellular carcinoma.
Portacaval shunt between splenic vein and left renal vein may relieve portal hypertension (see Color Image 29).

Enzyme markers of GI pathology

Serum enzyme	Major diagnostic use
Aminotransferases (AST and ALT)	Viral hepatitis Alcoholic hepatitis Myocardial infarction (AST)
GGT (γ-glutamyl transpeptidase)	Various liver diseases
Alkaline phosphatase	Obstructive liver disease (hepatocellular carcinoma), bone disease, bile duct disease
Amylase	Acute pancreatitis, mumps
Lipase	Acute pancreatitis
Ceruloplasmin (↓)	Wilson's disease

Reye's syndrome

Rare, often fatal childhood hepatoencephalopathy. Findings: fatty liver (microvesicular fatty change), hypoglycemia, coma. Associated with viral infection (especially VZV and influenza B) that has been treated with salicylates. **Aspirin is not recommended for children** (use acetaminophen, with caution).

Alcoholic liver disease

Hepatic steatosis: Short-term change with moderate alcohol intake. Reversible macrovesicular fatty change upon alcohol cessation (see Color Image 28).

Alcoholic hepatitis: Requires sustained, long-term consumption. Swollen and necrotic hepatocytes with neutrophilic infiltration. **Mallory bodies** (intracytoplasmic eosinophilic inclusions) are present.

Alcoholic cirrhosis: Final and irreversible form. Micronodular, irregularly shrunken liver with "hobnail" appearance (see Color Image 29). Sclerosis around central vein (zone III). Has manifestations of chronic liver disease (e.g., jaundice, hypoalbuminemia).

You're to**AST**ed with alcoholic hepatitis: **AST** > ALT (ratio usually > 1.5).
ALT > AST in viral hepatitis.

Hepatocellular carcinoma/hepatoma

Most common 1° malignant tumor of the liver in adults. ↑ incidence of hepatocellular carcinoma is associated with hepatitis B and C, Wilson's disease, hemochromatosis, α_1-antitrypsin deficiency, alcoholic cirrhosis, and carcinogens (e.g., aflatoxin in peanuts). Can present with tender hepatomegaly, ascites, polycythemia, and hypoglycemia.

Commonly spread by hematogenous dissemination.
Elevated **α-fetoprotein.** May lead to Budd-Chiari syndrome.

Budd-Chiari syndrome	Occlusion of IVC or hepatic veins with centrilobular congestion and necrosis, leading to congestive liver disease (hepatomegaly, ascites, abdominal pain, and eventual liver failure). May develop varices and have visible abdominal and back veins. Absence of JVD. Associated with polycythemia vera, pregnancy, and hepatocellular carcinoma.
α_1-antitrypsin deficiency	Misfolded gene product protein accumulates in hepatocellular ER. ↓ elastic tissue in lungs → emphysema. PAS-positive globules in liver. Autosomal recessive.
Jaundice	Normally, liver cells convert unconjugated (indirect) bilirubin into conjugated (direct) bilirubin. Direct bilirubin is water soluble and can be excreted into urine and by the liver into bile to be converted by gut bacteria to urobilinogen (some of which is reabsorbed). Some urobilinogen is also formed directly from heme metabolism.

Jaundice type	Hyperbilirubinemia	Urine bilirubin	Urine urobilinogen
Hepatocellular	Conjugated/unconjugated	↑	Normal/↓
Obstructive	Conjugated	↑	↓
Hemolytic	Unconjugated	Absent (acholuria)	↑

Hereditary hyperbilirubinemias

Gilbert's syndrome	Mildly ↓ UDP-glucuronyl transferase or ↓ bilirubin uptake. Asymptomatic. Elevated unconjugated bilirubin without overt hemolysis. Associated with stress.	No clinical consequences.
Crigler-Najjar syndrome, type I	Absent UDP-glucuronyl transferase. Presents early in life; patients die within a few years. Findings: jaundice, kernicterus (bilirubin deposition in brain), ↑ unconjugated bilirubin. Treatment: plasmapheresis and phototherapy.	Type II is less severe and responds to phenobarbital, which ↑ liver enzyme synthesis.
Dubin-Johnson syndrome	Conjugated hyperbilirubinemia due to defective liver excretion. Grossly black liver. Benign.	**Rotor's syndrome** is similar but even milder and does not cause black liver.

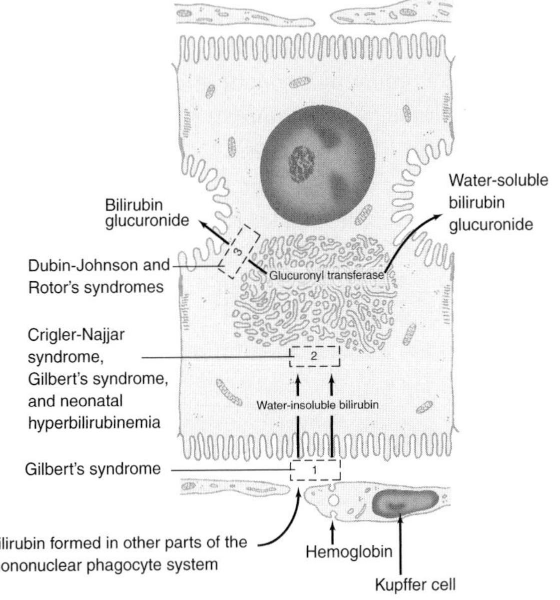

(Adapted, with permission, from Junqueira LC, Carneiro J, Kelley RO. *Basic Histology,* 9th ed. Stamford, CT: Appleton & Lange, 1999.)

Wilson's disease	Inadequate hepatic copper excretion and failure of copper to enter circulation as ceruloplasmin. Leads to copper accumulation, especially in liver, brain, cornea, kidneys, and joints. Also known as hepatolenticular degeneration.	Treat with penicillamine. Autosomal-recessive inheritance.
	Wilson's disease is characterized by: **A**sterixis **B**asal ganglia degeneration (parkinsonian symptoms) **C**eruloplasmin ↓, **C**irrhosis, **C**orneal deposits (Kayser-Fleischer rings—see Color Image 51), **C**opper accumulation, **C**arcinoma (hepatocellular), **C**horeiform movements **D**ementia	**ABCD.**
Hemochromatosis	Hemosiderosis is the deposition of hemosiderin (iron); hemochromatosis is the disease caused by this iron deposition (see Color Image 26). Classic triad of micronodular **C**irrhosis, **D**iabetes mellitus, and skin pigmentation → **"bronze" diabetes.** Results in **C**HF and ↑ risk of hepatocellular carcinoma. Disease may be 1° (autosomal recessive) or 2° to chronic transfusion therapy (e.g., β-thalassemia major). ↑ ferritin, ↑ iron, ↓ TIBC → ↑ transferrin saturation.	**H**emochromatosis **C**an **C**ause **D**eposits. Total body iron may reach 50 g, enough to set off metal detectors at airports. Treat hereditary hemochromatosis with repeated phlebotomy, deferoxamine. Associated with HLA-A3.
Primary sclerosing cholangitis	Both intra- and extrahepatic. Inflammation and fibrosis of bile ducts → alternating strictures and dilation with "beading" on ERCP. Concentric "onion skin" bile duct fibrosis. ↑ ALP. Associated with ulcerative colitis. Can lead to 2° biliary cirrhosis.	
Biliary cirrhosis		
Primary	Intrahepatic, autoimmune disorder; severe obstructive jaundice, steatorrhea, pruritus, hypercholesterolemia (xanthoma). ↑ ALP, ↑ **serum mitochondrial antibodies.** Associated with scleroderma and CREST syndrome.	
Secondary	Due to extrahepatic biliary obstruction. ↑ in pressure in intrahepatic ducts → injury/fibrosis. Often complicated by ascending cholangitis (bacterial infection), bile stasis, and "bile lakes." ↑ ALP, ↑ conjugated bilirubin.	

Gallstones (cholelithiasis)

Cystic duct
Hepatic duct
Stone in the common bile duct
Fibrosed gallbladder with gallstones
Pancreatic duct

Form when solubilizing bile acids and lecithin are overwhelmed by ↑ cholesterol and/or bilirubin.
2 types of stones:
1. **Cholesterol stones** (radiolucent with 10–20% opaque due to calcifications)—80% of stones. Associated with obesity, Crohn's disease, cystic fibrosis, advanced age, clofibrate, estrogens, multiparity, rapid weight loss, and Native American origin.
2. **Pigment stones** (radiopaque)—seen in patients with chronic RBC hemolysis, alcoholic cirrhosis, advanced age, and biliary infection.

Can cause ascending cholangitis, acute pancreatitis, bile stasis, cholecystitis.
Can also → **biliary colic**—gallstones interfere with bile flow, causing bile duct contraction. May present without pain (e.g., in diabetics).
Diagnose with ultrasound. Treat with cholecystectomy.

Risk factors (**4 F's**):
1. **F**emale
2. **F**at
3. **F**ertile
4. **F**orty

Charcot's triad of cholangitis:
1. Jaundice
2. Fever
3. RUQ pain

Cholecystitis

Inflammation of gallbladder. Can be infectious (e.g., CMV, *Cryptococcus*) or due to a gallstone complication. ↑ ALP if bile duct becomes involved (e.g., ascending cholangitis).

Acute pancreatitis

Autodigestion of pancreas by pancreatic enzymes.
Causes: **G**allstones, **E**thanol, **T**rauma, **S**teroids, **M**umps, **A**utoimmune disease, **S**corpion sting, **H**ypercalcemia/**H**yperlipidemia, **D**rugs (e.g., sulfa drugs).
Clinical presentation: epigastric abdominal pain radiating to back, anorexia, nausea.
Labs: elevated amylase, lipase (higher specificity).
Can lead to DIC, ARDS (pancreatic enzymes act on lung tissue), diffuse fat necrosis, hypocalcemia (Ca^{2+} collects in pancreatic calcium soap deposits), pseudocyst formation, hemorrhage, and infection.
Chronic pancreatitis can lead to pancreatic insufficiency → steatorrhea, fat-soluble vitamin deficiency, and diabetes mellitus.
Chronic calcifying pancreatitis is strongly associated with alcoholism (see Image 142).

GET SMASHeD.

Pancreatic adenocarcinoma

Prognosis averages 6 months or less; very aggressive; usually already metastasized at presentation; tumors more common in pancreatic head (→ obstructive jaundice) (see Image 134). ↑ risk in Jewish and African-American males. CEA and CA-19-9 tumor markers. Associated with cigarettes but not EtOH.

Often presents with:

1. Abdominal pain radiating to back
2. Weight loss (due to malabsorption and anorexia)
3. Migratory thrombophlebitis—redness and tenderness on palpation of extremities (Trousseau's syndrome)
4. Obstructive jaundice with palpable gallbladder (Courvoisier's sign) (see Image 141).

▶ GASTROINTESTINAL–PHARMACOLOGY

GI therapy

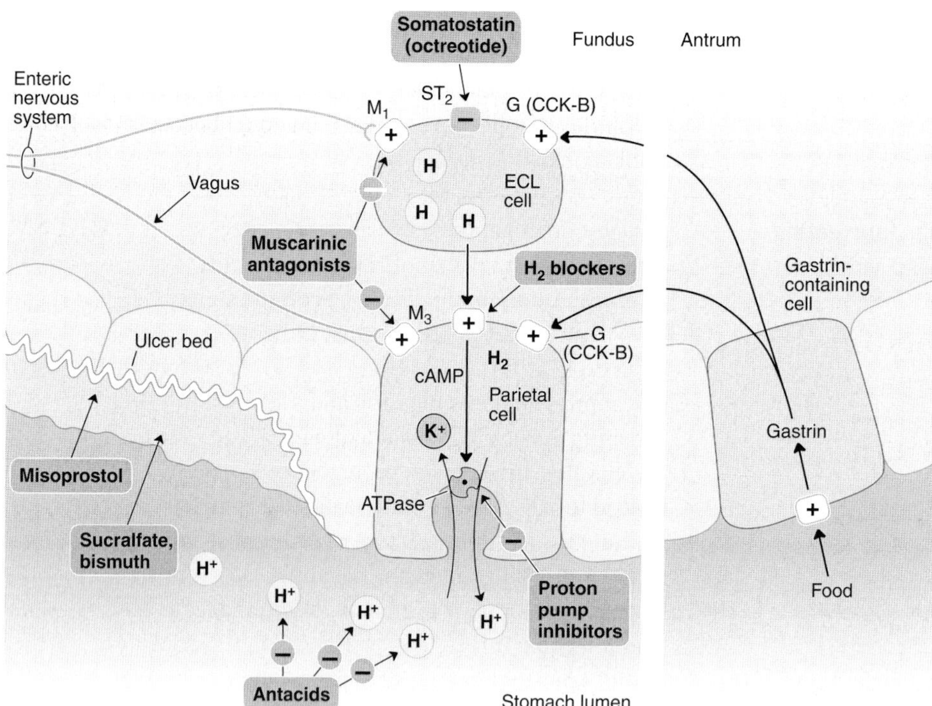

(Adapted, with permission, from Katzung BG, Trevor AJ. *USMLE Road Map: Pharmacology*, 1st ed. New York: McGraw-Hill, 2003: 159.)

Lymphocyte 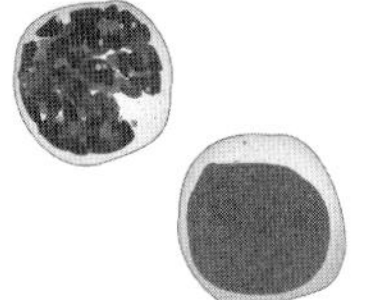	Round, densely staining nucleus. Small amount of pale cytoplasm. B lymphocytes produce antibodies. T lymphocytes manifest the cellular immune response as well as regulate B lymphocytes and macrophages.	
B lymphocyte 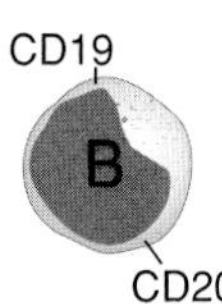	Part of humoral immune response. Arises from stem cells in bone marrow. Matures in marrow. Migrates to peripheral lymphoid tissue (follicles of lymph nodes, white pulp of spleen, unencapsulated lymphoid tissue). When antigen is encountered, B cells differentiate into plasma cells and produce antibodies. Has memory. Can function as an APC via MHC II.	**B** = **B**one marrow.
Plasma cell 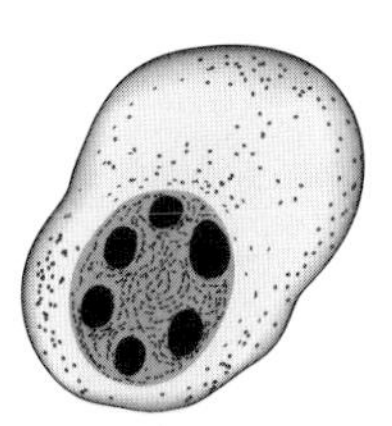	Off-center nucleus, clock-face chromatin distribution, abundant RER and well-developed Golgi apparatus. B cells differentiate into plasma cells, which produce large amounts of antibody specific to a particular antigen.	Multiple myeloma is a plasma cell neoplasm.
T lymphocyte 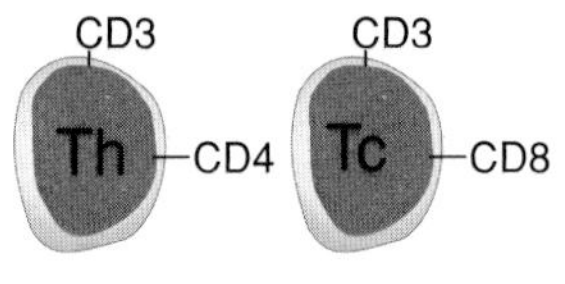	Mediates cellular immune response. Originates from stem cells in the bone marrow, but matures in the thymus. T cells differentiate into cytotoxic T cells (MHC I, CD8), helper T cells (MHC II, CD4), and suppressor T cells. The majority of circulating lymphocytes are T cells (80%).	**T** is for **T**hymus. **CD** is for **C**luster of **D**ifferentiation. **MHC × CD** = 8 (e.g., MHC 2 × CD4 = 8, and MHC 1 × CD8 = 8).

Coagulation cascade

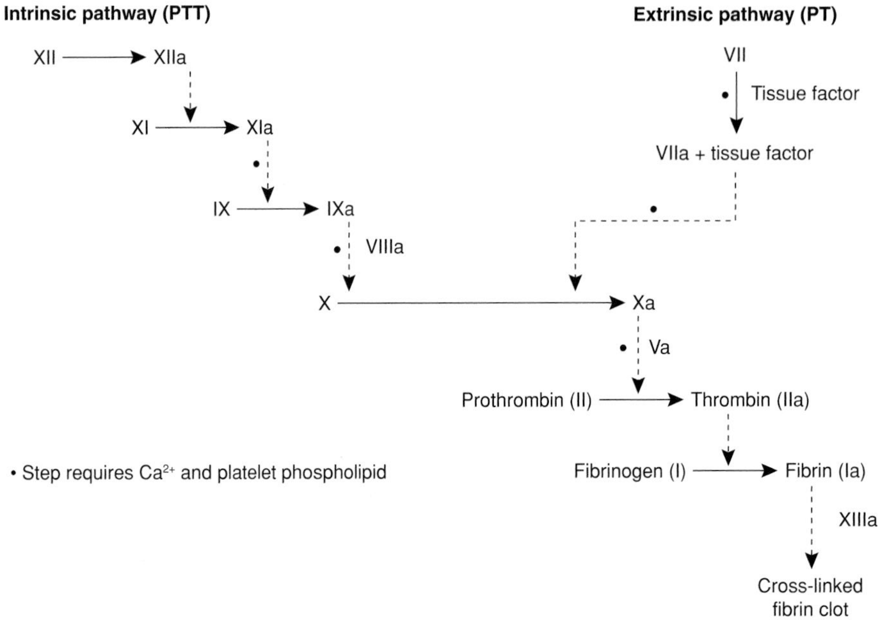

Coagulation factor inhibitors and fibrinolysis	Vitamin K–dependent factors = II, VII, IX, X, protein C, and protein S. Thrombomodulin activates protein C (protein S is a cofactor for protein C activation). Activated protein C → inactivation of Va and VIIIa. Antithrombin III—inactivates thrombin, IXa, Xa, and XIa; activated by heparin. tPA—generates plasmin from plasminogen, which cleaves fibrin clots.	Factor V Leiden mutation causes resistance to activated protein C.

Convergence of coagulation, complement, and kinin pathways

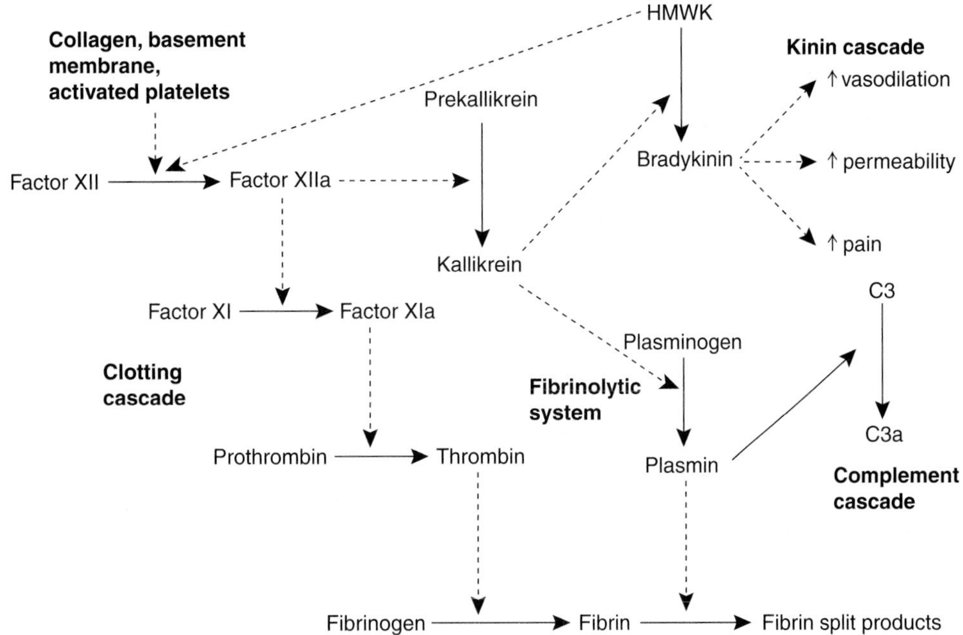

Note: Kallikrein activates bradykinin; ACE inactivates bradykinin.

Thrombogenesis

Platelet plug formation is a temporary repair. It occurs in 3 steps:

1. Platelet adhesion to exposed basement membrane—requires vWF
2. Aggregation—regulated as follows:
   a. TXA_2 released by platelets ↑ aggregation
   b. PGI_2 (prostacyclin) and NO released by endothelial cells ↓ aggregation
3. Swelling—ADP and Ca^{2+} release to strengthen plug → fibrin deposition

▶ HEMATOLOGY AND ONCOLOGY–PATHOLOGY

Blood groups

A	A antigen on RBC surface and B antibody in plasma.	Rh+ blood transfusions into an Rh– individual can result in massive IgG production.
B	B antigen on RBC surface and A antibody in plasma.	
AB	A and B antigens on RBC surface; no antibodies in plasma; "universal recipient."	Incompatible blood transfusions can cause immunologic response, hemolysis, renal failure, shock, and death.
O	Neither A nor B antigen on RBC surface; both antibodies in plasma; "universal donor."	

RBC forms

Biconcave	Normal.	
Spherocytes	Hereditary spherocytosis, autoimmune hemolysis.	
Elliptocyte	Hereditary elliptocytosis.	
Macro-ovalocyte	Megaloblastic anemia (also hypersegmented PMNs), marrow failure.	
Helmet cell, schistocyte	DIC, traumatic hemolysis.	
Sickle cell	Sickle cell anemia.	
Bite cell	G6PD deficiency.	
Teardrop cell	Myeloid metaplasia with myelofibrosis.	
Acanthocyte	Spiny appearance in abetalipoproteinemia.	
Target cell	**H**bC disease, **A**splenia, **L**iver disease, **T**halassemia.	"**HALT**," said the hunter to his **target.**
Poikilocytes	Nonuniform shapes in TTP/HUS, microvascular damage, DIC.	
Burr cell	TTP/HUS.	
Basophilic stippling	**T**halassemias, **A**nemia of chronic disease, **I**ron deficiency, **L**ead poisoning.	**TAIL.**

Anemia

Type	Etiology	Comments
Microcytic, hypochromic (MCV < 80)	Iron deficiency—↓ serum iron, ↑ TIBC, ↓ ferritin (intracellular iron stores) (see Color Image 20). Thalassemias—target cells (see Color Image 18). Lead poisoning, sideroblastic anemias.	Vitamin B_{12} and folate deficiencies are associated with hypersegmented PMNs. Unlike folate deficiency, vitamin B_{12} deficiency (e.g., pernicious anemia) is associated with neurologic problems.
Macrocytic (MCV > 100)	Megaloblastic—vitamin B_{12}/folate deficiency. Drugs that block DNA synthesis (e.g., sulfa drugs, phenytoin, AZT). Marked reticulocytosis (bigger than mature RBCs).	↓ serum haptoglobin and ↑ serum LDH indicate RBC hemolysis. Direct Coombs' test is used to distinguish between immune- vs. non-immune-mediated RBC hemolysis.
Normocytic, normochromic	Acute hemorrhage. Enzyme defects—G6PD deficiency (X-linked), PK deficiency (AR). RBC membrane defects (e.g., hereditary spherocytosis). Bone marrow disorders (e.g., aplastic anemia, leukemia). Hemoglobinopathies (e.g., sickle cell disease). Autoimmune hemolytic anemia. Anemia of chronic disease (ACD)—↓ TIBC, ↑ ferritin, ↑ storage iron in marrow macrophages.	

Lab values in anemia

	Iron deficiency	Chronic disease	Pregnancy/ OCP use	Hemo-chromatosis
Serum iron	↓ (1°)	↓	—	↑ (1°)
Transferrin/ TIBC (indirectly proportional to transferrin)	↑	↓*	↑ (1°)	↓
Ferritin	↓	↑ (1°)	—	↑
% transferrin saturation (serum Fe/TIBC)	↓↓	—	↓	↑↑

*Evolutionary reasoning—pathogens use circulating iron to thrive. The body has adapted a system in which iron is stored within the cells of the body and prevents pathogens from acquiring circulating iron.

Aplastic anemia	Pancytopenia characterized by severe anemia, neutropenia, and thrombocytopenia caused by failure or destruction of multipotent myeloid stem cells, with inadequate production or release of differentiated cell lines.
Causes	Radiation, benzene, chloramphenicol, alkylating agents, antimetabolites, viral agents (parvovirus B19, EBV, HIV), Fanconi's anemia, idiopathic (immune mediated, 1° stem cell defect). May follow acute hepatitis.
Symptoms	Fatigue, malaise, pallor, purpura, mucosal bleeding, petechiae, infection.
Pathologic features	Pancytopenia with normal cell morphology; hypocellular bone marrow with fatty infiltration. Diagnose with bone marrow biopsy.
Treatment	Withdrawal of offending agent, allogeneic bone marrow transplantation, RBC and platelet transfusion, G-CSF or GM-CSF.

Blood dyscrasias		
Sickle cell anemia	HbS mutation is a single amino acid replacement in β chain (substitution of normal glutamic acid with valine). Low O_2 or dehydration precipitates sickling. Heterozygotes (sickle cell trait) are relatively malaria resistant (balanced polymorphism). Complications in homozygotes (sickle cell disease) include aplastic crisis (due to parvovirus B19 infection), autosplenectomy, ↑ risk of encapsulated organism infection, *Salmonella* osteomyelitis, painful crisis (vaso-occlusive), renal papillary necrosis, and splenic sequestration crisis (see Color Image 21). Therapies for sickle cell anemia include hydroxyurea (↑ HbF) and bone marrow transplantation. HbC defect is a different β-chain mutation; patients with HbC or HbSC (1 of each mutant gene) have milder disease than do HbSS patients.	8% of African-Americans carry the HbS trait; 0.2% have the disease. Sickled cells are crescent-shaped RBCs. "Crew cut" on skull x-ray due to marrow expansion from ↑ erythropoiesis (also in thalassemias). Newborns—initially asymptomatic owing to ↑ HbF and ↓ HbS.
α-thalassemia	There are 4 α-globin genes. In α-thalassemia, the α-globin chain is underproduced (as a function of number of bad genes, 1–4). There is no compensatory ↑ of any other chains. HbH (β_4-tetramers, lacks 3 α-globin genes). Hb Barts (γ_4-tetramers, lacks all 4 α-globin genes) results in hydrops fetalis and intrauterine fetal death.	α-thalassemia is prevalent in Asia and Africa. β-thalassemia is prevalent in Mediterranean populations.
β-thalassemia	In β-thalassemia minor (heterozygote), the β chain is underproduced; in β-thalassemia major (homozygote), the β chain is absent. In both cases, fetal hemoglobin production is compensatorily ↑ but is inadequate. HbS/β-thalassemia heterozygote has mild to moderate disease (see Color Image 19).	β-thalassemia major results in severe anemia requiring blood transfusions. Cardiac failure due to 2° hemochromatosis. Marrow expansion ("crew cut" on skull x-ray) → skeletal deformities.

Hemolytic anemias	↑ serum bilirubin (jaundice, pigment gallstones), ↑ reticulocytes (marrow compensating for anemia).	
Autoimmune anemia	Mostly extravascular hemolysis (accelerated RBC destruction in liver Kupffer cells and spleen). **W**arm agglutinin (Ig**G**)—chronic anemia seen in SLE, in CLL, or with certain drugs (e.g., α-methyldopa). **Cold** agglutinin (Ig**M**)—acute anemia triggered by cold; seen with *Mycoplasma pneumoniae* infections or infectious mononucleosis. Erythroblastosis fetalis—seen in newborn due to Rh or other blood antigen incompatibility → mother's antibodies attack fetal RBCs.	Autoimmune hemolytic anemias are Coombs positive. Direct Coombs' test: anti-Ig Ab added to patient's RBCs agglutinate if RBCs are coated with Ig. Indirect Coombs' test: normal RBCs added to patient's serum agglutinate if serum has anti-RBC surface Ig. **W**arm weather is **GG**Great. **Cold** ice cream . . . **MMM**.
Hereditary spherocytosis	Intrinsic, extravascular hemolysis due to spectrin or ankyrin defect. RBCs are small and round with no central pallor → less membrane → ↑ MCHC, ↑ RDW. Howell-Jolly bodies present after splenectomy.	Coombs negative. Osmotic fragility test used to confirm.
Paroxysmal nocturnal hemoglobinuria	Intravascular hemolysis due to membrane defect → ↑ sensitivity of RBCs to the lytic activity of complement (impaired synthesis of GP I anchor in RBC membrane).	↑ urine hemosiderin.
Microangiopathic anemia	Intravascular hemolysis seen in DIC, TTP/HUS, SLE, or malignant hypertension.	Schistocytes (helmet cells) seen on blood smear.

DIC	Activation of coagulation cascade leading to microthrombi and global consumption of platelets, fibrin, and coagulation factors.	
Causes	**S**epsis (gram-negative), **T**rauma, **O**bstetric complications, acute **P**ancreatitis, **M**alignancy, **N**ephrotic syndrome, **T**ransfusion.	**STOP M**aking **N**ew **T**hrombi!
Lab findings	↑ PT, ↑ PTT, ↑ fibrin split products (D-dimers), ↓ platelet count. Helmet-shaped cells and schistocytes on blood smear.	

Bleeding disorders

Platelet abnormalities

Causes include:

1. ITP (peripheral platelet destruction, antiplatelet antibodies, ↑ megakaryocytes)
2. TTP (↑ platelet aggregation → thrombosis → schistocytes, ↑ LDH, neurologic and renal symptoms, fever)
3. DIC (schistocytes, ↑ fibrin split products)
4. Aplastic anemia
5. Drugs (e.g., immunosuppressive agents)

Microhemorrhage: mucous membrane bleeding, epistaxis, petechiae, purpura, ↑ bleeding time.

Coagulation factor defects

Coagulopathies include:

1. Hemophilia A (factor VIII deficiency)
2. Hemophilia B (factor IX deficiency)
3. von Willebrand's disease (mild; most common bleeding disorder; deficiency of von Willebrand factor → defect of platelet adhesion and ↓ factor VIII survival)

Macrohemorrhage: hemarthroses (bleeding into joints), easy bruising, ↑ PT and/or PTT.

Hemorrhagic disorders

Disorder	Platelet count	Bleeding time	PT	PTT
Thrombocytopenia	↓	↑	—	—
Hemophilia A or B	—	—	—	↑
von Willebrand's disease	—	↑	—	↑
DIC	↓	↑	↑	↑
Vitamin K deficiency	—	—	↑	↑
Bernard-Soulier disease	↓	↑	—	—
Glanzmann's thrombasthenia	—	↑	—	—

Bernard-Soulier disease = defect of platelet adhesion (↓ GP Ib).
Glanzmann's thrombasthenia = defect of platelet aGgregation (↓ GP IIb-IIIa).
Note: platelet count must reach a very low value (15,000–20,000/mm^3) before generalized bleeding occurs; thrombocytopenia = < 100,000/mm^3.
PT (extrinsic)—factors II, V, VII, and X.
PTT (intrinsic)—all factors except VII.

Reed-Sternberg cells

Distinctive tumor giant cell seen in Hodgkin's disease (see Color Image 25); binucleate or bilobed with the 2 halves as mirror images ("owl's eyes"). Necessary but not sufficient for a diagnosis of Hodgkin's disease. Variants include lacunar cells in nodular sclerosis variant.

Lymphomas

Hodgkin's	Non-Hodgkin's
Presence of Reed-Sternberg cells (RS cells are CD30+ and CD15+ B-cell origin)	Associated with HIV and immunosuppression
Localized, single group of nodes; extranodal rare; contiguous spread	Multiple, peripheral nodes; extranodal involvement common; noncontiguous spread
Constitutional ("B") signs/symptoms—low-grade fever, night sweats, weight loss	Majority involve B cells (except those of lymphoblastic T-cell origin)
Mediastinal lymphadenopathy	No hypergammaglobulinemia
50% of cases associated with EBV; bimodal distribution —young and old; more common in men except for nodular sclerosing type	Fewer constitutional signs/symptoms
Good prognosis = ↑ lymphocytes, ↓ RS	Peak incidence 20–40 years of age

Hodgkin's lymphoma

Type	RS	Lymphos	Prognosis	Comments
Nodular sclerosing (65–75%)	+	+++	Excellent	Most common; collagen banding; lacunar cells; women > men; primarily young adults.
Mixed cellularity (25%)	++++	+++	Intermediate	Numerous RS cells.
Lymphocyte predominant (6%)	+	++++	Excellent	< 35-year-old males.
Lymphocyte depleted (rare)	*	+	Poor	Older males with disseminated disease.

*RS high relative to lymphocytes.

Multiple myeloma

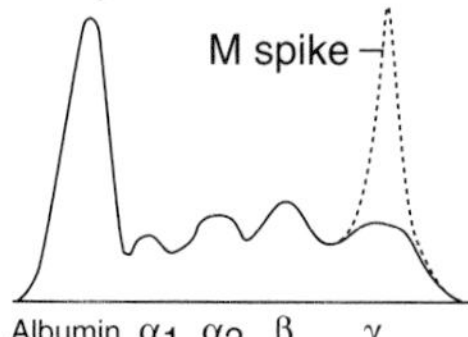

Monoclonal plasma cell ("fried-egg" appearance) cancer that arises in the marrow and produces large amounts of IgG (55%) or IgA (25%). Most common 1° tumor arising within bone in the elderly (> 40–50 years of age). Destructive bone lesions and consequent hypercalcemia. Renal insufficiency, ↑ susceptibility to infection, and anemia. Associated with 1° amyloidosis (AL) and punched-out lytic bone lesions on x-ray. Characterized by monoclonal immunoglobulin spike (M protein) on serum protein electrophoresis and Ig light chains in urine (Bence Jones protein). Blood smear shows RBCs stacked like poker chips (rouleaux formation). Compare with Waldenström's macroglobulinemia → M spike = IgM (→ hyperviscosity symptoms); no lytic bone lesions (see Color Image 23).

If asymptomatic, called monoclonal gammopathy of undetermined significance (MGUS).

Non-Hodgkin's lymphoma

Type	Occurs in	Cell type	Genetics	Comments
Small lymphocytic lymphoma	Adults	B cells		Like CLL with focal mass; low grade.
Follicular lymphoma (small cleaved cell)	Adults	B cells	t(14;18) *bcl*-2 expression	Most common (adult). Difficult to cure; indolent course; *bcl*-2 inhibits apoptosis.
Diffuse large cell lymphoma	Usually older adults, but 20% occur in children	80% B cells 20% T cells (mature)		Aggressive, but up to 50% are curable.
Mantle cell lymphoma	Adults	B cells	t(11;14)	Poor prognosis, CD5+.
Lymphoblastic lymphoma	Most often children	T cells (immature)		Most common in children; commonly presents with ALL and mediastinal mass; very aggressive T-cell lymphoma.
Burkitt's lymphoma	Most often children	B cells	t(8;14) c-*myc* gene moves next to heavy-chain Ig gene (14)	"Starry-sky" appearance (sheets of lymphocytes with interspersed macrophages); associated with EBV; jaw lesion in endemic form in Africa; pelvis or abdomen in sporadic form (see Color Image 24).

Chromosomal translocations

Translocation	Associated disorder	
t(9;22) (**Philadelphia** chromosome)	CML (*bcr-abl* hybrid)	**Philadelphia** Crea**ML** cheese.
t(8;14)	Burkitt's lymphoma (c-*myc* activation)	
t(14;18)	Follicular lymphomas (*bcl*-2 activation)	
t(15;17)	M3 type of AML (responsive to all-*trans* retinoic acid)	
t(11;22)	Ewing's sarcoma	
t(11;14)	Mantle cell lymphoma	

Leukemoid reaction	↑ with left shift (e.g., 80% bands) and ↑ leukocyte alkaline phosphatase.
Leukemias	General considerations— ↑ number of circulating leukocytes in blood; bone marrow infiltrates of leukemic cells; marrow failure can cause anemia (↓ RBCs), infections (↓ mature WBCs), and hemorrhage (↓ platelets); leukemic cell infiltrates in liver, spleen, and lymph nodes are common (see Color Image 22).
ALL	Children; lymphoblasts; TdT+ (marker of pre–T and pre–B cells); most responsive to therapy. May spread to CNS and testes.
AML	Auer rods; myeloblasts; adults.
CLL	Older adults (> 60 years of age); lymphadenopathy; hepatosplenomegaly; few symptoms; indolent course; ↑ smudge cells in peripheral blood smear; warm antibody autoimmune hemolytic anemia; very similar to SLL (small lymphocytic lymphoma).
CML	Defined by the Philadelphia chromosome (t[9;22], *bcr-abl*); myeloid stem cell proliferation; presents with ↑ neutrophils and metamyelocytes; splenomegaly; may accelerate to AML ("blast crisis"). Very low leukocyte alkaline phosphatase (vs. leukemoid reaction). Hairy cell leukemia—mature B-cell tumor in the elderly. Cells have filamentous, hair-like projections. Stains TRAP (tartrate-resistant acid phosphatase) positive.

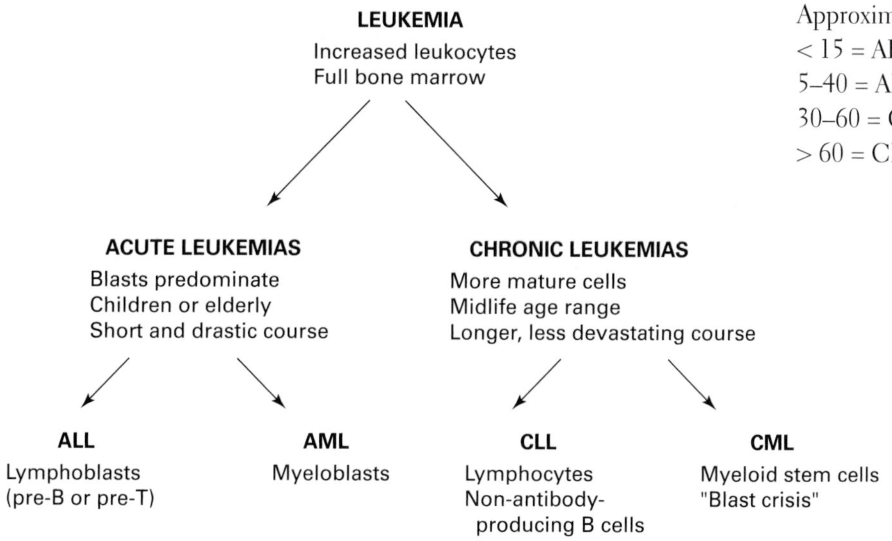

LEUKEMIA
Increased leukocytes
Full bone marrow

Approximate ages:
< 15 = ALL
5–40 = AML
30–60 = CML
> 60 = CLL

ACUTE LEUKEMIAS
Blasts predominate
Children or elderly
Short and drastic course

ALL
Lymphoblasts
(pre-B or pre-T)

AML
Myeloblasts

CHRONIC LEUKEMIAS
More mature cells
Midlife age range
Longer, less devastating course

CLL
Lymphocytes
Non-antibody-producing B cells

CML
Myeloid stem cells
"Blast crisis"

Auer bodies (rods)	Auer rods are peroxidase-positive cytoplasmic inclusions in granulocytes and myeloblasts. Primarily seen in acute promyelocytic leukemia (M3). Treatment of AML M3 can release Auer rods → DIC.
Histiocytosis X	Caused by Langerhans cells from the monocyte lineage that infiltrate the lung. Birbeck granules ("tennis rackets" on EM). Primarily affects young adults. Worse with smoking.

Heparin		
Mechanism	Catalyzes the activation of antithrombin III, ↓ thrombin and Xa. Short half-life.	
Clinical use	Immediate anticoagulation for pulmonary embolism, stroke, angina, MI, DVT. Used during pregnancy (does not cross placenta). Follow PTT.	
Toxicity	Bleeding, thrombocytopenia (HIT), osteoporosis, drug-drug interactions. For rapid reversal of heparinization, use **protamine sulfate** (positively charged molecule that acts by binding negatively charged heparin).	
Notes	Newer **low-molecular-weight heparins** (enoxaparin) act more on Xa, have better bioavailability and 2–4 times longer half-life. Can be administered subcutaneously and without laboratory monitoring. Not easily reversible. Heparin-induced thrombocytopenia (HIT)—heparin binds platelets, causing autoantibody production that destroys platelets and overactivates the remaining ones, resulting in a thrombocytopenic, hypercoagulable state.	
Lepirudin, bivalirudin	Hirudin derivatives; directly inhibit thrombin. Used as an alternative to heparin for anticoagulating patients with HIT.	
Warfarin (Coumadin)		
Mechanism	Interferes with normal synthesis and γ-carboxylation of vitamin K–dependent clotting factors II, VII, IX, and X and protein C and S. Metabolized by the cytochrome P-450 pathway. Affects **EX**trinsic pathway and ↑ **PT.** Long half-life.	The **EX-P**a**T**riot went to **WAR**(farin).
Clinical use	Chronic anticoagulation. Not used in pregnant women (because warfarin, unlike heparin, can cross the placenta). Follow PT/INR values.	
Toxicity	Bleeding, teratogenic, skin/tissue necrosis, drug-drug interactions.	

Heparin vs. warfarin

	Heparin	Warfarin
Structure	Large anionic polymer, acidic	Small lipid-soluble molecule
Route of administration	Parenteral (IV, SC)	Oral
Site of action	Blood	Liver
Onset of action	Rapid (seconds)	Slow, limited by half-lives of normal clotting factors
Mechanism of action	Activates antithrombin III, which ↓ the action of IIa (thrombin) and Xa	Impairs the synthesis of vitamin K–dependent clotting factors II, VII, IX, and X (vitamin K antagonist)
Duration of action	Acute (hours)	Chronic (days)
Inhibits coagulation in vitro	Yes	No
Treatment of acute overdose	Protamine sulfate	IV vitamin K and fresh frozen plasma
Monitoring	PTT (intrinsic pathway)	PT/INR (extrinsic pathway)
Crosses placenta	No	Yes (teratogenic)

Thrombolytics

Streptokinase, urokinase, tPA (alteplase), APSAC (anistreplase).

Mechanism Directly or indirectly aid conversion of plasminogen to plasmin, the major fibrinolytic enzyme, which cleaves thrombin and fibrin clots. ↑ PT, ↑ PTT, no change in platelet count.

Clinical use Early MI, early ischemic stroke.

Toxicity Bleeding. Contraindicated in patients with active bleeding, history of intracranial bleeding, recent surgery, known bleeding diatheses, or severe hypertension. Treat toxicity with aminocaproic acid, an inhibitor of fibrinolysis.

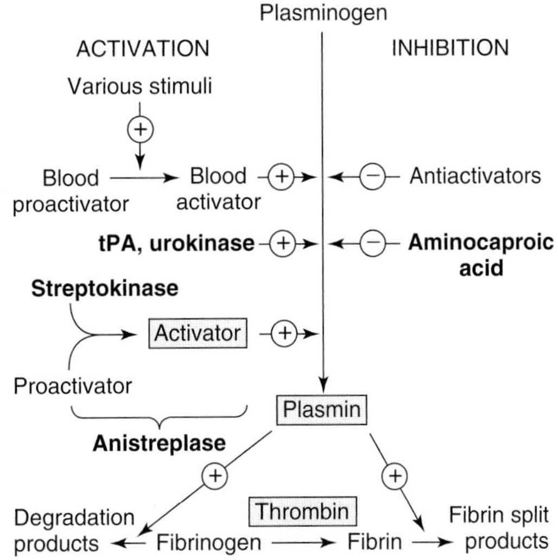

(Adapted, with permission, from Katzung BG. *Basic and Clinical Pharmacology,* 7th ed. Stamford, CT: Appleton & Lange, 1997: 550.)

Mechanism of antiplatelet interaction

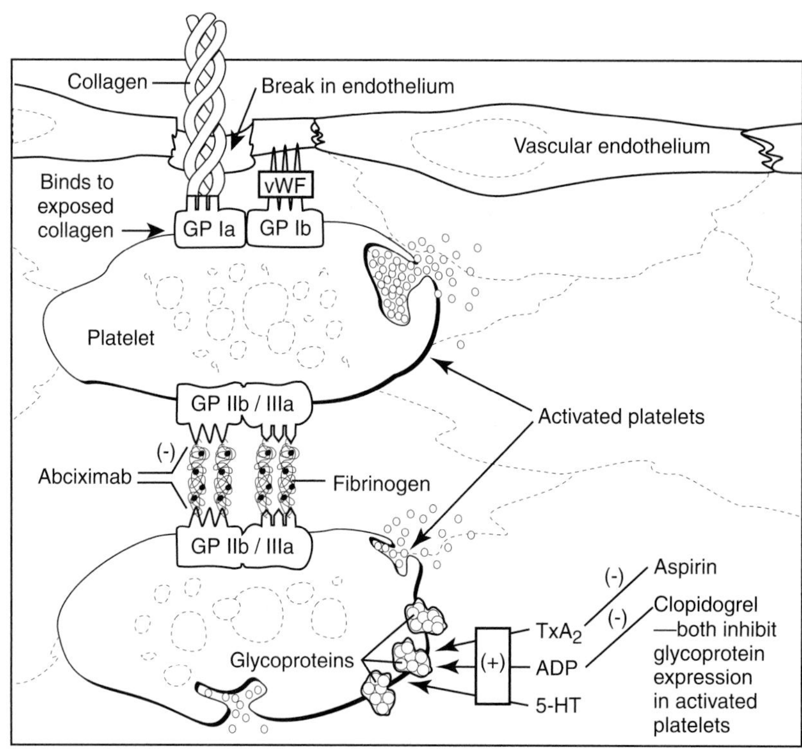

Aspirin (ASA)

Mechanism	Acetylates and irreversibly inhibits cyclooxygenase (both COX-1 and COX-2) to prevent conversion of arachidonic acid to thromboxane A_2. ↑ bleeding time. No effect on PT, PTT.
Clinical use	Antipyretic, analgesic, anti-inflammatory, antiplatelet drug.
Toxicity	Gastric ulceration, bleeding, hyperventilation, Reye's syndrome, tinnitus (CN VIII).

Clopidogrel, ticlopidine

Mechanism	Inhibit platelet aggregation by irreversibly blocking ADP receptors. Inhibit fibrinogen binding by preventing glycoprotein IIb/IIIa expression.
Clinical use	Acute coronary syndrome; coronary stenting. ↓ incidence or recurrence of thrombotic stroke.
Toxicity	Neutropenia (ticlopidine).

Abciximab

Mechanism	Monoclonal antibody that binds to the glycoprotein receptor IIb/IIIa on activated platelets, preventing aggregation.
Clinical use	Acute coronary syndromes, percutaneous transluminal coronary angioplasty.
Toxicity	Bleeding, thrombocytopenia.

Cancer drugs—site of action

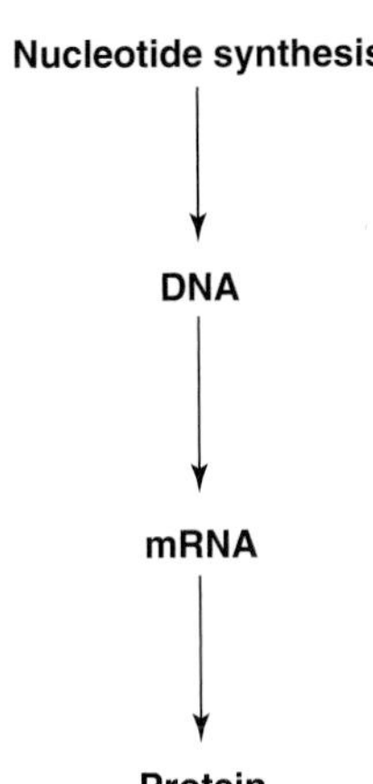

1. Methotrexate + 5-FU— ↓ thymidine synthesis
2. 6-MP— ↓ purine synthesis
3. Cytarabine
4. Alkylating agents + cisplatin—DNA cross-linkage
5. Dactinomycin + doxorubicin—DNA intercalation
6. Bleomycin—strand breakage + DNA intercalation
7. Etoposide—strand breakage
8. Steroids
9. Tamoxifen
10. Vinca alkaloids—inhibit microtubule formation
11. Paclitaxel—inhibits microtubule disassembly

Cell cycle specific—antimetabolites (MTX, 5-FU, 6-MP), etoposide, bleomycin, vinca alkaloids, paclitaxel.

Cell cycle nonspecific—alkylating agents, antibiotics (dactinomycin, doxorubicin).

Cancer drugs—cell cycle

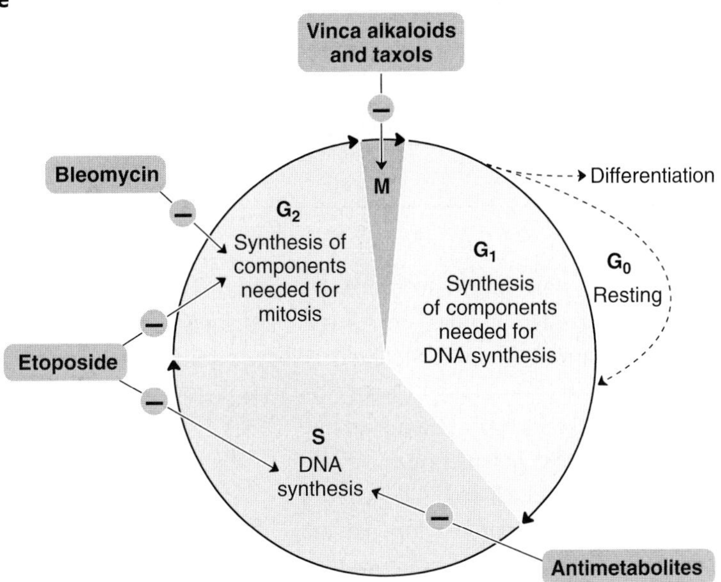

(Adapted, with permission, from Katzung BG, Trevor AJ. *USMLE Road Map: Pharmacology*, 1st ed. New York: McGraw-Hill, 2003: 133.)

Methotrexate (MTX)

Mechanism	S-phase-specific antimetabolite. Folic acid analog that inhibits dihydrofolate reductase, resulting in ↓ dTMP and therefore ↓ DNA and protein synthesis.
Clinical use	Leukemias, lymphomas, choriocarcinoma, sarcomas. Abortion, ectopic pregnancy, rheumatoid arthritis, psoriasis.
Toxicity	Myelosuppression, which is reversible with leucovorin (folinic acid) "rescue." Macrovesicular fatty change in liver. Mucositis.

5-fluorouracil (5-FU)

Mechanism	S-phase-specific antimetabolite. Pyrimidine analog bioactivated to 5F-dUMP, which covalently complexes folic acid. This complex inhibits thymidylate synthase, resulting in ↓ dTMP and same effects as MTX.
Clinical use	Colon cancer and other solid tumors, basal cell carcinoma (topical). Synergy with MTX.
Toxicity	Myelosuppression, which is NOT reversible with leucovorin; photosensitivity. Can "rescue" with thymidine.

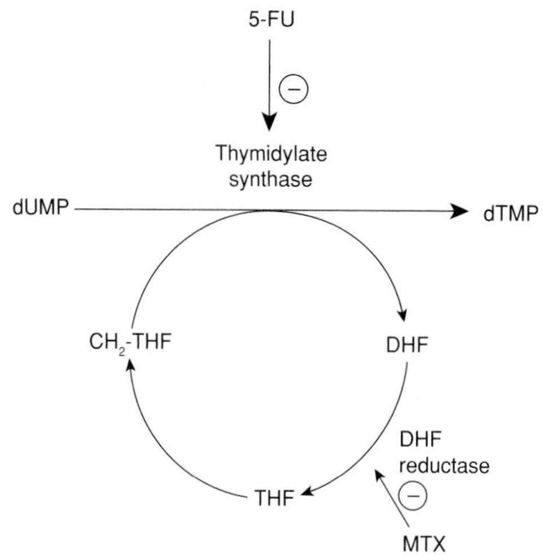

6-mercaptopurine (6-MP)

Mechanism	Blocks de novo purine synthesis. Activated by HGPRTase.
Clinical use	Leukemias, lymphomas (not CLL or Hodgkin's).
Toxicity	Bone marrow, GI, liver. Metabolized by xanthine oxidase; thus ↑ toxicity with allopurinol.

Cytarabine (ara-C)

Mechanism	Inhibits DNA polymerase.
Clinical use	AML.
Toxicity	Leukopenia, thrombocytopenia, megaloblastic anemia.

Cyclophosphamide, ifosfamide

Mechanism	Alkylating agents; covalently x-link (interstrand) DNA at guanine N-7. Require bioactivation by liver.
Clinical use	Non-Hodgkin's lymphoma, breast and ovarian carcinomas. Also immunosuppressants.
Toxicity	Myelosuppression; hemorrhagic cystitis, which can be partially prevented with mesna.

Nitrosoureas	Carmustine, lomustine, semustine, streptozocin.
Mechanism	Alkylate DNA. Require bioactivation. Cross blood-brain barrier → CNS.
Clinical use	Brain tumors (including glioblastoma multiforme).
Toxicity	CNS toxicity (dizziness, ataxia).

Cisplatin, carboplatin

Mechanism	Act like alkylating agents.
Clinical use	Testicular, bladder, ovary, and lung carcinomas.
Toxicity	Nephrotoxicity and acoustic nerve damage.

Busulfan

Mechanism	Alkylates DNA.
Clinical use	CML.
Toxicity	Pulmonary fibrosis, hyperpigmentation.

Doxorubicin (Adriamycin), daunorubicin

Mechanism	Generate free radicals and noncovalently intercalate in DNA (creating breaks in DNA strand to ↓ replication).
Clinical use	Part of the **A**BVD combination regimen for Hodgkin's and for myelomas, sarcomas, and solid tumors (breast, ovary, lung).
Toxicity	Cardiotoxicity; also myelosuppression and marked alopecia. Toxic extravasation.

Dactinomycin (actinomycin D)

Mechanism	Intercalates in DNA.	**ACT**inomycin D is used for childhood tumors (children **ACT** out).
Clinical use	Wilms' tumor, Ewing's sarcoma, rhabdomyosarcoma.	
Toxicity	Myelosuppression.	

Bleomycin

Mechanism	Induces formation of free radicals, which cause breaks in DNA strands.
Clinical use	Testicular cancer, lymphomas (part of the A**B**VD regimen for Hodgkin's).
Toxicity	Pulmonary fibrosis, skin changes, but minimal myelosuppression.

Hydroxyurea

Mechanism	Inhibits **R**ibonucleotide **R**eductase → ↓ DNA **S**ynthesis (**S**-phase specific).
Clinical use	Melanoma, CML, sickle cell disease.
Toxicity	Bone marrow suppression, GI upset.

Etoposide (VP-16)

Mechanism	G_2-phase-specific agent that inhibits topoisomerase II and ↑ DNA degradation.
Clinical use	Small cell carcinoma of the lung and prostate, testicular carcinoma.
Toxicity	Myelosuppression, GI irritation, alopecia.

Prednisone

Mechanism	May trigger apoptosis. May even work on nondividing cells.
Clinical use	Most commonly used glucocorticoid in cancer chemotherapy. Used in CLL, Hodgkin's lymphomas (part of the MO**P**P regimen). Also an immunosuppressant used in autoimmune diseases.
Toxicity	Cushing-like symptoms; immunosuppression, cataracts, acne, osteoporosis, hypertension, peptic ulcers, hyperglycemia, psychosis.

Tamoxifen, raloxifene

Mechanism	Receptor antagonists in breast, agonists in bone; block the binding of estrogen to estrogen receptor–positive cells.
Clinical use	Breast cancer. Also useful to prevent osteoporosis.
Toxicity	Tamoxifen may ↑ the risk of endometrial carcinoma via partial agonist effects; "hot flashes." Raloxifene does not cause endometrial carcinoma because it is an endometrial antagonist.

Trastuzumab (Herceptin)

Mechanism	Monoclonal antibody against HER-2 (*erb*-B2). Helps kill breast cancer cells that overexpress HER-2, possibly through antibody-dependent cytotoxicity.
Clinical use	Metastatic breast cancer.
Toxicity	Cardiotoxicity.

Imatinib (Gleevec)

Mechanism	Philadelphia chromosome *bcr-abl* tyrosine kinase inhibitor.
Clinical use	CML, GI stromal tumors.
Toxicity	Fluid retention.

Vincristine, vinblastine

Mechanism	M-phase-specific alkaloids that bind to tubulin and block polymerization of microtubules so that mitotic spindle cannot form. Microtubules are the **vines** of your cells.
Clinical use	Part of the MOPP (**O**ncovin [vincristine]) regimen for lymphoma, Wilms' tumor, choriocarcinoma.
Toxicity	Vincristine—neurotoxicity (areflexia, peripheral neuritis), paralytic ileus. Vin**BLAST**ine **BLAST**s **B**one marrow (suppression).

Paclitaxel, other taxols

Mechanism	M-phase-specific agents that bind to tubulin and hyperstabilize polymerized microtubules so that mitotic spindle cannot break down (anaphase cannot occur).
Clinical use	Ovarian and breast carcinomas.
Toxicity	Myelosuppression and hypersensitivity.

HIGH-YIELD SYSTEMS

Musculoskeletal and Connective Tissue

"I just use my muscles like a conversation piece, like someone walking a cheetah down 42nd Street."

—Arnold Schwarzenegger

"There's 215 bones in the human body. That's one."

—Sarah Connor in *Terminator 2: Judgment Day*

Vignette	Question	Answer
Soccer player who was kicked in the leg suffered a damaged medial meniscus.	What else is likely to have been damaged?	Anterior cruciate ligament (remember the "unhappy triad").
Gymnast dislocates her shoulder anteriorly.	What nerve is most likely to have been damaged?	Axillary nerve (C5, C6).
X-ray shows bilateral hilar lymphadenopathy.	What is the diagnosis?	Sarcoidosis.
25-year-old woman presents with a low-grade fever, a rash across her nose that gets worse when she is out in the sun, and widespread edema.	You are concerned about what disease?	SLE.
85-year-old man presents with acute knee pain and swelling. X-ray shows joint space without erosion.	What is the diagnosis, and what would you find on aspiration?	Pseudogout; rhomboid calcium pyrophosphate crystals.
Patient describes ↓ prick sensation on the lateral aspect of her leg and foot.	A deficit in what muscular action can also be expected?	Dorsiflexion and eversion of the foot (common peroneal nerve).
Elderly woman presents with arthritis, pain, numbness, and tingling over the lateral digits of her right hand. On exam, she has wasting of the thenar eminence.	What is the diagnosis?	Carpal tunnel syndrome, median nerve compression.
20-year-old dancer reports ↓ plantar flexion and ↓ sensation over the back of her thigh, calf, and lateral half of her foot.	What spinal nerve is involved?	Tibial (L4–S3).
Teen falls while rollerblading and hurts his elbow. He can't feel the medial part of his palm.	Which nerve and what injury?	Ulnar nerve due to broken medial condyle.
Field hockey player presents to the ER after falling on her arm during practice. X-ray shows midshaft break of the humerus.	Which nerve and which artery are most likely damaged?	The radial nerve and deep brachial artery, which run together.

Epidermis layers

From surface to base: stratum Corneum, stratum Lucidum, stratum Granulosum, stratum Spinosum, stratum Basalis.

Californians Like Girls in String Bikinis.

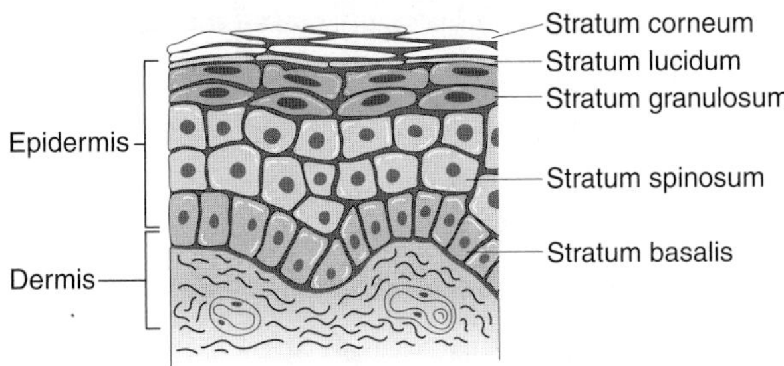

Epithelial cell junctions

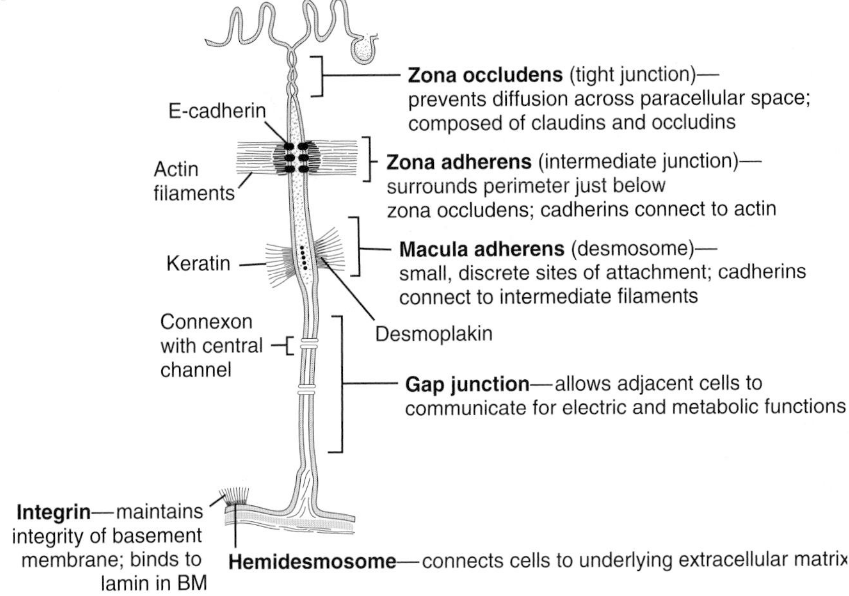

Unhappy triad/ knee injury

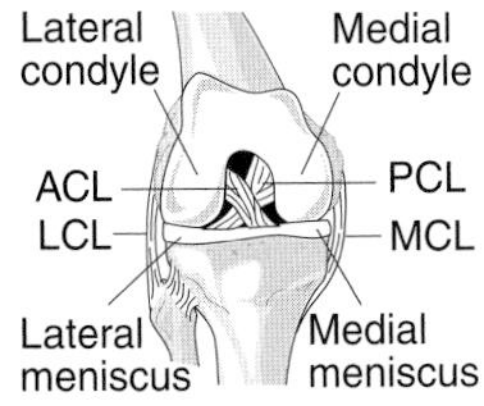

This common football injury (caused by clipping from the lateral side) consists of damage to medial collateral ligament (MCL), medial meniscus, and anterior cruciate ligament (ACL).

PCL = posterior cruciate ligament. LCL = lateral collateral ligament.

"Anterior" and "posterior" in ACL and PCL refer to sites of **tibial** attachment.

Positive anterior drawer sign indicates tearing of the ACL.

Abnormal passive abduction indicates a torn MCL.

Rotator cuff muscles

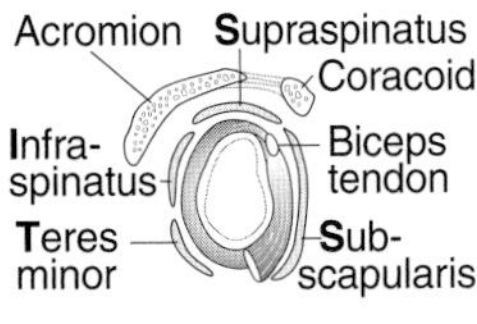

Shoulder muscles that form the rotator cuff:

Supraspinatus—helps deltoid abduct arm.

Infraspinatus—laterally rotates arm.

Teres minor—adducts and laterally rotates arm.

Subscapularis—medially rotates and adducts arm.

SItS (small t is for teres minor).

Brachial plexus

1. Waiter´s tip (Erb's palsy)
2. Claw hand (Klumpke's palsy)
3. Wrist drop
4. Winged scapula
5. Deltoid paralysis
6. Saturday night palsy (wrist drop)
7. Difficulty flexing elbow, variable sensory loss
8. ↓ thumb function, Pope´s blessing
9. Intrinsic muscles of hand, claw hand

Rad = radial nerve
Ax = axillary nerve
LT = long thoracic nerve
MC = musculocutaneous nerve
Med = median nerve
Uln = ulnar nerve

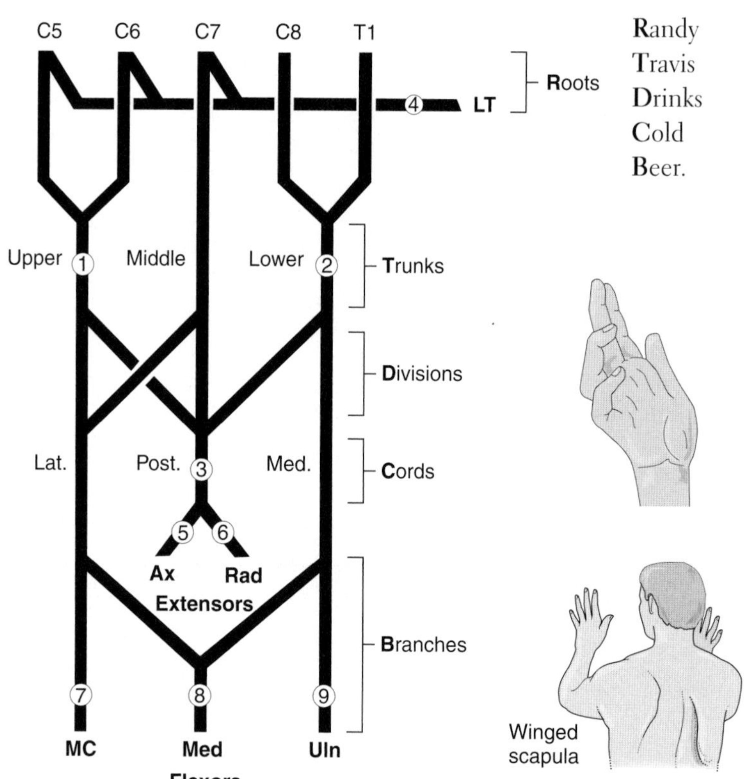

Clavicle fracture is relatively common—brachial plexus is protected from injury by subclavius muscle.

Upper extremity nerves

Common injury	Extensor/flexor	Motor deficit	Sensory deficit
Shoulder dislocation	Extensor	Can't abduct arm > 90°	
Midshaft humerus fracture	Extensor Flexor	Wrist drop Can't flex at elbow	Posterior arm and dorsal hand (excluding fingertips as well as little and ½ of ring fingers) Lateral arm
Supracondylar humerus fracture or wrist swelling/fracture (carpal tunnel syndrome)	Flexor (abduction and opposition of thumb)	Can't flex fingers; can't abduct/oppose thumb	Palmar aspect (and dorsal tips) of thumb, index, middle, and ½ of ring fingers
Fracture at medial epicondyle of humerus or wrist fracture	Flexor (adduction of thumb and both abduction and adduction of fingers)	Claw hand—can't adduct thumb; can't abduct or adduct fingers	Palmar and dorsal aspect of little finger and ½ of ring finger

Erb-Duchenne palsy 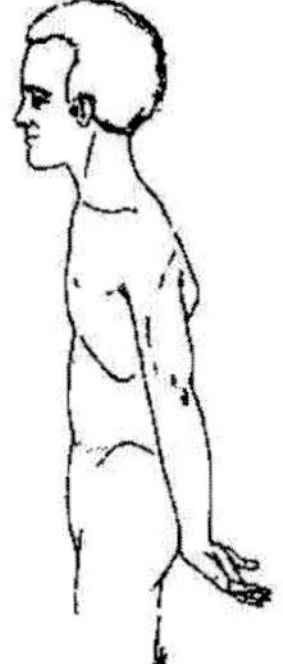	Traction or tear of the upper trunk of the brachial plexus (C5 and C6 roots); follows blow to shoulder or trauma during delivery. Findings: limb hangs by side (paralysis of abductors), medially rotated (paralysis of lateral rotators), forearm is pronated (loss of biceps).	"Waiter's tip" owing to appearance of arm.
Thoracic outlet syndrome (Klumpke's palsy)	An embryologic defect; can compress subclavian artery and inferior trunk of brachial plexus (C8, T1), resulting in thoracic outlet syndrome: 1. Atrophy of the thenar and hypothenar eminences 2. Atrophy of the interosseous muscles 3. Sensory deficits on the medial side of the forearm and hand 4. Disappearance of the radial pulse upon moving the head toward the opposite side	

Radial nerve

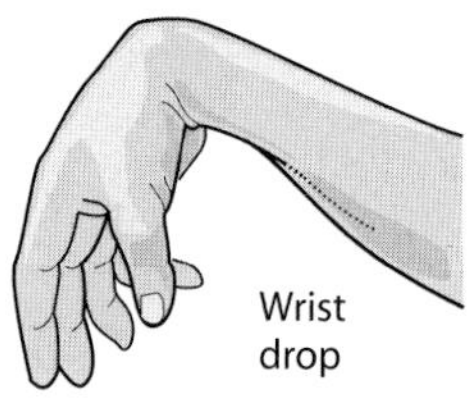

Known as the "great extensor nerve." Provides innervation of the **B**rachioradialis, **E**xtensors of the wrist and fingers, **S**upinator, and **T**riceps.

Radial nerve innervates the **BEST**!
To **SUP**inate is to move as if carrying a bowl of **SOUP**.

Hand muscles

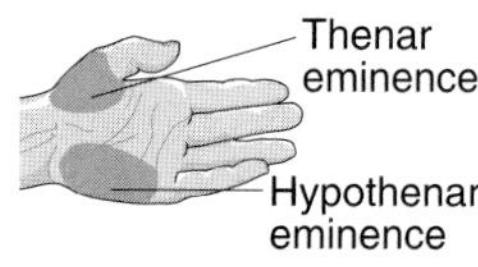

Thenar—**O**pponens pollicis, **A**bductor pollicis brevis, **F**lexor pollicis brevis.
Hypothenar—**O**pponens digiti minimi, **A**bductor digiti minimi, **F**lexor digiti minimi.
Dorsal interosseous muscles—abduct the fingers.
Palmar interosseous muscles—adduct the fingers.
Lumbrical muscles—flex at the MP joint.

Both groups perform the same functions: **O**ppose, **A**bduct, and **F**lex (**OAF**).

DAB = **D**orsals **AB**duct.
PAD = **P**almars **AD**duct.

Lower extremity nerves

Nerve name	Cause of injury	Motor deficit	Sensory deficit
Obturator	Anterior hip dislocation	Can't adduct thigh	Medial thigh
Femoral	Pelvic fracture	Can't flex thigh or extend leg	Anterior thigh and medial leg
Common peroneal	Trauma to lateral aspect of leg or fibula neck fracture	Can't evert or dorsiflex foot; can't extend toes	Anterolateral leg and dorsal aspect of foot
Tibial	Knee trauma	Can't invert or plantarflex foot; can't flex toes	Sole of foot
Superior gluteal	Posterior hip dislocation or polio	Can't abduct thigh (positive Trendelenburg sign)	
Inferior gluteal	Posterior hip dislocation	Can't jump, climb stairs, or rise from seated position	

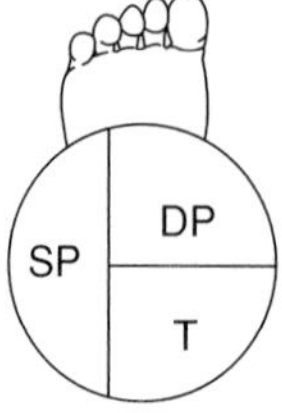

PED = **P**eroneal **E**verts and **D**orsiflexes; if injured, foot drop**PED**.

TIP = **T**ibial **I**nverts and **P**lantarflexes; if injured, can't stand on **TIP**toes.

Muscle conduction to contraction

A.

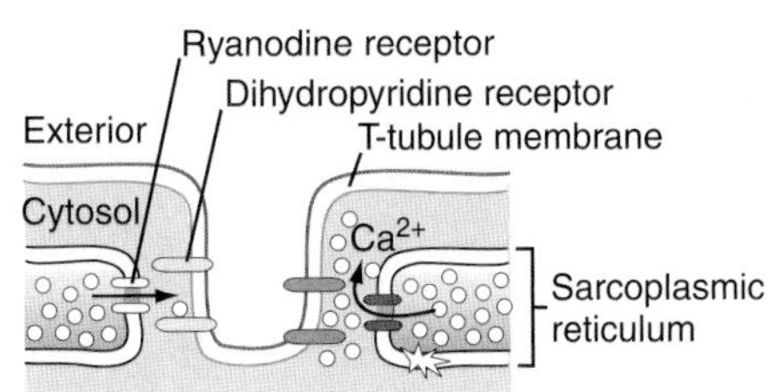

B.

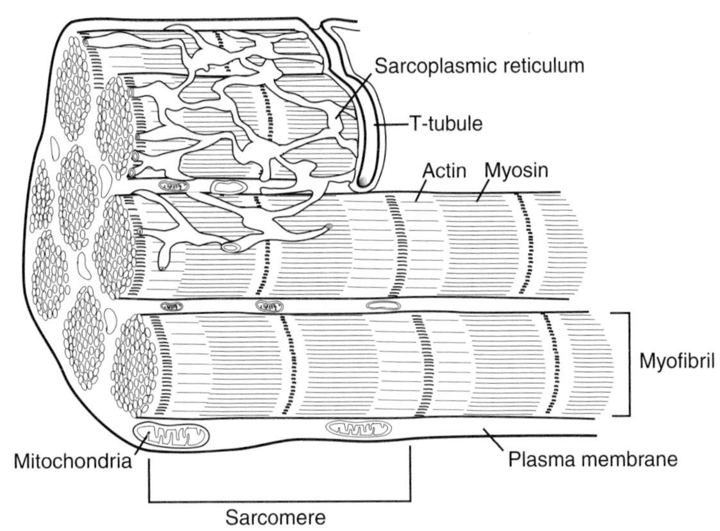

C.

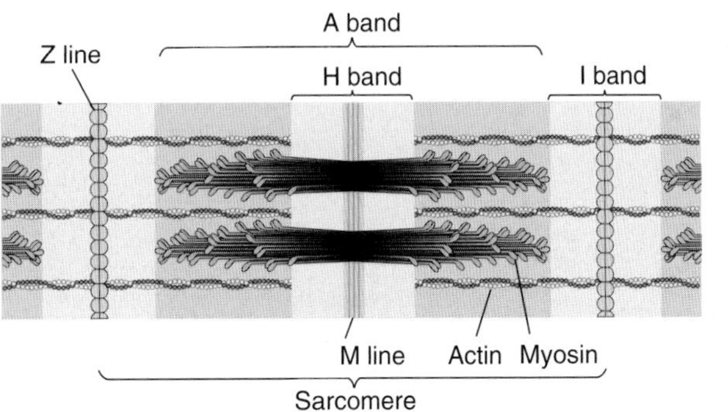

A band = length of myosin, I band = only actin, H band = only myosin, Z line = actin attachment, M line = myosin attachment.

Action potential:

1. Action potential depolarization opens voltage-gated Ca^{2+} channels, inducing neurotransmitter release.
2. Postsynaptic ligand binding leads to muscle cell depolarization in the motor end plate.
3. Depolarization travels along muscle cell and down the T-tubule.
4. Depolarization of the voltage-sensitive dihydropyridine receptor, coupled to the ryanodine receptor on the sarcoplasmic reticulum, induces a conformational change causing Ca^{2+} release (calcium-induced calcium release).
5. Released Ca^{2+} binds to troponin C, causing a conformational change that moves tropomyosin out of the myosin-binding groove on actin filaments.
6. Myosin releases bound ADP and is displaced on the actin filament (power stroke). Contraction results in H- and I band shortening, but the A band remains the same length (**A** band is **A**lways the same length).

Skeletal and cardiac muscle contraction

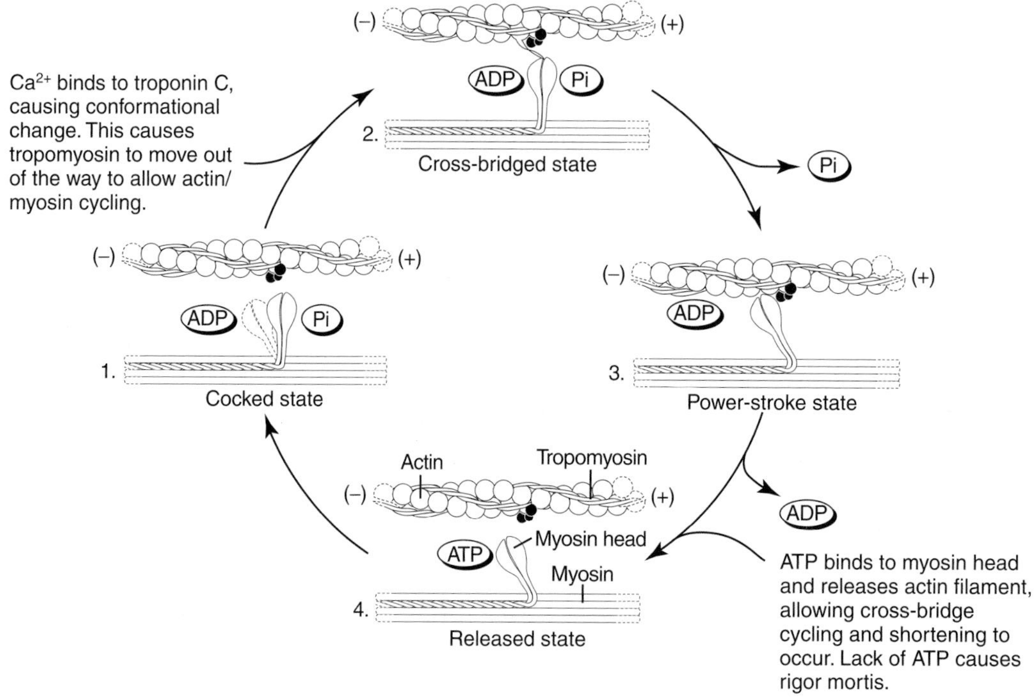

Smooth muscle contraction

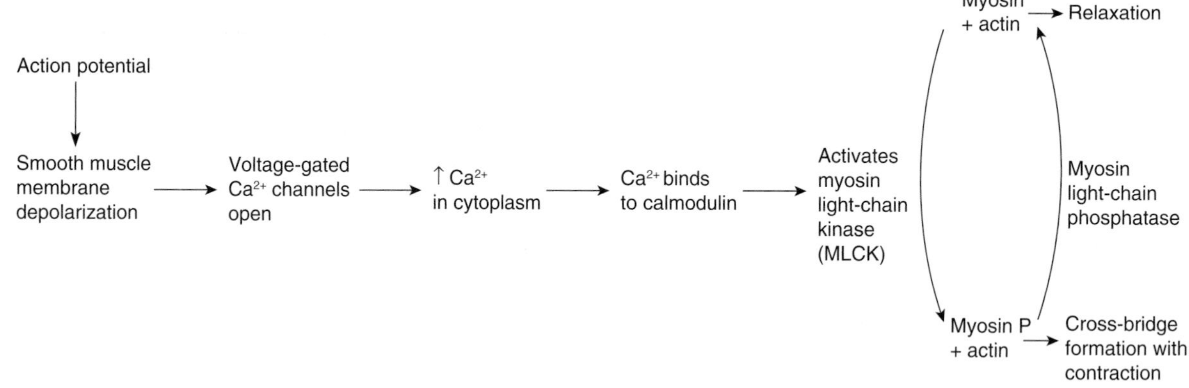

Bone formation

Endochondral ossification	Longitudinal bone growth. Cartilaginous model of bone is first made by chondrocytes. Osteoclasts and osteoblasts later replace with woven bone and remodel to lamellar bone.	Osteoblast source—mesenchymal stem cells in periosteum.
Membranous ossification	Flat bone growth (skull, facial bones, and axial skeleton). Woven bone formed directly without cartilage. Later remodeled to lamellar bone.	

Achondroplasia	Autosomal-dominant trait. Failure of longitudinal bone growth → short limbs. Membranous ossification is not affected. Impaired cartilage maturation in growth plate caused by fibroblast growth factor receptor mutation. Normal life span and fertility.	
Osteoporosis	Reduction of bone mass in spite of normal bone mineralization. Sparse trabeculae.	Vertebral crush fractures—acute back pain, loss of height, kyphosis.
Type I	Postmenopausal; ↑ bone resorption due to ↓ estrogen levels. Estrogen replacement is controversial as prophylaxis (side effects).	Distal radius (Colles') fractures, vertebral wedge fractures.
Type II	Senile osteoporosis—affects men and women > 70 years. 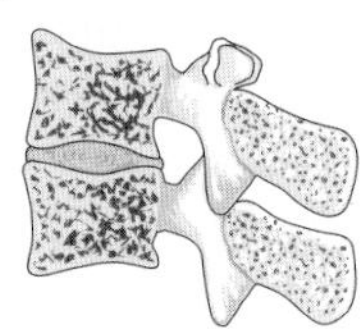 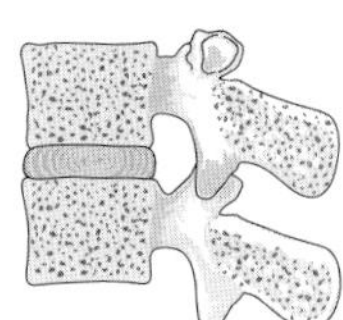 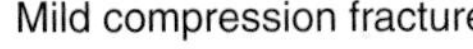 Mild compression fracture / Normal vertebra	Prophylaxis: exercise and calcium ingestion before age 30. Treatment: estrogen and/or calcitonin; bisphosphonates or pulsatile PTH for severe cases. Glucocorticoids are contraindicated.
Osteopetrosis (marble bone disease)	Failure of normal bone resorption → thickened, dense bones. Bone defect is due to abnormal function of osteoclasts. Serum calcium, phosphate, and **alkaline phosphatase** are **normal.** ↓ marrow space leads to anemia, thrombocytopenia, infection. Genetic deficiency of carbonic anhydrase II. X-rays shows "Erlenmeyer flask" bones that flare out. Can result in cranial nerve impingement and palsies due to narrowed foramina.	
Osteomalacia/rickets	Defective mineralization/calcification of osteoid → soft bones. Vitamin D deficiency in adults → ↓ calcium levels → ↑ secretion of PTH, ↓ in serum phosphate. Reversible when vitamin D is replaced. Vitamin D deficiency in childhood causes rickets.	
Osteitis fibrosa cystica	Caused by hyperparathyroidism. Characterized by "brown tumors" (cystic spaces lined by osteoclasts, filled with fibrous stroma and sometimes blood). High serum calcium, low serum phosphorus, and high ALP.	
Paget's disease (osteitis deformans)	Abnormal bone architecture caused by ↑ in both osteoblastic and osteoclastic activity. Possibly viral in origin. Serum calcium, phosphorus, and PTH levels are normal. ↑ **ALP.** Mosaic bone pattern; long bone chalk-stick fractures. ↑ blood flow from ↑ arteriovenous shunts may cause high-output CHF. Can lead to osteogenic sarcoma.	Hat size can be ↑; hearing loss is common due to auditory foramen narrowing.

Polyostotic fibrous dysplasia	Bone is replaced by fibroblasts, collagen, and irregular bony trabeculae. Affects many bones. **McCune-Albright syndrome** is a form of polyostotic fibrous dysplasia characterized by multiple unilateral bone lesions associated with endocrine abnormalities (precocious puberty) and unilateral pigmented skin lesions (café-au-lait spots/"coast of Maine" spots).

Primary bone tumors	
Benign	
Osteoma	Associated with Gardner's syndrome (FAP). New piece of bone grows on another piece of bone, often in the skull.
Osteoid osteoma	Interlacing trabeculae of woven bone surrounded by osteoblasts. < 2 cm and found in proximal tibia and femur. Most common in men < 25 years of age.
Osteoblastoma	Same morphologically as osteoid osteoma, but larger and found in vertebral column.
Giant cell tumor (osteoclastoma)	Occurs most commonly at epiphyseal end of long bones. Peak incidence 20–40 years of age. Locally aggressive benign tumor often around the distal femur, proximal tibial region (knee). Characteristic "double bubble" or "soap bubble" appearance on x-ray. Spindle-shaped cells with multinucleated giant cells.
Osteochondroma (exostosis)	Most common benign bone tumor. Mature bone with cartilaginous cap. Usually in men < 25 years of age. Commonly originates from long metaphysis. Malignant transformation to chondrosarcoma is rare.
Enchondroma	Benign cartilaginous neoplasm found in intramedullary bone. Usually distal extremities (vs. chondrosarcoma).
Malignant	
Osteosarcoma (osteogenic sarcoma)	2nd most common 1° malignant tumor of bone (after multiple myeloma). Peak incidence in men 10–20 years of age. Commonly found in the metaphysis of long bones, often around distal femur, proximal tibial region (knee). Predisposing factors include Paget's disease of bone, bone infarcts, radiation, and familial retinoblastoma. Codman's triangle or sunburst pattern (from elevation of periosteum) on x-ray. Poor prognosis.
Ewing's sarcoma	Anaplastic small blue cell malignant tumor. Most common in boys < 15. Extremely aggressive with early mets, but responsive to chemotherapy. Characteristic "**onion**-skin" appearance in bone ("going out for **Ewings** and **onion** rings"). Commonly appears in diaphysis of long bones, pelvis, scapula, and ribs. 11;22 translocation.
Chondrosarcoma	Malignant cartilaginous tumor. Most common in men aged 30–60. Usually located in pelvis, spine, scapula, humerus, tibia, or femur. May be of 1° origin or from osteochondroma. Expansile glistening mass within the medullary cavity.

Primary bone tumor locations

	Benign	Malignant
Epiphysis	Giant cell tumor (osteoclastoma)	—
Metaphysis	Osteochondroma	Osteosarcoma
Diaphysis	Osteoid osteoma	Ewing's sarcoma
Intramedullary	Enchondroma	Chondrosarcoma

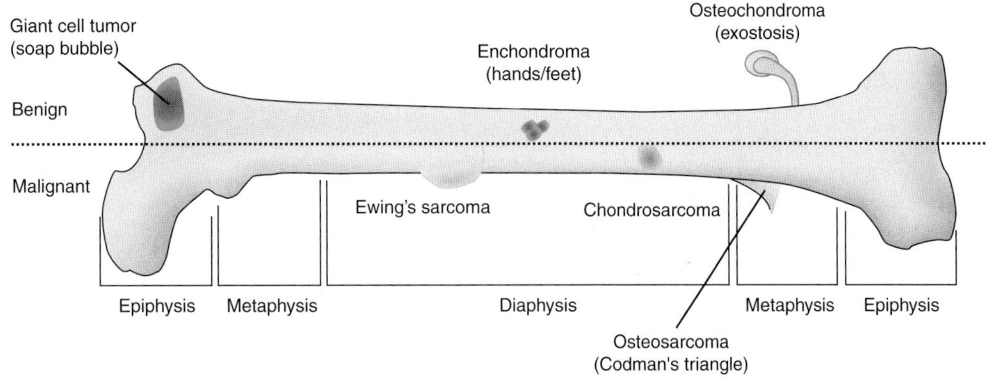

Osteoarthritis

Mechanical—wear and tear of joints leads to destruction of articular cartilage (see Image 144), subchondral cysts, sclerosis, osteophytes, eburnation, Heberden's nodes (DIP), and Bouchard's nodes (PIP).

Predisposing factors: age, obesity, joint deformity.

Classic presentation: pain in weight-bearing joints after use (e.g., at the end of the day), improving with rest. No systemic symptoms.

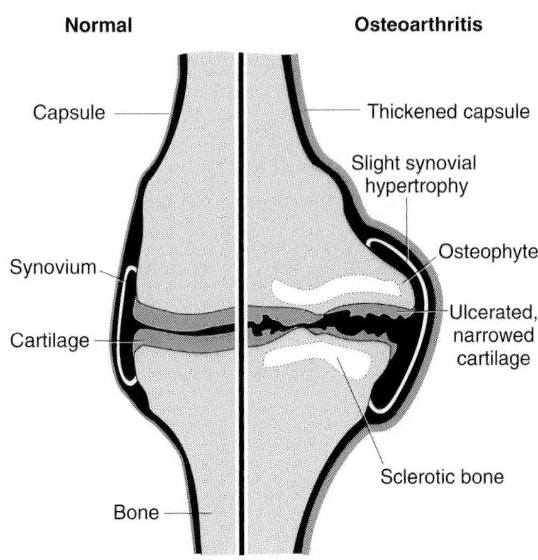

(Adapted, with permission, from Stobo J et al. *The Principles and Practice of Medicine,* 23rd ed. Stamford, CT: Appleton & Lange, 1996: 241.)

Rheumatoid arthritis

Autoimmune—inflammatory disorder affecting synovial joints, with pannus formation in joints (MCP, PIP), subcutaneous rheumatoid nodules, ulnar deviation, subluxation (see Color Image 56).

Females > males. 80% of RA patients have positive rheumatoid factor (anti-IgG antibody). Strong association with HLA-DR4.

Classic presentation: morning stiffness improving with use, symmetric joint involvement, and systemic symptoms (fever, fatigue, pleuritis, pericarditis).

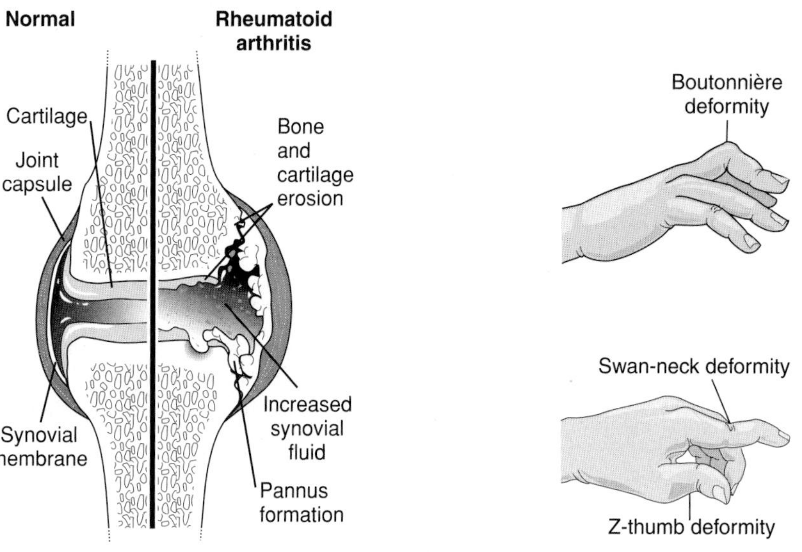

Sjögren's syndrome

Classic triad:

1. Xerophthalmia (dry eyes, conjunctivitis)
2. Xerostomia (dry mouth, dysphagia)
3. Arthritis

Parotid enlargement, ↑ risk of B-cell lymphoma, dental caries. Autoantibodies to ribonucleoprotein antigens, SS-A (Ro), SS-B (La).

Predominantly affects females between 40 and 60 years of age.

Associated with rheumatoid arthritis.

Sicca syndrome—dry eyes, dry mouth, nasal and vaginal dryness, chronic bronchitis, reflux esophagitis.

Gout

Symptoms: Asymmetric joint distribution. Joint is swollen, red, and painful. Classic manifestation is painful MTP joint of the big toe (podagra). Tophus formation (often on external ear or Achilles tendon). Acute attack tends to occur after alcohol consumption or a large meal.

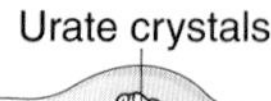

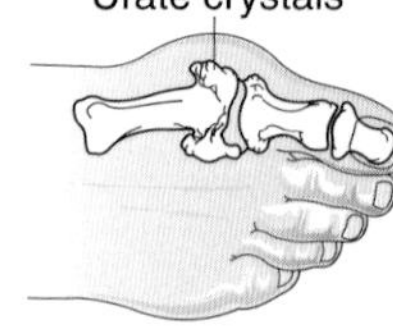

Findings: Precipitation of monosodium urate crystals into joints due to hyperuricemia, which can be caused by Lesch-Nyhan syndrome, PRPP excess, ↓ excretion of uric acid (e.g., thiazide diuretics), ↑ cell turnover, or von Gierke's disease. Crystals are needle shaped and **negatively birefringent** (see Color Image 54). More common in men.

Treatment: Allopurinol, probenecid, colchicine, and NSAIDs.

Pseudogout	Caused by deposition of calcium pyrophosphate crystals within the joint space. Forms basophilic, rhomboid crystals that are **weakly positively birefringent.** Usually affects large joints (classically the knee). > 50 years old; both sexes affected equally. No treatment. Gout—crystals are ye**ll**ow when parallel (||) to the light. Pseudogout—crystals are yellow when perpendicular (⊥) to the light. **P**seudogout is **P**ositively birefringent.	
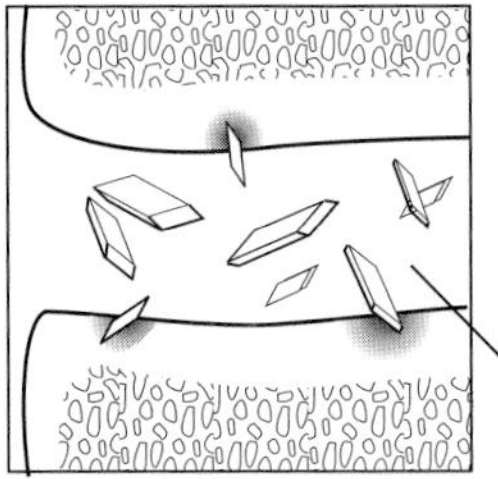		
Infectious arthritis		
Septic	*S. aureus*, *Streptococcus*, and *Neisseria gonorrhoeae* are common. **Gonococcal arthritis** presents as a monoarticular, migratory arthritis with an asymmetrical pattern. Affected joint is swollen, red, and painful.	
Chronic	TB (from mycobacterial dissemination) and Lyme disease.	
Seronegative spondylo-arthropathies	Arthritis without rheumatoid factor (no anti-IgG antibody). Strong association with HLA-B27 (gene that codes for HLA MHC I). Occurs more often in males.	
Ankylosing spondylitis	Chronic inflammatory disease of spine and sacroiliac joints → ankylosis (stiff spine), uveitis, and aortic regurgitation.	Bamboo spine.
Reiter's syndrome	Classic triad: 1. Conjunctivitis and anterior uveitis 2. Urethritis 3. Arthritis	"Can't **see,** can't **pee,** can't climb a **tree.**" Post-GI or chlamydia infections.
Psoriatic arthritis	Joint pain and stiffness associated with psoriasis. Asymmetric and patchy involvement. Dactylitis ("sausage fingers") is commonly observed. "Pencil and cup" deformity on x-ray. Seen in fewer than ⅓ of patients with psoriasis.	

Systemic lupus erythematosus

90% are female and between ages 14 and 45. Most common and severe in black females. Symptoms include fever, fatigue, weight loss, nonbacterial verrucous endocarditis, hilar adenopathy, and Raynaud's phenomenon (see Color Image 52). Wire-loop lesions in kidney with immune complex deposition (with nephrotic syndrome); death from renal failure and infections. False positives on syphilis tests (RPR/VDRL) due to antiphospholipid antibodies. Lab tests detect presence of:

1. Antinuclear antibodies (ANA)—sensitive, but not specific for SLE
2. Antibodies to double-stranded DNA (anti-dsDNA)—very specific, poor prognosis
3. Anti-Smith antibodies (anti-Sm)—very specific, but not prognostic
4. Antihistone antibodies—drug-induced lupus

Malar rash

I'M DAMN SHARP:
- **I**mmunoglobulins (anti-dsDNA, anti-Sm, antiphospholipid)
- **M**alar rash
- **D**iscoid rash
- **A**ntinuclear antibody
- **M**ucositis (oropharyngeal ulcers)
- **N**eurologic disorders
- **S**erositis (pleuritis, pericarditis)
- **H**ematologic disorders
- **A**rthritis
- **R**enal disorders
- **P**hotosensitivity

Sarcoidosis

Characterized by immune-mediated, widespread noncaseating granulomas and elevated serum ACE levels. Common in black females.

Associated with restrictive lung disease, bilateral hilar lymphadenopathy, erythema nodosum, Bell's palsy, epithelial granulomas containing microscopic Schaumann and asteroid bodies, uveoparotitis, and hypercalcemia (due to elevated conversion of vitamin D to its active form in epithelioid macrophages) (see Color Image 104).

GRAIN:
- **G**ammaglobulinemia
- **R**heumatoid arthritis
- **A**CE increase
- **I**nterstitial fibrosis
- **N**oncaseating granulomas

Polymyalgia rheumatica

Symptoms	Pain and stiffness in shoulders and hips, often with fever, malaise, and weight loss. Does not cause muscular weakness. Occurs in patients > 50 years of age; associated with temporal (giant cell) arteritis.
Findings	↑ ESR, normal CK.
Treatment	Prednisone.

Polymyositis/dermatomyositis

Symptoms	**Polymyositis**—progressive symmetric proximal muscle weakness caused by CD8+ T-cell-induced injury to myofibers. Muscle biopsy with evidence of inflammation is diagnostic. **Dermatomyositis**—similar to polymyositis, but also involves heliotrope rash, "shawl and face" rash and ↑ risk of malignancy.
Findings	Labs for polymyositis/dermatomyositis show ↑ CK, ↑ aldolase, and positive ANA, anti-Jo-1.
Treatment	Steroids.

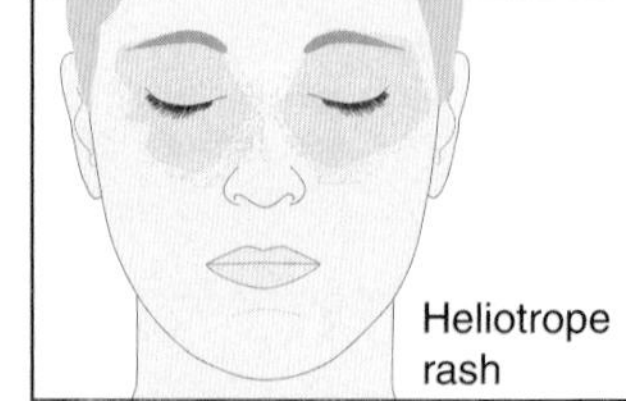

NMJ diseases	
Myasthenia gravis	Most common NMJ disorder. Autoantibodies to postsynaptic AChR cause ptosis, diplopia, and general weakness. Associated with thymoma. Symptoms worsen with muscle use. Reversal of symptoms occurs with AChE inhibitors.
Lambert-Eaton syndrome	Autoantibodies to presynaptic Ca^{2+} channel results in ↓ ACh release leading to proximal muscle weakness. Associated with paraneoplastic diseases (small cell lung cancer). Symptoms improve with muscle use. No reversal of symptoms with AChE inhibitors alone.
Mixed connective tissue disease	Raynaud's phenomenon, arthralgias, myalgias, fatigue, and esophageal hypomotility. Antibodies to U1RNP. Responds to steroids.
Scleroderma (progressive systemic sclerosis—PSS)	Excessive fibrosis and collagen deposition throughout the body. Commonly sclerosis of skin, manifesting as puffy and taut skin with absence of wrinkles (see Color Image 53). Also sclerosis of kidneys, pulmonary, cardiovascular, and GI systems. 75% female. 2 major categories: 1. Diffuse scleroderma—widespread skin involvement, rapid progression, early visceral involvement. Associated with anti-Scl-70 antibody. 2. **CREST** syndrome—**C**alcinosis, **R**aynaud's phenomenon, **E**sophageal dysmotility, **S**clerodactyly, and **T**elangiectasia. Limited skin involvement, often confined to fingers and face. More benign clinical course. Associated with **anticentromere antibody.**
Soft tissue tumors	
Lipoma	Soft, well-encapsulated fat tumor. Benign. Simple excision is usually curative.
Liposarcoma	Malignant fat tumor that can be quite large. Will recur unless adequately excised.
Rhabdomyosarcoma	Most common soft tissue tumor of childhood. Malignant. Arises from skeletal muscle, most often in head/neck.
Dermatologic terminology	
Macule	Flat discoloration < 1 cm.
Patch	Macule > 1 cm.
Papule	Elevated skin lesion < 1 cm.
Plaque	Papule > 1 cm.
Vesicle	Small fluid-containing blister.
Wheal	Transient vesicle.
Bulla	Large fluid-containing blister.
Keloid	Irregular, raised lesion resulting from scar tissue hypertrophy (follows trauma to skin, especially in African-Americans).
Pustule	Blister containing pus.
Crust	Dried exudates from a vesicle, bulla, or pustule.
Hyperkeratosis	↑ thickness of stratum corneum.
Parakeratosis	Hyperkeratosis with retention of nuclei in stratum corneum (e.g., psoriasis).
Acantholysis	Separation of epidermal cells.
Acanthosis	Epidermal hyperplasia.
Dermatitis	Inflammation of the skin.

Skin disorders

Common disorders

Verrucae	Warts. Soft, tan-colored, cauliflower-like lesions. Epidermal hyperplasia, hyperkeratosis, koilocytosis. Verruca vulgaris on hands; condyloma acuminatum on genitals (caused by HPV).
Nevocellular nevus	Common mole. Benign.
Urticaria	Hives. Intensely pruritic wheals that form after mast cell degranulation.
Ephelis	Freckle. ↑ melanin pigment.
Atopic dermatitis (eczema)	Pruritic eruption, commonly on skin flexures. Often associated with other atopic diseases (asthma, allergic rhinitis).
Allergic contact dermatitis	Type IV hypersensitivity reaction that follows exposure to allergen. Lesions occur at site of contact.
Psoriasis	Papules and plaques with silvery scaling, especially on knees and elbows (see Color Image 65). Acanthosis with parakeratotic scaling (nuclei still in stratum corneum). ↑ stratum spinosum, ↓ stratum granulosum. **Auspitz sign** (bleeding spots when scales are scraped off). Can be associated with psoriatic arthritis.
Seborrheic keratosis	Flat, greasy, pigmented squamous epithelial proliferation with keratin-filled cysts (horn cysts). Looks "pasted on." Lesions occur on head, trunk, and extremities. Common benign neoplasm of older persons.

Pigmentation disorders

Albinism	Normal melanocyte number with ↓ melanin production.
Vitiligo	Irregular areas of complete depigmentation. Caused by a ↓ in melanocytes.
Melasma	Hyperpigmentation associated with pregnancy ("mask of pregnancy") or OCP use.

Infectious disorders

Impetigo	Very superficial skin infection. Usually from *S. aureus* or *S. pyogenes*. Highly contagious. **Honey-colored crusting.**
Cellulitis	Acute, painful spreading infection of dermis and subcutaneous tissues. Usually from *S. pyogenes* or *S. aureus*.
Necrotizing fasciitis	Deeper tissue injury, usually from anaerobic bacteria and *S. pyogenes*. Results in crepitus from methane and CO_2 production. "Flesh-eating bacteria."
Staphylococcal scalded skin syndrome (SSSS)	Exotoxin destroys keratinocyte attachments in the stratum granulosum only. Characterized by fever and generalized erythematous rash with sloughing of the upper layers of the epidermis. Seen in newborns and children.
Hairy leukoplakia	White, painless plaques on the tongue that cannot be scraped off. EBV mediated. Relatively specific for HIV.

Blistering disorders

Bullous pemphigoid	Autoimmune disorder with IgG antibody against hemidesmosomes (epidermal basement membrane; antibodies are "**bullow**" the epidermis); shows linear immunofluorescence. Similar to but less severe than pemphigus vulgaris—affects skin but spares oral mucosa (see Color Image 64).
Pemphigus vulgaris	Potentially fatal autoimmune skin disorder with IgG antibody against desmosomes; shows immunofluorescence throughout epidermis. Acantholysis—intraepidermal bullae involving the skin and oral mucosa (see Color Image 63).
Dermatitis herpetiformis	Pruritic papules and vesicles. Deposits of IgA at the tips of dermal papillae. Associated with celiac disease.

Skin disorders *(continued)*

Erythema multiforme	Associated with infections, drugs, cancers, and autoimmune disease. Presents with multiple types of lesions—macules, papules, vesicles, and target lesions (red papules with a pale central area).
Stevens-Johnson syndrome	Characterized by fever, bulla formation and necrosis, sloughing of skin, and a high mortality rate. Usually associated with adverse drug reaction.
Toxic epidermal necrolysis	Characteristics similar to Stevens-Johnson syndrome, but more severe with greater epidermal involvement.

Miscellaneous disorders

Lichen **p**lanus	**P**ruritic, **P**urple, **P**olygonal **P**apules. Sawtooth infiltrate of lymphocytes at dermal-epidermal junction.
Actinic keratosis	Premalignant lesions caused by sun exposure. Small, rough, erythematous or brownish papules. "Cutaneous horn." Risk of carcinoma is proportional to epithelial dysplasia.
Acanthosis nigricans	Hyperplasia of stratum spinosum. Associated with hyperlipidemia (e.g., from Cushing's disease, diabetes) and visceral malignancy.

Skin cancer

Squamous cell carcinoma	Very common. Associated with excessive exposure to sunlight and arsenic exposure. Commonly appear on hands and face. Locally invasive, but rarely metastasizes. Ulcerative red lesion. Histopathology: keratin "pearls" (see Color Image 60).	**Actinic keratosis** is a precursor to squamous cell carcinoma.
Basal cell carcinoma	Most common in sun-exposed areas of body. Locally invasive, but almost never metastasizes. Rolled edges with central ulceration. Gross pathology: pearly papules (see Color Image 62).	Basal cell tumors have "palisading" nuclei.
Melanoma	Common tumor with significant risk of metastasis. S-100 tumor marker. Associated with sunlight exposure; fair-skinned persons are at ↑ risk. **Depth** of tumor correlates with risk of metastasis. Dark with irregular borders (see Color Image 61).	Dysplastic nevus is a precursor to melanoma.

HIGH-YIELD SYSTEMS

MUSCULOSKELETAL

Arachidonic acid products

	Lipoxygenase pathway yields **L**eukotrienes.	**L** for **L**ipoxygenase and **L**eukotriene.
	LT**B**$_4$ is a neutrophil chemotactic agent.	Neutrophils arrive "**B4**" others.
	LTC$_4$, D$_4$, and E$_4$ function in bronchoconstriction, vasoconstriction, contraction of smooth muscle, and ↑ vascular permeability.	
	PGI$_2$ inhibits platelet aggregation and promotes vasodilation.	**P**latelet-**G**athering **I**nhibitor.

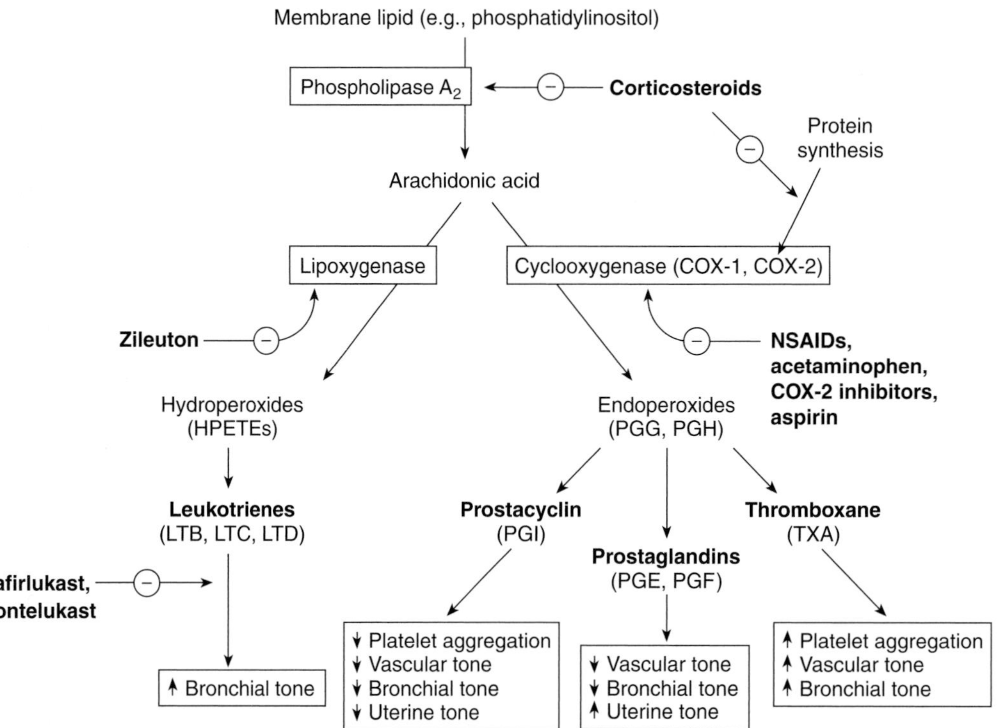

(Adapted, with permission, from Katzung BG, Trevor AJ. *Pharmacology: Examination & Board Review,* 5th ed. Stamford, CT: Appleton & Lange, 1998: 150.)

NSAIDs	Ibuprofen, naproxen, indomethacin, ketorolac.
Mechanism	Reversibly inhibit cyclooxygenase (both COX-1 and COX-2). Block prostaglandin synthesis.
Clinical use	Antipyretic, analgesic, anti-inflammatory. Indomethacin is used to close a PDA.
Toxicity	Renal damage, aplastic anemia, GI distress, ulcers.

COX-2 inhibitors (celecoxib)

Mechanism	Reversibly inhibit specifically the cyclooxygenase (COX) isoform 2, which is found in inflammatory cells and mediates inflammation and pain; spares COX-1, which helps maintain the gastric mucosa. Thus, should not have the corrosive effects of other NSAIDs on the GI lining.
Clinical use	Rheumatoid and osteoarthritis.
Toxicity	↑ risk of thrombosis. Sulfa allergy. Less toxicity to GI mucosa (lower incidence of ulcers, bleeding).

Acetaminophen

Mechanism	Reversibly inhibits cyclooxygenase, mostly in CNS. Inactivated peripherally.
Clinical use	Antipyretic, analgesic, but lacking anti-inflammatory properties.
Toxicity	Overdose produces hepatic necrosis; acetaminophen metabolite depletes glutathione and forms toxic tissue adducts in liver. N-acetylcysteine is antidote—regenerates glutathione.

Gout drugs

Colchicine	Acute gout. Depolymerizes microtubules, impairing leukocyte chemotaxis and degranulation. GI side effects, especially if given orally. (Note: indomethacin is less toxic, more commonly used in acute gout.)
Probenecid	Chronic gout. Inhibits reabsorption of uric acid in PCT (also inhibits secretion of penicillin).
Allopurinol	Chronic gout. Inhibits xanthine oxidase, ↓ conversion of xanthine to uric acid. Also used in lymphoma and leukemia to prevent tumor lysis–associated urate nephropathy. Interacts with azathioprine and 6-MP.

Probenecid and allopurinol should not be used to treat an acute episode of gout.

Do not give salicylates.

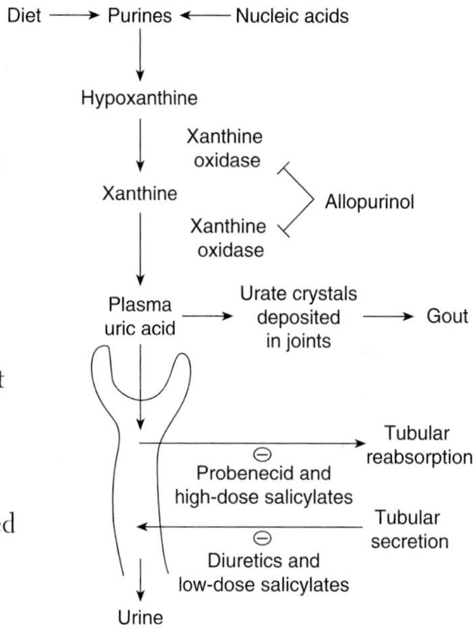

Etanercept

Mechanism	Recombinant form of human TNF receptor that binds TNF.	Etaner**CEPT** is a TNF decoy re**CEPT**or.
Clinical use	Rheumatoid arthritis, psoriasis, ankylosing spondylitis.	

Infliximab

Mechanism	Anti-TNF antibody.	**INFLIX**imab **INFLIX** pain on TNF.
Clinical use	Crohn's disease, rheumatoid arthritis, ankylosing spondylitis.	
Toxicity	Predisposes to infections (reactivation of latent TB).	

NOTES

Neurology

"Estimated amount of glucose used by an adult human brain each day, expressed in M&Ms: 250."

—Harper's Index

"He has two neurons held together by a spirochete."

—Anonymous

Patient presents with ↓ pain and temperature sensation over the lateral aspects of both arms.	What is the lesion?	Syringomyelia.
Penlight in patient's right eye produces bilateral pupillary constriction. When moved to the left eye, there is paradoxical dilatation.	What is the defect?	Atrophy of the left optic nerve.
Woman involved in a motor vehicle accident cannot turn her head to the left and has right shoulder droop.	What structure is damaged?	Right CN XI (runs through the jugular foramen with CN IX and X), innervating the sternocleidomastoid and trapezius muscles.
Man presents with 1 wild, flailing arm.	Where is the lesion?	Contralateral subthalamic nucleus (hemiballismus).
Patient with cortical lesion does not know that he has a disease.	Where is the lesion?	Right parietal lobe.
Patient's tongue protrudes toward the left side, and patient exhibits a right-sided spastic paralysis.	Where is the lesion?	Left medulla, CN XII.
Patient cannot blink his right eye or seal his lips.	What is the diagnosis, and which nerve is affected?	Bell's palsy; CN VII.
Woman presents with headache, visual disturbance, galactorrhea, and amenorrhea.	What is the diagnosis?	Prolactinoma.
43-year-old man experiences dizziness and tinnitus. CT shows an enlarged internal acoustic meatus.	What is the diagnosis?	Schwannoma.
25-year-old woman presents with sudden monocular vision loss and slightly slurred speech. She has a history of weakness and paresthesias that have resolved.	What is the diagnosis?	Multiple sclerosis.
10-year-old child "spaces out" in class (e.g., stops talking midsentence and then continues as if nothing had happened). During spells, the child has a slight quivering of the lips.	What is the diagnosis?	Absence seizures.

▪ 23-year-old woman crashes her motorcycle. She initially feels fine, but minutes later she loses consciousness. At the ER, a CT shows an intracranial hemorrhage that does not cross suture lines.	Which bone and vessel were injured during the crash?	Middle meningeal artery and temporal bone, resulting in an epidural hematoma.
▪ 38-year-old man with a history of Marfan's syndrome and hypertension presents with a severe headache. A spinal tap reveals blood in the CSF.	What is the cause of the man's head pain?	Subarachnoid hemorrhage resulting from a ruptured berry aneurysm.
▪ 78-year-old man with Alzheimer's disease falls and presents 3 days later with severe headache and vomiting.	What structures were damaged by the fall?	Bridging veins, resulting in subdural hematoma.

CNS/PNS supportive cells

Astrocytes—physical support, repair, K^+ metabolism; help maintain blood-brain barrier. Astrocyte marker—GFAP.
Ependymal cells—inner lining of ventricles; make CSF.
Microglia—macrophages of the brain.
Oligodendroglia—central myelin production.
Schwann cells—peripheral myelin production.
Microglia, like **M**acrophages, originate from **M**esoderm. All other CNS/PNS supportive cells originate from ectoderm.

Astrocyte

Oligodendrocyte

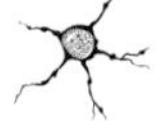

Microglia

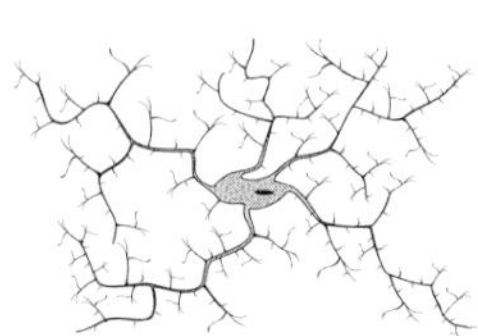

CNS phagocytes. Mesodermal origin. Not readily discernible in Nissl stains. Have small irregular nuclei and relatively little cytoplasm.
Microglia $\xrightarrow{\text{tissue damage}}$ large ameboid phagocytic cells.

HIV-infected microglia fuse to form multinucleated giant cells in the CNS.

Oligodendroglia

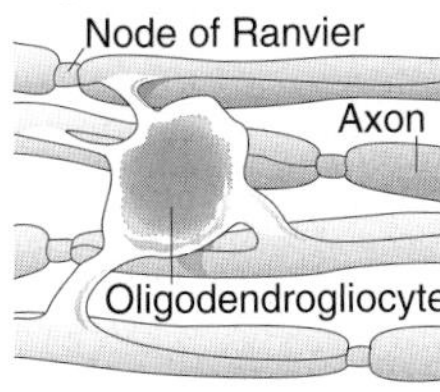

Each oligodendrocyte myelinates multiple CNS axons, up to 30 each. In Nissl stains, they appear as small nuclei with dark chromatin and little cytoplasm. Predominant type of glial cell in white matter.

These cells are destroyed in multiple sclerosis.
Look like fried eggs on H&E staining (see Color Image 49).

Schwann cells

Each Schwann cell myelinates only 1 PNS axon. Also promote axonal regeneration. Derived from neural crest.

Acoustic neuroma is an example of a schwannoma.
Acoustic neuromas are typically located in the internal acoustic meatus (CN VIII).

Peripheral nerve layers

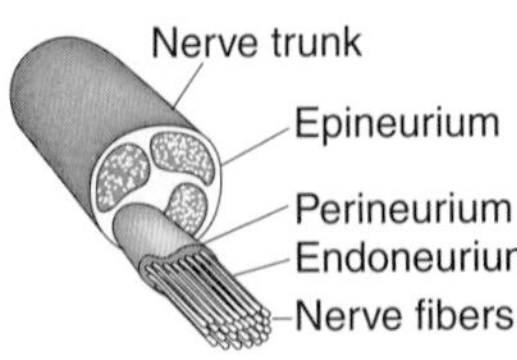

Endoneurium invests single nerve fiber.
Perineurium (permeability barrier) surrounds a fascicle of nerve fibers.
Epineurium (dense connective tissue) surrounds entire nerve (fascicles and blood vessels).

Perineurium—Permeability barrier; must be rejoined in microsurgery for limb reattachment.
Endo = inner.
Peri = around.
Epi = outer.

Neurotransmitters—locations of synthesis

NE	Locus ceruleus.
Dopamine	Ventral tegmentum and SNc.
5-HT	Raphe nucleus.
ACh	Basal nucleus of Meynert.

Blood-brain barrier 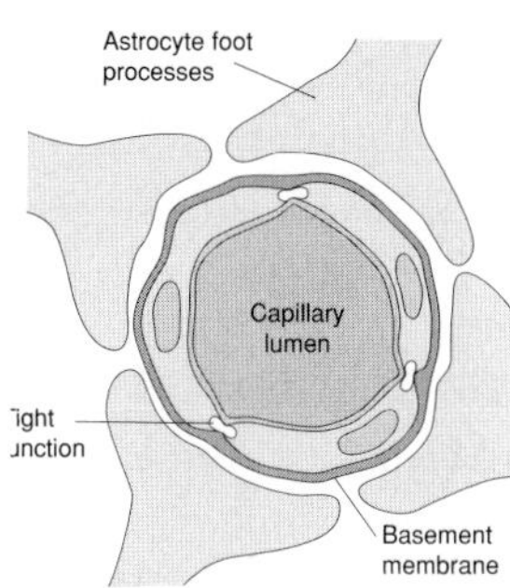 	Formed by 3 structures: 1. Tight junctions between nonfenestrated capillary endothelial cells 2. Basement membrane 3. Astrocyte processes Glucose and amino acids cross slowly by carrier-mediated transport mechanism. Nonpolar/lipid-soluble substances cross rapidly via diffusion. A few specialized brain regions with fenestrated capillaries and no blood-brain barrier allow molecules in the blood to affect brain function (e.g., area postrema—vomiting after chemo) or neurosecretory products to enter circulation (e.g., neurohypophysis—ADH release).	Other barriers include: 1. Blood-testis barrier 2. Maternal-fetal blood barrier of placenta Infarction destroys endothelial cell tight junctions → vasogenic edema.
Hypothalamus functions	**T**hirst and water balance (supraoptic nucleus). **A**denohypophysis control via releasing factors. **N**eurohypophysis and median eminence release hormones synthesized in hypothalamic nuclei. **H**unger (lateral area—destruction → anorexia and starvation) and satiety (ventromedial area—destruction → hyperphagia and obesity). **A**utonomic regulation (**A**nterior hypothalamus regulates p**A**rasympathetic; posterior hypothalamus regulates sympathetic) and circadian rhythms (suprachiasmatic nucleus). **T**emperature regulation (posterior hypothalamus regulates heat conservation and production when cold; **A**nterior hypothalamus coordinates **C**ooling when hot). **S**exual urges and emotions (**S**eptal nucleus—destruction → rage).	The hypothalamus wears **TAN HATS.** If you zap your **ventromedial** nucleus, you grow **ven**trally and **medial**ly. You need **sleep** to be **charismatic** (chiasmatic). If you zap your **P**osterior hypothalamus, you become a **P**oikilotherm (cold-blooded, like a snake). **A/C** = anterior cooling.
Posterior pituitary (neurohypophysis)	Receives hypothalamic axonal projections from supraoptic (ADH) and paraventricular (oxytocin) nuclei.	Oxytocin: *oxys* = quick; *tocos* = birth. **A**denohypophysis = **A**nterior pituitary.

Thalamus	Major relay for ascending sensory information that ultimately reaches the cortex. **L**ateral geniculate nucleus (LGN)—visual. **M**edial geniculate nucleus (MGN)—auditory. Ventral posterior nucleus, lateral part (VPL)—body sensation (proprioception, pressure, pain, touch, vibration via dorsal columns, spinothalamic tract). Ventral posterior nucleus, medial part (VPM)—facial sensation (via CN V). Ventral anterior/lateral (VA/VL) nuclei—motor.	**L**ateral for **L**ight. **M**edial for **M**usic. You put **M**akeup on your face, and the sensory info is relayed through the VP**M**. Motor is anterior to sensation in the thalamus, just like the cortex. Blood supply—posterior communicating, posterior cerebral, and anterior choroidal arteries.

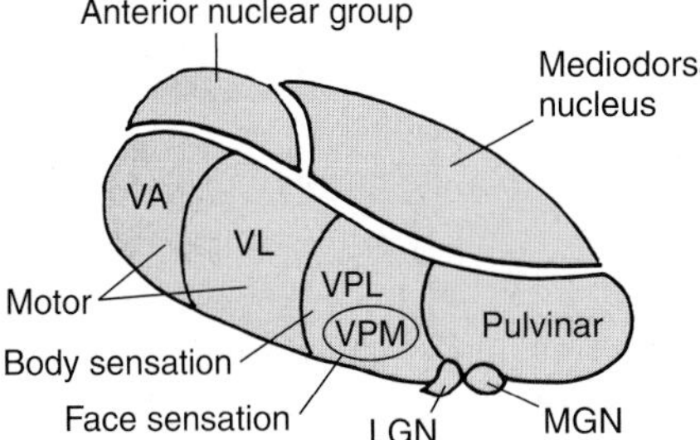

Limbic system	Includes cingulate gyrus, hippocampus, fornix, and mammillary bodies. Responsible for **F**eeding, **F**leeing, **F**ighting, **F**eeling, and sex.	The famous **5 F's.**
Cerebellar nerves	Climbing and mossy fibers—input to cerebellum. Purkinje fibers—output of cerebellum.	

Basal ganglia Important in voluntary movements and making postural adjustments.

■ stimulatory
■ inhibitory

SNc Substantia nigra pars compacta
GPe Globus pallidus externus
GPi Globus pallidus internus
STN Subthalamic nucleus
D1 Dopamine D1 receptor
D2 Dopamine D2 receptor

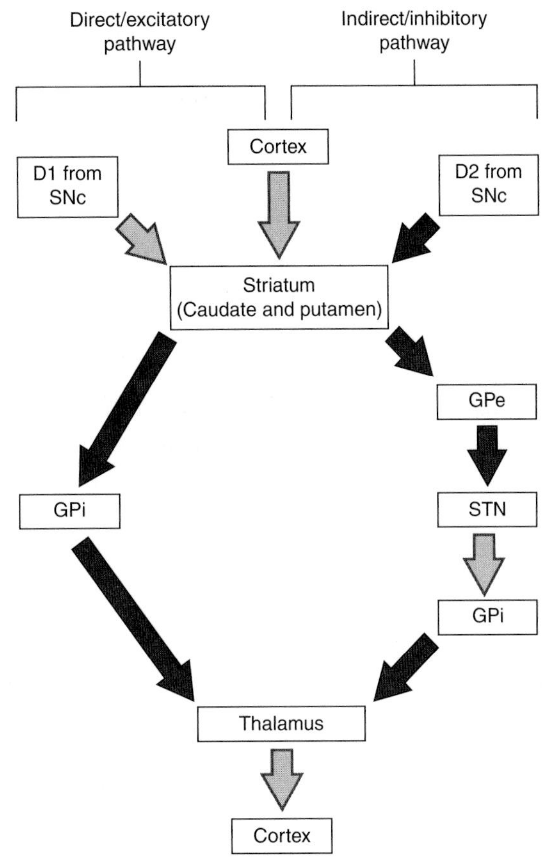

The SNc's dopamine binds to D1 receptors in the excitatory pathway, stimulating the excitatory pathway (↑ motion). Therefore, loss of dopamine in Parkinson's inhibits the excitatory pathway (↓ motion).

The SNc's dopamine binds to D2 receptors in the inhibitory pathway, inhibiting the inhibitory pathway (↑ motion). Therefore, loss of dopamine in Parkinson's excites (i.e., disinhibits) the inhibitory pathway (↓ motion).

Cerebral cortex functions

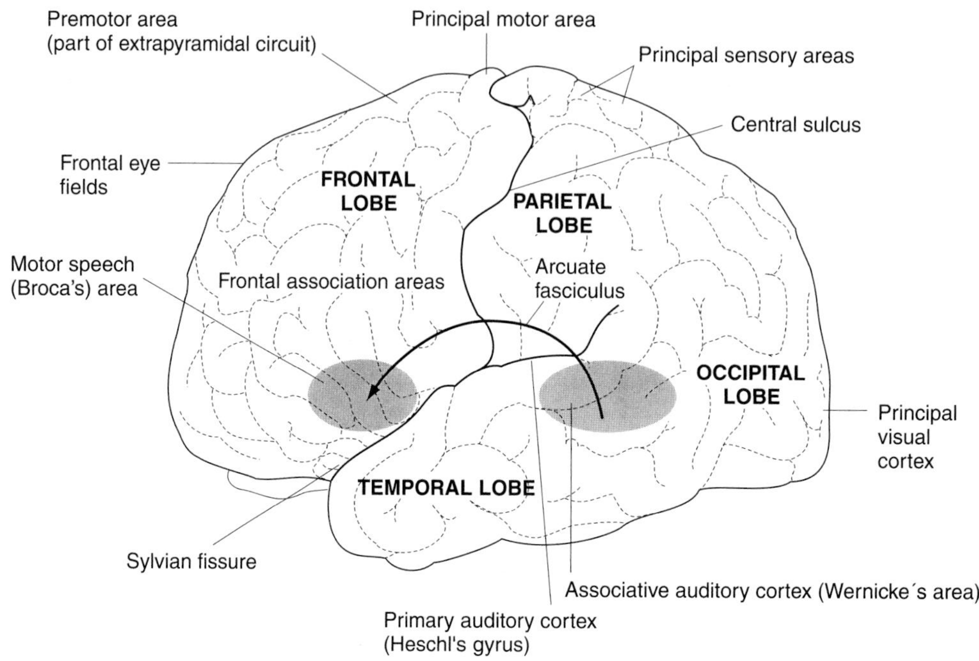

Frontal lobe functions	"Executive functions"—planning, inhibition, concentration, orientation, language, abstraction, judgment, motor regulation, mood. Lack of social judgment is most notable in frontal lobe lesion.	Damage = Disinhibition (e.g., Phineas Gage).

Homunculus

Topographical representation of sensory and motor areas in the cerebral cortex. Use to localize lesion (e.g., in blood supply) leading to specific defects.

For example, lower extremity deficit in sensation or movement indicates involvement of the anterior cerebral artery.

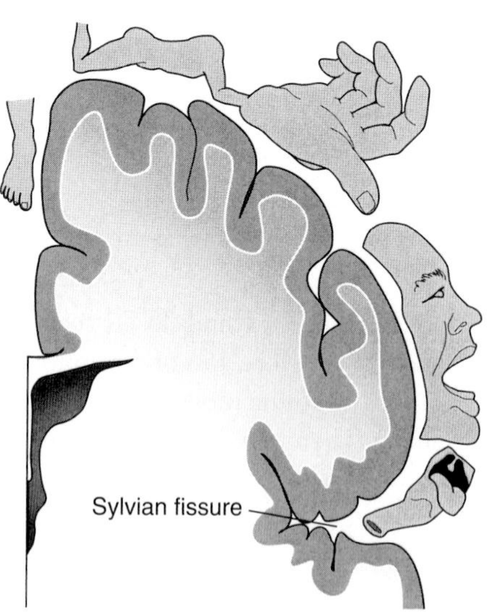

Motor homunculus

Cerebral arteries—cortical distribution

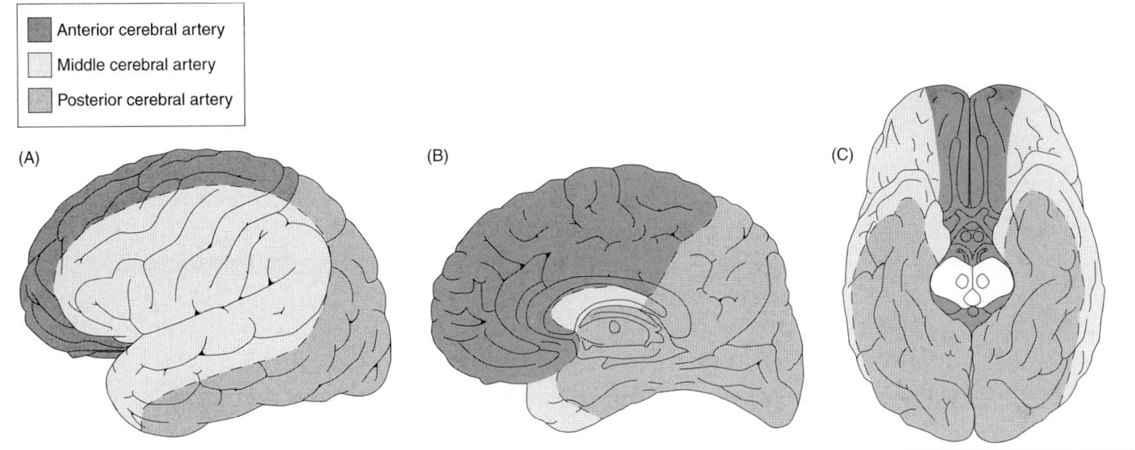

Circle of Willis

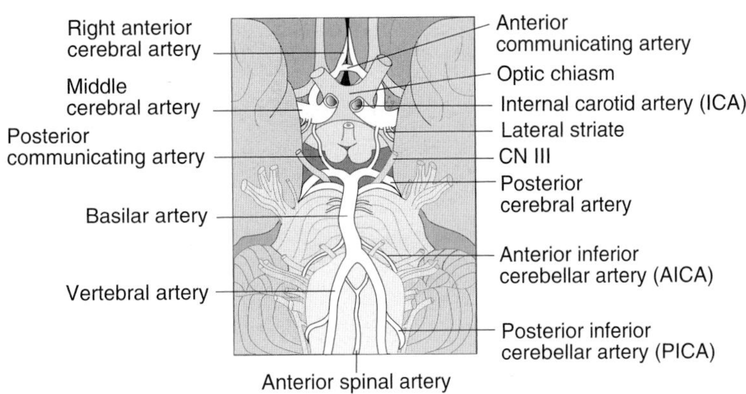

Anterior cerebral artery—supplies medial surface of the brain, leg-foot area of motor and sensory cortices.

Middle cerebral artery—supplies lateral aspect of brain, trunk-arm-face area of motor and sensory cortices, Broca's and Wernicke's speech areas.

Anterior communicating artery—most common site of circle of Willis aneurysm; lesions may cause visual field defects.

Posterior communicating artery—common area of aneurysm; causes CN III palsy.

Lateral striate—divisions of middle cerebral artery; "arteries of stroke"; supply internal capsule, caudate, putamen, globus pallidus.

In general, stroke of anterior circle → general sensory and motor dysfunction, aphasia; stroke of posterior circle → cranial nerve deficits (vertigo, visual deficits), coma, cerebellar deficits (ataxia).

Dural venous sinuses Venous sinuses run in the dura mater where its meningeal and periosteal layers separate. Cerebral veins → venous sinuses → internal jugular vein.

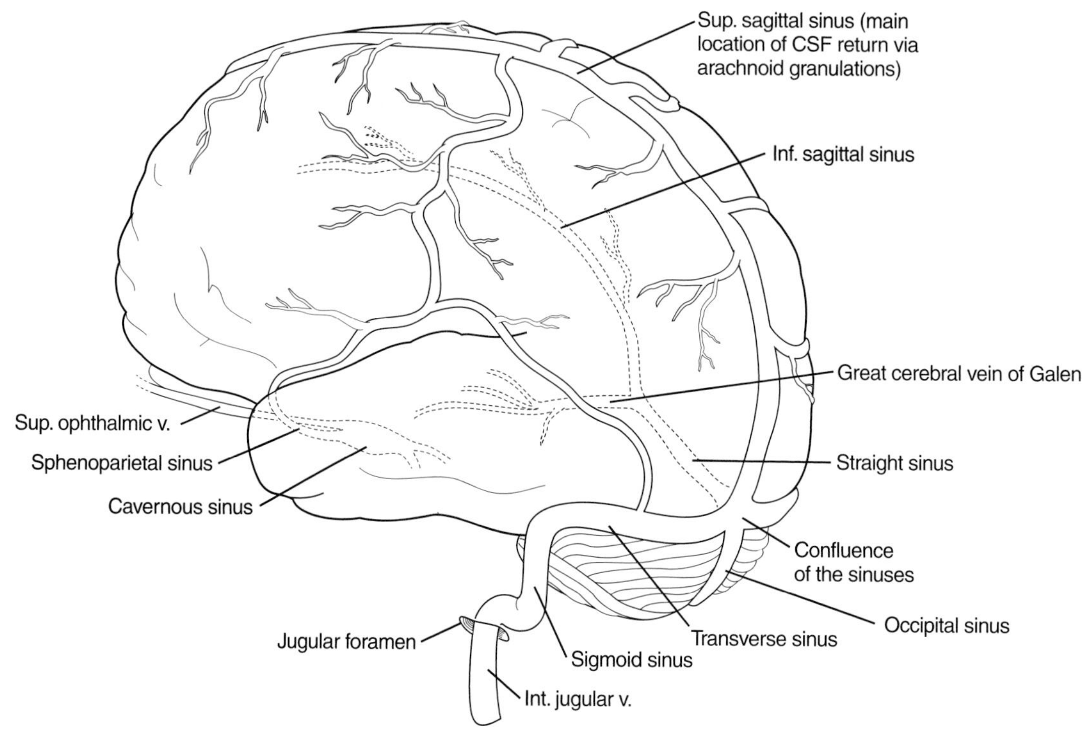

(Adapted, with permission, from White JS. *USMLE Road Map: Gross Anatomy,* 1st ed. New York: McGraw-Hill, 2003.)

Ventricular system

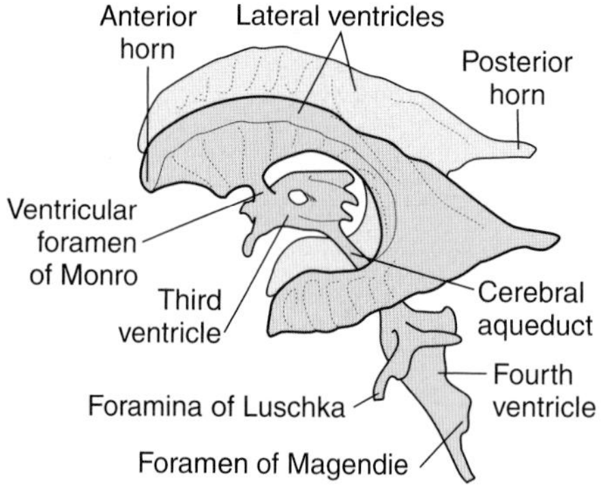

CSF is made by ependymal cells lining the ventricles; it is reabsorbed by venous sinus arachnoid granulations.

Hydrocephalus—accumulation of excess CSF in the ventricular system. Caused by impaired flow or reabsorption, choroid tumor, or ependymoma.

Lateral ventricle → 3rd ventricle via foramen of Monro.
3rd ventricle → 4th ventricle via cerebral aqueduct.
4th ventricle → subarachnoid space via:
Foramina of **L**uschka = **L**ateral.
Foramen of **M**agendie = **M**edial.

Spinal nerves	There are 31 spinal nerves altogether: 8 cervical, 12 thoracic, 5 lumbar, 5 sacral, 1 coccygeal. For C1–C7, nerves exit via intervertebral foramina above the corresponding vertebra. Nerves C8 and below exit below.	31, just like 31 flavors! Vertebral disk herniation usually occurs between L5 and S1.
Spinal cord lower extent	In adults, spinal cord extends to lower border of L1–L2; subarachnoid space extends to lower border of S2. Lumbar puncture is usually performed in L3–L4 or L4–L5 interspaces, at level of cauda equina.	To keep the cord **alive**, keep the spinal needle between **L3 and L5.**
Lumbar puncture Cauda equina Spinous process L3 L4 L4/5 disk L5 Needle in subarachnoid space	CSF obtained from lumbar subarachnoid space between L4 and L5 (at the level of iliac crests). Structures pierced as follows: 1. Skin/superficial fascia 2. Ligaments (supraspinous, interspinous, ligamentum flavum) 3. Epidural space 4. Dura mater 5. Subdural space 6. Arachnoid 7. Subarachnoid space—CSF	**Pia** is not **pierc**ed.

Spinal cord and associated tracts

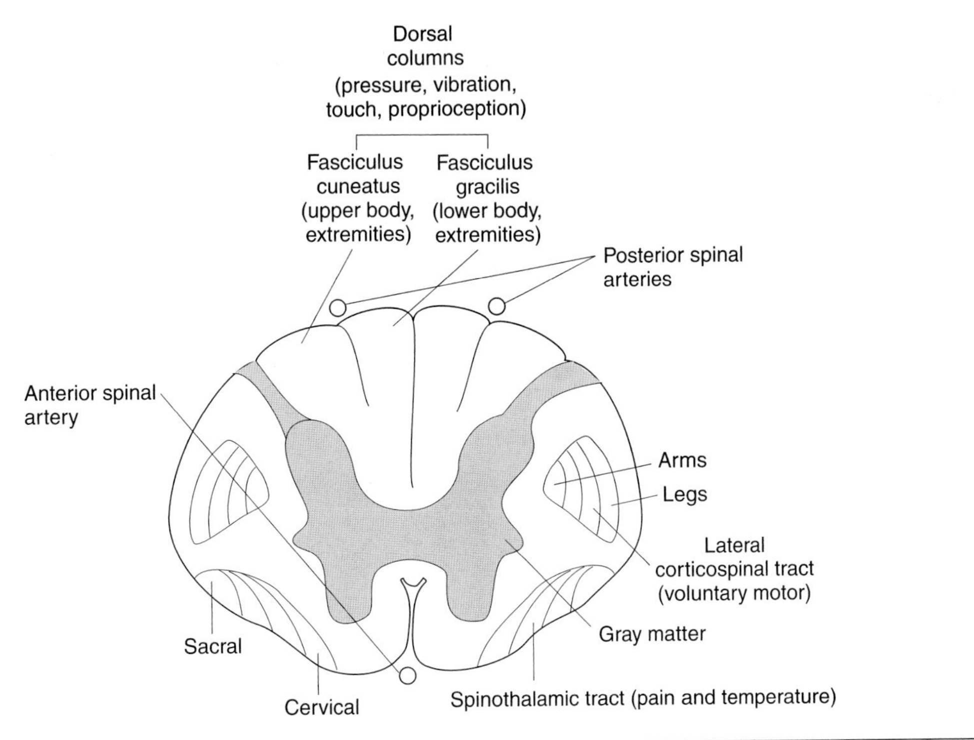

Spinal tract anatomy and functions

Tract and function	1st-order neuron	Synapse 1	2nd-order neuron	Synapse 2	3rd-order neuron
Dorsal column—medial lemniscal pathway (ascending pressure, vibration, touch, and proprioceptive sensation)	Sensory nerve ending → cell body in dorsal root ganglion → enters spinal cord, ascends ipsilaterally in dorsal column	Nucleus cuneatus or gracilis (medulla)	Decussates in medulla → ascends contralaterally in medial lemniscus	VPL of thalamus	Sensory cortex
Spinothalamic tract (ascending pain and temperature sensation)	Sensory nerve ending (A-delta and C fibers) (cell body in dorsal root ganglion) → enters spinal cord	Ipsilateral gray matter (spinal cord)	Decussates at anterior white commissure → ascends contralaterally	VPL of thalamus	Sensory cortex
Lateral corticospinal tract (descending voluntary movement of contralateral limbs)	**Upper motor neuron:** cell body in 1° motor cortex → descends ipsilaterally until decussating at caudal medulla (pyramidal decussation)→ descends contralaterally	Cell body of anterior horn (spinal cord)	**Lower motor neuron:** Leaves spinal cord	Neuromuscular junction	

Dorsal column organization

Fasciculus gracilis = legs.
Fasciculus cuneatus = arms.

Dorsal column is organized as you are, with hands at sides—arms outside and legs inside.

Clinically important landmarks

Pudendal nerve block (to relieve pain of pregnancy)—ischial spine.
Appendix—⅔ of the way from the umbilicus to the anterior superior iliac spine (McBurney's point).
Lumbar puncture—iliac crest.

Landmark dermatomes

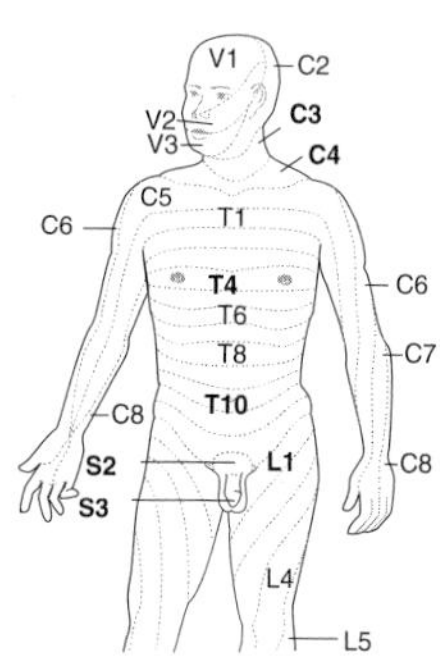

C2 is the posterior half of a skull "cap."
C3 is a high turtleneck shirt.
C4 is a low-collar shirt.
T4 is at the nipple.
T7 is at the xiphoid process.
T10 is at the umbilicus (important for early appendicitis pain referral).
L1 is at the inguinal ligament.
L4 includes the kneecaps.
S2, S3, S4 erection and sensation of penile and anal zones.

Gallbladder pain referred to the right shoulder via the phrenic nerve.
T4 at the **teat pore.**

T10 at the belly but**TEN.**

L1 is **IL** (**I**nguinal **L**igament).
Down on **L4s (all fours).**
"**S2, 3, 4** keep the penis off the floor."

Spindle muscle control

Muscle spindle	In parallel with muscle fibers. Muscle stretch → intrafusal stretch → stimulates Ia afferent→ stimulates α motor neuron → reflex muscle (extrafusal) contraction.	Muscle spindles monitor muscle length (help you pick up a heavy suitcase when you didn't know how heavy it was). Golgi Tendon organs monitor muscle Tension (make you drop a heavy suitcase you've been holding too long).
Gamma loop	CNS stimulates γ motor neuron → contracts intrafusal fiber → ↑ sensitivity of reflex arc.	

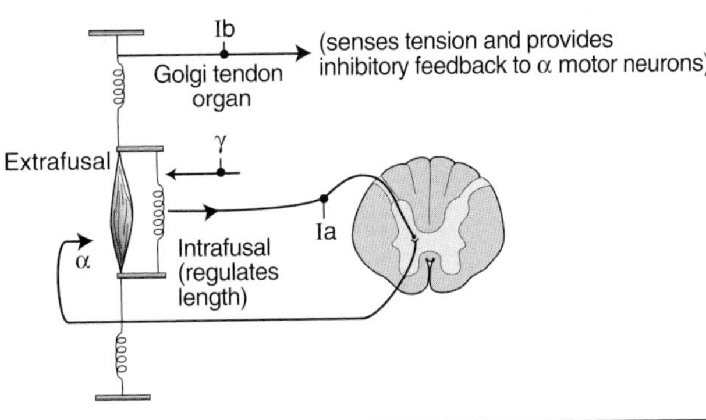

Clinical reflexes

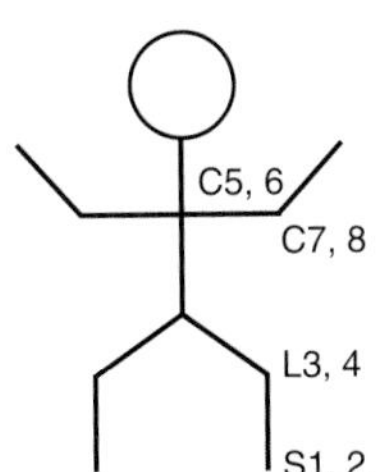

Biceps = C5 nerve root.
Triceps = C7 nerve root.
Patella = L4 nerve root.
Achilles = S1 nerve root.
Babinski—dorsiflexion of the big toe and fanning of other toes; sign of UMN lesion, but normal reflex in 1st year of life.

Reflexes count up in order:
S1, 2
L3, 4
C5, 6
C7, 8

Primitive reflexes

1. Moro reflex—extension of limbs when startled
2. Rooting reflex—nipple seeking
3. Palmar reflex—grasps objects in palm
4. Babinski reflex—large toe dorsiflexes with plantar stimulation

Normally disappear within 1st year. May reemerge following frontal lobe lesion.

Brain stem—ventral view

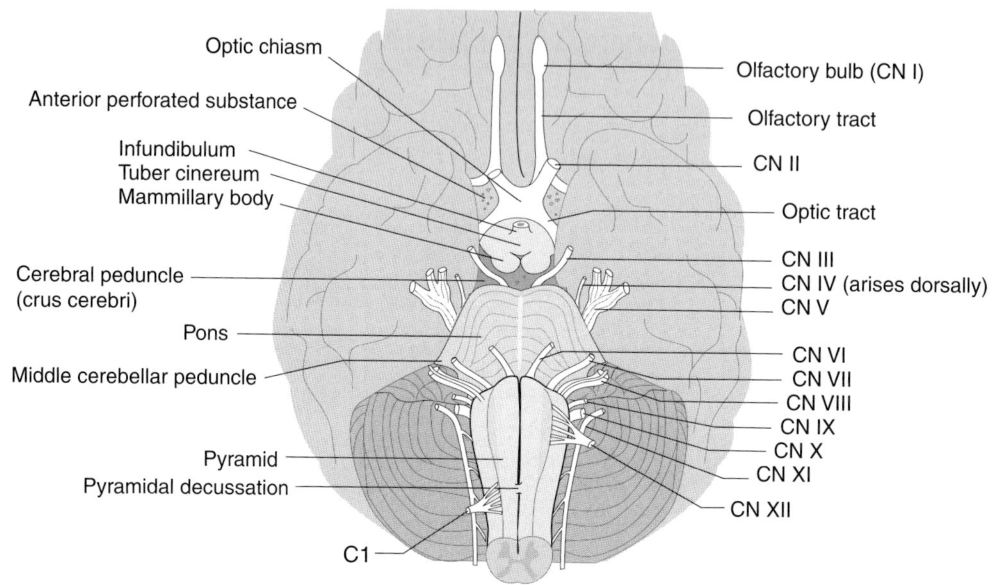

CNs that lie medially at brain stem: III, VI, XII. $3(\times 2) = 6(\times 2) = 12$.

Brain stem—dorsal view (cerebellum removed)

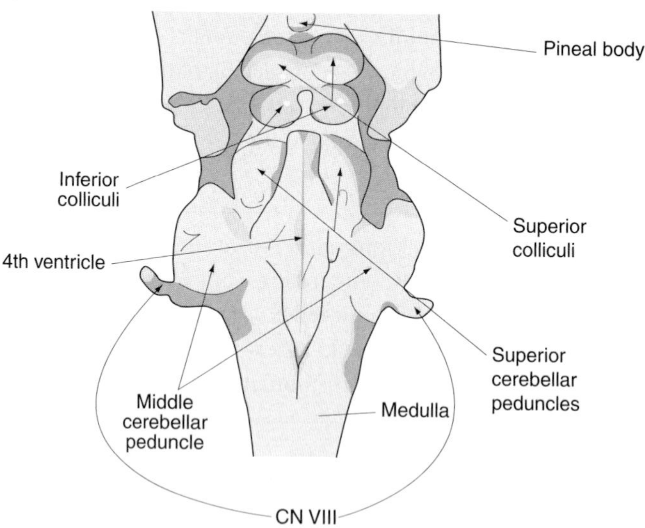

Pineal gland—melatonin secretion, circadian rhythms.

Superior colliculi—conjugate vertical gaze center.

Inferior colliculi—auditory.

Parinaud syndrome—paralysis of conjugate vertical gaze due to lesion in superior colliculi (e.g., pinealoma).

Your eyes are **above** your ears, and the superior colliculus (visual) is **above** the inferior colliculus (auditory).

Cranial nerves

Nerve	CN	Function	Type	Mnemonic
Olfactory	I	Smell (only CN without thalamic relay to cortex)	Sensory	Some
Optic	II	Sight	Sensory	Say
Oculomotor	III	Eye movement, pupil constriction, accommodation, eyelid opening (levator palpebrae)	Motor	Marry
Trochlear	IV	Eye movement	Motor	Money
Trigeminal	V	Mastication, facial sensation	Both	But
Abducens	VI	Eye movement (arises from contralateral nuclei)	Motor	My
Facial	VII	Facial movement, taste from anterior 2/3 of tongue, lacrimation, salivation (submandibular and sublingual glands), eyelid closing (orbicularis oculi), stapedius muscle in ear	Both	Brother
Vestibulocochlear	VIII	Hearing, balance	Sensory	Says
Glossopharyngeal	IX	Taste from posterior 1/3 of tongue, swallowing, salivation (parotid gland), monitoring carotid body and sinus chemo- and baroreceptors, and stylopharyngeus	Both	Big
Vagus	X	Taste from epiglottic region, swallowing, palate elevation, talking, coughing, thoracoabdominal viscera, monitoring aortic arch chemo- and baroreceptors	Both	Brains
Accessory	XI	Head turning, shoulder shrugging	Motor	Matter
Hypoglossal	XII	Tongue movement	Motor	Most

Cranial nerve nuclei

Located in tegmentum portion of brain stem (between dorsal and ventral portions).

1. Midbrain—nuclei of CN III, IV
2. Pons—nuclei of CN V, VI, VII, VIII
3. Medulla—nuclei of CN IX, X, XI, XII

Lateral nuclei = sensory.
Medial nuclei = Motor.

Reflexes and cranial nerves

Cranial nerve reflex	Afferent	Efferent
Corneal	V_1	VII
Lacrimation	V_1	VII
Jaw jerk	V_3 (sensory)	V_3 (motor)
Pupillary	II	III
Gag	IX	IX, X

Vagal nuclei

Nucleus Solitarius	Visceral Sensory information (e.g., taste, baroreceptors, gut distention).	VII, IX, X.
Nucleus aMbiguus	Motor innervation of pharynx, larynx, and upper esophagus (e.g., swallowing, palate elevation).	IX, X, XI.
Dorsal motor nucleus	Sends autonomic (parasympathetic) fibers to heart, lungs, and upper GI.	

Cranial nerve and vessel pathways

Cribriform plate (CN I).

Middle cranial fossa (CN II–VI)—through sphenoid bone:

1. Optic canal (CN II, ophthalmic artery, central retinal vein)
2. Superior orbital fissure (CN III, IV, V_1, VI, ophthalmic vein)
3. Foramen **R**otundum (CN V_2)
4. Foramen **O**vale (CN V_3)
5. Foramen spinosum (middle meningeal artery)

Posterior cranial fossa (CN VII–XII)—through temporal or occipital bone:

1. Internal auditory meatus (CN VII, VIII)
2. Jugular foramen (CN IX, X, XI, jugular vein)
3. Hypoglossal canal (CN XII)
4. Foramen magnum (spinal roots of CN XI, brain stem, vertebral arteries)

Divisions of CN V exit owing to **S**tanding **R**oom **O**nly.

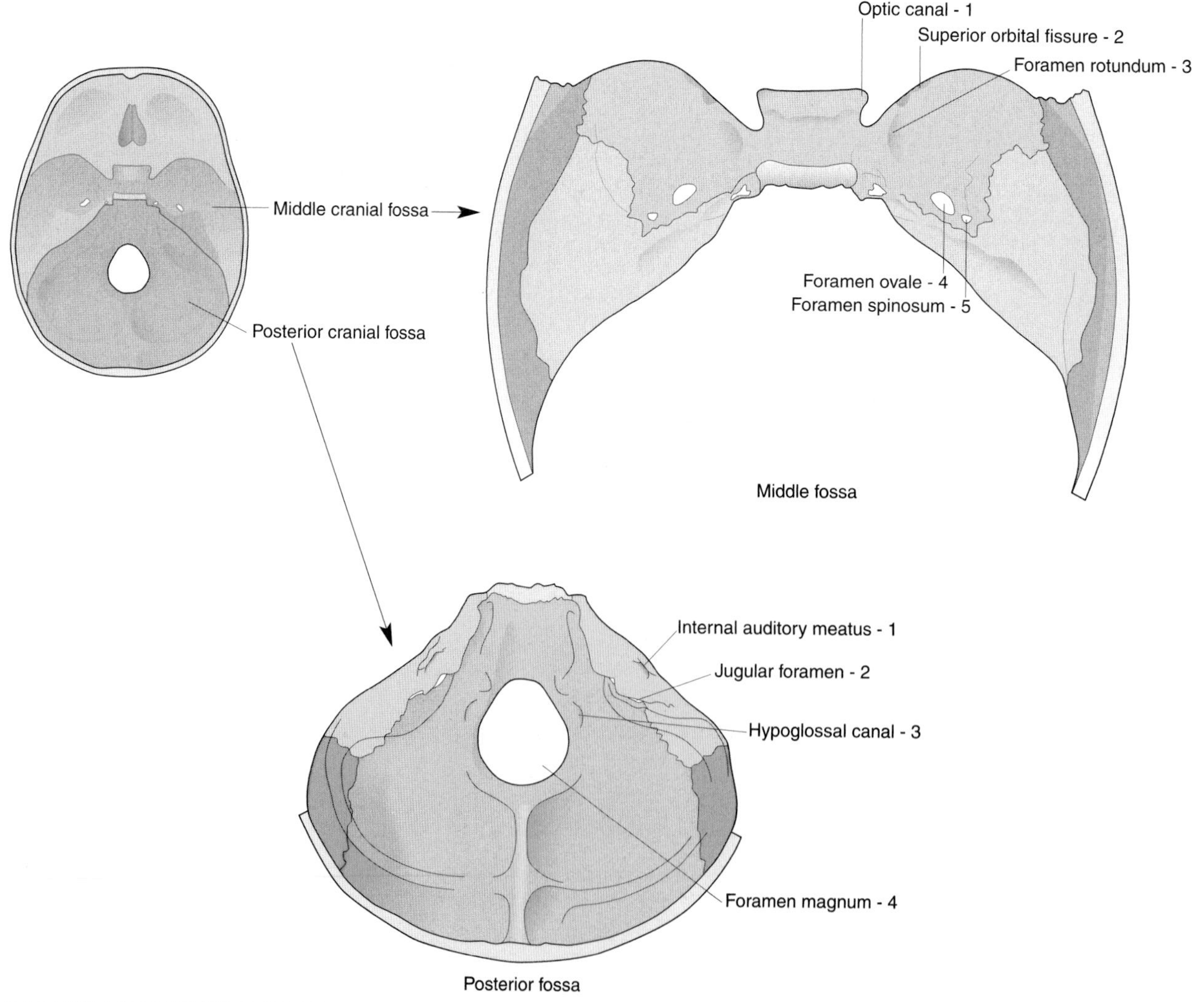

Cavernous sinus	A collection of venous sinuses on either side of the pituitary. Blood from eye and superficial cortex → cavernous sinus → internal jugular vein. CN III, IV, V_1, V_2, and VI and postganglionic sympathetic fibers en route to the orbit all pass through the cavernous sinus. Only CN VI is "free-floating." Cavernous portion of internal carotid artery is also here.	The nerves that control extraocular muscles (plus V_1 and V_2) pass through the cavernous sinus. Cavernous sinus syndrome (e.g., due to mass effect)—ophthalmoplegia, ophthalmic and maxillary sensory loss.

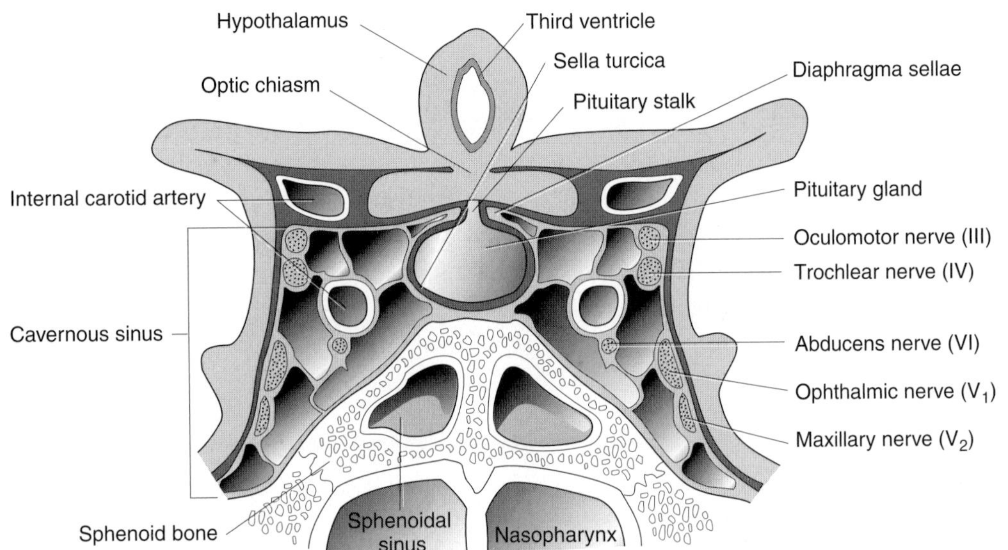

(Adapted, with permission, from Stobo J et al. *The Principles and Practice of Medicine,* 23rd ed. Stamford, CT: Appleton & Lange, 1996: 277.)

KLM sounds: kuh, la, mi	Kuh-kuh-kuh tests palate elevation (CN X—vagus). La-la-la tests tongue (CN XII—hypoglossal). Mi-mi-mi tests lips (CN VII—facial).	Say it aloud.
Mastication muscles	3 muscles close jaw: **M**asseter, te**M**poralis, **M**edial pterygoid. 1 opens: lateral pterygoid. All are innervated by the trigeminal nerve (V_3).	**M**'s **M**unch. **L**ateral **L**owers (when speaking of pterygoids with respect to jaw motion).
Muscles with *glossus*	All muscles with root *glossus* in their names (**except palatoglossus**, innervated by vagus nerve) are innervated by hypo*glossal* nerve.	*Palat*: vagus nerve. *Glossus*: hypo*glossal* nerve.
Muscles with *palat*	All muscles with root *palat* in their names (**except tensor veli palatini**, innervated by mandibular branch of CN V) are innervated by vagus nerve.	*Palat*: vagus nerve (except **TENS**or, who was too **TENSE**).

Sensory corpuscles

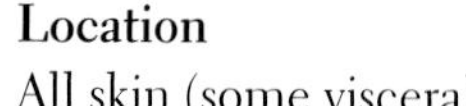

Receptor type	Location	Senses	
Free nerve endings (C, Aδ fibers)	All skin (some viscera)	Pain and temperature	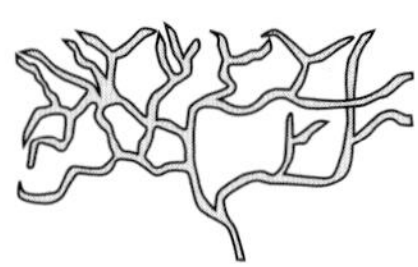
Meissner's corpuscles	Glabrous (hairless) skin—40% of fingertip receptors	Dynamic fine touch (e.g., manipulation)	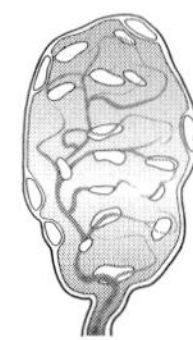
Pacinian corpuscles	Deep skin layers, ligaments, and joints—15% of fingertip receptors	Vibration	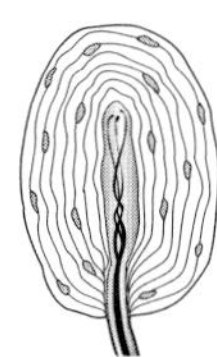
Merkel's disks (cup-shaped)	Hair follicles—25% of fingertip receptors	Static touch (e.g., shapes, edges, textures)	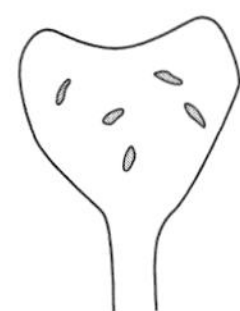

Inner ear

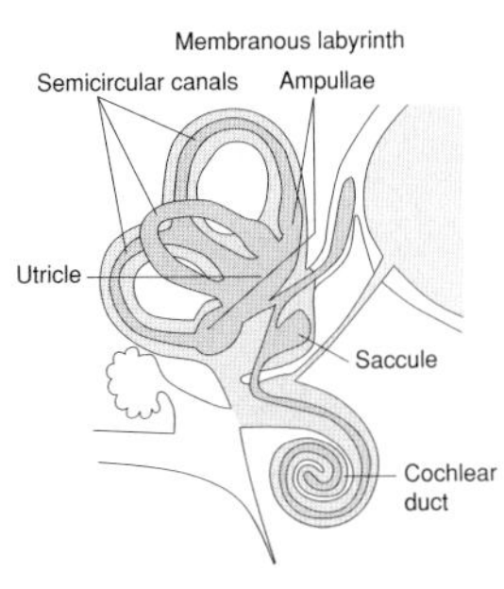

Consists of a series of tubes in the temporal bone (bony labyrinth) filled with perilymph (Na^+ rich, similar to ECF) that includes cochlea, vestibule, and semicircular canals.

Within the bony labyrinth is a 2nd series of tubes (membranous labyrinth) filled with endolymph (K^+ rich, similar to ICF) that includes cochlear duct (within the cochlea), utricle and saccule (within the vestibule), and semicircular canals. Hair cells (located within the organ of Corti) are the sensory elements in both vestibular apparatus (spatial orientation) and cochlea (hearing).

Hearing loss:

1. Conductive—negative Rinne (bone conduction > air conduction); Weber localizes to affected ear.
2. Sensorineural—positive Rinne (air conduction > bone conduction); Weber localizes to normal ear.

Peri—think outside of cell (Na^+).
Endo—think inside of cell (K^+).
Endolymph is made by the stria vascularis.
Utricle and saccule contain maculae—detect linear acceleration.
Semicircular canals contain **A**mpullae—detect **A**ngular acceleration.
Cochlear membrane = scuba flipper: narrow/stiff at the base (high frequency) and wide/flexible at the apex (low frequency).

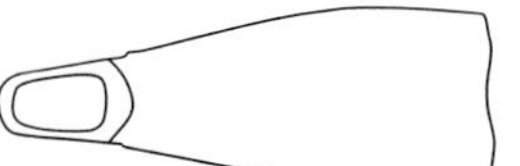

Hearing loss in the elderly—high frequency → low frequency.

Eye and retina

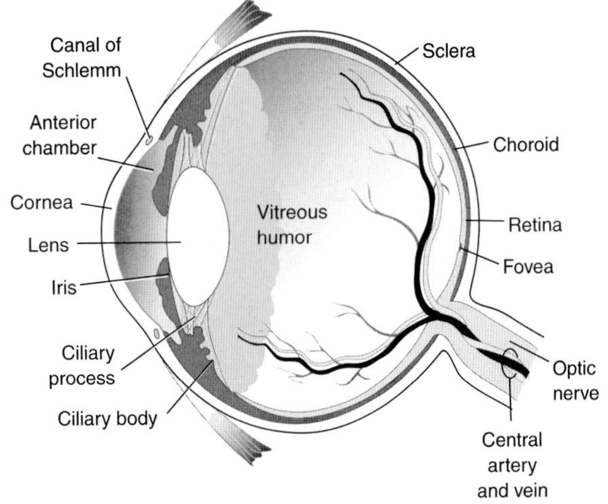

Extraocular muscles and nerves

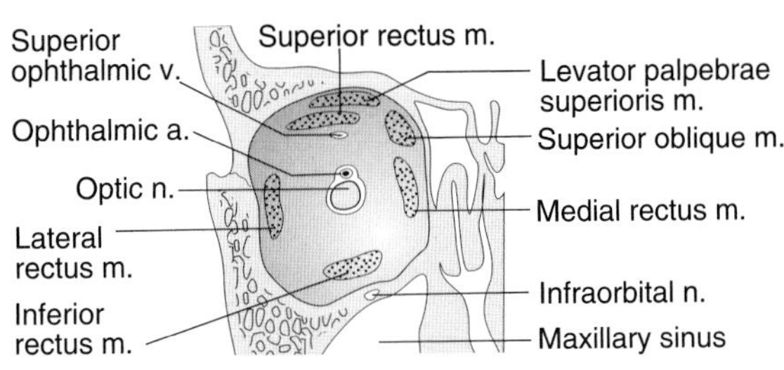

(Note: inferior oblique not in plane of diagram)

CN III damage—eye looks down and out,
CN IV damage—diplopia with downward gaze.
CN VI damage—medially directed eye.

CN VI innervates the **L**ateral **R**ectus.
CN IV innervates the **S**uperior **O**blique.
CN III innervates the **R**est.
The "chemical formula" $LR_6SO_4R_3$.
The superior oblique abducts, intorts, depresses.

HIGH-YIELD SYSTEMS

NEUROLOGY

Testing extraocular muscles

To test the function of each muscle, have the patient look in the following directions (i.e., to test SO, have patient depress eye from adducted position):

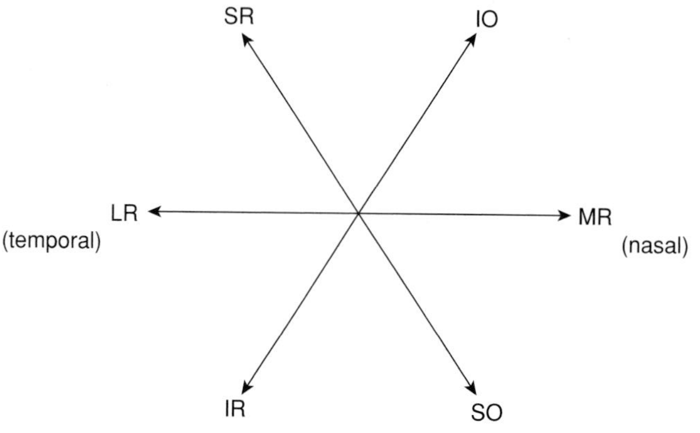

Pupillary light reflex

Light in either retina sends a signal via CN II to pretectal nuclei (dashed lines) in midbrain that activate bilateral Edinger-Westphal nuclei; pupils contract bilaterally (consensual reflex).

Note that the illumination of 1 eye results in bilateral pupillary constriction.

Marcus Gunn phenomenon—afferent pupillary defect (e.g., due to optic nerve damage or retinal detachment).

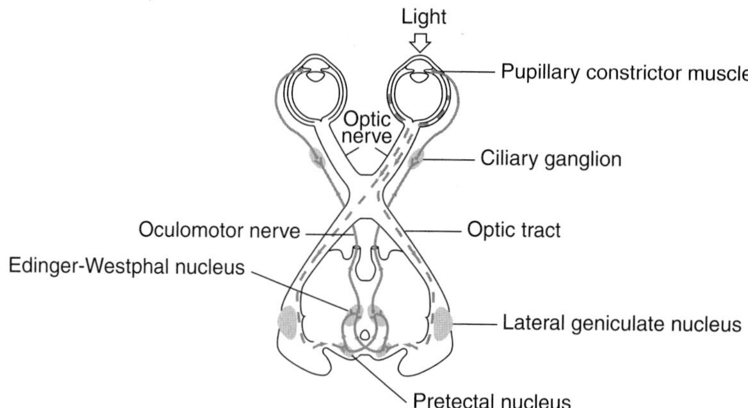

(Adapted, with permission, from Simon RP et al. *Clinical Neurology,* 3rd ed. Stamford, CT: Appleton & Lange, 1996.)

Visual field defects

1. Right anopia
2. Bitemporal hemianopia
3. Left homonymous hemianopia
4. Left upper quadrantic anopia (right temporal lesion)
5. Left lower quadrantic anopia (right parietal lesion)
6. Left hemianopia with macular sparing
7. Central scotoma (macular degeneration)

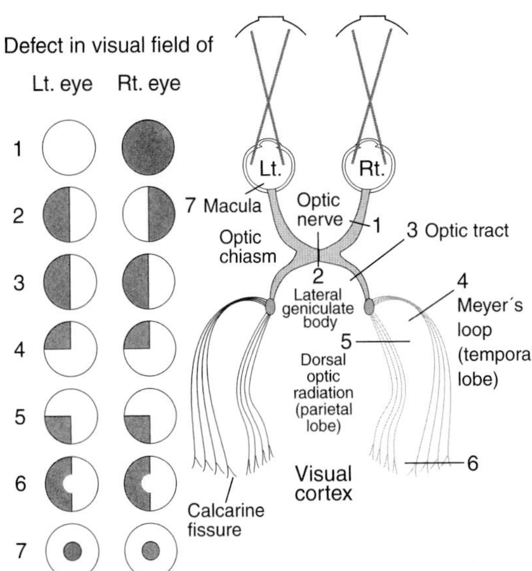

Note: When an image hits 1° visual cortex, it is upside down and left-right reversed.

Internuclear ophthalmoplegia (MLF syndrome)

Lesion in the medial longitudinal fasciculus (MLF). Results in medial rectus palsy on attempted lateral gaze. Nystagmus in abducting eye. Convergence is normal. MLF syndrome is seen in many patients with multiple sclerosis.

MLF = MS.

When looking left, the left nucleus of CN VI fires, which contracts the left lateral rectus and stimulates the contralateral (right) nucleus of CN III via the right MLF to contract the right medial rectus.

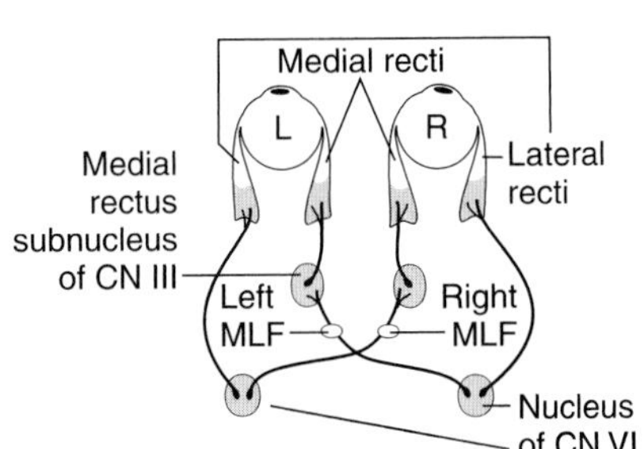

Looking to the right with left MLF damage

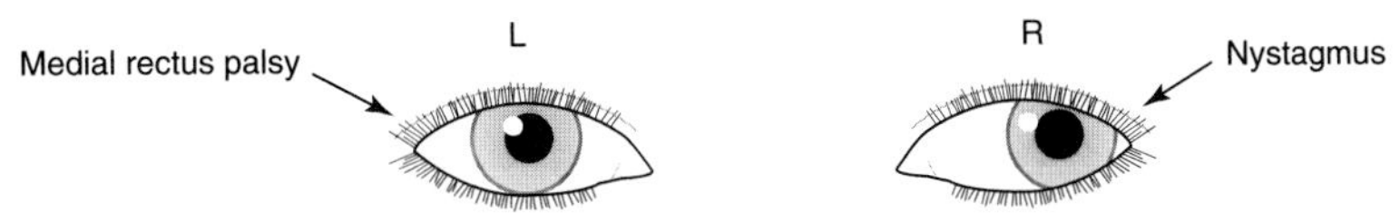

Neural tube defects

Associated with low folic acid intake during pregnancy. Elevated α-fetoprotein in amniotic fluid and maternal serum.

Spina bifida occulta—failure of bony spinal canal to close, but no structural herniation. Usually seen at lower vertebral levels. Dura is intact.

Meningocele—meninges herniate through spinal canal defect.

Meningomyelocele—meninges and spinal cord herniate through spinal canal defect.

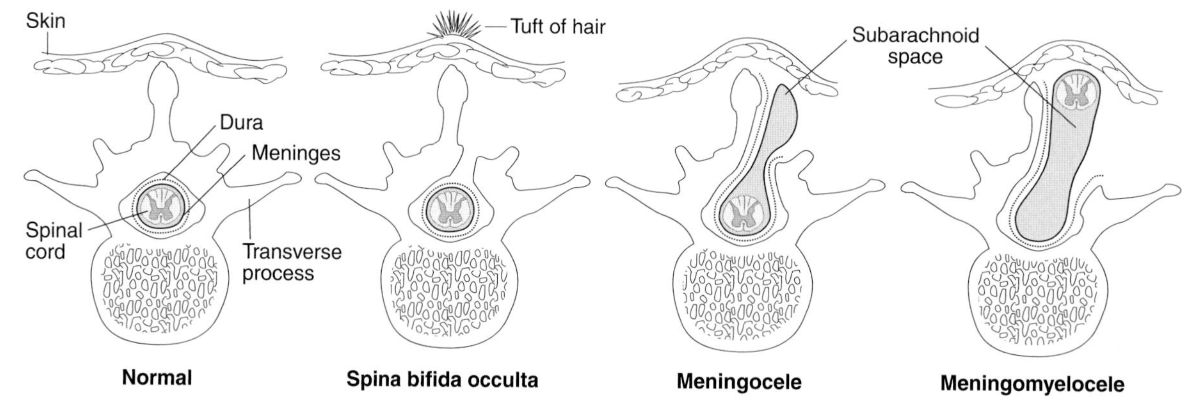

Regional specification of developing brain

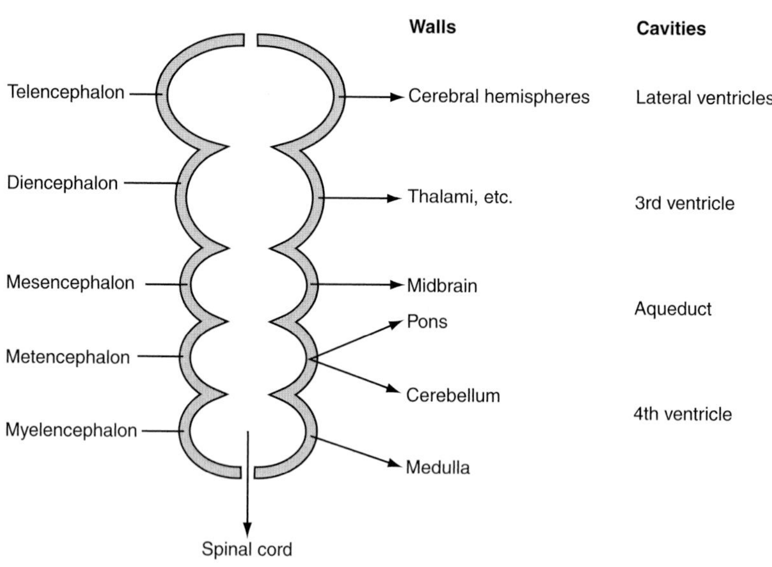

Forebrain anomalies

Anencephaly	Malformation of anterior end of neural tube; no brain/calvarium, elevated AFP, polyhydramnios (no swallowing center in brain).
Holoprosencephaly	↓ separation of hemispheres across midline; results in cyclopia; associated with Patau's syndrome and severe fetal alcohol syndrome.

Motor neuron signs

Sign	UMN lesion	LMN lesion
Weakness	+	+
Atrophy	–	+
Fasciculation	–	+
Reflexes	↑	↓
Tone	↑	↓
Babinski	+	–
Spastic paralysis	+	–

Lower MN = everything **lowered** (less muscle mass, ↓ muscle tone, ↓ reflexes, downgoing toes).
Upper MN = everything **up** (tone, DTRs, toes).
Upgoing Babinski is normal in infants.

Spinal cord lesions

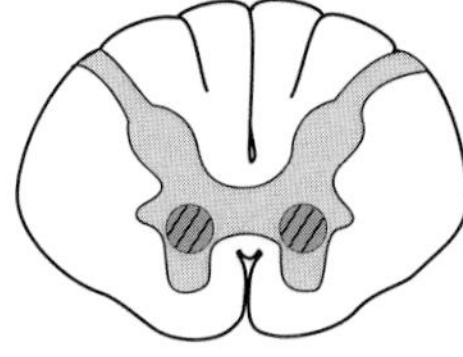

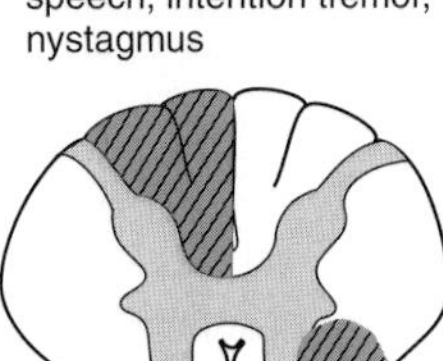

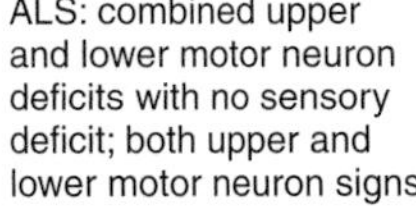

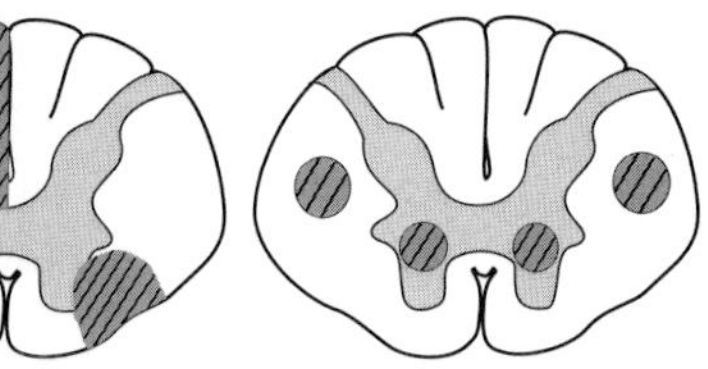

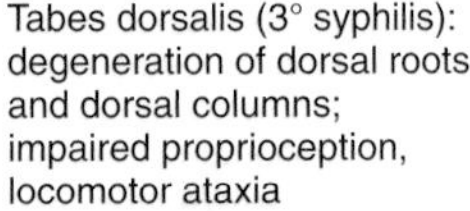

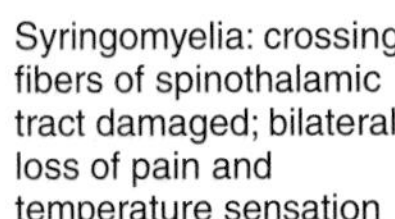

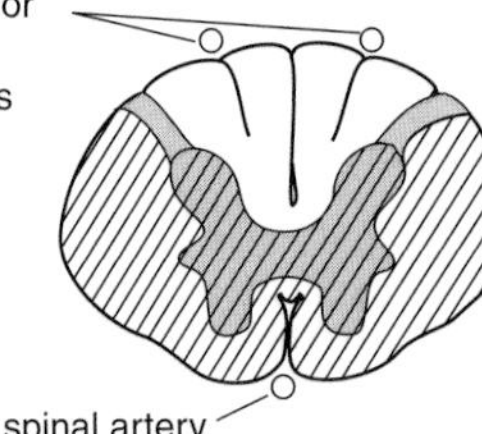

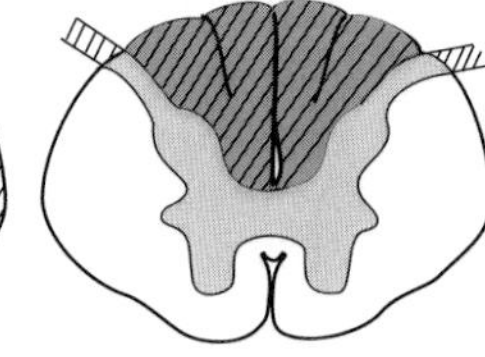

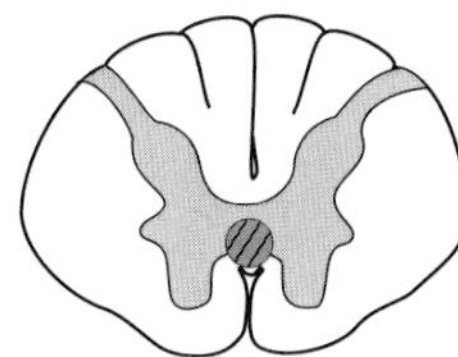

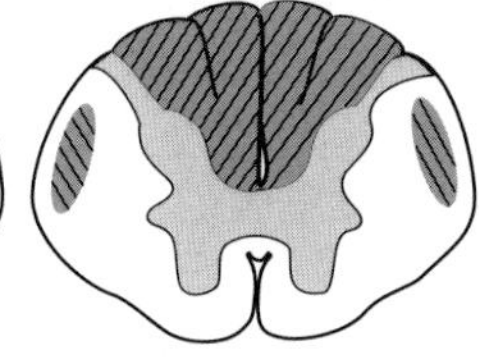

Syringomyelia

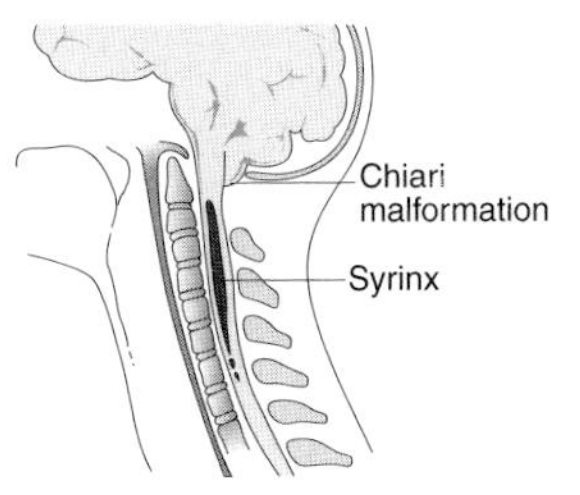

Enlargement of the central canal of spinal cord. Crossing fibers of spinothalamic tract are damaged. Bilateral loss of pain and temperature sensation in upper extremities with preservation of touch sensation.

Syrinx (Greek) = tube, as in syringe.
Often presents in patients with Arnold-Chiari malformation.
Most common at C8–T1.

Tabes dorsalis

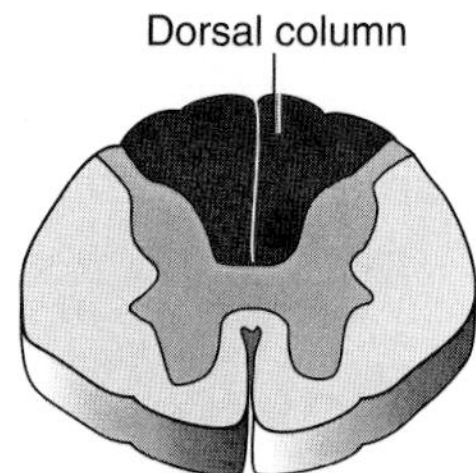

Degeneration of dorsal columns and dorsal roots due to 3° syphilis, resulting in impaired proprioception and locomotor ataxia. Associated with Charcot's joints, shooting (lightning) pain (see Color Image 12), Argyll Robertson pupils (reactive to accommodation but not to light), and absence of DTRs.

Argyll Robertson pupils are also known as "prostitute's pupils" because they accommodate but do not react.

Brown-Séquard syndrome

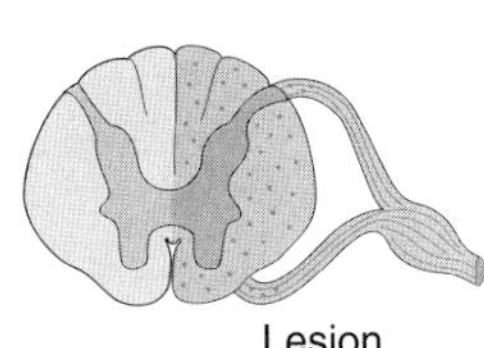

Hemisection of spinal cord. Findings:

1. Ipsilateral UMN signs (corticospinal tract) below lesion
2. Ipsilateral loss of tactile, vibration, proprioception sense (dorsal column) below lesion
3. Contralateral pain and temperature loss (spinothalamic tract) below lesion
4. Ipsilateral loss of all sensation at level of lesion
5. LMN signs (e.g., flaccid paralysis) at level of lesion

If lesion occurs above T1, presents with Horner's syndrome.

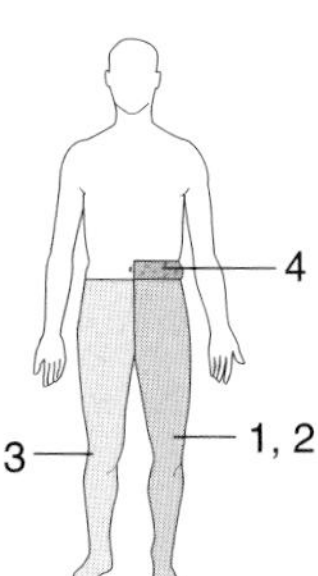

Horner's syndrome	Sympathectomy of face: 1. **P**tosis (slight drooping of eyelid) 2. **A**nhidrosis (absence of sweating) and flushing (rubor) of affected side of face 3. **M**iosis (pupil constriction) Associated with lesion of spinal cord above T1 (e.g., Pancoast's tumor, Brown-Séquard syndrome [cord hemisection], late-stage syringomyelia).	**PAM** is **horny** (Horner's).

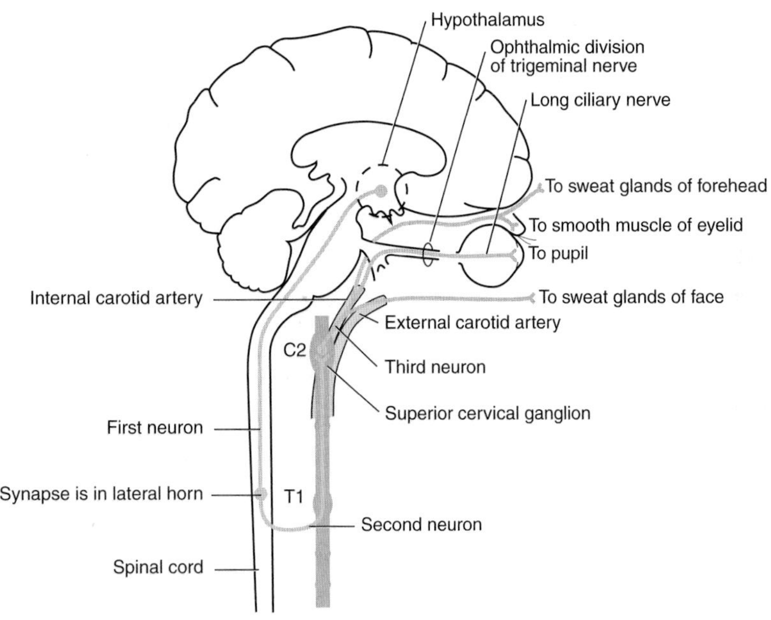

The 3-neuron oculosympathetic pathway above projects from the hypothalamus to the intermediolateral column of the spinal cord, then to the superior cervical (sympathetic) ganglion, and finally to the pupil, the smooth muscle of the eyelids, and the sweat glands of the forehead and face. Interruption of these pathways results in Horner's syndrome.

Brain lesions

Area of lesion	Consequence	
Broca's area	Motor (nonfluent/expressive) aphasia with good comprehension	**BRO**ca's is **BRO**ken speech.
Wernicke's area	Sensory (fluent/receptive) aphasia with poor comprehension	**W**ernicke's is **W**ordy but makes no sense.
Arcuate fasciculus	Conduction aphasia; poor repetition with good comprehension, fluent speech	Connects Wernicke's to Broca's area.
Amygdala (bilateral)	Klüver-Bucy syndrome (hyperorality, hypersexuality, disinhibited behavior)	
Frontal lobe	Personality changes and deficits in concentration, orientation, and judgment; may have reemergence of primitive reflexes	
Right parietal lobe	Spatial neglect syndrome (agnosia of the contralateral side of the world)	
Reticular activating system	Reduced levels of arousal and wakefulness (e.g., coma)	
Mammillary bodies (bilateral)	Wernicke-Korsakoff syndrome	
Basal ganglia	May result in tremor at rest, chorea, or athetosis	
Cerebellar hemisphere	Intention tremor, limb ataxia. Damage to the cerebellum results in ipsilateral deficits.	Cerebellar hemispheres are **laterally** located—affect **lateral** limbs.
Cerebellar vermis	Truncal ataxia, dysarthria	Vermis is **centrally** located—affects **central** body.
Subthalamic nucleus	Contralateral hemiballismus	
Hippocampus	Anterograde amnesia—can't make new memories	
Parapontine reticular formation (PPRF)	Eyes look toward side of lesion	
Frontal eye fields	Eyes look away from lesion	

Chorea	Sudden, jerky, purposeless movements. Characteristic of basal ganglia lesion (e.g., Huntington's disease).	*Chorea* = dancing (Greek). Think choral dancing or choreography.
Athetosis	Slow, writhing movements, especially of fingers. Characteristic of basal ganglia lesion.	*Athetos* = not fixed (Greek). Think snakelike.
Hemiballismus	Sudden, wild flailing of 1 arm. Characteristic of contralateral subthalamic nucleus lesion. Loss of inhibition of thalamus through globus pallidus.	Half ballistic (as in throwing a baseball).
Aphasia		
Broca's	Nonfluent aphasia with intact comprehension. Broca's area—inferior frontal gyrus.	**Bro**ca's **Bro**ken **Boca.**
Wernicke's	Fluent aphasia with impaired comprehension. Wernicke's area—superior temporal gyrus.	**W**ernicke's is **W**ordy but makes no sense. **W**ernicke's = "**W**hat?"

Degenerative diseases

Cerebral cortex	**Alzheimer's disease**—most common cause of dementia in the elderly. Associated with senile plaques (extracellular, β-amyloid core) and neurofibrillary tangles (intracellular, abnormally phosphorylated tau protein; tangles correlate with degree of dementia). Down syndrome patients are at ↑ risk of developing Alzheimer's. Familial form (10%) associated with genes on chromosomes 1, 14, 19 (*APOE4* allele), and 21 (p-*App* gene) (see Color Image 41).	Multi-infarct dementia is the 2nd most common cause of dementia in the elderly. May cause amyloid angiopathy → intracranial hemorrhage. Alzheimer's—diffuse cortical atrophy.
	Pick's disease (frontotemporal dementia)—dementia, aphasia, parkinsonian aspects; associated with Pick bodies (intracellular, aggregated tau protein).	Pick's—frontotemporal lobe atrophy.
	Lewy body dementia—parkinsonism with dementia and hallucinations. Caused by α-synuclein defect.	
	Creutzfelt-Jakob disease (CJD)—rapidly progressive (weeks to months) dementia with myoclonus, spongiform cortex; associated with prions.	
Basal ganglia and brain stem	**Huntington's disease**—autosomal-dominant inheritance, chorea, dementia. Atrophy of caudate nucleus (loss of GABAergic neurons). Triplet repeat defect causes genetic anticipation. Degeneration of caudate leads to enlarged lateral ventricles on CT.	Chromosome 4—expansion of CAG repeats. **CAG**—**C**audate loses **A**Ch and **G**ABA.
	Parkinson's disease—associated with Lewy bodies (composed of α-synuclein) and depigmentation of the substantia nigra pars compacta (loss of dopaminergic neurons). Rare cases have been linked to exposure to MPTP, a contaminant in illicit street drugs.	**TRAP** = **T**remor (at rest), cogwheel **R**igidity, **A**kinesia, and **P**ostural instability (you are **TRAP**ped in your body).
Spinocerebellar	**Olivopontocerebellar atrophy; Friedreich's ataxia.**	
Motor neuron	**Amyotrophic lateral sclerosis (ALS)**—associated with **both** LMN and UMN signs; no sensory deficit. Can be caused by defect in superoxide dismutase 1 (SOD1).	Commonly known as Lou Gehrig's disease.
	Werdnig-Hoffmann disease (infantile spinal muscular atrophy)—autosomal-recessive inheritance; presents at birth as a "floppy baby," tongue fasciculations; median age of death 7 months. Associated with degeneration of anterior horns. LMN involvement only.	
	Polio—follows infection with poliovirus; LMN signs. Associated with degeneration of anterior horns.	

Poliomyelitis	Caused by poliovirus, which is transmitted by the fecal-oral route. Replicates in the oropharynx and small intestine before spreading through the bloodstream to the CNS, where it leads to the destruction of cells in the anterior horn of the spinal cord, leading in turn to LMN destruction.	
Symptoms	Malaise, headache, fever, nausea, abdominal pain, sore throat. Signs of LMN lesions—muscle weakness and atrophy, fasciculations, fibrillation, and hyporeflexia.	
Findings	CSF with lymphocytic pleocytosis with slight elevation of protein (with no change in CSF glucose). Virus recovered from stool or throat.	
Demyelinating and dysmyelinating diseases	**Multiple sclerosis (MS)**—↑ prevalence with ↑ distance from the equator; periventricular plaques (areas of oligodendrocyte loss and reactive gliosis) with preservation of axons; ↑ protein (IgG) in CSF. Many patients have a relapsing-remitting course. Patients can present with optic neuritis (sudden loss of vision), MLF syndrome (internuclear ophthalmoplegia), hemiparesis, hemisensory symptoms, or bladder/bowel incontinence (see Color Image 47). **Progressive multifocal leukoencephalopathy (PML)**—associated with JC virus and seen in 2–4% of AIDS patients (reactivation of latent viral infection). **Acute disseminated (postinfectious) encephalomyelitis.** **Metachromatic leukodystrophy**—an autosomal-recessive lysosomal storage disease; arylsulfatase A deficiency. **Guillain-Barré syndrome** (see below).	Classic triad of **MS** is a **SIN**: **S**canning speech **I**ntention tremor, **I**ncontinence, **I**nternuclear ophthalmoplegia **N**ystagmus Most often affects women in their 20s and 30s; more common in whites. Treatment: β-interferon or immunosuppressant therapy.
Guillain-Barré syndrome (acute idiopathic polyneuritis)	Inflammation and demyelination of peripheral nerves and motor fibers of ventral roots (sensory effect less severe than motor), causing symmetric ascending muscle weakness beginning in distal lower extremities. Facial paralysis in 50% of cases. Autonomic function may be severely affected (e.g., cardiac irregularities, hypertension, or hypotension). Almost all patients survive; the majority recover completely after weeks to months. Findings: elevated CSF protein with normal cell count ("albuminocytologic dissociation"). Elevated protein → papilledema.	Associated with infections → autoimmune attack of peripheral myelin due to molecular mimicry (e.g., *Campylobacter jejuni* or herpesvirus infection), inoculations, and stress, but no definitive link to pathogens. Respiratory support is critical until recovery. Additional treatment: plasmapheresis, IV immune globulins.

Seizures	Partial seizures—1 area of the brain. 1. Simple partial (consciousness intact)—motor, sensory, autonomic, psychic 2. Complex partial (impaired consciousness) Generalized seizures—diffuse. 1. Absence (petit mal)—blank stare 2. Myoclonic—quick, repetitive jerks 3. Tonic-clonic (grand mal)—alternating stiffening and movement 4. Tonic—stiffening 5. Atonic—"drop" seizures—falls to floor; commonly mistaken for fainting	Epilepsy is a disorder of recurrent seizures (febrile seizures are not epilepsy). Partial seizures can secondarily generalize. Causes of seizures by age: Children—genetic, infection, trauma, congenital, metabolic. Adults—tumors, trauma, stroke, infection. Elderly—stroke, tumor, trauma, metabolic, infection.
Intracranial hemorrhage		
Epidural hematoma	Rupture of middle meningeal artery (branch of maxillary artery), often 2° to fracture of temporal bone. Lucid interval (see Color Image 44).	CT shows "biconvex disk" not crossing suture lines.
Subdural hematoma	Rupture of bridging veins. Venous bleeding (less pressure) with delayed onset of symptoms. Seen in elderly individuals, alcoholics, blunt trauma, shaken baby (predisposing factors—brain atrophy, shaking, whiplash) (see Color Image 43).	Crescent-shaped hemorrhage that crosses suture lines.
Subarachnoid hemorrhage	Rupture of an aneurysm (usually berry aneurysm) or an AVM. Patients complain of "worst headache of my life." Bloody or yellow (xanthochromic) spinal tap.	
Parenchymal hematoma	Caused by hypertension, amyloid angiopathy, diabetes mellitus, and tumor.	
Berry aneurysms	Berry aneurysms occur at the bifurcations in the circle of Willis. Most common site is bifurcation of the anterior communicating artery. Rupture (most common complication) leads to hemorrhagic stroke/subarachnoid hemorrhage. Associated with adult polycystic kidney disease, Ehlers-Danlos syndrome, and Marfan's syndrome. Other risk factors: advanced age, hypertension, smoking, race (higher risk in blacks) (see Color Image 46). Charcot-Bouchard microaneurysms—associated with chronic hypertension; affects small vessels.	

Hydrocephalus	Normal pressure (communicating) hydrocephalus—enlarged ventricles with normal opening pressure on lumbar puncture. Classic triad of dementia, gait problems, urinary incontinence. Caused by impaired absorption of CSF by arachnoid granulations. Obstructive (noncommunicating) hydrocephalus—caused by structural blockage of CSF circulation within the ventricular system (e.g., stenosis of the aqueduct of Sylvius).
Neurocutaneous disorders	Sturge-Weber syndrome—congenital disorder with port-wine stains and ipsilateral leptomeningeal angioma. Can cause glaucoma, seizures, hemiparesis, and mental retardation. Tuberous sclerosis—hamartomas in CNS, skin, organs; cardiac rhabdomyoma, renal angiomyolipoma, subependymal giant cell astrocytoma, MR, seizures, ash leaf spots, sebaceous adenoma, shagreen patch. Neurofibromatosis—café-au-lait spots, Lisch nodules (iris), neurofibromas in skin. von Hippel–Lindau disease—autosomal-dominant disorder with cavernous hemangiomas in skin, mucosa, organs; renal cell carcinoma, hemangioblastoma in retina, brain stem, cerebellum.

Primary brain tumors — Clinical presentation due to mass effects (e.g., seizures, dementia, focal lesions); 1° brain tumors rarely undergo metastasis. The majority of adult 1° tumors are supratentorial, while the majority of childhood 1° tumors are infratentorial. Note: half of adult brain tumors are metastases; usually present at the gray-white junction.

Tumor	Description	Features
Adult peak incidence		
Glioblastoma multiforme (grade IV astrocytoma)	Most common 1° brain tumor. Prognosis grave; < 1-year life expectancy. Found in cerebral hemispheres. Can cross corpus callosum ("butterfly glioma") (see Color Image 48). Stain astrocytes for GFAP.	"Pseudopalisading" pleomorphic tumor cells—border central areas of necrosis and hemorrhage.
Meningioma	2nd most common 1° brain tumor. Most often occurs in convexities of hemispheres and parasagittal region. Arises from arachnoid cells external to brain. Resectable.	Spindle cells concentrically arranged in a whorled pattern; **psammoma bodies** (laminated calcifications).
Schwannoma	3rd most common 1° brain tumor. Schwann cell origin; often localized to CN VIII → acoustic schwannoma. Resectable.	Bilateral schwannoma found in neurofibromatosis type 2.
Oligodendroglioma	Relatively rare, slow growing. Most often in frontal lobes. Chicken-wire capillary pattern (see Color Image 49).	Oligodendrocytes = "fried egg" cells—round nuclei with clear cytoplasm. Often calcified in oligodendroglioma.
Pituitary adenoma	Prolactin secreting is most common form. Bitemporal hemianopia (due to pressure on optic chiasm) and hyper- or hypopituitarism are sequelae.	Rathke's pouch.
Childhood peak incidence		
Pilocytic (low-grade) astrocytoma	Usually well circumscribed. In children, most often found in posterior fossa. Benign; good prognosis.	Rosenthal fibers—eosinophilic, corkscrew fibers.
Medulloblastoma	Highly malignant cerebellar tumor. A form of primitive neuroectodermal tumor (PNET). Can compress 4th ventricle, causing hydrocephalus.	Rosettes or perivascular pseudorosette pattern of cells. Radiosensitive.
Ependymoma	Ependymal cell tumors most commonly found in 4th ventricle. Can cause hydrocephalus. Poor prognosis.	Characteristic perivascular pseudorosettes. Rod-shaped blepharoplasts (basal ciliary bodies) found near nucleus.
Hemangioblastoma	Most often cerebellar; associated with von Hippel–Lindau syndrome when found with retinal angiomas. Can produce EPO → 2° polycythemia.	Foamy cells and high vascularity are characteristic.
Craniopharyngioma	Benign childhood tumor, confused with pituitary adenoma (can also cause bitemporal hemianopia). Most common childhood supratentorial tumor.	Derived from remnants of Rathke's pouch. Calcification is common (tooth enamel–like).

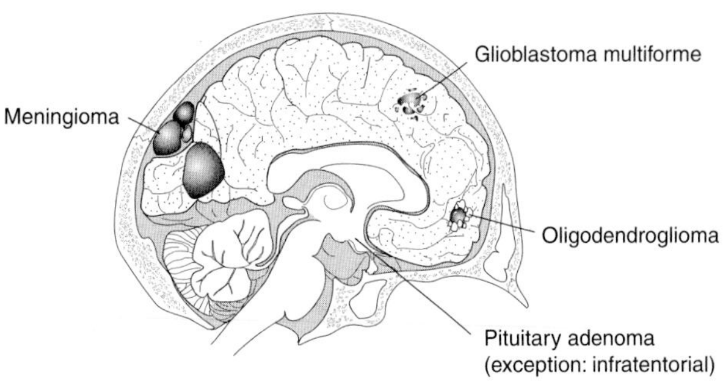

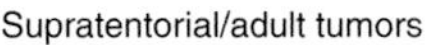
Supratentorial/adult tumors

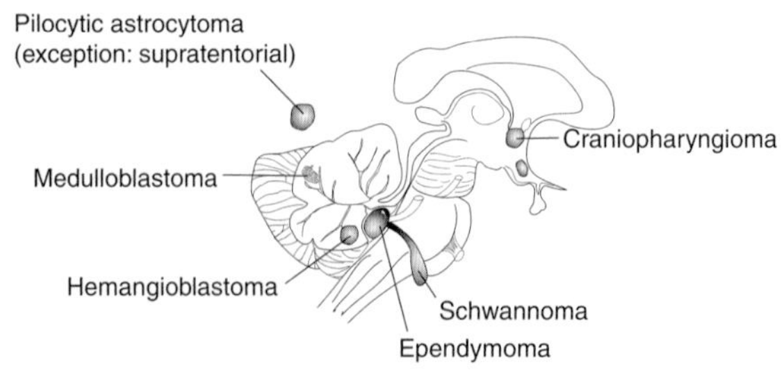

Infratentorial/childhood tumors

Posterior fossa malformations	Arnold-Chiari—small posterior fossa, downward displacement of cerebellum, medulla deformity; associated with tonsillar herniation. Chiari I—low-lying cerebellum obstructs CSF flow and compresses medulla; cerebellar tonsils descend through foramen magnum. Frequently asymptomatic; correctable with surgery. Chiari II—cerebellar vermis and medulla descend through foramen magnum; fatal Dandy-Walker—large posterior fossa; absent cerebellum with cyst in its place.
Cranial nerve and cerebellar lesions	CN XII lesion (LMN)—tongue deviates **toward** side of lesion (lick your wounds). CN V motor lesion—jaw deviates **toward** side of lesion. Unilateral lesion of cerebellum—patient tends to fall **toward** side of lesion. CN X lesion—uvula deviates **away** from side of lesion. CN XI lesion—weakness turning head to contralateral side of lesion. Shoulder droop on side of lesion.

Facial lesions

UMN lesion	Lesion of motor cortex or connection between cortex and facial nucleus. Contralateral paralysis of lower face only.	**AL**exander **Bell** with **STD**: **A**IDS, **L**yme, **S**arcoid, **T**umors, **D**iabetes.
LMN lesion	Ipsilateral paralysis of upper and lower face.	
Bell's palsy	Complete destruction of the facial nucleus itself or its branchial efferent fibers (facial nerve proper). Peripheral ipsilateral facial paralysis with inability to close eye on involved side. Only lower face is affected, since upper face has contralateral and ipsilateral innervation by CN VII. Can occur idiopathically; gradual recovery in most cases. Seen as a complication in **A**IDS, **L**yme disease, **S**arcoidosis, **T**umors, **D**iabetes.	

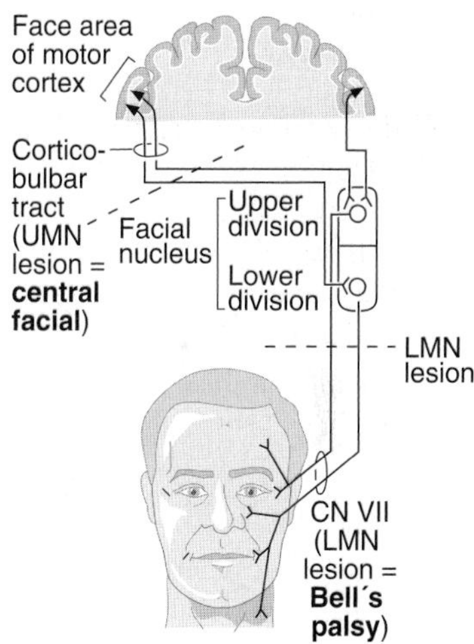

Herniation syndromes

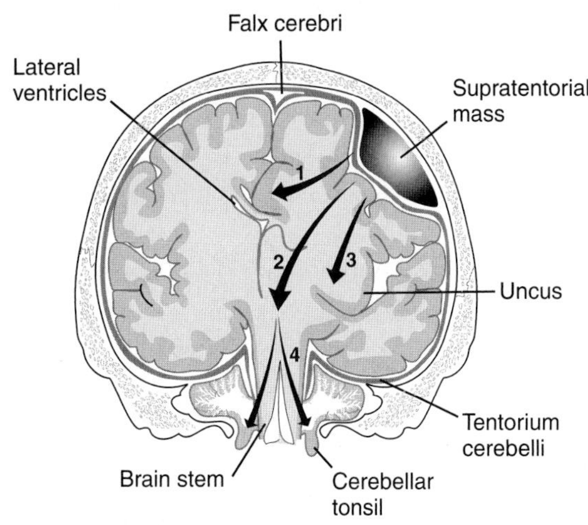

(Adapted, with permission, from Simon RP et al. *Clinical Neurology*, 4th ed. Stamford, CT: Appleton & Lange, 1999: 314.)

1. Cingulate (subfalcine) herniation under falx cerebri	Can compress anterior cerebral artery.
2. Downward transtentorial (central) herniation	Coma and death result when these herniations compress the brain stem.
3. Uncal herniation	Uncus = medial temporal lobe.
4. Cerebellar tonsillar herniation into the foramen magnum	

Uncal herniation

Clinical signs	Cause
Ipsilateral dilated pupil/ptosis	Stretching of CN III
Contralateral homonymous hemianopia	Compression of ipsilateral posterior cerebral artery
Ipsilateral paresis	Compression of contralateral crus cerebri (Kernohan's notch); this is a "false localizing" sign
Duret hemorrhages—paramedian artery rupture	Caudal displacement of brain stem

▶ NEUROLOGY–PHARMACOLOGY

Opioid analgesics	Morphine, fentanyl, codeine, heroin, methadone, meperidine, dextromethorphan.
Mechanism	Act as agonists at opioid receptors (mu = morphine, delta = enkephalin, kappa = dynorphin) to modulate synaptic transmission.
Clinical use	Pain, cough suppression (dextromethorphan), diarrhea (loperamide and diphenoxylate), acute pulmonary edema, maintenance programs for addicts (methadone).
Toxicity	Addiction, **respiratory depression,** constipation, miosis (**pinpoint pupils**), additive **CNS depression** with other drugs. Tolerance does not develop to miosis and constipation. Toxicity treated with naloxone or naltrexone (opioid receptor antagonist).

Epilepsy drugs

	PARTIAL		GENERALIZED				
	Simple	Complex	Tonic-Clonic	Absence	Status	Mechanism	Notes
Phenytoin	✓	✓	1st line		1st line for prophylaxis	↑ Na^+ channel inactivation	
Carbamazepine	✓	✓	1st line			↑ Na^+ channel inactivation	1st line for trigeminal neuralgia
Lamotrigine	✓	✓	✓			Blocks voltage-gated Na^+ channels	
Gabapentin	✓	✓	✓			↑ GABA release	Also used for peripheral neuropathy
Topiramate	✓	✓	✓			Blocks Na^+ channels, ↑ GABA action	
Phenobarbital	✓	✓	✓			↑ $GABA_A$ action	1st line in pregnant women, children
Valproic acid	✓	✓	1st line	✓		↑ Na^+ channel inactivation, ↑ GABA concentration	Also used for myoclonic seizures
Ethosuximide				1st line		Blocks thalamic T-type Ca^{2+} channels	
Benzodiazepines (diazepam or lorazepam)					1st line for acute	↑ $GABA_A$ action	Also used for seizures of eclampsia (1st line to prevent seizures of eclampsia is $MgSO_4$)

Epilepsy drug toxicities

- Benzodiazepines — Sedation, tolerance, dependence.
- Carbamazepine — Diplopia, ataxia, blood dyscrasias (agranulocytosis, aplastic anemia), liver toxicity, teratogenesis, induction of cytochrome P-450.
- Ethosuximide — GI distress, fatigue, headache, urticaria, Stevens-Johnson syndrome.
- Phenobarbital — Sedation, tolerance, dependence, induction of cytochrome P-450.
- Phenytoin — Nystagmus, diplopia, ataxia, sedation, gingival hyperplasia, hirsutism, megaloblastic anemia, teratogenesis, SLE-like syndrome, induction of cytochrome P-450.
- Valproic acid — GI distress, rare but fatal hepatotoxicity (measure LFTs), neural tube defects in fetus (spina bifida), tremor, weight gain. Contraindicated in pregnancy.
- Lamotrigine — Stevens-Johnson syndrome.
- Gabapentin — Sedation, ataxia.
- Topiramate — Sedation, mental dulling, kidney stones, weight loss.

EFGH—**E**thosuximide, **F**atigue, **GI**, **H**eadache.

Stevens-Johnson syndrome—prodrome of malaise and fever followed by rapid onset of erythematous/purpuric macules (oral, ocular, genital). Skin lesions progress to epidermal necrosis and sloughing.

Phenytoin		
Mechanism	Use-dependent blockade of Na^+ channels; inhibition of glutamate release from excitatory presynaptic neuron.	
Clinical use	Tonic-clonic seizures. Also a class IB antiarrhythmic.	
Toxicity	Nystagmus, ataxia, diplopia, sedation, SLE-like syndrome, induction of cytochrome P-450. Chronic use produces gingival hyperplasia in children, peripheral neuropathy, hirsutism, megaloblastic anemia (↓ folate absorption), and malignant hyperthermia (rare); teratogenic (fetal hydantoin syndrome).	
Barbiturates	Phenobarbital, pentobarbital, thiopental, secobarbital.	
Mechanism	Facilitate $GABA_A$ action by ↑ **duration** of Cl^- channel opening, thus ↓ neuron firing.	Barbi**DURAT**e (↑ **DURAT**ion). Contraindicated in porphyria.
Clinical use	Sedative for anxiety, seizures, insomnia, induction of anesthesia (thiopental).	
Toxicity	Dependence, additive CNS depression effects with alcohol, respiratory or cardiovascular depression (can lead to death), drug interactions owing to induction of liver microsomal enzymes (cytochrome P-450). Treat overdose with symptom management (assist respiration, ↑ BP).	
Benzodiazepines	Diazepam, lorazepam, triazolam, temazepam, oxazepam, midazolam, chlordiazepoxide, alprazolam.	
Mechanism	Facilitate $GABA_A$ action by ↑ **frequency** of Cl^- channel opening. Most have long half-lives and active metabolites.	**FRE**nzodiazepines (↑ **FRE**quency). Short acting = **TOM** Thumb = **T**riazolam, **O**xazepam, **M**idazolam.
Clinical use	Anxiety, spasticity, status epilepticus (lorazepam and diazepam), detoxification (especially alcohol withdrawal–DTs), night terrors, sleepwalking.	
Toxicity	Dependence, additive CNS depression effects with alcohol. Less risk of respiratory depression and coma than with barbiturates. Treat overdose with flumazenil (competitive antagonist at GABA receptor).	
Anesthetics—general principles	CNS drugs must be lipid soluble (cross the blood-brain barrier) or be actively transported. Drugs with ↓ solubility in blood = rapid induction and recovery times. Drugs with ↑ solubility in lipids = ↑ potency = $\frac{1}{MAC}$ where MAC = minimal alveolar concentration. Examples: N_2O has low blood and lipid solubility, and thus fast induction and low potency. Halothane, in contrast, has ↑ lipid and blood solubility, and thus high potency and slow induction.	

Inhaled anesthetics	Halothane, enflurane, isoflurane, sevoflurane, methoxyflurane, nitrous oxide.
Mechanism	Mechanism unknown.
Effects	Myocardial depression, respiratory depression, nausea/emesis, ↑ cerebral blood flow (↓ cerebral metabolic demand).
Toxicity	Hepatotoxicity (halothane), nephrotoxicity (methoxyflurane), proconvulsant (enflurane), malignant hyperthermia (rare).

Intravenous anesthetics		
Barbiturates	Thiopental—high potency, high lipid solubility, rapid entry into brain. Used for induction of anesthesia and short surgical procedures. Effect terminated by redistribution from brain. ↓ cerebral blood flow.	**B. B. K**ing on **OPIATES PROPO**ses **FOOL**ishly.
Benzodiazepines	Midazolam most common drug used for endoscopy; used adjunctively with gaseous anesthetics and narcotics. May cause severe postoperative respiratory depression, ↓ BP (treat overdose with flumazenil), and amnesia.	
Arylcyclohexylamines (**K**etamine)	PCP analogs that act as dissociative anesthetics. Cardiovascular stimulants. Cause disorientation, hallucination, and bad dreams. ↑ cerebral blood flow.	
Opiates	Morphine, fentanyl used with other CNS depressants during general anesthesia.	
Propofol	Used for rapid anesthesia induction and short procedures. Less postoperative nausea than thiopental.	

Local anesthetics	Esters—procaine, cocaine, tetracaine; amides—lIdocaIne, mepIvacaIne, bupIvacaIne (amIdes have 2 **I**'s in name).
Mechanism	Block Na^+ channels by binding to specific receptors on inner portion of channel. Preferentially bind to activated Na^+ channels, so most effective in rapidly firing neurons. 3° amine local anesthetics penetrate membrane in uncharged form, then bind to ion channels as charged form.
Principle	1. In infected (acidic) tissue, alkaline anesthetics are charged and cannot penetrate membrane effectively. Therefore, more anesthetic is needed in these cases. 2. Order of nerve blockade—small-diameter fibers > large diameter. Myelinated fibers > unmyelinated fibers. Overall, size factor predominates over myelination such that small myelinated fibers > small unmyelinated fibers > large myelinated fibers > large unmyelinated fibers. Order of loss—pain (lose first) > temperature > touch > pressure (lose last). 3. Except for cocaine, given with vasoconstrictors (usually epinephrine) to enhance local action—↓ bleeding, ↑ anesthesia by ↓ systemic concentration.
Clinical use	Minor surgical procedures, spinal anesthesia. If allergic to esters, give amides.
Toxicity	CNS excitation, severe cardiovascular toxicity (bupivacaine), hypertension, hypotension, and arrhythmias (cocaine).

Neuromuscular blocking drugs	Used for muscle paralysis in surgery or mechanical ventilation. Selective for motor (vs. autonomic) nicotinic receptor.
Depolarizing	Succinylcholine (complications include hypercalemia and hyperkalemia). Reversal of blockade: Phase I (prolonged depolarization)—no antidote. Block potentiated by cholinesterase inhibitors. Phase II (repolarized but blocked)—antidote consists of cholinesterase inhibitors (e.g., neostigmine).
Nondepolarizing	Tubocurarine, atracurium, mivacurium, pancuronium, vecuronium, rocuronium. Competitive—compete with ACh for receptors. Reversal of blockade—neostigmine, edrophonium, and other cholinesterase inhibitors.

Dantrolene	Used in the treatment of **malignant hyperthermia**, which is caused by the concomitant use of inhalation anesthetics (except N_2O) and succinylcholine. Also used to treat **neuroleptic malignant syndrome** (a toxicity of antipsychotic drugs). Mechanism: prevents the release of Ca^{2+} from the sarcoplasmic reticulum of skeletal muscle.

Parkinson's disease drugs

Parkinsonism is due to loss of dopaminergic neurons and excess cholinergic activity.

Strategy	Agents	
Agonize dopamine receptors	**Br**omocriptine (ergot alkaloid and partial dopamine agonist), pramipexole, ropinirole	**BALSA:** **B**romocriptine **A**mantadine **L**evodopa (with carbidopa) **S**elegiline (and COMT inhibitors) **A**ntimuscarinics
↑ dopamine	**A**mantadine (may ↑ dopamine release); also used as an antiviral against influenza A and rubella; toxicity = ataxia L-dopa/carbidopa (converted to dopamine in CNS)	
Prevent dopamine breakdown	**S**elegiline (selective MAO type B inhibitor); entacapone, tolcapone (COMT inhibitors)	
Curb excess cholinergic activity	**Benz**tropine (**A**ntimuscarinic; improves tremor and rigidity but has little effect on bradykinesia)	↓ your tremor before you drive your Mercedes-**BENZ.**

For essential or familial tremors, use a β-blocker.

L-dopa (levodopa)/carbidopa

Mechanism	↑ level of dopamine in brain. Unlike dopamine, L-dopa can cross blood-brain barrier and is converted by dopa decarboxylase in the CNS to dopamine.
Clinical use	Parkinsonism.
Toxicity	Arrhythmias from peripheral conversion to dopamine. Long-term use can → dyskinesia following administration, akinesia between doses. Carbidopa, a peripheral decarboxylase inhibitor, is given with L-dopa in order to ↑ the bioavailability of L-dopa in the brain and to limit peripheral side effects.

Selegiline	
Mechanism	Selectively inhibits MAO-B, thereby ↑ the availability of dopamine.
Clinical use	Adjunctive agent to L-dopa in treatment of Parkinson's disease.
Toxicity	May enhance adverse effects of L-dopa.

Sumatriptan	
Mechanism	5-HT_{1D} agonist. Causes vasoconstriction. Half-life < 2 hours.
Clinical use	Acute migraine, cluster headache attacks.
Toxicity	Coronary vasospasm, mild tingling (contraindicated in patients with CAD or Prinzmetal's angina), hypertensive emergencies.

NOTES

HIGH-YIELD PRINCIPLES IN

Psychiatry

"What a terrible thing to have lost one's mind. Or not to have a mind at all. How true that is."

—Dan Quayle

Vignette	Question	Answer
■ Person demands only the best and most famous doctor in town.	What is the personality disorder?	Narcissistic personality disorder.
■ Nurse has episodes of hypoglycemia; blood analysis reveals no elevation in C-peptide.	What is the diagnosis?	Factitious disorder; surreptitious insulin.
■ 55-year-old businessman complains of lack of successful sexual contacts with women and lack of ability to reach a full erection. Two years ago he had a heart attack.	What might be the cause of his problem?	Fear of sudden death during intercourse.
■ 15-year-old girl of normal height and weight for her age has enlarged parotid glands but no other complaints. The mother confides that she found laxatives in the daughter's closet.	What is the diagnosis?	Bulimia.
■ Man on several medications, including antidepressants and antihypertensives, has mydriasis and becomes constipated.	What is the cause of his symptoms?	TCAs (anticholinergic effects).
■ Woman on MAO inhibitor has hypertensive crisis after a meal.	What did she ingest?	Tyramine (wine or cheese).
■ 3-year-old child presents with retinal detachment.	What is the most likely diagnosis, and what must you do?	Child abuse. Report it!
■ Homeless man admitted for pneumonia complains of bugs crawling on his skin (formication).	What is the most likely diagnosis?	Delirium tremens 2° to alcohol withdrawal.
■ Vietnam veteran becomes paralyzed upon hearing airplane engines.	What is the most likely diagnosis?	PTSD.
■ Unconscious teenager is rushed to the ER. He has pinpoint pupils and is seizing.	What is the most likely diagnosis?	Opioid overdose.

Infant deprivation effects	Long-term deprivation of affection results in: 1. ↓ muscle tone 2. Poor language skills 3. Poor socialization skills 4. Lack of basic trust 5. Anaclitic depression 6. Weight loss 7. Physical illness Severe deprivation can result in infant death.	The **4 W's: Weak, Wordless, Wanting** (socially), **Wary.** Deprived babies say **Wah, Wah, Wah, Wah.** Deprivation for > 6 months can lead to irreversible changes.
Anaclitic depression	Depression in an infant attributable to continued separation from caregiver—can result in failure to thrive. Infant becomes withdrawn and unresponsive.	
Regression in children	Children regress to younger behavior under conditions of stress such as physical illness, punishment, birth of a new sibling, or fatigue (e.g., bedwetting in a previously toilet-trained child when hospitalized).	
Childhood and early-onset disorders	**Attention-deficit hyperactivity disorder (ADHD)**—limited attention span and hyperactivity. Children are emotionally labile, impulsive, and prone to accidents. Normal intelligence. Treatment: methylphenidate (Ritalin). **Conduct disorder**—continued behavior violating social norms. After 18 years of age, diagnosed as antisocial personality disorder. **Oppositional defiant disorder**—child is noncompliant in the absence of criminality. **Tourette's syndrome**—motor/vocal tics and involuntary profanity. Associated with OCD. Onset at < 18 years of age. Treatment: haloperidol. **Separation anxiety disorder**—fear of loss of attachment figure leading to factitious physical complaints to avoid going to school. Common onset at 7–8 years of age.	
Pervasive developmental disorders	**Autistic disorder**—patients have severe communication problems and difficulty forming relationships. Characterized by repetitive behavior, unusual abilities (savants), and usually below-normal intelligence. Treatment: ↑ communication and social skills. **Asperger's disorder**—a milder form of autism involving problems with social relationships and repetitive behavior. Children are of normal intelligence and lack verbal or cognitive deficits. **Rett's disorder**—X-linked disorder seen only in girls (affected males die in utero). Characterized by loss of development and mental retardation appearing at approximately age 4. Stereotyped hand-wringing. **Childhood disintegrative disorder**—marked regression in multiple areas of functioning after at least 2 years of apparently normal development. Significant loss of expressive or receptive language, social skills or adaptive behavior, bowel or bladder control, play, or motor skills. Onset at 2–10 years of age.	

Child abuse

	Physical abuse	Sexual abuse
Evidence	Healed fractures on x-ray, cigarette burns, subdural hematomas, multiple bruises, retinal hemorrhage or detachment	Genital/anal trauma, STDs, UTIs
Abuser	Usually female and the 1° caregiver	Known to victim, usually male
Epidemiology	~3000 deaths/year in the United States	Peak incidence 9–12 years of age

Neurotransmitter changes with disease

Anxiety—↑ NE, ↓ GABA, ↓ serotonin (5-HT).
Depression—↓ NE and ↓ serotonin (5-HT).
Alzheimer's dementia—↓ ACh.
Huntington's disease—↓ GABA, ↓ ACh.
Schizophrenia—↑ dopamine.
Parkinson's disease—↓ dopamine, ↑ ACh.

Orientation

Patient's ability to know who he or she is, what date and time it is, and what his or her present circumstances are.

Deficits in orientation:

1. Anosognosia—lack of awareness that one is ill
2. Autotopagnosia—inability to locate one's own body parts
3. Depersonalization—body seems unreal or dissociated

Order of loss: 1st—time; 2nd—place; last—person.

Amnesia types

*Antero*grade amnesia—inability to remember things that occurred after a CNS insult (no new memory).

Korsakoff's amnesia—classic anterograde amnesia that is caused by thiamine deficiency. Leads to bilateral destruction of the mammillary bodies. Seen in alcoholics, and associated with confabulations.

*Retro*grade amnesia—inability to remember things that occurred before a CNS insult.

Delirium

Waxing and waning level of consciousness; rapid ↓ in attention span and level of arousal—disorganized thinking, hallucinations, illusions, misperceptions, disturbance in sleep-wake cycle, cognitive dysfunction.

The most common psychiatric illness on medical and surgical floors. Often reversible. Abnormal EEG.

Deli**RIUM** = changes in senso**RIUM.**

Check for drugs with anticholinergic effects.

Dementia

Gradual ↓ in cognition—memory deficits, aphasia, apraxia, agnosia, loss of abstract thought, behavioral/personality changes, impaired judgment. Patient is alert; no change in level of consciousness.

↑ incidence with age. More often gradual onset.

De**MEM**tia is characterized by **MEM**ory loss. Commonly irreversible.

In elderly patients, depression may present like dementia (pseudodementia). Normal EEG.

Hallucination vs. illusion vs. delusion vs. loose association	Hallucinations are perceptions in the absence of external stimuli. Illusions are misinterpretations of actual external stimuli. Delusions are false beliefs not shared with other members of culture/subculture that are firmly maintained in spite of obvious proof to the contrary. Loose associations are disorders in the form of thought (the way ideas are tied together).
Dissociative fugue	Abrupt change in geographic location with inability to recall past, confusion about personal identity, or assumption of a new identity. Leads to distress or impairment. Not the result of substance abuse or general medical condition.
Hallucination types	Visual and auditory hallucinations are common in schizophrenia. Olfactory hallucination often occurs as an aura of a psychomotor epilepsy. Gustatory hallucination is rare. Tactile hallucination (e.g., formication—the sensation of ants crawling on one's skin) is common in DTs. Also seen in cocaine abusers ("cocaine bugs"). Hypna**GO**gic hallucination occurs while **GO**ing to sleep. Hypnopompic hallucination occurs while waking from sleep.
Schizophrenia	Periods of psychosis and disturbed behavior with a decline in functioning lasting > 6 months (1–6 months—schizophreniform disorder; < 1 month—brief psychotic disorder, usually stress related). Diagnosis requires 2 or more of the following (1–4 are "positive symptoms"): 1. Delusions 2. Hallucinations—often auditory 3. Disorganized thought (loose associations) 4. Disorganized or catatonic behavior 5. "Negative symptoms"—flat affect, social withdrawal, lack of motivation, lack of speech or thought Genetic factors outweigh environmental factors in the etiology of schizophrenia. Lifetime prevalence—1.5% (males = females, blacks = whites). Presents earlier in men. 5 subtypes: 1. Disorganized (with regard to speech, behavior, and affect) 2. Catatonic (automatisms) 3. Paranoid (delusions) 4. Undifferentiated (elements of all types) 5. Residual Schizoaffective disorder—schizophrenia plus a major depressive, manic, or mixed (both) episode. 2 subtypes: bipolar or depressive.

Manic episode

Distinct period of abnormally and persistently elevated, expansive, or irritable mood lasting at least 1 week.

During mood disturbance, 3 or more of the following are present:

1. **D**istractibility
2. **I**rresponsibility—seeks pleasure without regard to consequences (hedonistic)
3. **G**randiosity—inflated self-esteem
4. **F**light of ideas—racing thoughts
5. ↑ in goal-directed **A**ctivity/psychomotor **A**gitation
6. ↓ need for **S**leep
7. **T**alkativeness or pressured speech

Maniacs **DIG FAST.**

Hypomanic episode

Like manic episode except mood disturbance is not severe enough to cause marked impairment in social and/or occupational functioning or to necessitate hospitalization; there are no psychotic features.

Bipolar disorder

6 separate criteria sets exist for bipolar disorders with combinations of manic (bipolar I), hypomanic (bipolar II), and depressed episodes. 1 manic or hypomanic episode defines bipolar disorder. Lithium is drug of choice.

Cyclothymic disorder is a milder form lasting at least 2 years.

Major depressive episode

Characterized by at least 5 of the following for 2 weeks, including either depressed mood or anhedonia:

1. **S**leep disturbance
2. Loss of **I**nterest (anhedonia)
3. **G**uilt or feelings of worthlessness
4. Loss of **E**nergy
5. Loss of **C**oncentration
6. Change in **A**ppetite/weight
7. **P**sychomotor retardation or agitation
8. **S**uicidal ideations
9. Depressed mood

SIG E CAPS.

SIG is short for *signatura* (Latin for "directions"). Depressed patients are **directed** to take Energy **CAPS**ules.

Lifetime prevalence of major depressive episode—5–12% male, 10–25% female.

Major depressive disorder, recurrent—requires 2 or more episodes with a symptom-free interval of 2 months.

Dysthymia is a milder form of depression lasting at least 2 years.

Sleep patterns of depressed patients

Patients with depression typically have the following changes in their sleep stages:

1. ↓ slow-wave sleep
2. ↓ REM latency
3. ↑ REM early in sleep cycle
4. ↑ total REM sleep
5. Repeated nighttime awakenings
6. Early-morning awakening (important screening question)

Risk factors for suicide completion	**S**ex (male), **A**ge (teenager or elderly), **D**epression, **P**revious attempt, **E**thanol or drug use, loss of **R**ational thinking, **S**ickness (medical illness, 3 or more prescription medications), **O**rganized plan, **N**o spouse (divorced, widowed, or single, especially if childless), **S**ocial support lacking. Women try more often; men succeed more often.	SAD PERSONS.
Electroconvulsive therapy	Treatment option for major depressive disorder refractory to other treatment. Produces a painless seizure. Major adverse effects of ECT are disorientation, anterograde and retrograde amnesia.	
Panic disorder	Recurrent periods of intense fear and discomfort peaking in 10 minutes with 4 of the following: **P**alpitations, **P**aresthesias, **A**bdominal distress, **N**ausea, **I**ntense fear of dying or losing control, l**I**ght-headedness, **C**hest pain, **C**hills, **C**hoking, dis**C**onnectedness, **S**weating, **S**haking, **S**hortness of breath. Panic is described in context of occurrence (e.g., panic disorder with agoraphobia). High incidence during Step 1 exam.	PANICS.
Specific phobia	Fear that is excessive or unreasonable and interferes with normal routine. **Cued** by presence or anticipation of a specific object or situation. Person recognizes fear is excessive (insight), yet exposure provokes an anxiety response. Can treat with systematic desensitization. Examples include: 1. Gamophobia (*gam* = gamete)—fear of marriage 2. Algophobia (*alg* = pain)—fear of pain 3. Acrophobia (*acro* = height)—fear of heights 4. Agoraphobia (*agora* = open market)—fear of being in public place or situation from which escape may be difficult	
Post-traumatic stress disorder	Persistent reexperiencing of a previous traumatic event in the life of the patient as nightmares or flashbacks. Response involves intense fear, helplessness, or horror. Leads to avoidance of stimuli associated with the trauma and persistently ↑ arousal. **Disturbance lasts > 1 month** and causes distress or social/occupational impairment. PTSD often follows acute stress disorder, which lasts up to 2–4 weeks.	
Other anxiety disorders	**Adjustment disorder**—emotional symptoms (anxiety, depression) causing impairment following an identifiable psychosocial stressor (e.g., divorce, moving) and lasting < 6 months. **Generalized anxiety disorder**—uncontrollable anxiety for at least 6 months that is unrelated to a specific person, situation, or event. Sleep disturbance, fatigue, and difficulty concentrating are common.	
Malingering	Patient consciously fakes or claims to have a disorder in order to attain a specific 2° gain (e.g., avoiding work, obtaining drugs). Complaints cease after gain (vs. factitious disorder).	

Factitious disorder	Consciously creates symptoms in order to assume "sick role" and to get medical attention (1° gain). **Munchausen's syndrome** is manifested by a chronic history of multiple hospital admissions and willingness to receive invasive procedures. **Munchausen's syndrome by proxy** is seen when illness in a child is caused by the parent. Motivation is to assume a sick role by proxy. A form of child abuse and must be reported.	
Somatoform disorders	Both illness production and motivation are unconscious drives. More common in women. Several types: 1. **Conversion**—motor or sensory symptoms (e.g., paralysis, pseudoseizure) that suggest neurologic or physical disorder, but tests and physical exam are negative; often follows an acute stressor; patient may be unconcerned about symptoms 2. **Pain disorder**—prolonged pain that is not explained completely by illness 3. **Hypochondriasis**—preoccupation with and fear of having a serious illness in spite of medical reassurance 4. **Somatization disorder**—variety of complaints in multiple organ systems with no identifiable underlying physical findings 5. **Body dysmorphic disorder**—preoccupation with minor or imagined physical flaws; patients often seek cosmetic surgery 6. **Pseudocyesis**—false belief of being pregnant associated with objective physical signs of pregnancy	
Gain: 1°, 2°, 3°	1° gain—what the symptom does for the patient's internal psychic economy. 2° gain—what the symptom gets the patient (sympathy, attention). 3° gain—what the caretaker gets (like an MD on an interesting case).	
Personality	Personality trait—an enduring pattern of perceiving, relating to, and thinking about the environment and oneself that is exhibited in a wide range of important social and personal contexts. Personality disorder—when these patterns become inflexible and maladaptive, causing impairment in social or occupational functioning or subjective distress; person is usually not aware of problem. Disordered patterns must be stable by early adulthood; not usually diagnosed in children.	
Cluster A personality disorders	Odd or eccentric; cannot develop meaningful social relationships. No psychosis; genetic association with schizophrenia. Types: 1. Paranoid—distrust and suspiciousness; projection is main defense mechanism 2. Schizoid—voluntary social withdrawal, limited emotional expression, content with social isolation, unlike avoidant 3. Schizotypal—interpersonal awkwardness, odd beliefs or magical thinking, eccentric appearance	**"Weird."**

Cluster B personality disorders	Dramatic, emotional, or erratic; genetic association with mood disorders and substance abuse. Types: 1. Antisocial—disregard for and violation of rights of others, criminality; males > females; conduct disorder if < 18 years 2. Borderline—unstable mood and interpersonal relationships, impulsiveness, sense of emptiness; females > males; splitting is a major defense mechanism 3. Histrionic—excessive emotionality, attention seeking, sexually provocative, overly concerned with appearance 4. Narcissistic—grandiosity, sense of entitlement; may react to criticism with rage; may demand "top" physician/best health care	**"Wild"** (**B**ad to the **B**one). Anti**SOC**ial = **SOC**iopath.
Cluster C personality disorders	Anxious or fearful; genetic association with anxiety disorders. Types: 1. Avoidant—sensitive to rejection, socially inhibited, timid, feelings of inadequacy 2. Obsessive-compulsive—preoccupation with order, perfectionism, and control 3. Dependent—submissive and clinging, excessive need to be taken care of, low self-confidence	**"Worried"** (**C**hattering teeth).
Schizo-	Keeping "schizo-" straight: **Schizoid** < **Schizotypal** (schizoid + odd thinking) < **Schizophrenic** (greater odd thinking than schizotypal) < **Schizoaffective** (schizophrenia + mood disorder) Schizophrenia time course: < 1 mo—brief psychotic disorder, usually stress related. 1–6 mo—schizophreniform disorder. > 6 mo—schizophrenia.	

HIGH-YIELD PRINCIPLES

PSYCHIATRY

Eating disorders	**Anorexia nervosa**—abnormal eating habits (excessive dieting), body image distortion, and ↑ exercise. Severe weight loss, metatarsal stress fractures, amenorrhea, anemia, and electrolyte disturbances can follow. Seen primarily in adolescent girls. Commonly coexists with depression. **Bulimia nervosa**—binge eating followed by self-induced vomiting or use of laxatives. Body weight is normal. Parotitis, enamel erosion, electrolyte disturbances, alkalosis, dorsal hand calluses from inducing vomiting (Russell's sign).
Substance dependence	Maladaptive pattern of substance use defined as 3 or more of the following signs in 1 year: 1. Tolerance—need more to achieve same effect 2. Withdrawal 3. Substance taken in larger amounts or over longer time than desired 4. Persistent desire or attempts to cut down 5. Significant energy spent obtaining, using, or recovering from substance 6. Important social, occupational, or recreational activities reduced because of substance use 7. Continued use in spite of knowing the problems that it causes
Substance abuse	Maladaptive pattern leading to clinically significant impairment or distress. Symptoms have NEVER met criteria for substance dependence. 1. Recurrent use resulting in failure to fulfill major obligations at work, school, or home 2. Recurrent use in physically hazardous situations 3. Recurrent substance-related legal problems 4. Continued use in spite of persistent problems caused by use
Withdrawal	Behavioral, physiologic, and cognitive state caused by cessation or reduction of heavy and prolonged substance use. A substance-specific syndrome with signs and symptoms often opposite to those seen in intoxication and not attributable to another medical condition.

Signs and symptoms of substance abuse

Drug	Intoxication	Withdrawal
Alcohol	Disinhibition, emotional lability, slurred speech, ataxia, coma, blackouts. Serum γ-glutamyltransferase (GGT)—sensitive indicator of alcohol use.	Tremor, tachycardia, hypertension, malaise, nausea, seizures, delirium tremens (DTs), tremulousness, agitation, hallucinations
Opioids	CNS depression, nausea and vomiting, constipation, pupillary constriction (pinpoint pupils), seizures (overdose is life-threatening).	Anxiety, insomnia, anorexia, sweating, dilated pupils, piloerection ("cold turkey"), fever, rhinorrhea, nausea, stomach cramps, diarrhea ("flulike" symptoms), yawning
Amphetamines	Psychomotor agitation, impaired judgment, pupillary dilation, hypertension, tachycardia, euphoria, prolonged wakefulness and attention, cardiac arrhythmias, delusions, hallucinations, fever.	Post-use "crash," including depression, lethargy, headache, stomach cramps, hunger, hypersomnolence
Cocaine	Euphoria, psychomotor agitation, impaired judgment, tachycardia, pupillary dilation, hypertension, hallucinations (including tactile), paranoid ideations, angina, sudden cardiac death.	Post-use "crash," including severe depression and suicidality, hypersomnolence, fatigue, malaise, severe psychological craving
PCP	Belligerence, impulsiveness, fever, psychomotor agitation, vertical and horizontal nystagmus, tachycardia, ataxia, homicidality, psychosis, delirium.	Recurrence of intoxication symptoms due to reabsorption in GI tract; sudden onset of severe, random, homicidal violence
LSD	Marked anxiety or depression, delusions, visual hallucinations, flashbacks, pupillary dilation.	
Marijuana	Euphoria, anxiety, paranoid delusions, perception of slowed time, impaired judgment, social withdrawal, ↑ appetite, dry mouth, hallucinations.	Can be detected in urine up to 1 month after last use
Barbiturates	Low safety margin, respiratory depression.	Anxiety, seizures, delirium, life-threatening cardiovascular collapse
Benzodiazepines	Greater safety margin. Amnesia, ataxia, somnolence, minor respiratory depression. Additive effects with alcohol.	Rebound anxiety, seizures, tremor, insomnia
Caffeine	Restlessness, insomnia, ↑ diuresis, muscle twitching, cardiac arrhythmias.	Headache, lethargy, depression, weight gain
Nicotine	Restlessness, insomnia, anxiety, arrhythmias.	Irritability, headache, anxiety, weight gain, craving

Heroin addiction

Approximately 500,000 U.S. addicts. Look for track marks (needle sticks in veins).

Users at risk for hepatitis, abscesses, overdose, hemorrhoids, AIDS, and right-sided endocarditis.

Naloxone and naltrexone competitively inhibit opioids and are used in cases of overdose.

Methadone (long-acting oral opiate) is used for heroin detoxification or long-term maintenance.

Alcoholism

Physiologic tolerance and dependence with symptoms of withdrawal (tremor, tachycardia, hypertension, malaise, nausea, DTs) when intake is interrupted. Continued drinking despite medical and social contraindications and life disruptions.

Treatment: disulfiram to condition the patient to abstain from alcohol use. Supportive treatment of other systemic manifestations. Alcoholics Anonymous and other peer support groups are helpful in sustaining abstinence.

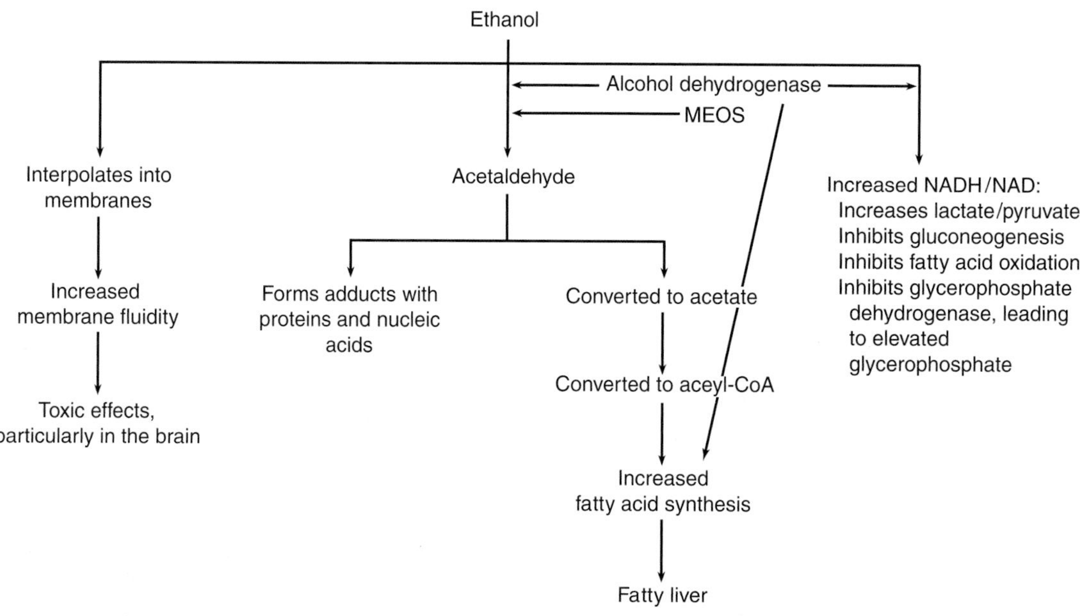

Delirium tremens

Life-threatening alcohol withdrawal syndrome that peaks 2–5 days after last drink.
In order of appearance—autonomic system hyperactivity (tachycardia, tremors, anxiety), psychotic symptoms (hallucinations, delusions), confusion.
Treat with benzodiazepines.

Complications of alcoholism

Alcoholic cirrhosis	Micronodular cirrhosis with jaundice, hypoalbuminemia, coagulation factor deficiencies, and portal hypertension, leading to peripheral edema and ascites, encephalopathy, neurologic manifestations (e.g., asterixis, flapping tremor of the hands), and esophageal varices.
Wernicke-Korsakoff syndrome	Caused by vitamin B_1 (thiamine) deficiency; common in malnourished alcoholics. Triad of confusion, ophthalmoplegia, and ataxia (Wernicke's encephalopathy). May progress to memory loss, confabulation, personality change (Korsakoff's psychosis; irreversible). Associated with periventricular hemorrhage/necrosis, especially in mammillary bodies. Treatment: IV vitamin B_1 (thiamine).
Mallory-Weiss syndrome	Longitudinal lacerations at the gastroesophageal junction caused by excessive vomiting. Often presents with hematemesis. Associated with pain in contrast to esophageal varices.
Other	Hepatitis, pancreatitis, peripheral neuropathy, testicular atrophy, hyperestrinism.

Intelligence quotient	Stanford-Binet and Wechsler are the most famous tests of intelligence quotient (IQ). Stanford-Binet calculates IQ as mental age/chronological age × 100. Wechsler Adult Intelligence Scale uses 11 subtests (6 verbal, 5 performance). Mean is defined at 100, with standard deviation of 15. IQ < 70 (or 2 standard deviations below the mean) is one of the criteria for diagnosis of mental retardation (MR). IQ < 40—severe MR. IQ < 20—profound MR. IQ scores are correlated with genetic factors and are highly correlated with school achievement. Intelligence tests are objective (not projective) tests.	
Classical conditioning	Learning in which a natural response (salivation) is elicited by a conditioned, or learned, stimulus (bell) that previously was presented in conjunction with an unconditioned stimulus (food).	Pavlov's classical experiments with dogs—ringing the bell provoked salivation.
Operant conditioning	Learning in which a particular action is elicited because it produces a reward. Positive reinforcement—desired reward produces action (mouse presses button to get food). Negative reinforcement—removal of aversive stimulus elicits behavior (mouse presses button to avoid shock). Do not confuse with punishment. Punishment—application of aversive stimulus to extinguish unwanted behavior.	
Reinforcement schedules	Pattern of reinforcement determines how quickly a behavior is learned or extinguished.	
Continuous	Reward received after every response. Rapidly extinguished.	Think vending machine—stop using it if it does not deliver.
Variable ratio	Reward received after random number of responses. Slowly extinguished.	Think slot machine—continue to play even if it rarely rewards.
Transference and countertransference		
Transference	Patient projects feelings about formative or other important persons onto physician (e.g., psychiatrist = parent).	
Countertransference	Doctor projects feelings about formative or other important persons onto patient.	
Structural theory of the mind	Freud's 3 structures of the mind.	
Id	Primal urges, sex, and aggression. The id "drives"; Instinct. (I want it.)	
Ego	Mediator between the unconscious mind and the external world. The ego "resists." (Deals with the conflict. Take it and you will get in trouble.)	
Superego	Moral values, conscience; can lead to self-blame and attacks on ego. (You know you can't have it. Taking it is wrong.)	
Topographic theory of the mind	Conscious—what you are aware of. Preconscious—what you are able to make conscious with effort (e.g., your phone number). Unconscious—what you are not aware of; the central goal of Freudian psychoanalysis is to make the patient aware of what is hidden in his/her unconscious.	
Oedipus complex	Repressed sexual feelings of a child for the opposite-sex parent, accompanied by rivalry with same-sex parent. First described by Freud.	

Social learning (modeling) Behavior acquired by watching others and assimilating actions into one's own repertoire.

Ego defenses All ego defenses are automatic and unconscious reactions to psychological stress.

Immature—more primitive

Acting out	Unacceptable feelings and thoughts are expressed through actions.	Tantrums.
Dissociation	Temporary, drastic change in personality, memory, consciousness, or motor behavior to avoid emotional stress.	Extreme forms can result in multiple personalities (dissociative identity disorder).
Denial	Avoidance of awareness of some painful reality.	A common reaction in newly diagnosed AIDS and cancer patients.
Displacement	Process whereby avoided ideas and feelings are transferred to some neutral person or object (vs. projection).	Mother yells at child because she is angry at her husband.
Fixation	Partially remaining at a more childish level of development (vs. regression).	Men fixating on sports games.
Identification	Modeling behavior after another person who is more powerful (though not necessarily admired).	Abused child becomes an abuser.
Isolation	Separation of feelings from ideas and events.	Describing murder in graphic detail with no emotional response.
Projection	An unacceptable internal impulse is attributed to an external source.	A man who wants another woman thinks his wife is cheating on him.
Rationalization	Proclaiming logical reasons for actions actually performed for other reasons, usually to avoid self-blame.	After getting fired, claiming that the job was not important anyway.
Reaction formation	Process whereby a warded-off idea or feeling is replaced by an (unconsciously derived) emphasis on its opposite.	A patient with libidinous thoughts enters a monastery.
Regression	Turning back the maturational clock and going back to earlier modes of dealing with the world.	Seen in children under stress (e.g., bedwetting) and in patients on dialysis (e.g., crying).
Repression	Involuntary withholding of an idea or feeling from conscious awareness.	The basic mechanism underlying all others.
Splitting	Belief that people are either all good or all bad.	A patient says that all the nurses are cold and insensitive but that the doctors are warm and friendly.

Mature—less primitive

Altruism	Guilty feelings alleviated by unsolicited generosity toward others.	Mafia boss makes large donation to charity.
Humor	Appreciating the amusing nature of an anxiety-provoking or adverse situation.	Nervous medical student jokes about the boards.
Sublimation	Process whereby one replaces an unacceptable wish with a course of action that is similar to the wish but does not conflict with one's value system.	Aggressive impulses used to succeed in business ventures.
Suppression	Voluntary (unlike repression) withholding of an idea or feeling from conscious awareness.	Choosing not to think about the USMLE until the week of the exam.

Mature women wear a **SASH**: **S**ublimation, **A**ltruism, **S**uppression, **H**umor.

Treatment for selected psychiatric conditions

Psychiatric condition	Drug
Alcohol withdrawal	Benzodiazepines
Anorexia/bulimia	SSRIs
Anxiety	Barbiturates Benzodiazepines Buspirone MAO inhibitors
ADHD	Methylphenidate (Ritalin) Amphetamine
Atypical depression	MAO inhibitors
Bipolar disorder	Mood stabilizers: Lithium Valproic acid Carbamazepine
Depression	SSRIs TCAs
Depression with insomnia	Trazodone Mirtazapine
Obsessive-compulsive disorder	SSRIs
Panic disorder	TCAs Buspirone
Schizophrenia	Antipsychotics
Tourette's syndrome	Antipsychotics (haloperidol)

Antipsychotics (neuroleptics) Thioridazine, haloperidol, fluphenazine, chlorpromazine (haloperidol + "-azine"s).

Mechanism	Most antipsychotics block dopamine D_2 receptors (excess dopamine effects connected with schizophrenia).	Low potency: thioridazine, chlorpromazine—non-neurologic side effects.
Clinical use	Schizophrenia, psychosis, acute mania, Tourette's syndrome.	High potency: haloperidol, trifluoperazine—neurologic side effects.
Toxicity	Extrapyramidal system (EPS) side effects, endocrine side effects (e.g., dopamine receptor antagonism → hyperprolactinemia → galactorrhea), and side effects arising from blocking muscarinic (dry mouth, constipation), α (hypotension), and histamine (sedation) receptors. **Neuroleptic malignant syndrome**—rigidity, myoglobinuria, autonomic instability, hyperpyrexia (treat with dantrolene and dopamine agonists). **Tardive dyskinesia**—stereotypic oral-facial movements probably due to dopamine receptor sensitization; results of long-term antipsychotic use.	Evolution of EPS side effects: 4 h acute dystonia 4 d akinesia 4 wk akathisia 4 mo tardive dyskinesia (often irreversible) Dystonia—muscle spasm, stiffness, oculogyric crisis. Akinesia—parkinsonian symptoms. Akathisia—restlessness.

Atypical antipsychotics	**Clo**zapine, **ol**anzapine, **risper**idone, quetiapine, aripiprazole, ziprasidone.	It's not **atypical** for **old clos**ets to **risper.**
Mechanism	Block 5-HT_2 and dopamine receptors.	
Clinical use	Treatment of schizophrenia; useful for positive and negative symptoms. **Olanzapine** is also used for OCD, anxiety disorder, depression, mania, Tourette's syndrome.	
Toxicity	Fewer extrapyramidal and anticholinergic side effects than other antipsychotics. **Clozapine** may cause agranulocytosis (requires weekly WBC monitoring).	

Lithium		
Mechanism	Not established; possibly related to inhibition of phosphoinositol cascade.	LMNOP: **L**ithium side effects— **M**ovement (tremor) **N**ephrogenic diabetes insipidus Hyp**O**thyroidism **P**regnancy problems
Clinical use	Mood stabilizer for bipolar affective disorder; blocks relapse and acute manic events.	
Toxicity	Tremor, hypothyroidism, polyuria (ADH antagonist causing nephrogenic diabetes insipidus), teratogenesis. Narrow therapeutic window requiring close monitoring of serum levels.	

Buspirone	
Mechanism	Stimulates 5-HT_{1A} receptors
Clinical use	Anxiolysis for generalized anxiety disorder. Does not cause sedation or addiction. Does not interact with alcohol.

Antidepressants

1. SSRIs
2. Heterocyclic antidepressants (includes tricyclics)
3. MAOIs

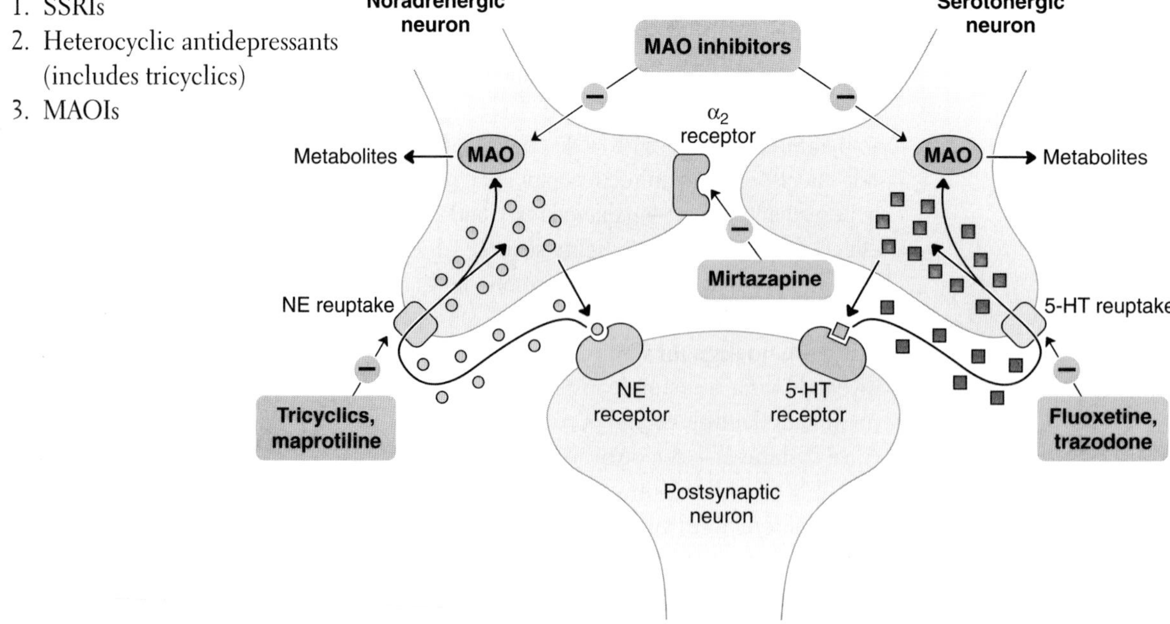

(Adapted, with permission, from Katzung BG, Trevor AJ. *USMLE Road Map: Pharmacology*, 1st ed. New York: McGraw-Hill, 2003: 80.)

SSRIs	Fluoxetine, sertraline, paroxetine, citalopram.	
Mechanism	Serotonin-specific reuptake inhibitors.	It normally takes 2–3 weeks for antidepressants to have an effect.
Clinical use	Endogenous depression, OCD.	
Toxicity	Fewer than TCAs. GI distress, sexual dysfunction (anorgasmia). "Serotonin syndrome" with MAO inhibitors—hyperthermia, muscle rigidity, cardiovascular collapse.	

Tricyclic antidepressants	Imipramine, amitriptyline, desipramine, nortriptyline, clomipramine, doxepin, amoxapine.
Mechanism	Block reuptake of NE and serotonin.
Clinical use	Major depression, bedwetting (imipramine), OCD (clomipramine).
Side effects	Sedation, α-blocking effects, atropine-like (anticholinergic) side effects (tachycardia, urinary retention). 3° TCAs (amitriptyline) have more anticholinergic effects than do 2° TCAs (nortriptyline). Desipramine is the least sedating.
Toxicity	**Tri-C**'s: **C**onvulsions, **C**oma, **C**ardiotoxicity (arrhythmias); also respiratory depression, hyperpyrexia. Confusion and hallucinations in elderly due to anticholinergic side effects (use nortriptyline).

Other antidepressants		
Bupropion (Wellbutrin)	Also used for smoking cessation. Mechanism not well known. Toxicity: stimulant effects (tachycardia, insomnia), headache, seizure in bulimic patients. Does not cause sexual side effects.	You need **BU**tane in your **VEIN**s to **MUR**der for a **MAP** of Alca**TRAZ**.
Venlafaxine	Also used in generalized anxiety disorder. Inhibits serotonin, NE, and dopamine reuptake. Toxicity: stimulant effects, sedation, nausea, constipation, ↑ BP.	
Mirtazapine	α_2 antagonist (↑ release of NE and serotonin) and potent 5-HT_2 and 5-HT_3 receptor antagonist. Toxicity: sedation, ↑ appetite, weight gain, dry mouth.	
Maprotiline	Blocks NE reuptake. Toxicity: sedation, orthostatic hypotension.	
Trazodone	Primarily inhibit serotonin reuptake. Toxicity: sedation, nausea, priapism, postural hypotension.	

Monoamine oxidase (MAO) inhibitors	Phenelzine, tranylcypromine.
Mechanism	Nonselective MAO inhibition → ↑ levels of amine neurotransmitters.
Clinical use	Atypical depression (i.e., with mood reactivity, sensitivity to rejection, hypersomnia), anxiety, hypochondriasis.
Toxicity	Hypertensive crisis with tyramine ingestion (in many foods) and β-agonists; CNS stimulation. Contraindication with SSRIs or meperidine (to prevent serotonin syndrome).

Methylphenidate (Ritalin)	
Mechanism	↑ presynaptic NE vesicular release (like amphetamines). However, the mechanism for relieving ADHD symptoms is not known.
Clinical use	ADHD.

NOTES

HIGH-YIELD SYSTEMS

Renal

"But I know all about love already. I know precious little about kidneys."
—Aldous Huxley, *Antic Hay*

"This too shall pass. Just like a kidney stone."
—Hunter Madsen

- 3-year-old boy presents with facial edema, malaise, and proteinuria. — What is the appropriate treatment? — Steroids for minimal change disease.
- Woman presents with UTI positive for *Proteus vulgaris*. — What type of kidney stone is she at risk for? — Ammonium magnesium phosphate (struvite).
- Patient describes a 2-year history of acetaminophen use. — What is she at risk for? — Renal papillary necrosis.
- X-ray film shows massively enlarged kidneys bilaterally. — What is the diagnosis? — Adult polycystic kidney disease.
- Patient taking enalapril complains of constant coughing. — What is an appropriate alternative drug? — Losartan—angiotensin II receptor blocker.
- Patient with CHF needs diuretic therapy but has a sulfa allergy. — What is an appropriate alternative drug? — Ethacrynic acid.
- Patient is diagnosed with a horseshoe kidney. — What artery keeps it low in the abdomen? — IMA.
- Patient presents with hypertension, hypokalemia, metabolic alkalosis, and low plasma renin. — What is the diagnosis, and how do you treat it? — Conn's syndrome (1° hyperaldosteronism). Treat with spironolactone.

Kidney anatomy and glomerular structure

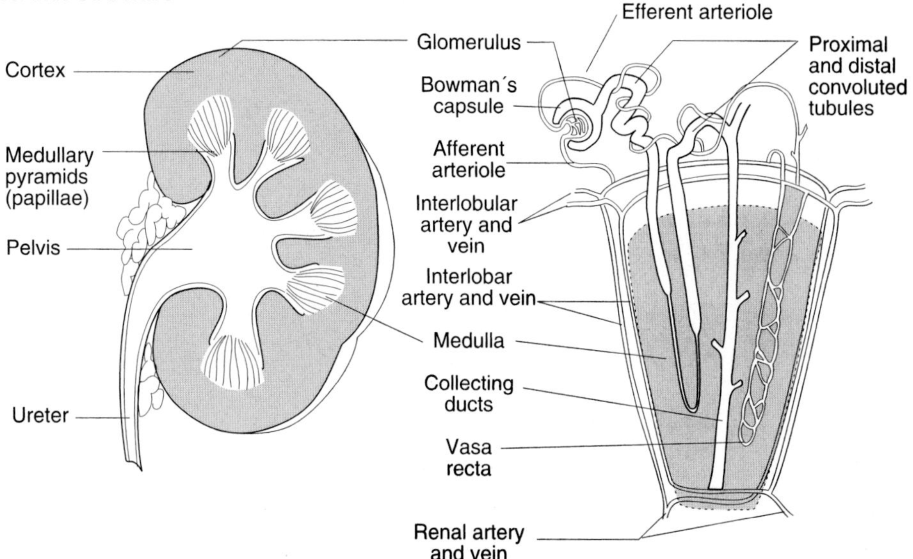

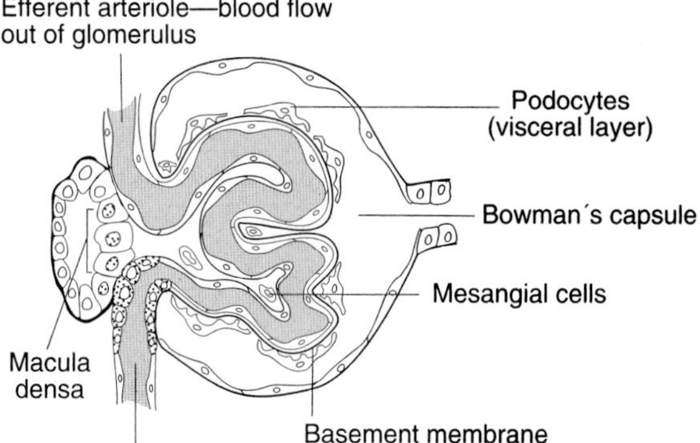

The left kidney is taken during transplantation because it has a longer renal vein.

(Adapted, with permission, from McPhee S et al. *Pathophysiology of Disease: An Introduction to Clinical Medicine,* 3rd ed. New York: McGraw-Hill, 2000: 384.)

Ureters: course	Ureters pass **under** uterine artery and **under** ductus deferens (retroperitoneal).	Water (ureters) **under** the bridge (artery, ductus deferens).

Fluid compartments

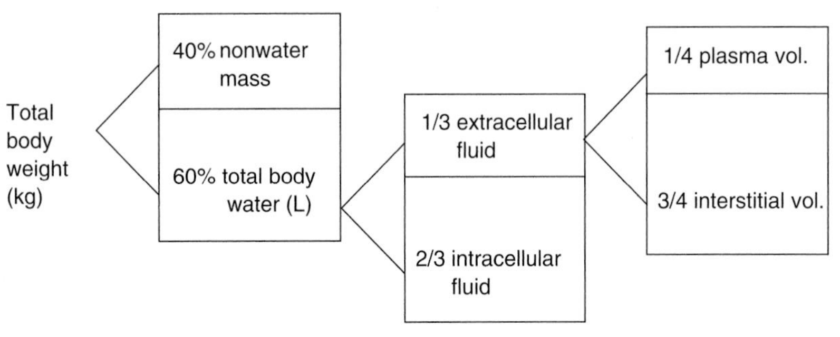

ECF: ↑ NaCl, ↓ K^+.
ICF: ↑ K^+, ↓ NaCl.
TBW – ECF = ICF.
ECF – PV = interstitial volume.
60–40–20 rule (% of body weight):
- 60% total body water
- 40% ICF
- 20% ECF

Plasma volume measured by radiolabeled albumin.
Extracellular volume measured by inulin.
Osmolarity = 290 mOsm.

Renal clearance

$C_x = U_xV/P_x$ = volume of plasma from which the substance is completely cleared per unit time.
If C_x < GFR, then there is net tubular reabsorption of X.
If C_x > GFR, then there is net tubular secretion of X.
If C_x = GFR, then there is no net secretion or reabsorption.

Be familiar with calculations.
C_x = clearance of X.
U_x = urine concentration of X.
P_x = plasma concentration of X.
V = urine flow rate.

Glomerular filtration barrier

Responsible for filtration of plasma according to size and net charge.
Composed of:
1. Fenestrated capillary endothelium (size barrier)
2. Fused basement membrane with heparan sulfate (negative charge barrier)
3. Epithelial layer consisting of podocyte foot processes

The charge barrier is lost in **nephrotic syndrome,** resulting in albuminuria, hypoproteinemia, generalized edema, and hyperlipidemia.

Glomerular filtration rate

Inulin can be used to calculate GFR because it is freely filtered and is neither reabsorbed nor secreted.
$GFR = U_{inulin} \times V/P_{inulin} = C_{inulin}$
$= K_f [(P_{GC} - P_{BS}) - (\pi_{GC} - \pi_{BS})]$.
(GC = glomerular capillary; BS = Bowman's space.)
π_{BS} normally equals zero.

Creatinine clearance is an approximate measure of GFR.

Effective renal plasma flow

ERPF can be estimated using PAH because it is both filtered and actively secreted in the proximal tubule. All PAH entering the kidney is excreted.
$ERPF = U_{PAH} \times V/P_{PAH} = C_{PAH}$.
RBF = RPF/(1 – Hct).
ERPF underestimates true RPF by ~10%.

Filtration

Filtration fraction = GFR/RPF.

Filtered load = GFR × plasma concentration.

GFR can be estimated with creatinine.

RPF is best estimated with PAH.

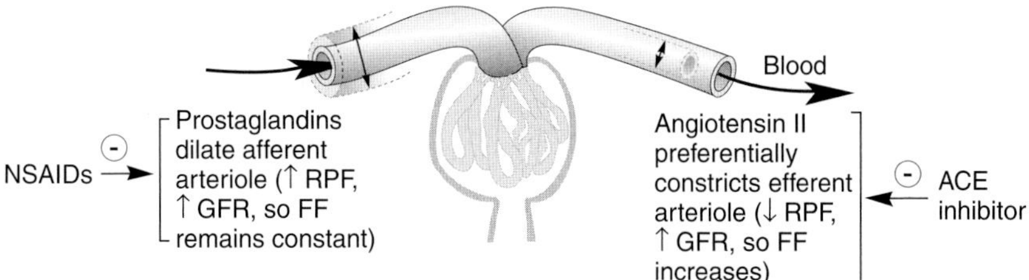

Changes in renal function

Effect	RPF	GFR	FF (GFR/RPF)
Afferent arteriole constriction	↓	↓	NC
Efferent arteriole constriction	↓	↑	↑
↑ plasma protein concentration	NC	↓	↓
↓ plasma protein concentration	NC	↑	↑
Constriction of ureter	NC	↓	↓

Free water clearance

Ability to dilute urine. Given urine flow rate, urine osmolarity, and plasma osmolarity, be able to calculate free water clearance:

$C_{H_2O} = V - C_{osm}$.

V = urine flow rate; $C_{osm} = U_{osm}V/P_{osm}$.

With ADH: $C_{H_2O} < 0$.

Without ADH: $C_{H_2O} > 0$.

Isotonic urine: $C_{H_2O} = 0$.

Glucose clearance

Glucose at a normal plasma level is completely reabsorbed in proximal tubule.

At plasma glucose of 200 mg/dL, glucosuria begins (threshold). At 350 mg/dL, transport mechanism is saturated (T_m).

Glucosuria is an important clinical clue to diabetes mellitus.

Amino acid clearance

Reabsorption by at least 3 distinct carrier systems, with competitive inhibition within each group. 2° active transport occurs in proximal tubule and is saturable.

Nephron physiology

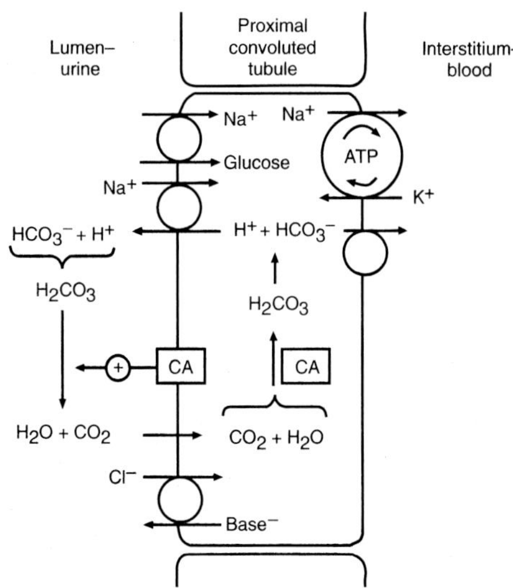

A. Early proximal convoluted tubule—"workhorse of the nephron." Contains brush border. Reabsorbs **all** of the glucose and amino acids and **most** of the bicarbonate, sodium, and water. Isotonic absorption. Secretes ammonia, which acts as a buffer for secreted H^+.

B. Thin descending loop of Henle—passively reabsorbs water via medullary hypertonicity (impermeable to sodium). Makes urine hypertonic.

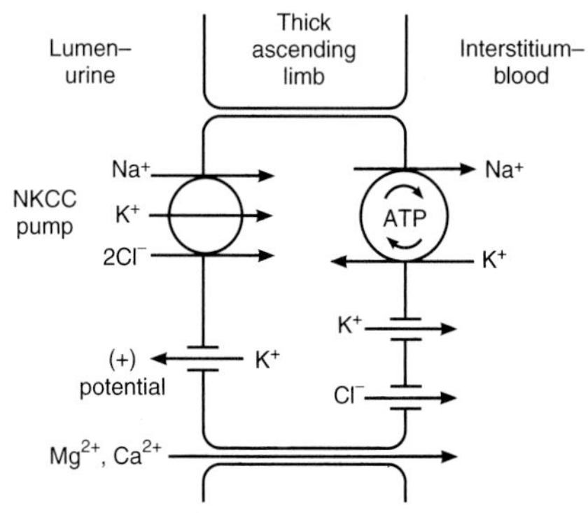

C. Thick ascending loop of Henle—actively reabsorbs Na^+, K^+, and Cl^- and indirectly induces the reabsorption of Mg^{2+} and Ca^{2+}. Impermeable to H_2O. Diluting segment. Makes urine hypotonic.

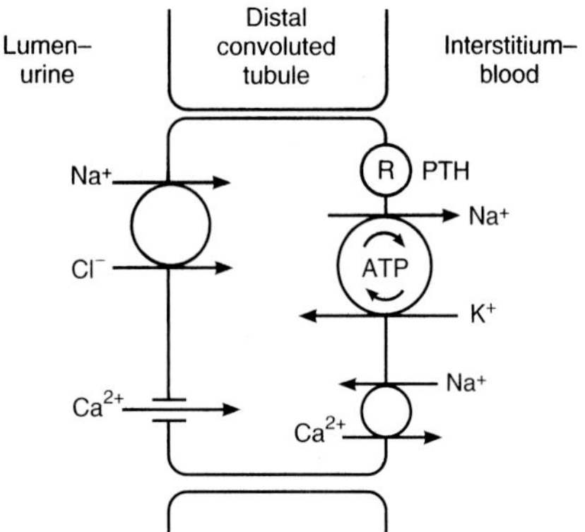

D. Early distal convoluted tubule—actively reabsorbs Na^+, Cl^-. Reabsorption of Ca^{2+} is under the control of PTH. Diluting segment. Makes urine hypotonic.

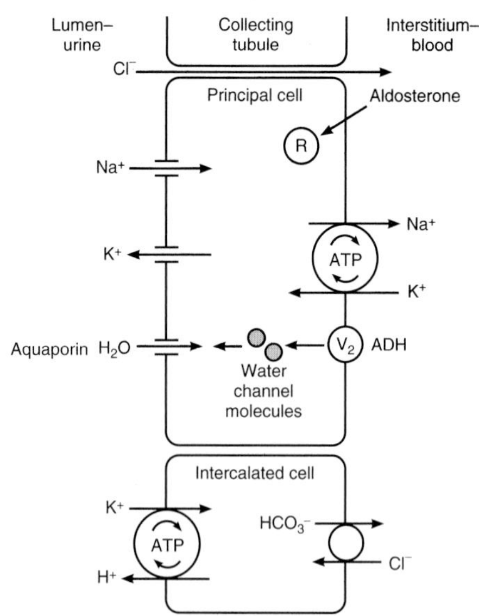

E. Collecting tubules—reabsorb Na^+ in exchange for secreting K^+ or H^+ (regulated by aldosterone). Reabsorption of water is regulated by ADH (vasopressin). Osmolarity of medulla can reach 1200 mOsm/L H_2O.

Relative concentrations along renal tubule

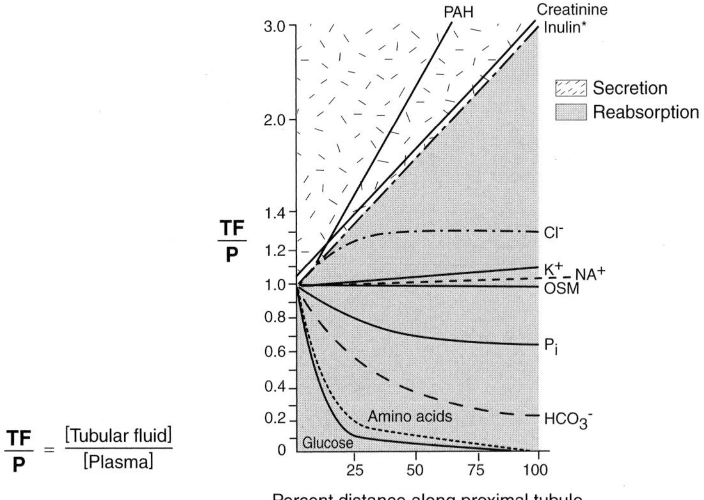

$\frac{TF}{P} = \frac{[\text{Tubular fluid}]}{[\text{Plasma}]}$

* Neither secreted nor reabsorbed; concentration increases as water is reabsorbed.

(Adapted, with permission, from Ganong WF. *Review of Medical Physiology,* 22nd ed. New York: McGraw-Hill, 2005.)

Renin-angiotensin system

Mechanism	Renin is released by the kidneys upon sensing ↓ BP and cleaves angiotensinogen (from the liver) to angiotensin I. Angiotensin I is then cleaved by angiotensin-converting enzyme (ACE), primarily in the lung capillaries, to angiotensin II.
Actions of angiotensin II	1. Potent vasoconstriction 2. Release of aldosterone from adrenal cortex 3. Release of ADH from posterior pituitary 4. Stimulates hypothalamus → ↑ thirst Overall, angiotensin II serves to ↑ intravascular volume and ↑ BP. ANP released from atria may act as a "check" on the renin-angiotensin system (e.g., in heart failure). ↓ renin and ↑ GFR.

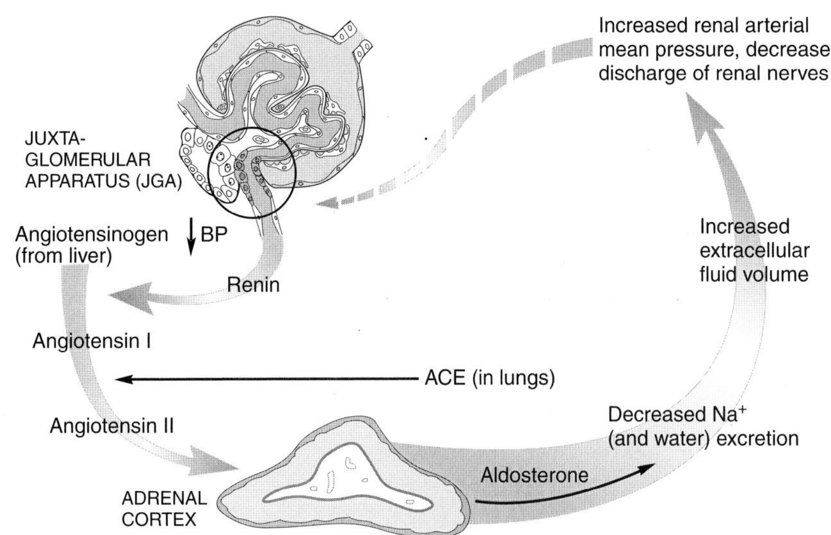

(Adapted, with permission, from Ganong WF. *Review of Medical Physiology,* 22nd ed. New York: McGraw-Hill, 2005.)

Juxtaglomerular apparatus (JGA)	JGA—JG cells (modified smooth muscle of afferent arteriole) and macula densa (Na^+ sensor, part of the distal convoluted tubule). JG cells secrete renin (leading to ↑ angiotensin II and aldosterone levels) in response to ↓ renal blood pressure, ↓ Na^+ delivery to distal tubule, and ↑ sympathetic tone.	JGA defends glomerular filtration rate via the renin-angiotensin system. *Juxta* = close by.
Kidney endocrine functions	1. Endothelial cells of peritubular capillaries secrete erythropoietin in response to hypoxia 2. Conversion of 25-OH vitamin D to 1,25-$(OH)_2$ vitamin D by 1α-hydroxylase, which is activated by PTH 3. JG cells secrete renin in response to ↓ renal arterial pressure and ↑ renal sympathetic discharge (β_1 effect) 4. Secretion of prostaglandins that vasodilate the afferent arterioles to ↑ GFR 25-OH vitamin D → 1,25-OH vitamin D (1α-hydroxylase; stimulated by PTH)	NSAIDs can cause acute renal failure in high vasoconstrictive states by inhibiting the renal production of prostaglandins, which keep the afferent arterioles vasodilated to maintain GFR.

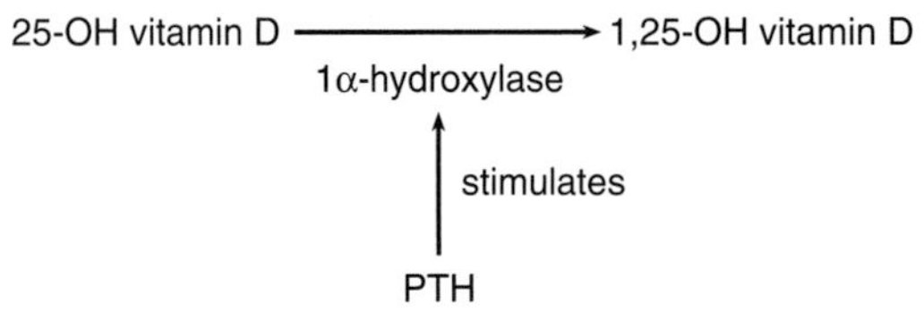

Hormones acting on kidney

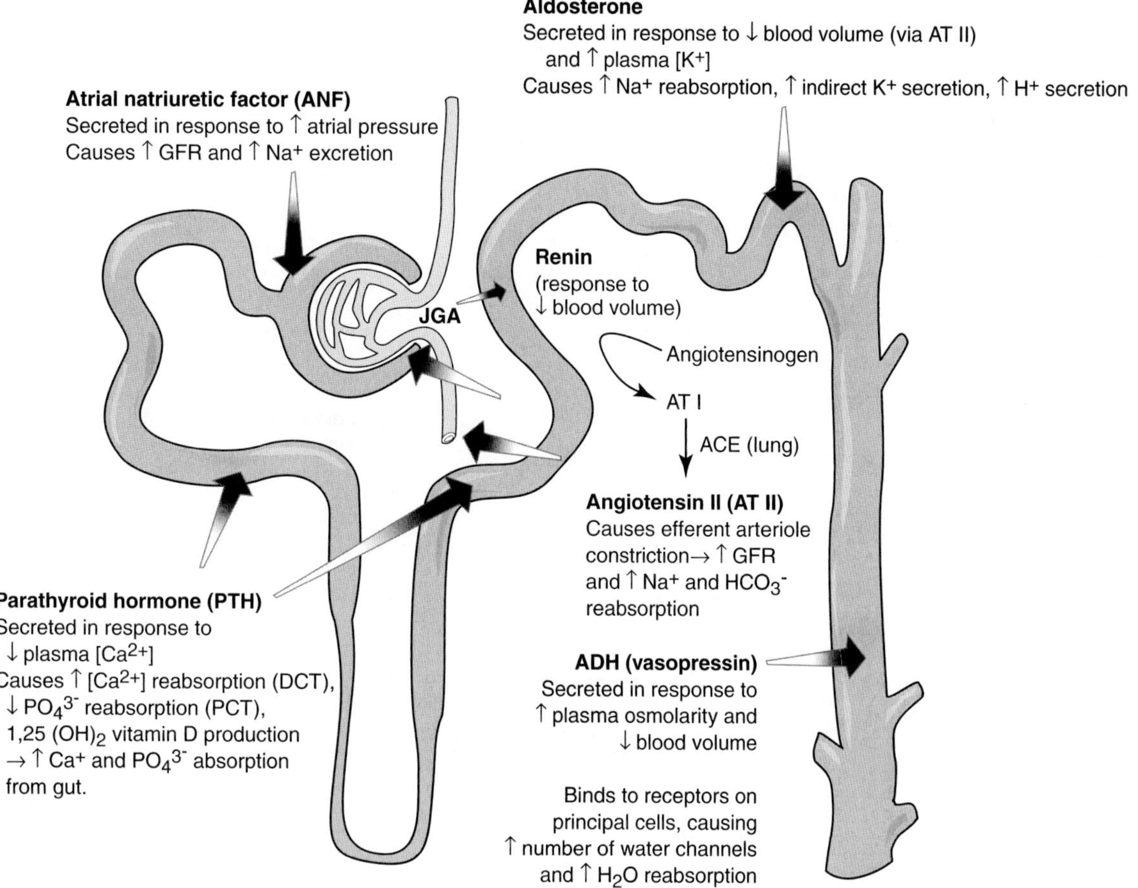

Acid-base physiology

	pH	P_{CO_2}	$[HCO_3^-]$	Compensatory response
Metabolic acidosis	↓	↓	**↓**	Hyperventilation
Metabolic alkalosis	↑	↑	**↑**	Hypoventilation
Respiratory acidosis	↓	**↑**	↑	↑ renal $[HCO_3^-]$ reabsorption
Respiratory alkalosis	↑	**↓**	↓	↓ renal $[HCO_3^-]$ reabsorption

Henderson-Hasselbalch equation: $pH = pKa + \log \frac{[HCO_3^-]}{0.03\ P_{CO_2}}$

Key: **↑ ↓** = 1° disturbance; ↓ ↑ = compensatory response.

HIGH-YIELD SYSTEMS

RENAL

Acidosis/alkalosis

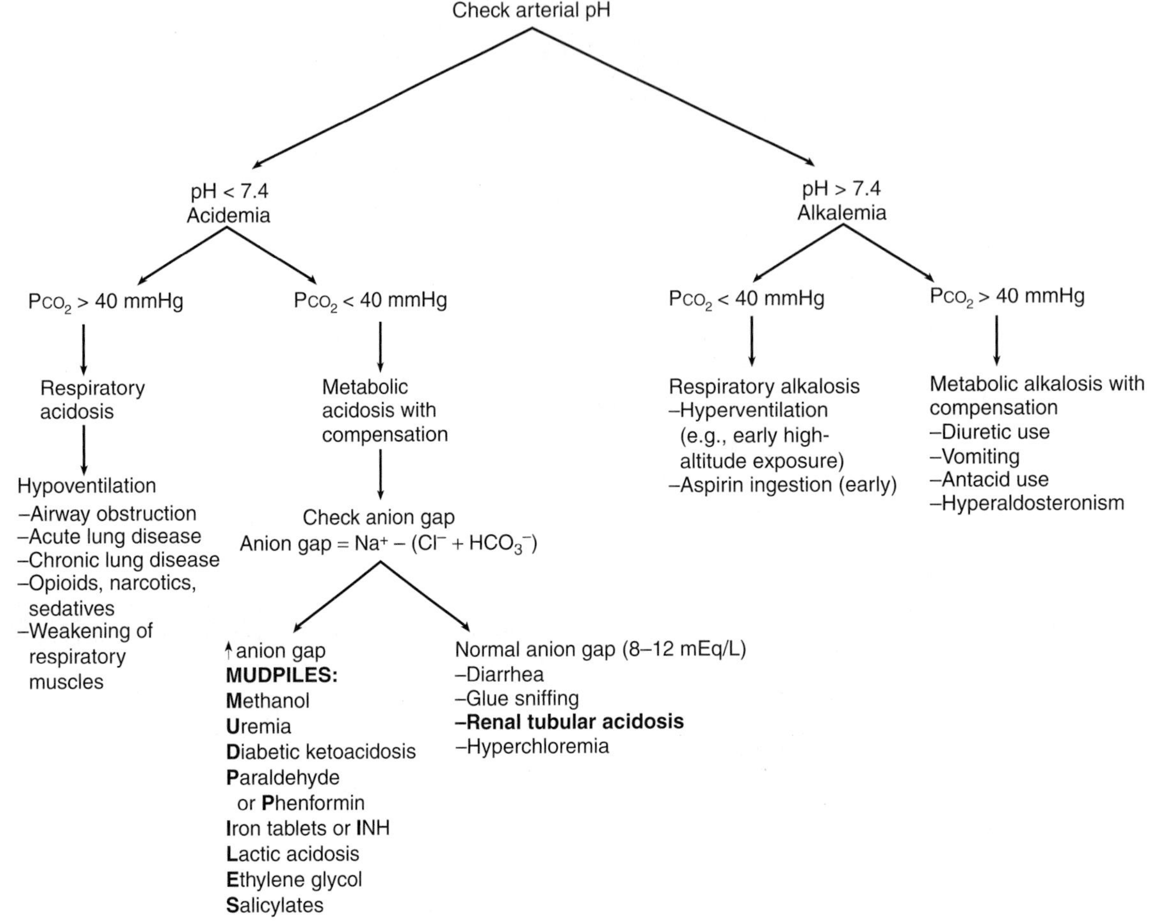

Renal tubular acidosis	
Type 1	Defect in H^+ pump → failure to acidify urine.
Type 2	Renal loss of bicarbonate.
Type 4	Hypoaldosteronism → hypokalemia → inhibition of ammonia excretion.

Acid-base compensations	The following formulas give appropriate compensations for a single disorder. If the formula does not match the actual values, suspect a mixed disorder.
Metabolic acidosis	Winter's formula: $P_{CO_2} = 1.5\ (HCO_3^-) + 8 \pm 2$.
Metabolic alkalosis	P_{CO_2} ↑ 0.7 mmHg for every ↑ 1 mEq/L HCO_3^-.
Respiratory acidosis	Acute— ↑ 1 mEq/L HCO_3^- for every ↑ 10 mmHg P_{CO_2}. Chronic— ↑ 3.5 mEq/L HCO_3^- for every ↑ 10 mmHg P_{CO_2}.
Respiratory alkalosis	Acute— ↓ 2 mEq/L HCO_3^- for every ↓ 10 mmHg P_{CO_2}. Chronic— ↓ 5 mEq/L HCO_3^- for every ↓ 10 mmHg P_{CO_2}.

Acid-base nomogram

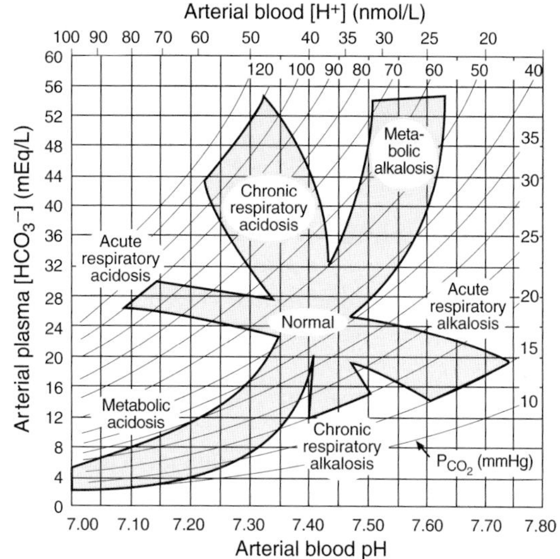

(Adapted, with permission, from Ganong WF. *Review of Medical Physiology,* 22nd ed. New York: McGraw-Hill, 2005: 734.)

▶ RENAL–PATHOLOGY

Potter's syndrome

Bilateral renal agenesis → oligohydramnios → limb deformities, facial deformities, pulmonary hypoplasia. Caused by malformation of ureteric bud.

Babies with Potter's can't "Pee" in utero.

Horseshoe kidney

Inferior poles of both kidneys fuse. As they ascend from pelvis during fetal development, horseshoe kidneys get trapped under inferior mesenteric artery and remain low in the abdomen. Kidney functions normally.

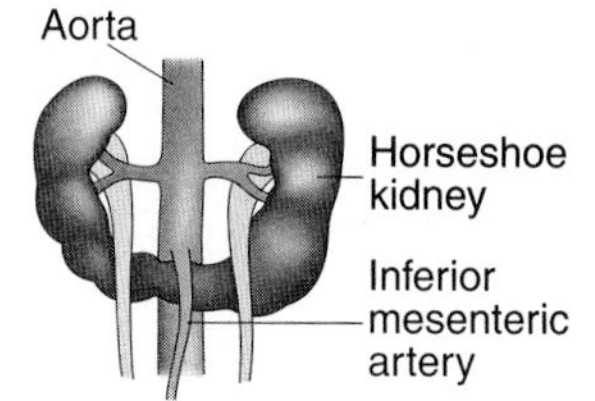

Casts

Casts in urine:

- RBC casts—glomerular inflammation (nephritic syndromes), ischemia, or malignant hypertension.
- WBC casts—tubulointerstitial disease, acute pyelonephritis, glomerular disorders.
- Granular ("muddy brown") casts—acute tubular necrosis.
- Waxy casts—advanced renal disease/CRF.
- Hyaline casts—nonspecific.

Presence of casts indicates that hematuria/pyuria is of renal origin.

Bladder cancer → RBCs, no casts.

Acute cystitis → WBCs, no casts.

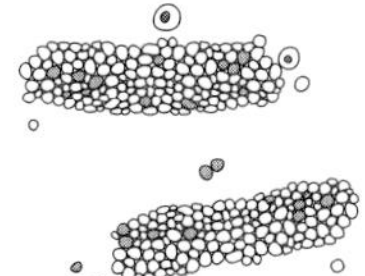

Red blood cell casts

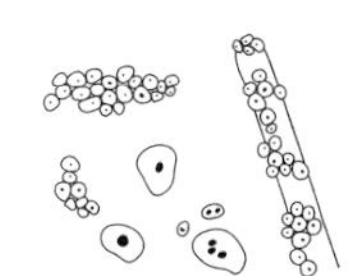

White blood cell casts

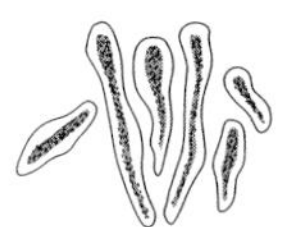

Hyaline casts

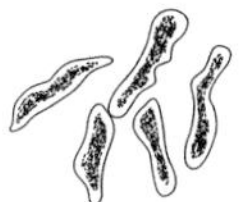

Granular casts

Glomerular pathology

NephrItic syndrome—hematuria, hypertension, oliguria, azotemia.	I = inflammation.
1. **Acute poststreptococcal glomerulonephritis**—LM: glomeruli enlarged and hypercellular, neutrophils, "lumpy-bumpy." EM: subepithelial humps. IF: granular pattern.	Most frequently seen in children. Peripheral and periorbital edema. Resolves spontaneously.
2. **Membranoproliferative glomerulonephritis**—EM: subendothelial humps, "tram track."	Slowly progresses to renal failure.
3. **Rapidly progressive (crescentic) glomerulonephritis**—LM and IF: crescent-moon shape.	Rapid course to renal failure. Number of crescents indicates prognosis.
4. **Goodpasture's syndrome (type II hypersensitivity)**—IF: linear pattern, anti-GBM antibodies.	Hemoptysis, hematuria.
5. **IgA nephropathy (Berger's disease)**—IF and EM: mesangial deposits of IgA.	Mild disease. Often postinfectious. Common cause of recurrent hematuria in young patients.
6. **Alport's syndrome**—split basement membrane.	Collagen IV mutation. Nerve deafness and ocular disorders.
NephrOtic syndrome—massive proteinuria (frothy urine), hypoalbuminemia, peripheral and periorbital edema, hyperlipidemia.	O = prOteinuria.
1. **Membranous glomerulonephritis**—LM: diffuse capillary and basement membrane thickening. IF: granular pattern. EM: "spike and dome."	Most common cause of adult nephrotic syndrome.
2. **Minimal change disease (lipoid nephrosis)**—LM: normal glomeruli. EM: foot process effacement (see Color Image 93).	Most common cause of childhood nephrotic syndrome. Responds well to steroids.
3. **Focal segmental glomerular sclerosis**—LM: segmental sclerosis and hyalinosis.	More severe disease in HIV patients.
4. **Diabetic nephropathy**—LM: Kimmelstiel-Wilson nodular lesions, basement membrane thickening (see Color Image 95).	
5. **SLE** (5 patterns of renal involvement)—LM: In membranous glomerulonephritis pattern, wire-loop lesion with subepithelial deposits.	
6. **Amyloidosis**—IF: Congo red stain, apple-green birefringence.	Associated with multiple myeloma, chronic conditions, TB, rheumatoid arthritis.

(LM = light microscopy; EM = electron microscopy; IF = immunofluorescence)

Glomerular histopathology

EP = epithelium with foot processes
US = urinary space
GBM = glomerular basement membrane
EN = fenestrated endothelium
MC = mesangial cells
EM = extracellular matrix

1 = subepithelial deposits (membranous nephropathy)
2 = large irregular subepithelial deposits or "humps" (acute glomerulonephritis)
3 = subendothelial deposits in lupus glomerulonephritis
4 = mesangial deposits (IgA nephropathy)
5 = antibody binding to GBM—smooth linear pattern on immunofluorescence (Goodpasture's)
6 = effacement of epithelial foot processes (common in all forms of glomerular injury with proteinuria)

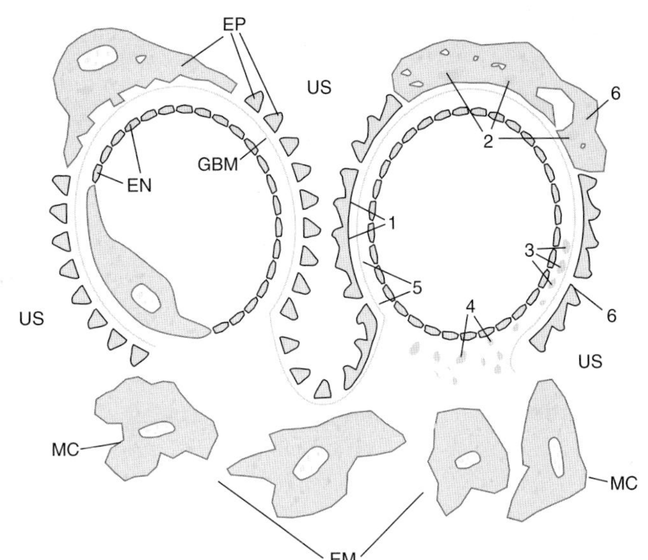

Kidney stones	Can lead to severe complications, such as hydronephrosis and pyelonephritis. 4 major types:	
Calcium	Most common kidney stones (75–85%). Calcium oxalate (see Color Image 97), calcium phosphate, or both. Conditions that cause hypercalcemia (cancer, ↑ PTH, ↑ vitamin D, milk-alkali syndrome) can lead to hypercalciuria and stones. Tend to recur.	Radiopaque. Oxalate crystals can result from antifreeze or vitamin C abuse.
Ammonium magnesium phosphate (**struvite**)	2nd most common kidney stone. Caused by infection with urease-positive bugs (*Proteus vulgaris, Staphylococcus, Klebsiella*). Can form **staghorn calculi** that can be a nidus for UTIs.	Radiopaque or radiolucent. Worsened by alkaluria.
Uric acid	Strong association with hyperuricemia (e.g., gout). Often seen as a result of diseases with ↑ cell turnover, such as leukemia and myeloproliferative disorders.	I can't see **U** on x-ray or CT.
Cystine	Most often 2° to cystinuria. Hexagonal shape.	Faintly radiopaque. Treat with alkalinization of urine.

Renal cell carcinoma

Most common renal malignancy. Invades IVC and spreads hematogenously. Most common in men ages 50–70. ↑ incidence with smoking and obesity. Associated with von Hippel–Lindau and gene deletion in chromosome 3. Originates in renal tubule cells → polygonal clear cells. Manifests clinically with hematuria, palpable mass, 2° polycythemia, flank pain, fever, and weight loss. Associated with paraneoplastic syndromes (ectopic EPO, ACTH, PTHrP, and prolactin) (see Color Image 98).

Wilms' tumor

Most common renal malignancy of early childhood (ages 2–4). Presents with huge, palpable flank mass, hemihypertrophy. Contains embryonic glomerular structures. Deletion of tumor suppression gene *WT1* on chromosome 11. Can be part of **WAGR** complex: **W**ilms' tumor, **A**niridia, **G**enitourinary malformation, and mental-motor **R**etardation.

Transitional cell carcinoma	Most common tumor of urinary tract system (can occur in renal calyces, renal pelvis, ureters, and bladder). Painless hematuria is suggestive of bladder cancer. Associated with problems in your Pee **SAC**: **P**henacetin, **S**moking, **A**niline dyes, and **C**yclophosphamide (see Color Image 90).
Pyelonephritis	
Acute	Affects cortex with relative sparing of glomeruli/vessels. White cell casts in urine are pathognomonic (see Color Image 89A). Presents with fever, CVA tenderness.
Chronic	Coarse, asymmetric corticomedullary scarring, blunted calyx. Tubules can contain eosinophilic casts (thyroidization of kidney) (see Color Image 89B).
Diffuse cortical necrosis	Acute generalized infarction of cortices of both kidneys. Likely due to a combination of vasospasm and DIC. Associated with obstetric catastrophes (e.g., abruptio placentae) and septic shock.
Drug-induced interstitial nephritis	Acute interstitial renal inflammation. Fever, rash, eosinophilia, hematuria 2 weeks after administration. Drugs (e.g., penicillin derivatives, NSAIDs, diuretics) act as haptens inducing hypersensitivity.
Acute tubular necrosis	Most common cause of acute renal failure. Reversible, but fatal if left untreated. Associated with renal ischemia (e.g., shock), crush injury (myoglobulinuria), toxins. Death most often occurs during initial oliguric phase. Recovery in 2–3 weeks. Loss of cell polarity, epithelial cell detachment, necrosis, granular ("muddy brown") casts. Three stages: inciting event → maintenance (low urine) → recovery.
Renal papillary necrosis	Associated with: 1. Diabetes mellitus 2. Acute pyelonephritis 3. Chronic phenacetin use (acetaminophen is phenacetin derivative) 4. Sickle cell anemia
Acute renal failure	Abrupt decline in renal function with ↑ creatinine and ↑ BUN over a period of several days. 1. Prerenal azotemia—↓ RBF (e.g., hypotension) → ↓ GFR. Na^+/H_2O and urea retained by kidney. 2. Intrinsic renal—generally due to acute tubular necrosis or ischemia/toxins. Patchy necrosis leads to debris obstructing tubule and fluid backflow across necrotic tubule → ↓ GFR. Urine has epithelial/granular casts. 3. Postrenal—outflow obstruction (stones, BPH, neoplasia). Develops only with bilateral obstruction.

Variable	Prerenal	Renal	Postrenal
Urine osmolality	> 500	< 350	< 350
Urine Na	< 10	> 20	> 40
Fe_{Na}	< 1%	> 2%	> 4%
BUN/Cr ratio	> 20	< 15	> 15

Consequences of renal failure	Failure to make urine and excrete nitrogenous wastes. Uremia—clinical syndrome marked by ↑ BUN and ↑ creatinine and associated symptoms. Consequences: 1. Anemia (failure of erythropoietin production) 2. Renal osteodystrophy (failure of active vitamin D production) 3. Hyperkalemia, which can lead to cardiac arrhythmias 4. Metabolic acidosis due to ↓ acid secretion and ↓ generation of HCO_3^- 5. Uremic encephalopathy 6. Sodium and H_2O excess → CHF and pulmonary edema 7. Chronic pyelonephritis 8. Hypertension	2 forms of renal failure—acute renal failure (often due to acute tubular necrosis) and chronic renal failure (e.g., due to hypertension and diabetes).

Fanconi's syndrome	Defect in proximal tubule transport of amino acids, glucose, phosphate, uric acid, protein, and electrolytes. Complications include rickets, osteomalacia, hypokalemia, metabolic acidosis.

Cysts

Adult polycystic kidney disease	Multiple, large, bilateral cysts that ultimately destroy the parenchyma. Presents with flank pain, hematuria, hypertension, urinary infection, progressive renal failure. Autosomal-dominant mutation in *APKD1*. Death from uremia or hypertension. Associated with polycystic liver disease, berry aneurysms, mitral valve prolapse.
Infantile polycystic kidney disease	Infantile presentation in parenchyma. Autosomal recessive. Associated with hepatic cysts and fibrosis.
Dialysis cysts	Cortical and medullary cysts resulting from long-standing dialysis.
Simple cysts	Benign, incidental finding. Cortex only.
Medullary cystic disease	Medullary cysts. Ultrasound shows small kidney. Poor prognosis.
Medullary sponge disease	Collecting duct cysts. Good prognosis.

Electrolyte disturbances

Electrolyte	Low serum concentration	High serum concentration
Na^+	Disorientation, stupor, coma	Neurologic: irritability, delirium, coma
Cl^-	2° to metabolic alkalosis, hypokalemia, hypovolemia, ↑ aldosterone	2° to non–anion gap acidosis
K^+	U waves on ECG, flattened T waves, arrhythmias, paralysis	Peaked T waves, wide QRS, arrhythmias
Ca^{2+}	Tetany, neuromuscular irritability	Delirium, renal stones, abdominal pain, not necessarily calciuria
Mg^{2+}	Neuromuscular irritability, arrhythmias	Delirium, ↓ DTRs, cardiopulmonary arrest
PO_4^{2-}	Low-mineral ion product causes bone loss, osteomalacia	High-mineral ion product causes metastatic calcification, renal stones, met calcifications

Diuretics: site of action

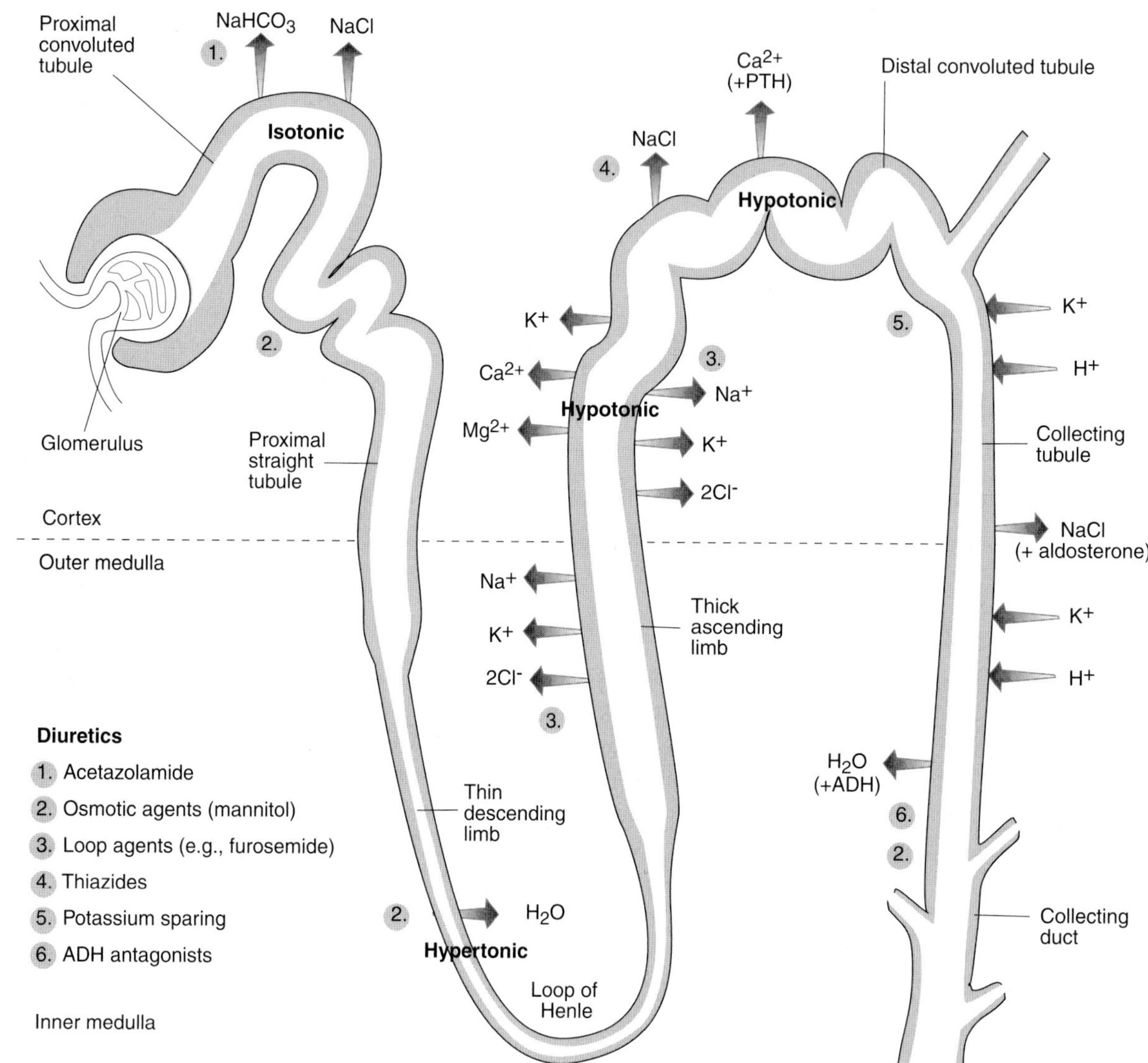

(Adapted, with permission, from Katzung BG. *Basic and Clinical Pharmacology,* 7th ed. Stamford, CT: Appleton & Lange, 1997: 243.)

HIGH-YIELD SYSTEMS

RENAL

Mannitol

Mechanism	Osmotic diuretic, ↑ tubular fluid osmolarity, producing ↑ urine flow.	
Clinical use	Shock, drug overdose, ↓ intracranial/intraocular pressure.	
Toxicity	Pulmonary edema, dehydration. Contraindicated in anuria, CHF.	

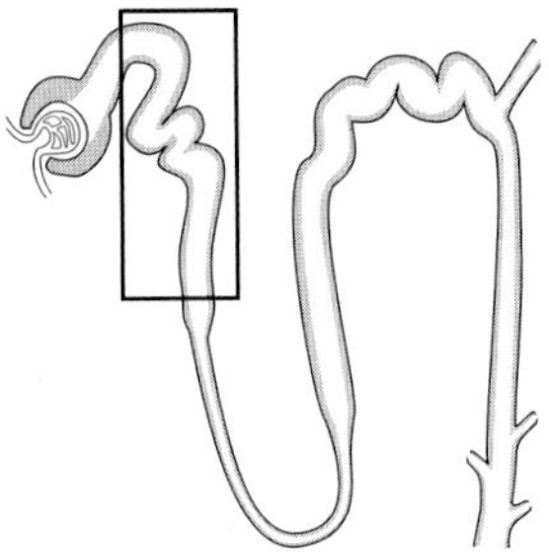

Acetazolamide

Mechanism	Carbonic anhydrase inhibitor. Causes self-limited $NaHCO_3$ diuresis and reduction in total-body HCO_3^- stores.	
Clinical use	Glaucoma, urinary alkalinization, metabolic alkalosis, altitude sickness.	
Toxicity	Hyperchloremic metabolic acidosis, neuropathy, NH_3 toxicity, sulfa allergy.	**ACID**azolamide causes **ACID**osis.

Furosemide

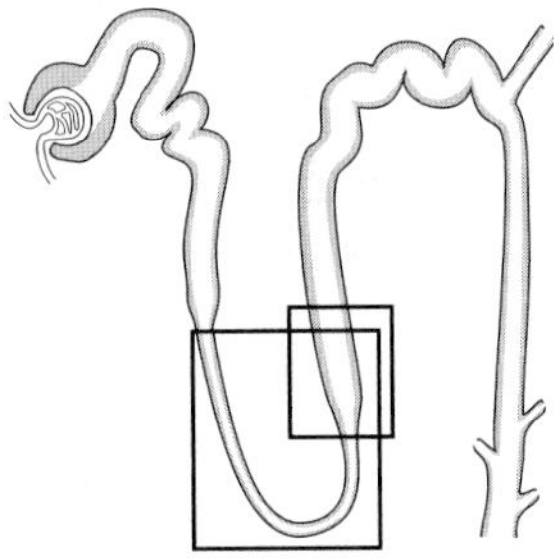

Mechanism	Sulfonamide loop diuretic. Inhibits cotransport system (Na^+, K^+, 2 Cl^-) of thick ascending limb of loop of Henle. Abolishes hypertonicity of medulla, preventing concentration of urine. ↑ Ca^{2+} excretion. **L**oops **L**ose calcium.	
Clinical use	Edematous states (CHF, cirrhosis, nephrotic syndrome, pulmonary edema), hypertension, hypercalcemia.	
Toxicity	**O**totoxicity, **H**ypokalemia, **D**ehydration, **A**llergy (sulfa), **N**ephritis (interstitial), **G**out.	**OH DANG!**

Ethacrynic acid

Mechanism	Phenoxyacetic acid derivative (NOT a sulfonamide). Essentially same action as furosemide.
Clinical use	Diuresis in patients allergic to sulfa drugs.
Toxicity	Similar to furosemide; can be used in hyperuricemia, acute gout (never used to treat gout).

Hydrochlorothiazide

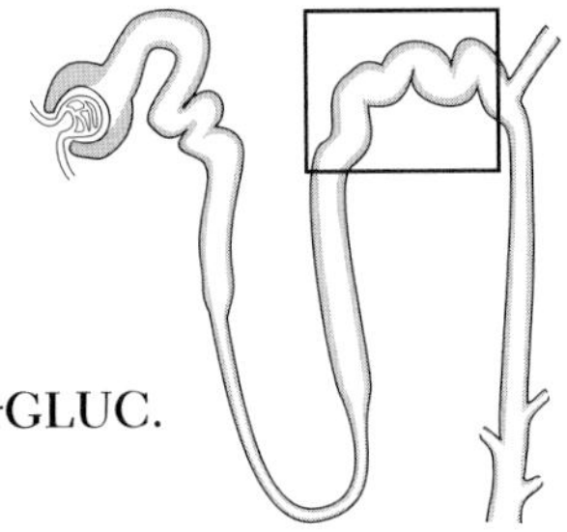

Mechanism	Thiazide diuretic. Inhibits NaCl reabsorption in early distal tubule, reducing diluting capacity of the nephron. ↓ Ca^{2+} excretion.	
Clinical use	Hypertension, CHF, idiopathic hypercalciuria, nephrogenic diabetes insipidus.	
Toxicity	Hypokalemic metabolic alkalosis, hyponatremia, hyper**G**lycemia, hyper**L**ipidemia, hyper**U**ricemia, and hyper**C**alcemia. Sulfa allergy.	Hyper**GLUC**.

K^+-sparing diuretics	Spironolactone, **T**riamterene, **A**miloride, eplerenone.	The K^+ **STA**ys.
Mechanism	Spironolactone is a competitive aldosterone receptor antagonist in the cortical collecting tubule. Triamterene and amiloride act at the same part of the tubule by blocking Na^+ channels in the CCT.	
Clinical use	Hyperaldosteronism, K^+ depletion, CHF.	
Toxicity	Hyperkalemia, endocrine effects (e.g., spironolactone causes gynecomastia, antiandrogen effects).	

Diuretics: electrolyte changes	
Urine NaCl	↑ (all diuretics—carbonic anhydrase inhibitors, loop diuretics, thiazides, K^+-sparing diuretics).
Urine K^+	↑ (all except K^+-sparing diuretics).
Blood pH	↓ (acidemia)—carbonic anhydrase inhibitors, K^+-sparing diuretics; ↑ (alkalemia)—loop diuretics, thiazides.
Urine Ca^+	↑ loop diuretics, ↓ thiazides.

ACE inhibitors	Captopril, enalapril, lisinopril.	
Mechanism	Inhibit angiotensin-converting enzyme, reducing levels of angiotensin II and preventing inactivation of bradykinin, a potent vasodilator. **Renin release is** ↑ due to loss of feedback inhibition.	**Losartan** is an angiotensin II receptor antagonist. It is **not** an ACE inhibitor and does not cause cough.
Clinical use	Hypertension, CHF, diabetic renal disease.	
Toxicity	**C**ough, **A**ngioedema, **P**roteinuria, **T**aste changes, hyp**O**tension, **P**regnancy problems (fetal renal damage), **R**ash, **I**ncreased renin, **L**ower angiotensin II. Also **hyperkalemia.** Avoid with bilateral renal artery stenosis.	**CAPTOPRIL.**

HIGH-YIELD SYSTEMS

Reproductive

"Artificial insemination is when the farmer does it to the cow instead of the bull."

—Student essay

▶ REPRODUCTIVE—HIGH-YIELD CLINICAL VIGNETTES

■ 24-year-old man develops testicular cancer.	Metastatic spread first occurs to what site?	Para-aortic lymph nodes (recall descent of testes during development).
■ Woman with a previous cesarean section has a scar in her lower uterus close to the opening of the os.	What is she at ↑ risk for?	Placenta previa.
■ Obese woman presents with hirsutism and ↑ levels of serum testosterone.	What is the diagnosis?	Polycystic ovarian syndrome.
■ Pregnant woman at 16 weeks of gestation presents with an atypically large abdomen.	What is the diagnosis?	High hCG; hydatidiform mole.
■ 55-year-old postmenopausal woman is on tamoxifen therapy.	What is she at ↑ risk of acquiring?	Endometrial carcinoma.

Gonadal drainage		
Venous drainage	Left ovary/testis → left gonadal vein → left renal vein → IVC. Right ovary/testis → right gonadal vein → IVC.	Just as the left adrenal vein makes an extra stop at the left renal vein before the IVC.
Lymphatic drainage	Ovaries/testes → para-aortic lymph nodes.	

Ligaments of the uterus		
Suspensory ligament of ovaries	Contains the ovarian vessels.	
Transverse cervical (cardinal) ligament	Contains the uterine vessels.	
Round ligament of uterus	Contains no important structures. Travels through the inguinal canal and attaches distally to the labia majora.	**Round** like the number of structures it carries: **0**.
Broad ligament	Contains the round ligaments of the uterus and ovaries and the fallopian tubes.	

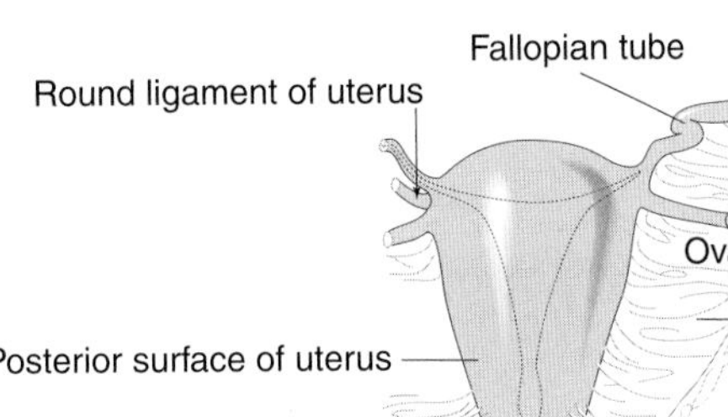

Autonomic innervation of the male sexual response	Erection is mediated by the **P**arasympathetic nervous system. Nitric oxide is vasodilator. Emission is mediated by the **S**ympathetic nervous system. Ejaculation is mediated by visceral and somatic nerves.	**P**oint and **S**hoot.
Derivation of sperm parts	Acrosome is derived from the Golgi apparatus and flagellum (tail) from one of the centrioles. **M**iddle piece (neck) has **M**itochondria. **F**eeds on **F**ructose.	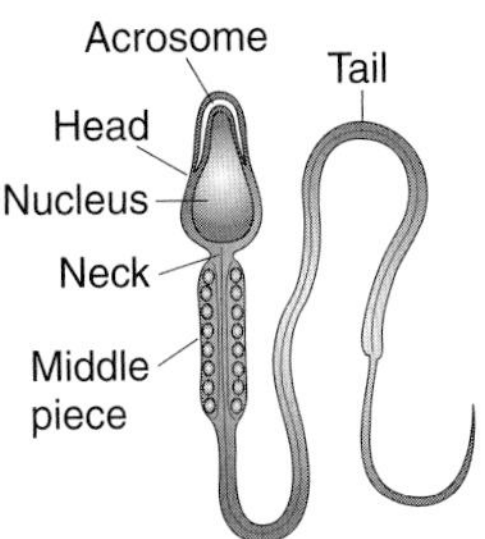

Sperm development

Spermatogenesis begins at puberty with spermatogonia (type A and type B). Full development takes 2 months. Spermatogenesis occurs in Seminiferous tubules.

Blood-testis barrier is a physical barrier in the testis between the tissues responsible for spermatogenesis and the bloodstream (to avoid autoimmune response).

SEVEN UP:
- Seminiferous tubules
- Epididymis
- Vas deferens
- Ejaculatory ducts
- (Nothing)
- Urethra
- Penis

Sertoli cells
- Support Sperm
- Synthesis.

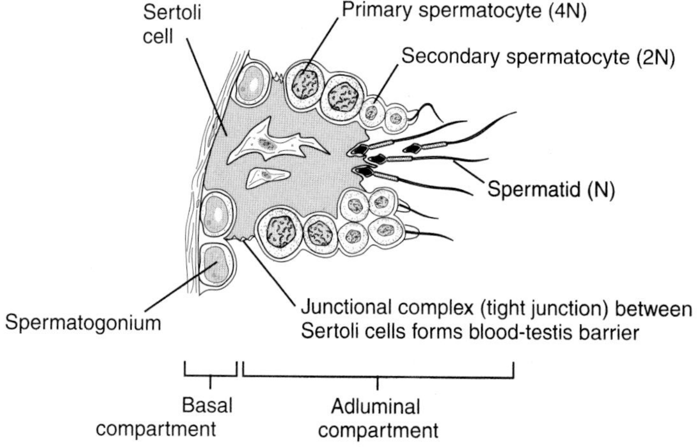

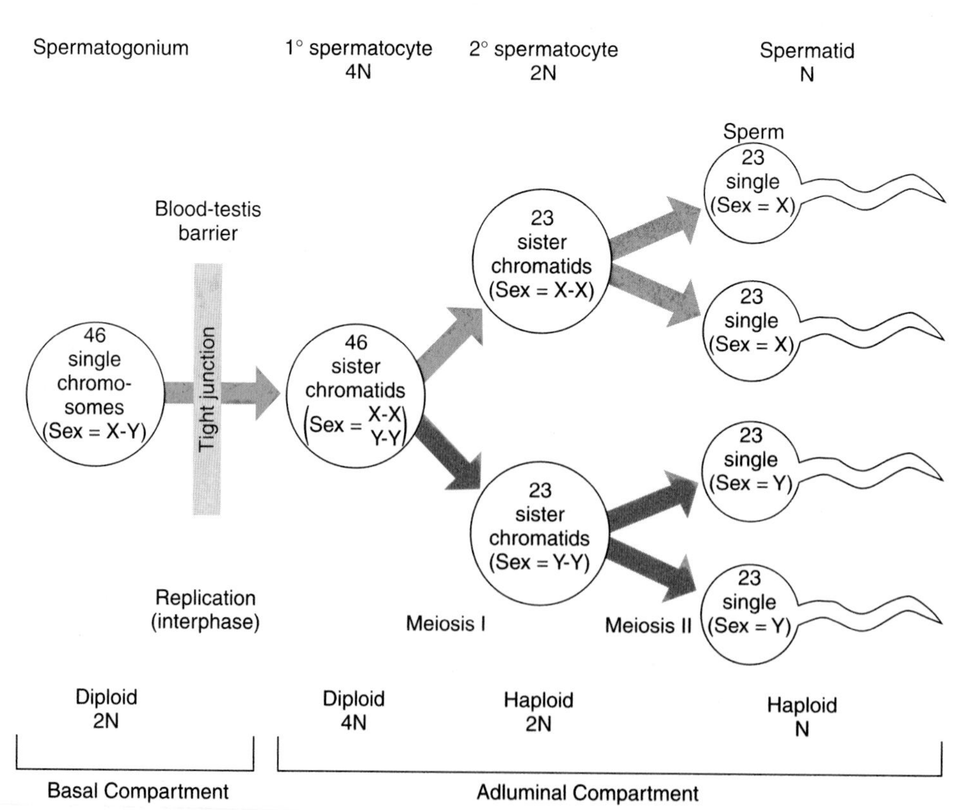

Male spermatogenesis

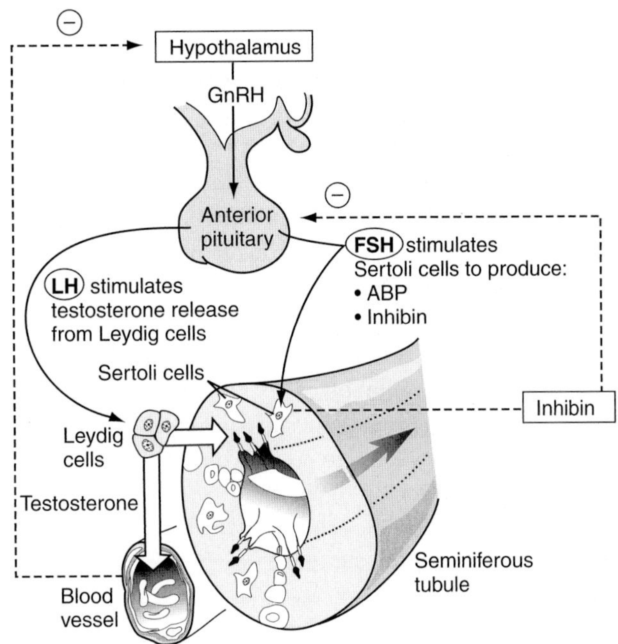

PRODUCTS	FUNCTIONS OF PRODUCTS
Androgen-binding protein (ABP)	Ensures that testosterone in seminiferous tubule is high
Inhibin	Inhibits FSH
Testosterone	Differentiates male genitalia, has anabolic effects on protein metabolism, maintains gametogenesis, maintains libido, inhibits GnRH, and fuses epiphyseal plates in bone

FSH → **S**ertoli cells → **S**perm production
LH → **L**eydig cell → testosterone

Androgens

Testosterone, dihydrotestosterone (DHT), androstenedione.

Source

DHT and testosterone (testis), androstenedione (adrenal).

Potency—DHT > testosterone > androstenedione.

Targets

Prostate, seminal vesicles, epididymis, liver, muscle, brain, skin.

Testosterone is converted to DHT by the enzyme 5α-reductase, which is inhibited by finasteride.

Function

1. Differentiation of wolffian duct system into internal gonadal structures
2. 2° sexual characteristics and growth spurt during puberty, close epiphyseal plates
3. Required for normal spermatogenesis
4. Anabolic effects—↑ muscle size, ↑ RBC production
5. ↑ libido

Testosterone and androstenedione are converted to estrogen in adipose tissue and Sertoli cells by enzyme aromatase.

Estrogen		
Source	Ovary (17β-estradiol), placenta (estriol), blood (aromatization).	Potency—estradiol > estrone > estriol.
Function	1. Growth of follicle 2. Endometrial proliferation 3. Development of genitalia 4. Stromal development of breast 5. Female fat distribution 6. Hepatic synthesis of transport proteins (↑ synthesis of sex hormone–binding globulin) 7. Feedback inhibition of FSH and LH 8. LH surge (estrogen negative feedback on LH secretion switches to positive from negative just before LH surge) 9. ↑ myometrial excitability 10. ↑ HDL, ↓ LDL	Pregnancy: 50-fold ↑ in estradiol and estrone 1000-fold ↑ in estriol (indicator of fetal well-being)

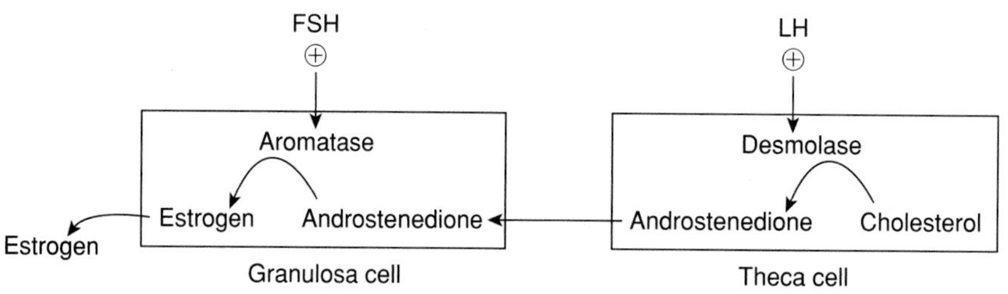

Progesterone		
Source	Corpus luteum, placenta, adrenal cortex, testes.	Elevation of progesterone is indicative of ovulation.
Function	1. Stimulation of endometrial glandular secretions and spiral artery development 2. Maintenance of pregnancy 3. ↓ myometrial excitability 4. Production of thick cervical mucus, which inhibits sperm entry into the uterus 5. ↑ body temperature 6. Inhibition of gonadotropins (LH, FSH) 7. Uterine smooth muscle relaxation (preventing contractions)	Progesterone Prepares for Pregnancy.

Menstrual cycle

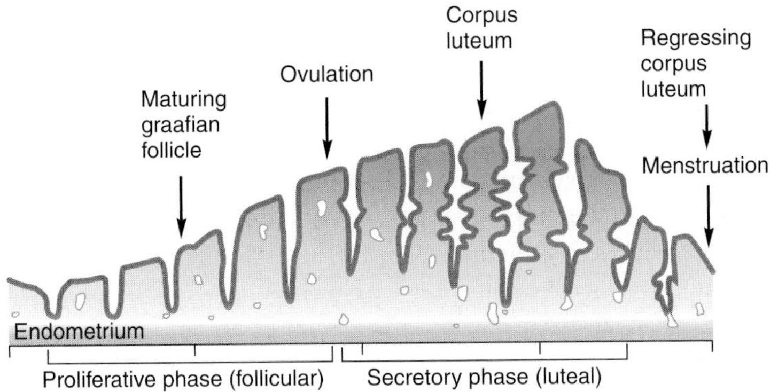

Follicular growth is fastest during 2nd week of proliferative phase.

Estrogen stimulates endometrial proliferation.

Progesterone maintains endometrium to support implantation.

↓ progesterone leads to ↓ fertility.

Follicular phase can vary in length. Luteal phase is usually a constant 14 days. Ovulation day = menstruation day 14.

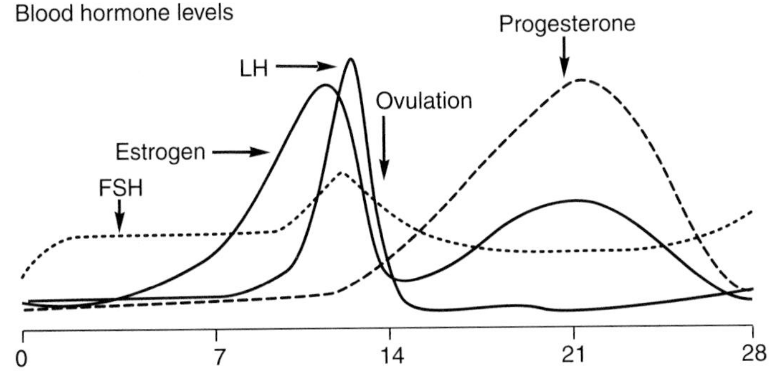

Estrogen
↓
LH
↓
Ovulate
↓
Progesterone (from corpus luteum)
↓
Period

Ovulation

Estrogen surge day before ovulation.
Stimulates LH, inhibits FSH.
LH surge causes ovulation (rupture of follicle).
↑ temperature (progesterone induced).
Ferning of cervical mucosa.
Oral contraceptives prevent estrogen surge, LH surge → ovulation does not occur.

Mittelschmerz—blood from ruptured follicle causes peritoneal irritation that can mimic appendicitis.

Meiosis and ovulation

1° oocytes begin meiosis I during fetal life and complete meiosis I just prior to ovulation.
Meiosis I is arrested in pr**O**phase for years until **O**vulation (1° oocytes).
Meiosis II is arrested in **MET**aphase until fertilization (2° oocytes).

An egg **MET** a sperm.

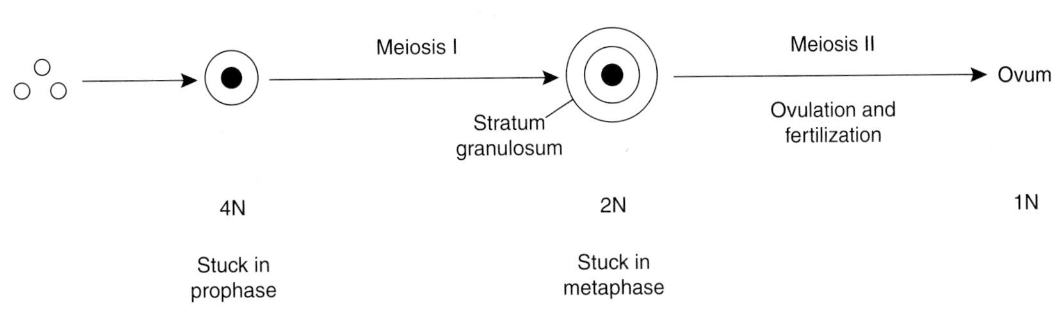

Pregnancy

Fertilization most commonly occurs in upper end of oviduct. Occurs within 1 day after ovulation.

Implantation occurs 6 days after fertilization. Trophoblasts secrete β-hCG, which is detectable in blood 1 week after conception and on home test in urine 2 weeks after conception.

↑ estrogen, progesterone, oxytocin, and prolactin at term (hCG peak is in 1st trimester).

Lactation—during pregnancy, estrogen inhibits prolactin and inhibits lactation. After labor, the ↓ in maternal estrogen induces lactation. Suckling is required to maintain milk production, since ↑ nerve stimulation ↑ oxytocin.

hCG

Source: Syncytiotrophoblast of placenta.

Function:
1. Maintains the corpus luteum (and thus progesterone) for the 1st trimester by acting like LH (otherwise no luteal cell stimulation, and abortion results). In the 2nd and 3rd trimester, the placenta synthesizes its own estriol and progesterone and the corpus luteum degenerates.
2. Used to detect pregnancy because it appears early in the urine (see above).
3. Elevated hCG in women with hydatidiform moles or choriocarcinoma.

Menopause

Cessation of estrogen production with age-linked decline in number of ovarian follicles. Average age of onset is 51 years (earlier in smokers).

Hormonal changes: ↓ estrogen, ↑↑ FSH, ↑ LH (no surge), ↑ GnRH.

Menopause causes **HAVOC**: **H**ot flashes, **A**trophy of the **V**agina, **O**steoporosis, **C**oronary artery disease.

Early menopause can indicate premature ovarian failure.

▶ REPRODUCTIVE–PATHOLOGY

Bicornuate uterus

Results from incomplete fusion of the paramesonephric ducts. Associated with urinary tract abnormalities and infertility.

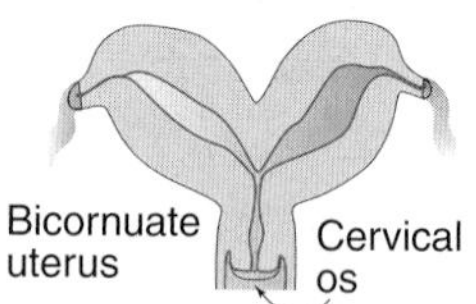

Congenital penile abnormalities

Hypospadias

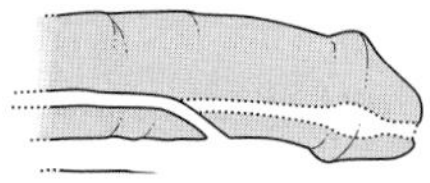

Hypospadias—abnormal opening of penile urethra on inferior (ventral) side of penis due to failure of urethral folds to close.

Epispadias

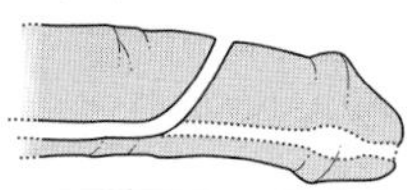

Epispadias—abnormal opening of penile urethra on superior (dorsal) side of penis due to faulty positioning of genital tubercle.

Hypospadias is more common than epispadias. Fix hypospadias to prevent UTIs.

Hypo is **below.**

Exstrophy of the bladder is associated with **E**pispadias.

When you have **E**pispadias, you hit your **E**ye when you p**EE**.

Sex chromosome disorders

Klinefelter's syndrome [male] (XXY), 1:850	Testicular atrophy, eunuchoid body shape, tall, long extremities, gynecomastia, female hair distribution. Presence of inactivated X chromosome (Barr body) (see Image 108). Common cause of hypogonadism seen in infertility workup.	Dysgenesis of seminiferous tubules → ↓ inhibin → ↑ FSH. Abnormal Leydig cell function → ↓ testosterone → ↑ LH → ↑ estrogen.
Turner's syndrome [female] **(XO)**, 1:3000	Short stature, ovarian dysgenesis (streak ovary), webbing of neck, preductal coarctation of the aorta, most common cause of 1° amenorrhea. No Barr body (see Image 109).	"Hugs and kisses" **(XO)** from Tina **Turner** (female). ↓ estrogen leads to ↑ LH and FSH.
Double Y males [male] (XYY), 1:1000	Phenotypically normal, very tall, severe acne, antisocial behavior (seen in 1–2% of XYY males). Normal fertility.	Observed with ↑ frequency among inmates of penal institutions.

Pseudo-hermaphroditism	Disagreement between the phenotypic (external genitalia) and gonadal (testes vs. ovaries) sex.
Female pseudo-hermaphrodite (XX)	Ovaries present, but external genitalia are virilized or ambiguous. Due to excessive and inappropriate exposure to androgenic steroids during early gestation (i.e., congenital adrenal hyperplasia or exogenous administration of androgens during pregnancy).
Male pseudo-hermaphrodite (XY)	Testes present, but external genitalia are female or ambiguous. Most common form is androgen insensitivity syndrome (testicular feminization).
True hermaphrodite (46,XX or 47,XXY)	Both ovary and testicular tissue present; ambiguous genitalia. Very rare.
Androgen insensitivity syndrome (46,XY)	Defect in androgen receptor resulting in normal-appearing female; female external genitalia with rudimentary vagina; uterus and uterine tubes generally absent; develops testes (often found in labia majora; surgically removed to prevent malignancy). Levels of testosterone, estrogen, and LH are all high.
5α-reductase deficiency	Unable to convert testosterone to DHT. Ambiguous genitalia until puberty, when ↑ testosterone causes masculinization of genitalia. Testosterone/estrogen levels are normal; LH is normal or ↑. "Penis at 12" (when testosterone production begins at puberty, it stimulates growth of external male genitalia).

Hydatidiform mole	A pathologic ovum ("empty egg"—ovum with no DNA) resulting in cystic swelling of chorionic villi and proliferation of chorionic epithelium (trophoblast). Most common precursor of choriocarcinoma. High β-hCG. "Honeycombed uterus," "cluster of grapes" appearance. Genotype of a **complete** mole is 46,XX and is **completely** paternal in origin (no maternal chromosomes). Complete moles have no associated fetus and commonly lead to an abnormally enlarged uterus. **PART**ial mole is made up of 3 or more **PARTS** (triploid or tetraploid); may contain fetal **PARTS.** Partial moles are less likely to be associated with excessive uterine size (see Color Image 74). Moles can lead to uterine rupture. Treat with dilatation and curettage and methotrexate. Monitor β-hCG.	Complete—2 sperm + empty egg. Partial—2 sperm + 1 egg.

Pregnancy-induced hypertension (preeclampsia-eclampsia)	Preeclampsia is the triad of hypertension, proteinuria, and edema; eclampsia is the addition of seizures to the triad. Affects 7% of pregnant women from 20 weeks' gestation to 6 weeks postpartum (before 20 weeks suggests molar pregnancy). ↑ incidence in patients with preexisting hypertension, diabetes, chronic renal disease, and autoimmune disorders. Etiology involves placental ischemia (lack of trophoblastic invasion of spiral arteries in myometrium). Can be associated with HELLP syndrome (**H**emolysis, **E**levated **L**FTs, **L**ow **P**latelets). Mortality due to cerebral hemorrhage and ARDS.
Clinical features	Headache, blurred vision, abdominal pain, edema of face and extremities, altered mentation, hyperreflexia; lab findings may include thrombocytopenia, hyperuricemia.
Treatment	Delivery of fetus as soon as viable. Otherwise bed rest, salt restriction, and monitoring and treatment of hypertension. For eclampsia, a medical emergency, IV magnesium sulfate and diazepam.

Pregnancy complications	**Abruptio placentae**—premature detachment of placenta from implantation site. **Painful** uterine bleeding (usually during 3rd trimester). Fetal death. May be associated with DIC. ↑ risk with smoking, hypertension, cocaine use.	Painful bleeding.
	Placenta accreta—defective decidual layer allows placenta to attach directly to myometrium. Predisposed by prior C-section or inflammation. May have massive hemorrhage after delivery.	Massive bleeding.
	Placenta previa—attachment of placenta to lower uterine segment. May occlude internal os. **Painless** bleeding in any trimester. Prior C-section predisposes.	Painless bleeding.
	Ectopic pregnancy—most often in fallopian tubes, predisposed by salpingitis (PID). Suspect with ↑ hCG and sudden lower abdominal pain; confirm with ultrasound. Often clinically mistaken for appendicitis.	Pain without bleeding.

Amniotic fluid abnormalities

Polyhydramnios	> 1.5–2 L of amniotic fluid; associated with esophageal/duodenal atresia, causing inability to swallow amniotic fluid, and with anencephaly.
Oligohydramnios	< 0.5 L of amniotic fluid; associated with bilateral renal agenesis or posterior urethral valves (in males) and resultant inability to excrete urine. Can give rise to Potter's syndrome.

Cervical pathology

Dysplasia and carcinoma in situ	Disordered epithelial growth; begins at basal layer of squamo-columnar junction and extends outward. Classified as CIN 1, CIN 2, or CIN 3 (carcinoma in situ), depending on extent of dysplasia. Associated with HPV **16, 18.** Vaccine—Gardasil (tetravalent). May progress slowly to invasive carcinoma.
Invasive carcinoma	Often squamous cell carcinoma. Pap smear can catch cervical dysplasia (koilocytes) before it progresses to invasive carcinoma. Lateral invasion can block ureters, causing renal failure.

Uterine pathology

Endometriosis	Non-neoplastic endometrial glands/stroma in abnormal locations outside the uterus. Characterized by cyclic bleeding (menstrual type) from ectopic endometrial tissue resulting in blood-filled "chocolate cysts." In ovary or on peritoneum. Manifests clinically as severe menstrual-related pain. Often results in infertility (see Color Image 77). Can be due to retrograde menstrual flow.
Adenomyosis	Endometriosis within the myometrium.
Endometrial hyperplasia	Abnormal endometrial gland proliferation usually caused by excess estrogen stimulation. ↑ risk for endometrial carcinoma. Most commonly manifests clinically as postmenopausal vaginal bleeding. Risk factors include anovulatory cycles, hormone replacement therapy, polycystic ovarian syndrome, and granulosa cell tumor.
Endometrial carcinoma	Most common gynecologic malignancy. Peak age 55–65 years of age. Clinically presents with vaginal bleeding. Typically preceded by endometrial hyperplasia. Risk factors include prolonged use of estrogen without progestins, obesity, diabetes, hypertension, nulliparity, and late menopause. Prognosis correlates with degree of myometrial invasion.
Leiomyoma (fibroid)	Most common of all tumors in females. Often presents with multiple tumors with well-demarcated borders. ↑ incidence in blacks. Benign smooth muscle tumor; malignant transformation is rare. Estrogen sensitive—tumor size ↑ with pregnancy and ↓ with menopause. Peak occurrence in women 20–40 years of age. May be asymptomatic or may cause abnormal uterine bleeding. Severe bleeding may lead to iron deficiency anemia. Does not progress to leiomyosarcoma (see Image 129). Whorled pattern of smooth muscle bundles.
Leiomyosarcoma	Bulky, irregularly shaped tumor with areas of necrosis and hemorrhage, typically arising de novo (not from leiomyoma). ↑ incidence in blacks. Highly aggressive tumor with tendency to recur. May protrude from cervix and bleed.

Gynecological tumor epidemiology	Incidence—endometrial > ovarian > cervical. Worst prognosis—ovarian > cervical > endometrial.

Polycystic ovarian syndrome

↑ LH, ↓ FSH, ↑ testosterone. ↑ LH production leads to anovulation, hyperandrogenism due to deranged steroid synthesis. Enlarged, bilateral cystic ovaries manifest clinically with amenorrhea, infertility, obesity, and hirsutism. Associated with insulin resistance. ↑ risk of endometrial cancer. Treat with weight loss, OCPs, gonadotropin analogs, clomiphene, or surgery.

Ovarian cysts

1. Follicular cyst—distention of unruptured graafian follicle. May be associated with hyperestrinism and endometrial hyperplasia.
2. Corpus luteum cyst—hemorrhage into persistent corpus luteum. Menstrual irregularity.
3. Theca-lutein cyst—often bilateral/multiple. Due to gonadotropin stimulation. Associated with choriocarcinoma and moles.
4. "Chocolate cyst"—blood-containing cyst from ovarian endometriosis. Varies with menstrual cycle.

Ovarian germ cell tumors

Type	Characteristics	Tumor markers
Dysgerminoma	Malignant, equivalent to male seminoma. Sheets of uniform cells.	hCG.
Choriocarcinoma	Rare but malignant; can develop during pregnancy in mother or baby. Large, hyperchromatic syncytiotrophoblastic cells. ↑ frequency of theca-lutein cysts.	hCG.
Yolk sac (endodermal sinus tumor)	Aggressive malignancy in ovaries (testes in boys) and sacrococcygeal area of young children.	AFP.
Teratoma	90% of ovarian germ cell tumors (see Images 130, 131). Contain cells from 2 or 3 germ layers. Mature teratoma ("dermoid cyst")—most frequent benign ovarian tumor. Immature teratoma—aggressively malignant. Struma ovarii—contains functional thyroid tissue. Can present as hyperthyroidism.	

Ovarian non–germ cell tumors	1. Serous cystadenoma—20% of ovarian tumors. Frequently bilateral, lined with fallopian tube–like epithelium. Benign. 2. Serous cystadenocarcinoma—50% ovarian tumors, malignant and frequently bilateral. 3. Mucinous cystadenoma—multilocular cyst lined by mucus-secreting epithelium. Benign. 4. Mucinous cystadenocarcinoma—malignant. Pseudomyxoma peritonei—intraperitoneal accumulation of mucinous material from ovarian or appendiceal tumor. 5. **B**renner tumor—**B**enign. Looks like **B**ladder. 6. Fibromas—bundles of spindle-shaped fibroblasts. Meigs' syndrome—triad of ovarian fibroma, ascites, and hydrothorax. Pulling sensation in groin. 7. Granulosa cell tumor—secretes estrogen → precocious puberty (kids). Can cause endometrial hyperplasia or carcinoma in adults. Call-Exner bodies—small follicles filled with eosinophilic secretions. 8. Krukenberg tumor—GI malignancy that metastasizes to ovaries, causing a mucin-secreting signet cell adenocarcinoma.	↑ CA-125 is general ovarian cancer marker. Risk factors—BRCA-1, HNPCC.
Vaginal carcinoma	1. Squamous cell carcinoma—2° to cervical SCC. 2. Clear cell adenocarcinoma—exposure to DES. 3. Sarcoma botryoides (rhabdomyosarcoma variant)—affects girls < 4 years of age; spindle-shaped tumor cells that are desmin positive.	

Breast tumors

Type	Characteristics
Benign tumors	1. Fibroadenoma—most common tumor < 25 years. Small, mobile, firm mass with sharp edges. ↑ size and tenderness with pregnancy. Not a precursor to breast cancer. 2. Intraductal papilloma—tumor of lactiferous ducts; presents with serous or bloody nipple discharge. 3. Phyllodes tumor—large, bulky mass of connective tissue and cysts. Tumor may have "leaflike" projections. Some may be malignant (cystosarcoma phyllodes).
Malignant tumors (carcinoma)	Common postmenopause. Arise from mammary duct epithelium or lobular glands. Overexpression of estrogen/progesterone receptors or *erb*-B2 (HER-2, an EGF receptor) is common; affects therapy and prognosis (give tamoxifen for ER/PR-positive tumors). Axillary lymph node involvement is the single most important prognostic factor. Histologic types: 1. **Noninvasive:** Ductal carcinoma in situ (DCIS)—early malignancy without basement membrane penetration. 2. **Invasive** (in descending order of incidence): a. Invasive ductal, no specific type (76%)—firm, fibrous mass. Worst and most invasive. Common. b. Invasive lobular (8%)—often multiple, bilateral, orderly rows of cells. c. Medullary (1.2%–10%)—fleshy, cellular, lymphocytic infiltrate. Good prognosis. d. Comedocarcinoma (1.6%)—ductal, caseous necrosis. e. Inflammatory—lymphatic involvement; red, swollen; peau d'orange (breast skin resembles orange peel). f. Paget's disease of the breast—eczematous patches on nipple. Paget cells—large cells with clear halo; suggest underlying carcinoma. Also seen on vulva. Risk factors: gender, age, early 1st menarche (< 12 years old), delayed 1st pregnancy (> 30 years old), late menopause (> 50 years old), family history of 1st-degree relative with breast cancer at a young age. Risk is NOT increased by fibroadenoma or nonhyperplastic cysts.

Common breast conditions		
Fibrocystic disease	Most common cause of "breast lumps" from age 25 to menopause. Presents with diffuse breast pain and multiple lesions, often bilateral. Usually does not indicate ↑ risk of carcinoma. Histologic types: 1. Fibrosis—hyperplasia of breast stroma. 2. Cystic—fluid filled, blue dome. 3. Sclerosing—↑ acini and intralobular fibrosis. 4. Epithelial hyperplasia—↑ in number of epithelial cell layers in terminal duct lobule. ↑ risk of carcinoma with atypical cells. Occurs in women > 30 years of age.	
Acute mastitis	Breast abscess; during breast-feeding, ↑ risk of bacterial infection through cracks in the nipple; S. *aureus* is the most common pathogen.	
Fat necrosis	A benign painless lump; forms as a result of injury to breast tissue.	
Gynecomastia	Results from hyperestrogenism (cirrhosis, testicular tumor, puberty, old age), Klinefelter's syndrome, or drugs (estrogen, marijuana, heroin, psychoactive drugs, **S**pironolactone, **D**igitalis, **C**imetidine, **A**lcohol, **K**etoconazole).	**S**ome **D**rugs **C**reate **A**wesome **K**nockers.

Prostate pathology	Prostatitis—dysuria, frequency, urgency, low back pain. Acute: bacterial (e.g., *E. coli*); chronic: bacterial or abacterial (most common).
Benign prostatic hyperplasia (not hypertrophy)	Common in men > 50 years of age. May be due to an age-related ↑ in estradiol with possible sensitization of the prostate to the growth-promoting effects of DHT. Characterized by a nodular enlargement of the periurethral (lateral and middle) lobes of the prostate gland, compressing the urethra into a vertical slit. Often presents with ↑ frequency of urination, nocturia, difficulty starting and stopping the stream of urine, and dysuria. May lead to distention and hypertrophy of the bladder, hydronephrosis, and UTIs. Not considered a premalignant lesion. ↑ free prostate-specific antigen (PSA).
Prostatic adenocarcinoma	Common in men > 50 years of age. Arises most often from the posterior lobe (peripheral zone) of the prostate gland and is most frequently diagnosed by digital rectal examination (hard nodule) and prostate biopsy. Prostatic acid phosphatase (PAP) and PSA are useful tumor markers (↑ total PSA, with ↓ fraction of free PSA). Osteoblastic metastases in bone may develop in late stages, as indicated by lower back pain and an ↑ in serum alkaline phosphatase and PSA.
Cryptorchidism	Undescended testis (one or both); lack of spermatogenesis due to ↑ body temperature; associated with ↑ risk of germ cell tumors. Prematurity ↑ the risk of cryptorchidism.

Testicular germ cell tumors	~95% of all testicular tumors.
Seminoma	Malignant; painless testicular enlargement; most common testicular tumor, mostly affecting males age 15–35. Large cells in lobules with watery cytoplasm and a "fried egg" appearance. Radiosensitive. Late metastasis, excellent prognosis.
Embryonal carcinoma	Malignant; painful; worse prognosis than seminoma. Often glandular/papillary morphology. Can differentiate to other tumors.
Yolk sac (endodermal sinus) tumor	Analogous to ovarian yolk sac tumor. Schiller-Duval bodies, primitive glomeruli (↑ AFP).
Choriocarcinoma	Malignant, ↑ hCG.
Teratoma	Unlike in females, mature teratoma in males is most often malignant.

Testicular non–germ cell tumors	5% of all testicular tumors. Mostly benign.
Leydig cell	Benign, contains Reinke crystals; usually androgen producing, gynecomastia in men, precocious puberty in boys.
Sertoli cell	Benign, androblastoma from sex cord stroma.
Testicular lymphoma	Most common testicular cancer in older men.

Tunica vaginalis lesions

Lesions in the serous covering of testis—present as testicular masses that can be transilluminated (vs. testicular tumors).

1. Varicocele—dilated vein in pampiniform plexus; can cause infertility; "bag of worms"
2. Hydrocele—↑ fluid 2° to incomplete fusion of processus vaginalis
3. Spermatocele—dilated epididymal duct

Penile pathology	
Carcinoma in situ	
Erythroplasia of Queyrat	Red velvety plaques, usually involving the glans; otherwise similar to Bowen's disease.
Bowenoid papulosis	Multiple papular lesions; affects younger age group than other subtypes; usually does not become invasive.
Bowen's disease	Gray, solitary, crusty plaque, usually on the shaft of the penis or on the scrotum; peak incidence in 5th decade of life; progresses to invasive SCC in < 10% of cases.
Squamous cell carcinoma (SCC)	Rare in circumcised men; uncommon in the United States and Europe, more common in Asia, Africa, and South America. Commonly associated with HPV.
Peyronie's disease	Bent penis due to acquired fibrous tissue formation.

Antiandrogens	Testosterone $\xrightarrow{5\alpha\text{-reductase}}$ DHT (more potent).	
Finasteride (Propecia)	A 5α-reductase inhibitor (↓ conversion of testosterone to dihydrotestosterone). Useful in BPH. Also promotes hair growth—used to treat male-pattern baldness.	To prevent male-pattern hair growth, give a drug that will encourage female breast growth.
Flutamide	A nonsteroidal competitive inhibitor of androgens at the testosterone receptor. Used in prostate carcinoma.	Ketoconazole and spironolactone are used in the treatment of polycystic ovarian syndrome to prevent hirsutism. Both have side effects of gynecomastia and amenorrhea.
Ketoconazole	Inhibits steroid synthesis.	
Spironolactone	Inhibits steroid binding.	

Leuprolide		
Mechanism	GnRH analog with agonist properties when used in pulsatile fashion; antagonist properties when used in continuous fashion.	**Leu**prolide can be used in **lieu** of GnRH.
Clinical use	Infertility (pulsatile), prostate cancer (continuous—use with flutamide), uterine fibroids.	
Toxicity	Antiandrogen, nausea, vomiting.	

Sildenafil, vardenafil		
Mechanism	Inhibit cGMP phosphodiesterase, causing ↑ cGMP, smooth muscle relaxation in the corpus cavernosum, ↑ blood flow, and penile erection.	Sildena**fil** and vardena**fil** **fill** the penis.
Clinical use	Treatment of erectile dysfunction.	
Toxicity	Headache, flushing, dyspepsia, impaired blue-green color vision. Risk of life-threatening hypotension in patients taking nitrates.	

Mifepristone (RU-486)	
Mechanism	Competitive inhibitor of progestins at progesterone receptors.
Clinical use	Termination of pregnancy. Administered with misoprostol (PGE_1).
Toxicity	Heavy bleeding, GI effects (nausea, vomiting, anorexia), abdominal pain.

Oral contraception (synthetic progestins, estrogen)	Advantages	Disadvantages
	Reliable (< 1% failure)	Taken daily
	↓ risk of endometrial and ovarian cancer	No protection against STDs
	↓ incidence of ectopic pregnancy	↑ triglycerides
	↓ pelvic infections	Depression, weight gain, nausea, hypertension
	Regulation of menses	Hypercoagulable state

Hormone replacement therapy (HRT)	Used for relief or prevention of menopausal symptoms (e.g., hot flashes, vaginal atrophy) and osteoporosis (due to diminished estrogen levels). Unopposed estrogen replacement therapy (ERT) ↑ the risk of endometrial cancer, so progesterone is added. Possible ↑ CV risk.

Dinoprostone — PGE_2 analog causing cervical dilation and uterine contraction, inducing labor.

Ritodrine/terbutaline — β_2-agonists that relax the uterus.

Anastrozole — Aromatase inhibitor used in postmenopausal women with breast cancer.

Testosterone (methyltestosterone)

- Mechanism — Agonist at androgen receptors.
- Clinical use — Treat hypogonadism and promote development of 2° sex characteristics; stimulation of anabolism to promote recovery after burn or injury; treat ER-positive breast cancer (exemestane).
- Toxicity — Causes masculinization in females; reduces intratesticular testosterone in males by inhibiting Leydig cells; leads to gonadal atrophy. Premature closure of epiphyseal plates. ↑ LDL, ↓ HDL.

Estrogens (ethinyl estradiol, DES, mestranol)

- Mechanism — Bind estrogen receptors.
- Clinical use — Hypogonadism or ovarian failure, menstrual abnormalities, HRT in postmenopausal women; use in men with androgen-dependent prostate cancer.
- Toxicity — ↑ risk of endometrial cancer, bleeding in postmenopausal women, clear cell adenocarcinoma of vagina in females exposed to DES in utero, ↑ risk of thrombi. Contraindications—ER-positive breast cancer.

Progestins

- Mechanism — Bind progesterone receptors, reduce growth, and ↑ vascularization of endometrium.
- Clinical use — Used in oral contraceptives and in the treatment of endometrial cancer and abnormal uterine bleeding.

Estrogen partial agonists (selective estrogen receptor modulators—SERMs)

- Clomiphene — Partial agonist at estrogen receptors in pituitary gland. Prevents normal feedback inhibition and ↑ release of LH and FSH from pituitary, which stimulates ovulation. Used to treat infertility and PCOS. May cause hot flashes, ovarian enlargement, multiple simultaneous pregnancies, and visual disturbances.
- Tamoxifen — Antagonist on breast tissue; used to treat and prevent recurrence of ER-positive breast cancer.
- Raloxifene — Agonist on bone; reduces reabsorption of bone; used to treat osteoporosis.

Respiratory

"There's so much pollution in the air now that if it weren't for our lungs, there'd be no place to put it all."

—Robert Orben

"Mars is essentially in the same orbit. Somewhat the same distance from the Sun, which is very important. We have seen pictures where there are canals, we believe, and water. If there is water, that means there is oxygen. If there is oxygen, that means we can breathe."

—Former Vice President Dan Quayle

Vignette	Question	Answer
Patient exhibits an extended expiratory phase.	What is the disease process?	Obstructive lung disease.
Tall, thin male teenager has abrupt-onset dyspnea and left-sided chest pain. There is hyperresonant percussion on the affected side, and breath sounds are diminished.	What is the diagnosis?	Spontaneous pneumothorax.
Young man is concerned about his wife's inability to conceive and her recurrent URIs. She has dextrocardia.	Which of her proteins is defective?	Dynein (Kartagener's).
The following lung volumes are obtained from an elderly smoker: FRC 5.0 L, IRV 1.5 L, IC 2.0 L, VC 3.5 L.	What is his TLC?	7.0 L.
Preterm infant has difficulty breathing. An x-ray reveals ↑ lung densities.	What is the diagnosis, and what could have prevented this condition?	Neonatal respiratory distress syndrome; administration of maternal steroids before birth to ↑ surfactant production.
25-year-old comatose man on ventilatory support following an automobile accident develops fever and dies. Autopsy reveals a pus-filled cavity in his right lung.	What is the likely etiology?	Aspiration of infective material leading to lung abscess.
52-year-old woman undergoing menopause is chronically tired.	What is the most likely diagnosis, and what changes have occurred in her oxygen content and saturation?	Anemia due to chronic blood loss. ↓ oxygen content; oxygen saturation unchanged.
Patient is shown to have hypoxia despite a normal chest x-ray.	What is the cause of the hypoxia, and what disease process does it mimic?	Pulmonary embolism. May be mistaken for an MI.
Patient is shown to have hypoxia and has an abnormal chest x-ray showing an enlarged heart.	What is the most likely cause of the hypoxia?	CHF.

Respiratory tree

Conducting zone	Consists of nose, pharynx, trachea, bronchi, bronchioles, and terminal bronchioles. Cartilage is present only in the trachea and bronchi. Brings air in and out. Warms, humidifies, filters air. Anatomic dead space. Walls of conducting airways contain smooth muscle.
Respiratory zone	Consists of respiratory bronchioles, alveolar ducts, and alveoli. Participates in gas exchange.

Pneumocytes

Pseudocolumnar ciliated cells extend to the respiratory bronchioles; goblet cells extend only to the terminal bronchioles.

Type I cells (97% of alveolar surfaces) line the alveoli. Squamous; thin for optimal gas diffusion.

Type II cells (3%) secrete pulmonary surfactant (dipalmitoyl phosphatidylcholine), which ↓ the alveolar surface tension. Cuboidal and clustered. Also serve as precursors to type I cells and other type II cells. Type II cells proliferate during lung damage.

Clara cells—nonciliated; columnar with secretory granules. Secrete component of surfactant; degrade toxins; act as reserve cells.

Mucus secretions are swept out of the lungs toward the mouth by ciliated cells.

A lecithin-to-sphingomyelin ratio of > 2.0 in amniotic fluid is indicative of fetal lung maturity.

Gas exchange barrier

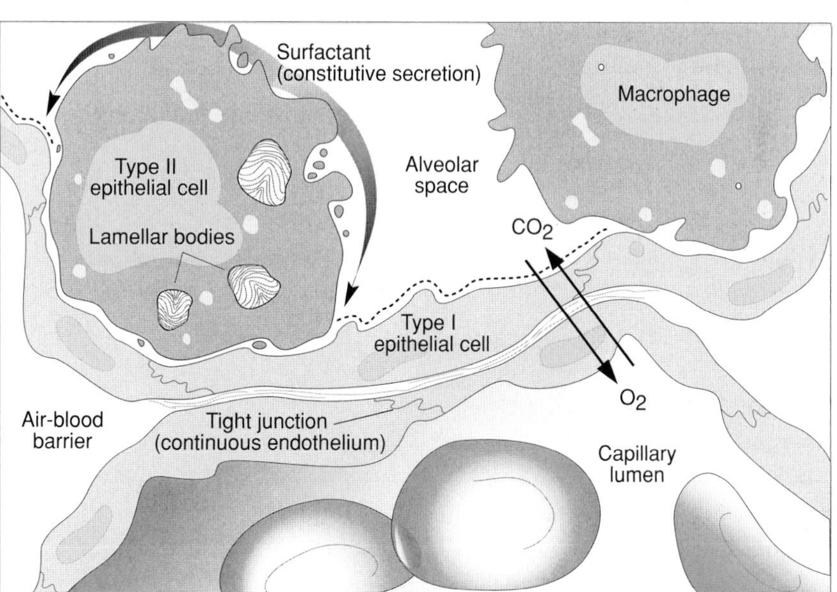

Bronchopulmonary segments

Each bronchopulmonary segment has a 3° (segmental) bronchus and 2 arteries (bronchial and pulmonary) in the center; veins and lymphatics drain along the borders.

Pulmonary arteries carry deoxygenated blood from the right side of the heart. Elastic walls maintain pulmonary arterial pressure at relatively constant levels throughout cardiac cycle.

Arteries run with Airways.

Lung relations	Right lung has 3 lobes; **L**eft has 2 lobes and **L**ingula (homologue of right middle lobe). Right lung is more common site for inhaled foreign body because the right main stem bronchus is wider and more vertical than the left.	Instead of a middle lobe, the left lung has a space occupied by the heart. The relation of the pulmonary artery to the bronchus at each lung hilus is described by **RALS**—**R**ight **A**nterior; **L**eft **S**uperior.

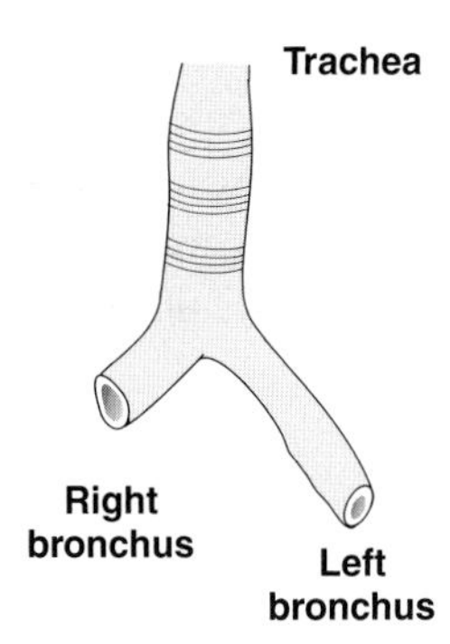

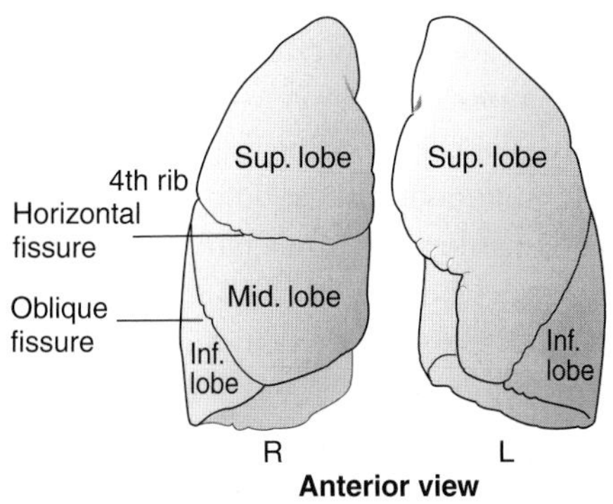

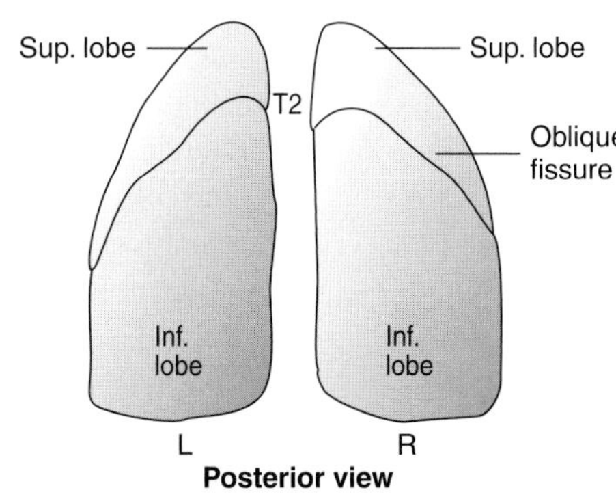

Diaphragm structures	Structures perforating diaphragm: At T8: IVC. At T10: esophagus, vagus (2 trunks). At T12: aorta (red), thoracic duct (white), azygous vein (blue). Diaphragm is innervated by **C3, 4,** and **5** (phrenic nerve). Pain from the diaphragm can be referred to the shoulder.	Number of letters = T level: **T8:** vena cava **T10:** (o)esophagus **T12:** aortic hiatus "**C3, 4, 5** keeps the diaphragm alive."

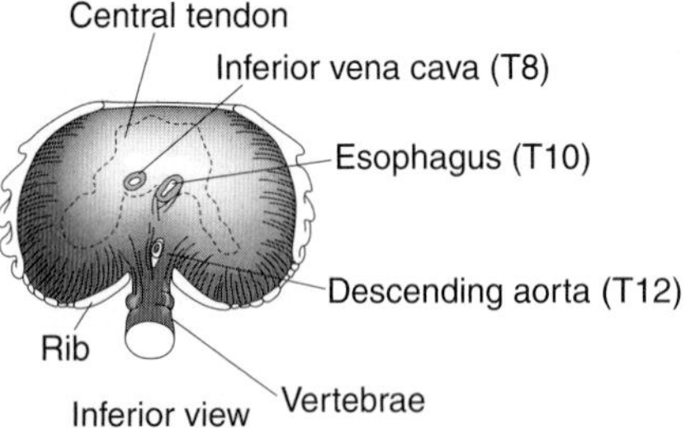

Muscles of respiration	Quiet breathing: Inspiration—diaphragm. Expiration—passive. Exercise: Inspiration—external intercostals, scalene muscles, sternomastoids. Expiration—rectus abdominis, internal and external obliques, transversus abdominis, internal intercostals.

Important lung products

1. Surfactant—produced by type II pneumocytes, ↓ alveolar surface tension, ↑ compliance, ↓ work of inspiration
2. Prostaglandins
3. Histamine ↑ bronchoconstriction
4. Angiotensin-converting enzyme (ACE)—angiotensin I → angiotensin II; inactivates bradykinin (ACE inhibitors ↑ bradykinin and cause cough, angioedema)
5. Kallikrein—activates bradykinin

Surfactant—dipalmitoyl phosphatidylcholine (lecithin) deficient in neonatal RDS.

Collapsing pressure = $\frac{2 \text{ (tension)}}{\text{radius}}$

Lung volumes

1. Residual volume (RV)—air in lung after maximal expiration
2. Expiratory reserve volume (ERV)—air that can still be breathed out after normal expiration
3. Tidal volume (TV)—air that moves into lung with each quiet inspiration, typically 500 mL
4. Inspiratory reserve volume (IRV)—air in excess of tidal volume that moves into lung on maximum inspiration
5. Vital capacity (VC)—TV + IRV + ERV
6. Functional residual capacity (FRC)—RV + ERV (volume in lungs after normal expiration)
7. Inspiratory capacity (IC)—IRV + TV
8. Total lung capacity—TLC = IRV + TV + ERV + RV

Vital capacity is everything but the residual volume.

A capacity is a sum of ≥ 2 volumes.

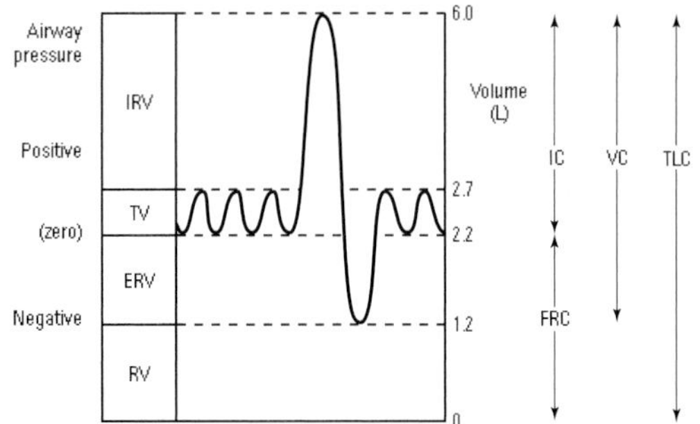

Determination of physiologic dead space

$$V_D = V_T \times \frac{(PaCO_2 - PeCO_2)}{PaCO_2}$$

V_D = physiologic dead space = anatomical dead space of conducting airways plus functional dead space in alveoli. Volume of inspired air that does not take part in gas exchange.

V_T = tidal volume.

$PaCO_2$ = arterial PCO_2, $PeCO_2$ = expired air PCO_2.

Oxygen-hemoglobin dissociation curve

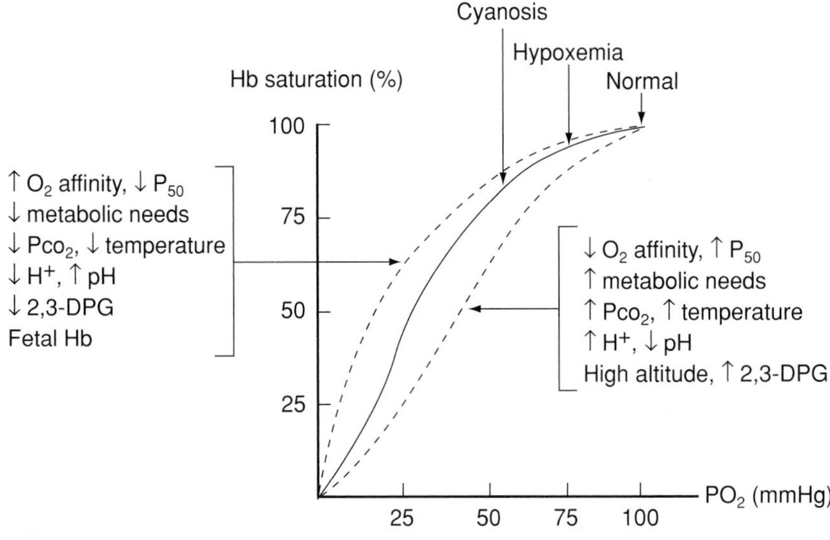

Sigmoidal shape due to positive cooperativity, i.e., hemoglobin can bind 4 oxygen molecules and has higher affinity for each subsequent oxygen molecule bound.

When curve shifts to the right, ↓ affinity of hemoglobin for O_2 (facilitates unloading of O_2 to tissue).

An ↑ in all factors (except pH) causes a shift of the curve to the right.

A ↓ in all factors (except pH) causes a shift of the curve to the left.

Fetal Hb has a higher affinity for oxygen than adult Hb, so its dissociation curve is shifted left.

Right shift—**CADET** face **right:**

CO_2
Acid/**A**ltitude
DPG (2,3-DPG)
Exercise
Temperature

Pulmonary circulation

Normally a low-resistance, high-compliance system. P_{O_2} and P_{CO_2} exert opposite effects on pulmonary and systemic circulation. A ↓ in Pa_{O_2} causes a hypoxic vasoconstriction that shifts blood away from poorly ventilated regions of lung to well-ventilated regions of lung.

1. Perfusion limited—O_2 (normal health), CO_2, N_2O. Gas equilibrates early along the length of the capillary. Diffusion can be ↑ only if blood flow ↑.
2. Diffusion limited—O_2 (emphysema, fibrosis), CO. Gas does not equilibrate by the time blood reaches the end of the capillary.

A consequence of pulmonary hypertension is cor pulmonale and subsequent right ventricular failure (jugular venous distention, edema, hepatomegaly).

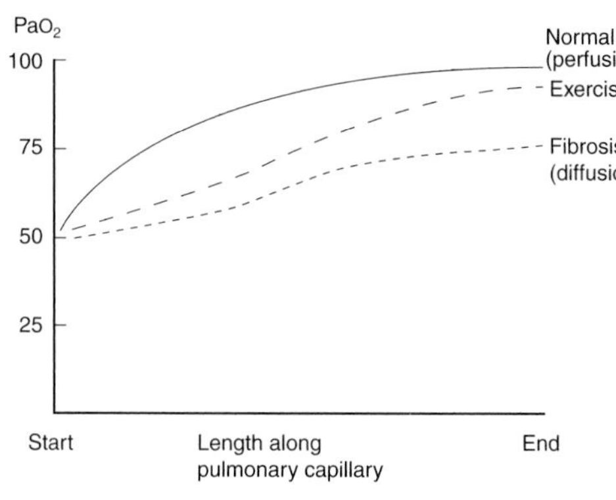

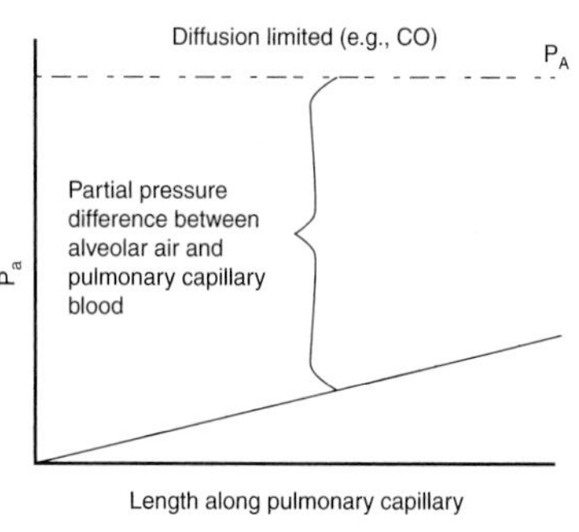

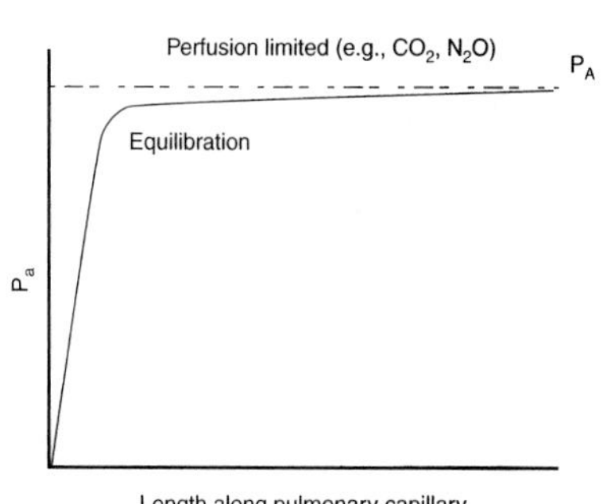

P_a = partial pressure of gas in pulmonary capillary blood
P_A = partial pressure of gas in alveolar air

CO poisoning

CO has 50 times greater affinity for hemoglobin than does oxygen. Causes ↓ oxygen-binding capacity with a left shift in the oxygen-hemoglobin dissociation curve. ↓ oxygen unloading in tissues.

Pulmonary hypertension

Normal pulmonary artery pressure = 10–14 mmHg; pulmonary hypertension ≥ 25 mmHg or > 35 mmHg during exercise.
1°—unknown etiology; poor prognosis.
2°—usually caused by COPD; can also be caused by L → R shunt.

Pulmonary vascular resistance (PVR)

$$PVR = \frac{P_{pulm\ artery} - P_{L\ atrium}}{\text{Cardiac output}}$$

Remember: $\Delta P = Q \times R$, so $R = \Delta P / Q$.
$R = 8\eta l / \pi r^4$

$P_{pulm\ artery}$ = pressure in pulmonary artery.
$P_{L\ atrium}$ = pulmonary wedge pressure.
η = the viscosity of inspired air; l = airway length; r = airway radius.

Oxygen content of blood

O_2 content = (O_2 binding capacity × % saturation) + dissolved O_2.
Normally 1 g Hb can bind 1.34 mL O_2; normal Hb amount in blood is 15 g/dL. Cyanosis results when Hb is < 5 g/dL.
O_2 binding capacity ≈ 20.1 mL O_2 / dL.
O_2 content of arterial blood ↓ as Hb falls, but O_2 saturation and arterial Po_2 do not.
Arterial Po_2 ↓ with chronic lung disease because physiologic shunt ↓ O_2 extraction ratio.
Oxygen delivery to tissues = cardiac output × oxygen content of blood.

Alveolar gas equation

$$PAo_2 = PIo_2 - \frac{PAco_2}{R}$$

Can normally be approximated:
$PAo_2 = 150 - Paco_2 / 0.8$

PAo_2 = alveolar Po_2 (mmHg).
PIo_2 = Po_2 in inspired air (mmHg).
$PAco_2$ = alveolar Pco_2 (mmHg).
R = respiratory quotient.
A-a gradient = $PAo_2 - Pao_2$ = 10–15 mmHg.
↑ A-a gradient may occur in hypoxemia; causes include shunting, V/Q mismatch, fibrosis (diffusion block).

V/Q mismatch

Ideally, ventilation is matched to perfusion (i.e., V/Q = 1) in order for adequate gas exchange to occur.
Lung zones:

1. Apex of the lung—V/Q = 3 (wasted ventilation)
2. Base of the lung—V/Q = 0.6 (wasted perfusion)

Both ventilation and perfusion are greater at the base of the lung than at the apex of the lung.

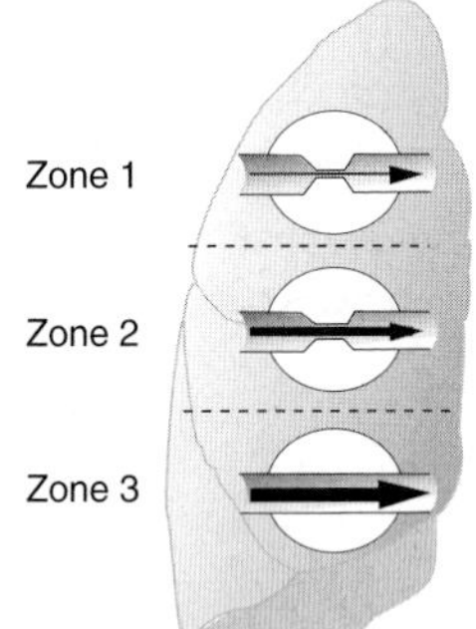

Apex: $P_A > P_a > P_v \rightarrow V/Q = 3$ (wasted ventilation)

$P_a > P_A > P_v$

Base: $P_a > P_v > P_A \rightarrow V/Q = 0.6$ (wasted perfusion); NOTE: both ventilation and perfusion are greater at the base of the lung than at the apex

With exercise (↑ cardiac output), there is vasodilation of apical capillaries, resulting in a V/Q ratio that approaches 1.
Certain organisms that thrive in high O_2 (e.g., TB) flourish in the apex.
V/Q → 0 = airway obstruction (shunt). In shunt, 100% O_2 does not improve Po_2.
V/Q → ∞ = blood flow obstruction (physiologic dead space). Assuming < 100% dead space, 100% O_2 improves Po_2.

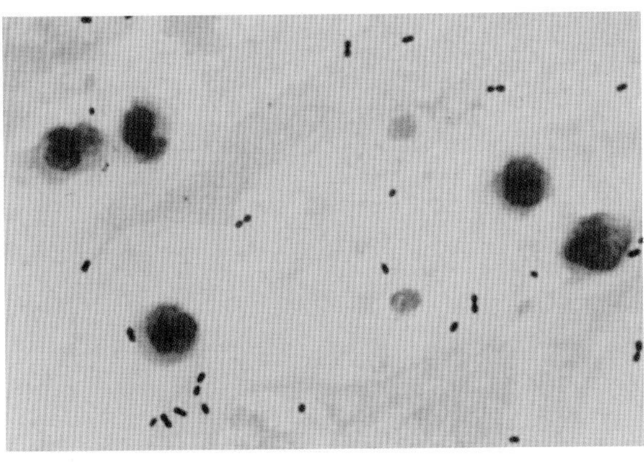

Color Image 1. *Streptococcus pneumoniae.* Sputum sample from a patient with pneumonia shows gram-positive diplococci.

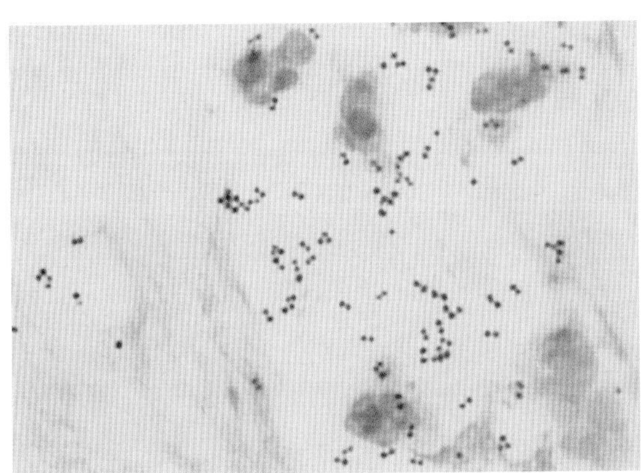

Color Image 3. *Staphylococcus aureus.* Sputum sample from another patient with pneumonia shows gram-positive cocci in clusters.

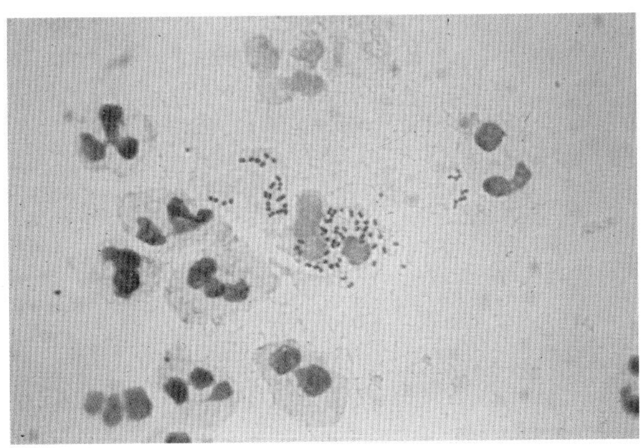

Color Image 4. *Neisseria gonorrhoeae.* Gram stain shows multiple gram-negative diplococci within polymorphonuclear leukocytes as well as in the extracellular areas of a smear from a urethral discharge. (Reproduced, with permission, from Wolff K et al. *Fitzpatrick's Color Atlas and Synopsis of Clinical Dermatology*, 5th ed. New York: McGraw-Hill, 2005: 906.)

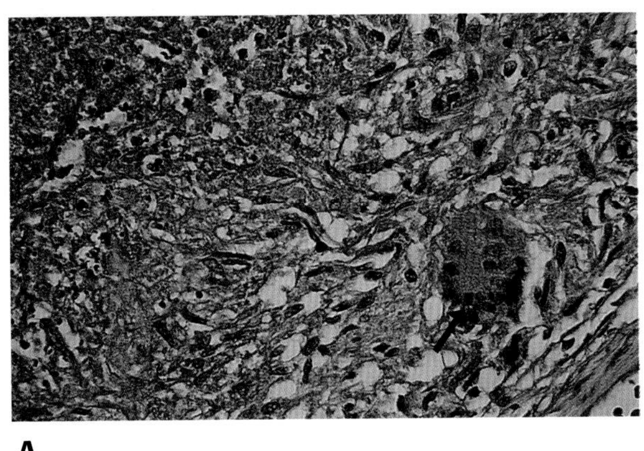

A

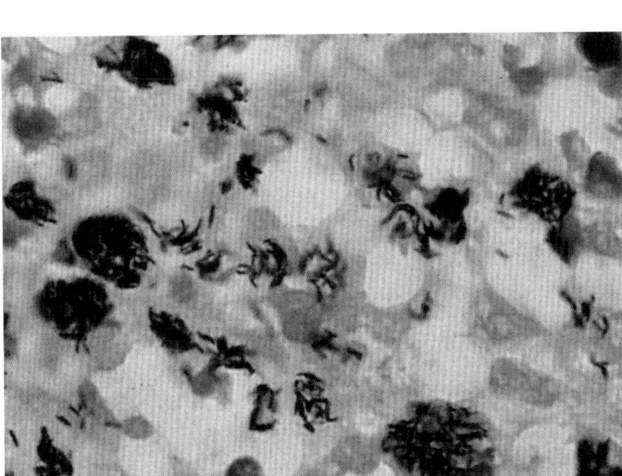

B

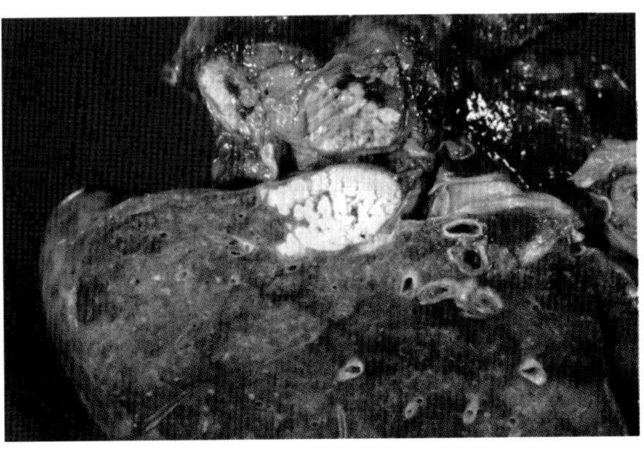

C

Color Image 2. *Mycobacterium tuberculosis* (A) is characterized by caseating granulomas containing Langhans' giant cells, which have a "horseshoe" pattern of nuclei (see arrow). Organisms **(B)** are identified by their red color on acid-fast staining ("red snappers"). **Miliary tuberculosis (C)** is seen here with large caseous lesions at the left medial upper lobe and miliary lesions in the surrounding hilar node. This life-threatening infection is caused by blood-borne dissemination of *Mycobacterium tuberculosis* to many organs from a quiescent site of infection.*

*Reproduced courtesy of the Pathology Education Instructional Resource Digital Library (http://peir.net) at the University of Alabama, Birmingham.

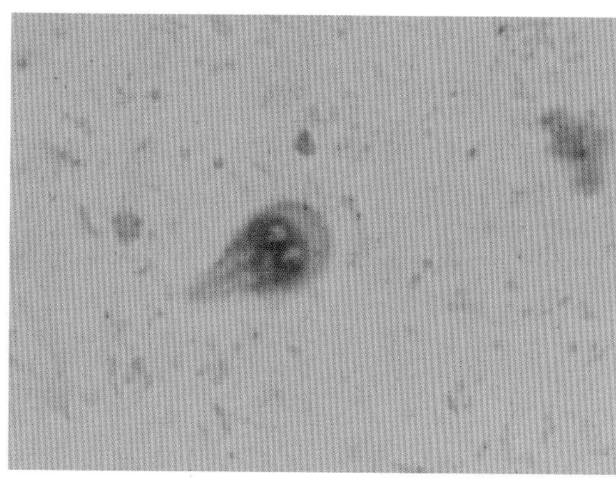

Color Image 5. ***Giardia lamblia,*** small intestine, microscopic. The trophozoite has a classic pear shape, with double nuclei giving an "owl's-eye" appearance.

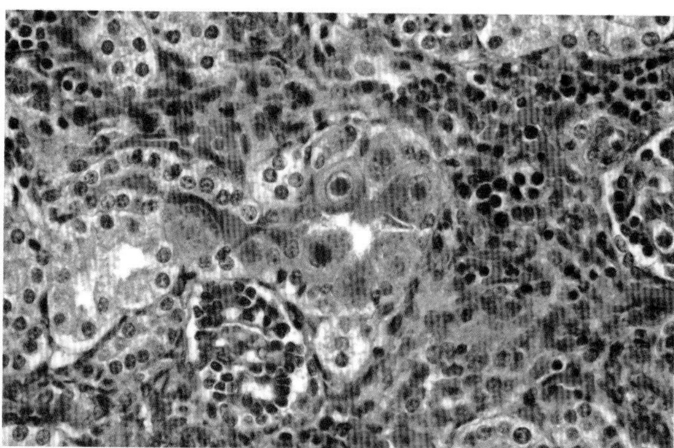

Color Image 6. Cytomegalovirus (CMV). Renal tubular cells in a neonate with congenital CMV infection show prominent Cowdry type A nuclear inclusions resembling owls' eyes. (Reproduced, with permission, from USMLERx.com.)

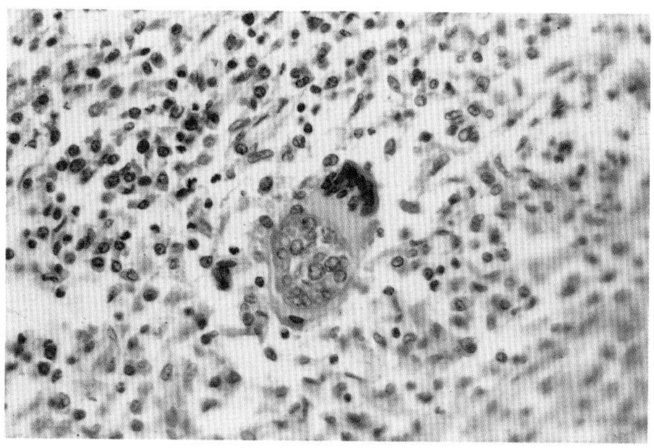

Color Image 7. Coccidioidomycosis. Endospores within a spherule in infected lung parenchyma. Initial infection usually resolves spontaneously, but when immunity is compromised, dissemination to almost any organ can occur. Endemic in the southwestern United States.

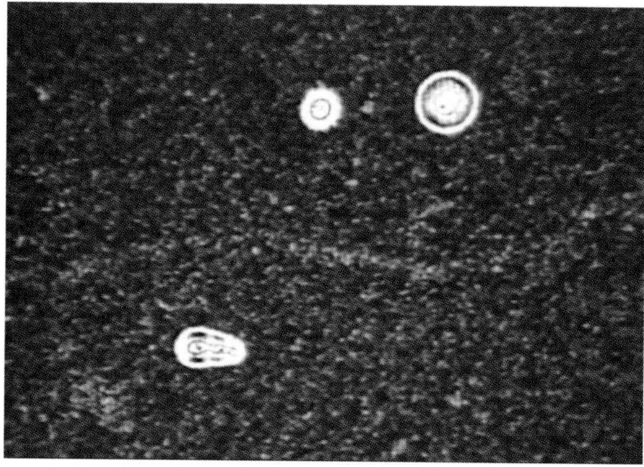

Color Image 8. ***Cryptococcus neoformans.*** The polysaccharide capsule is visible by India ink preparation in CSF from an AIDS patient with meningoencephalitis.*

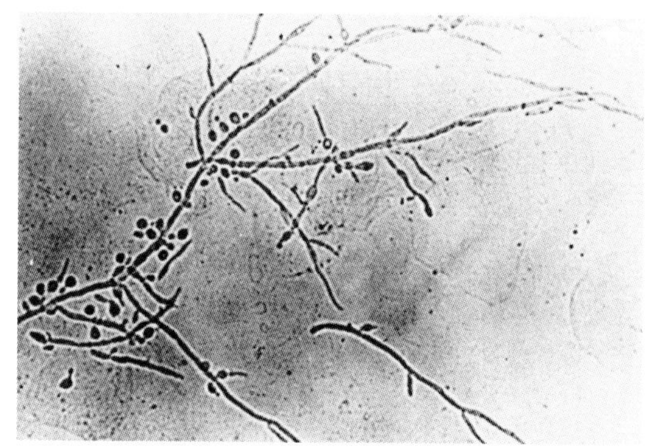

Color Image 9. ***Candida albicans.*** KOH preparation showing branched and budding *C. albicans.* (Reproduced, with permission, from DeCherney AH. *Current Obstetric and Gynecologic Diagnosis and Treatment*, 9th ed. New York: McGraw-Hill, 2003: 652.)

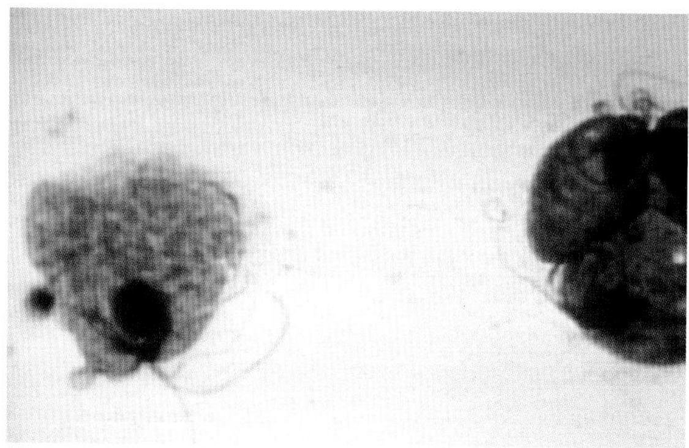

Color Image 10. ***Trichomonas vaginalis*** demonstrating trophozoites with flagellae.*

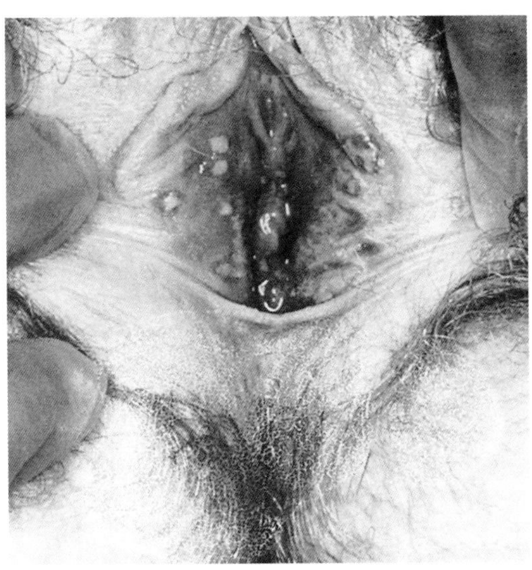

Color Image 11. Herpes genitalis. Ulcerating vesicles associated with HSV-2. (Reproduced, with permission, from DeCherney AH. *Current Obstetric and Gynecologic Diagnosis and Treatment,* 9th ed. New York: McGraw-Hill, 2003: 664.)

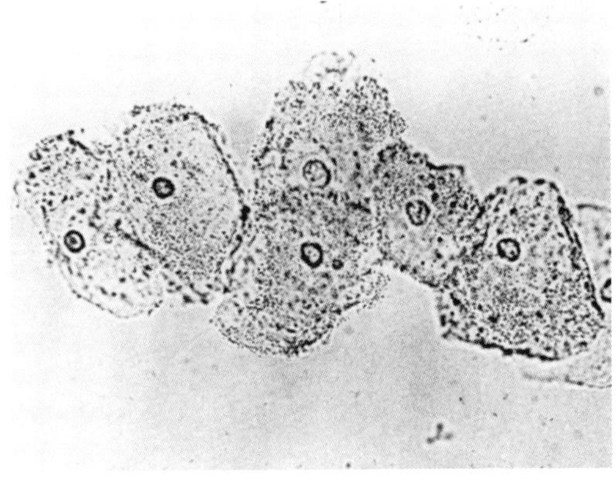

Color Image 13. Bacterial vaginosis. Saline wet mount of clue cells. Note the absence of inflammatory cells. (Reproduced, with permission, from DeCherney AH. *Current Obstetric and Gynecologic Diagnosis and Treatment,* 9th ed. New York: McGraw-Hill, 2003: 653.)

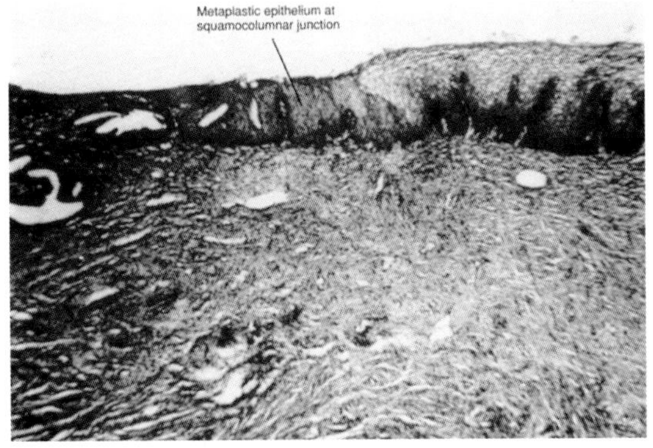

Color Image 14. Human papillomavirus. Metaplastic epithelium at the cervical squamocolumnar junction, associated with HPV. (Reproduced, with permission, from DeCherney AH. *Current Obstetric and Gynecologic Diagnosis and Treatment,* 9th ed. New York: McGraw-Hill, 2003: 683.)

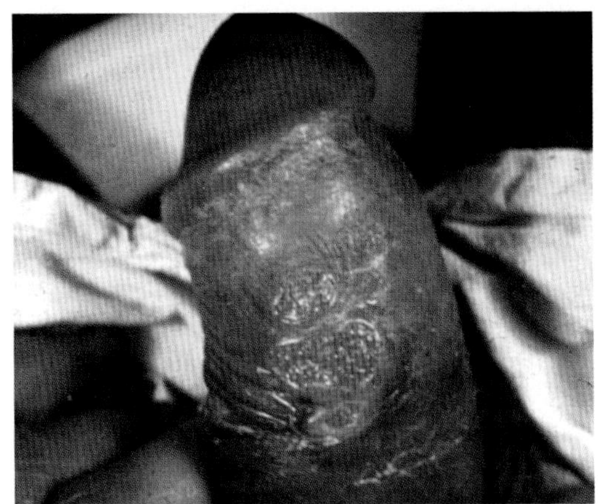

A

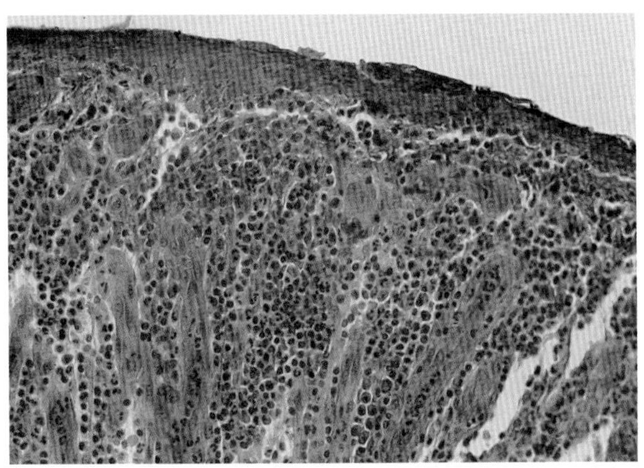

B

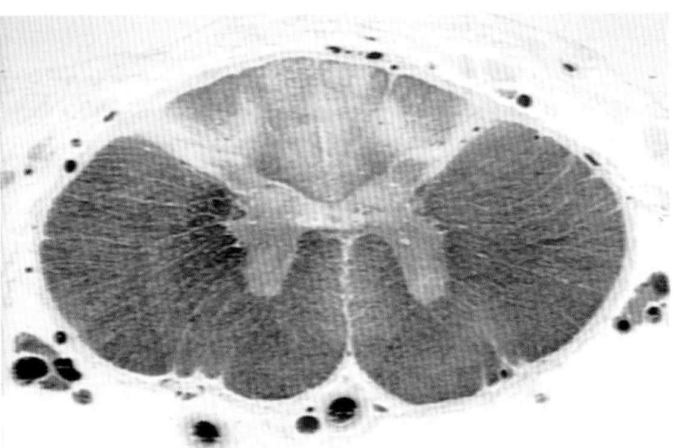

C

Color Image 12. Syphilis. (A) Chancre associated with primary syphilis. These ulcerative lesions are painless. **(B) Primary syphilis.** A dense infiltrate of plasma cells and dilated blood vessels can be seen. There is epidermal ulceration with crust; neutrophils are present within the predominantly plasmacytic infiltrate. **(C) Tabes dorsalis** resulting from progressive syphilis infection, thoracic spinal cord. Note degeneration of the dorsal columns and dorsal roots.* (Image B reproduced, with permission, from Hurwitz RM et al. *Pathology of the Skin: Atlas of Clinical-Pathological Correlation,* 2nd ed. Stamford, CT: Appleton & Lange, 1998.)

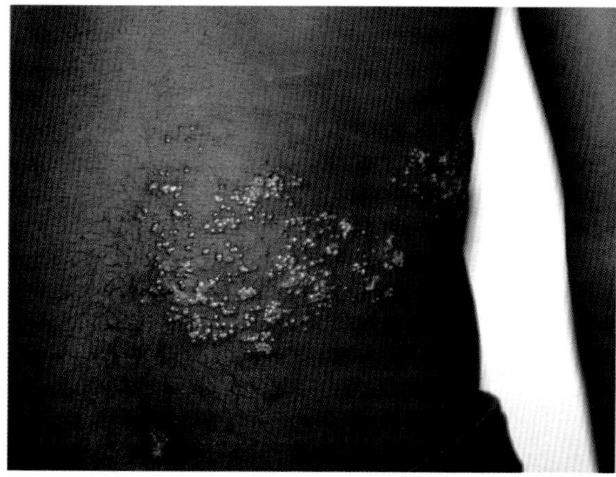

Color Image 15. Herpes zoster. Reactivation of virus spreads along the dermatomal distribution of infected nerves and can occur many years after initial infection. It is considered benign unless it affects an immunocompromised host or is a reinfection of the V_1 branch of the trigeminal nerve with eye/cornea involvement.*

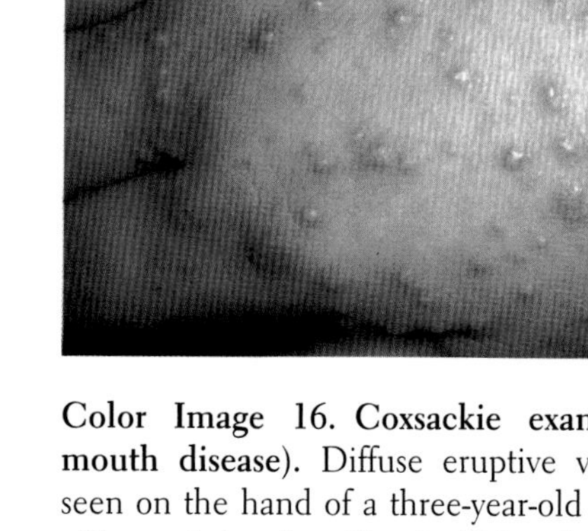

Color Image 16. Coxsackie exanthem (hand-foot-mouth disease). Diffuse eruptive vesiculopapules are seen on the hand of a three-year-old child. (Reproduced, with permission, from Hurwitz RM et al. *Pathology of the Skin: Atlas of Clinical-Pathological Correlation*, 2nd ed. Stamford, CT: Appleton & Lange, 1998.)

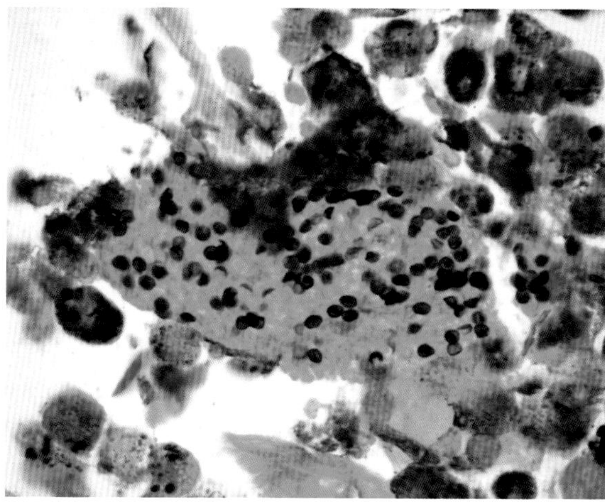

Color Image 17. *Pneumocystis carinii*. Special silver stain of lung epithelium shows numerous small, disk-shaped organisms. (Reproduced, with permission, from USMLERx.com.)

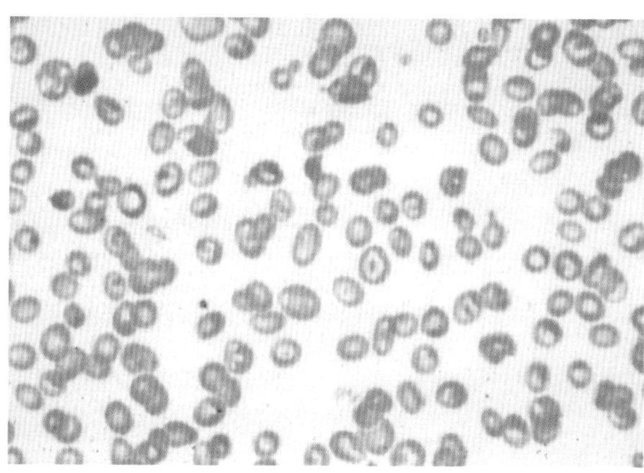

Color Image 18. Target cells. Due to an increase in surface area–to-volume ratio from iron deficiency anemia (decreased cell volume) or in obstructive liver disease (increased cell membrane).*

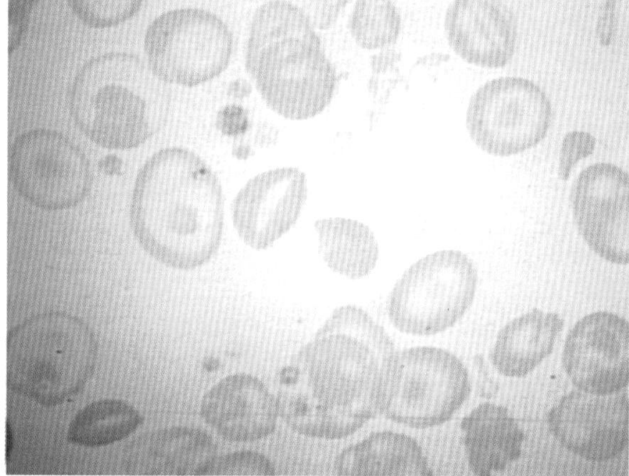

Color Image 19. Thalassemia major. A blood dyscrasia caused by a defect in β-chain synthesis in hemoglobin. Note the presence of target cells.*

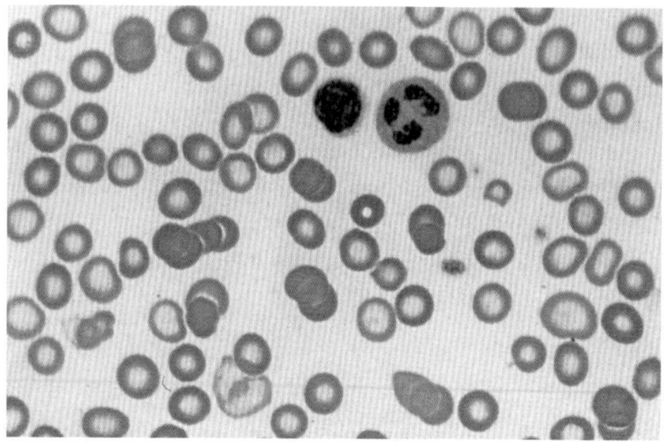

Color Image 20. Iron deficiency anemia. Microcytosis and hypochromia can be seen.

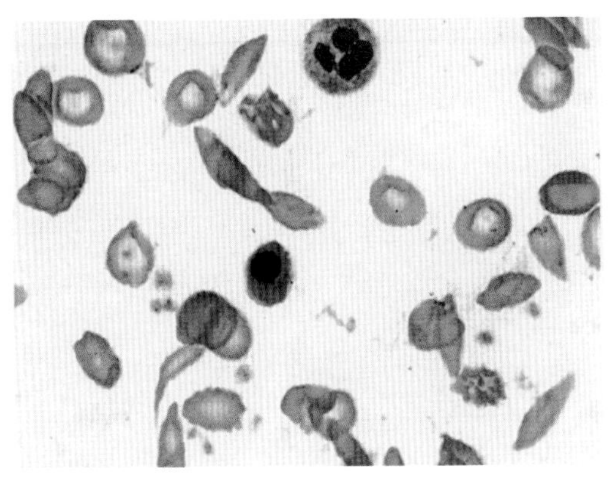

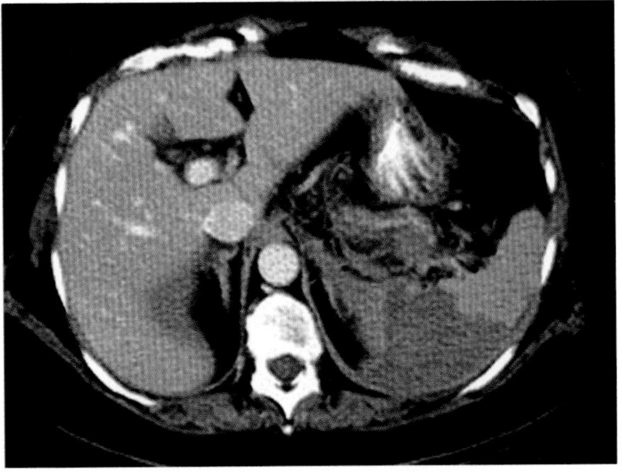

Color Image 21. Sickle cell anemia. (A) Sickle cell peripheral blood smear. Note the sickled cells as well as anisocytosis, poikilocytosis, and nucleated RBCs. **(B) Splenic infarction.** The splenic artery lacks collateral supply, making the spleen particularly susceptible to ischemic damage. Coagulative necrosis has occurred in a wedge shape along the pattern of vascular supply. Individual sickle cells cause generalized splenic infarcts that result in autosplenectomy by adolescence.*

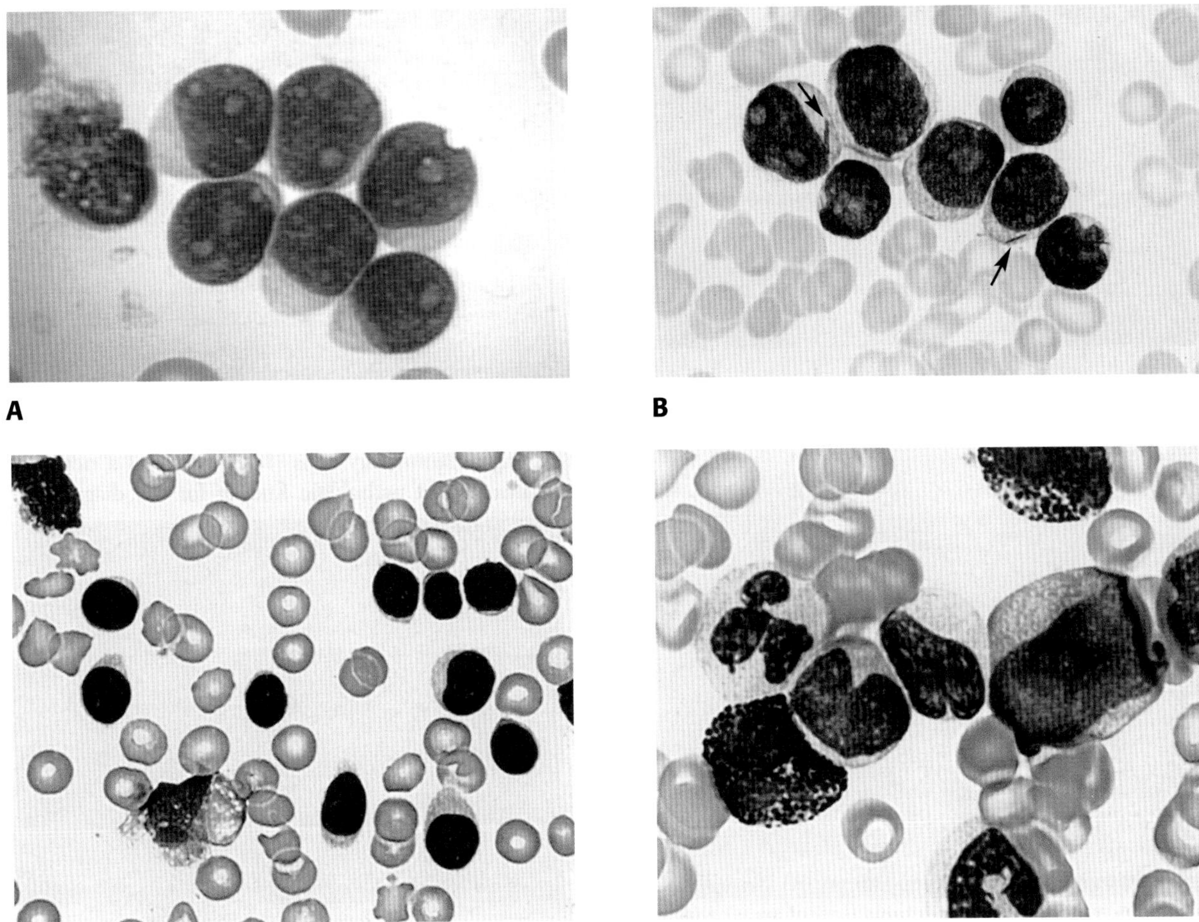

Color Image 22. Leukemia. (A) Acute lymphocytic leukemia, peripheral blood smear. Affects children less than 10 years of age. **(B) Acute myelocytic leukemia** with Auer rods (arrows), peripheral blood smear. Affects adolescents to young adults. **(C) Chronic lymphocytic leukemia,** peripheral blood smear. In CLL, the lymphocytes are excessively fragile. These lymphocytes are easily destroyed during slide preparation, forming "smudge cells." Affects individuals older than 60 years of age. **(D) Chronic myeloid leukemia,** peripheral blood smear. Promyelocytes and myelocytes are seen adjacent to a vascular structure. Affects individuals from 30 to 60 years of age.*

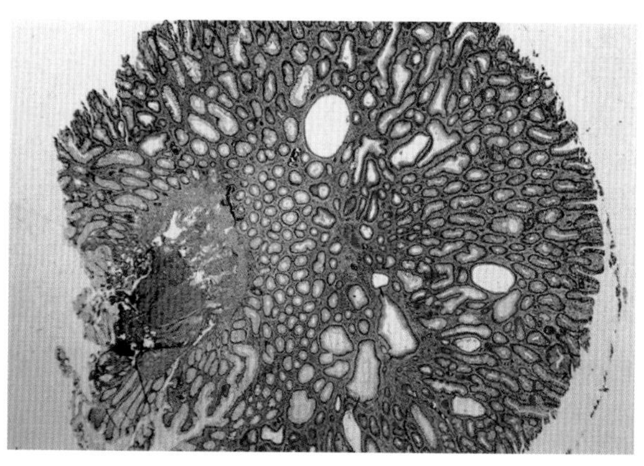

A

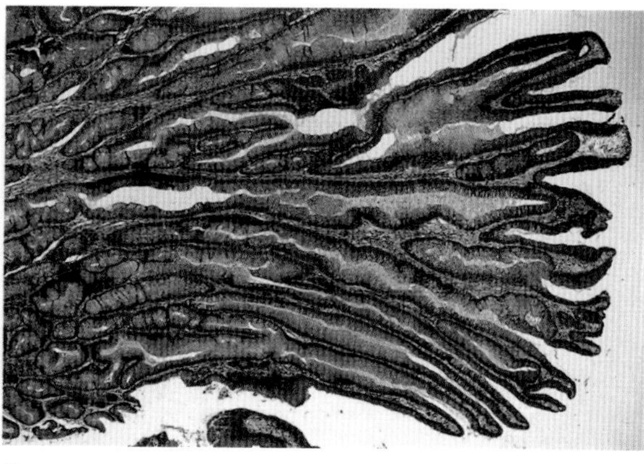

B

Color Image 30. Colonic polyps. Tubular adenomas (A) are smaller and rounded in morphology and have less malignant potential than do **villous adenomas (B)**, which are composed of long, fingerlike projections.

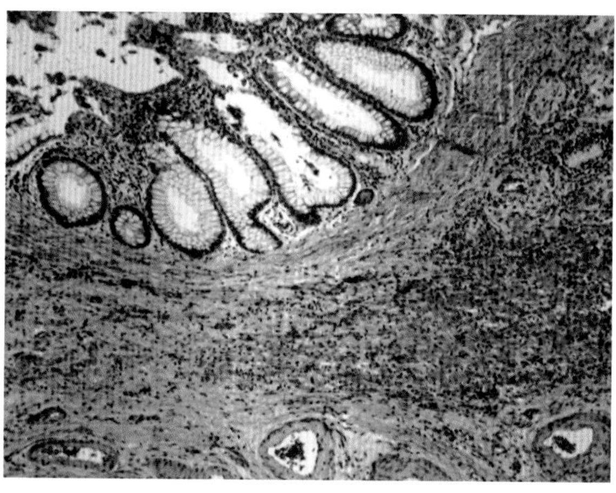

Color Image 31. Diverticulitis. Inflammation of the diverticula typically causes LLQ pain and can progress to perforation, peritonitis, abscess formation, or bowel stenosis. Note the presence of macrophages. Gut lumen is seen at the top of the photo.*

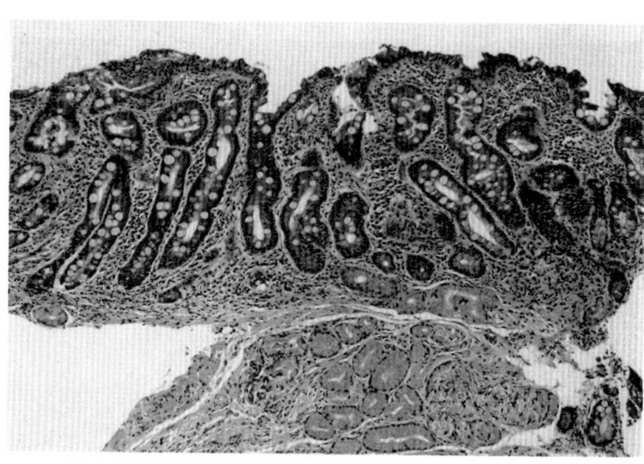

Color Image 32. Celiac sprue (gluten-sensitive enteropathy). Histology shows blunting of villi and crypt hyperplasia.

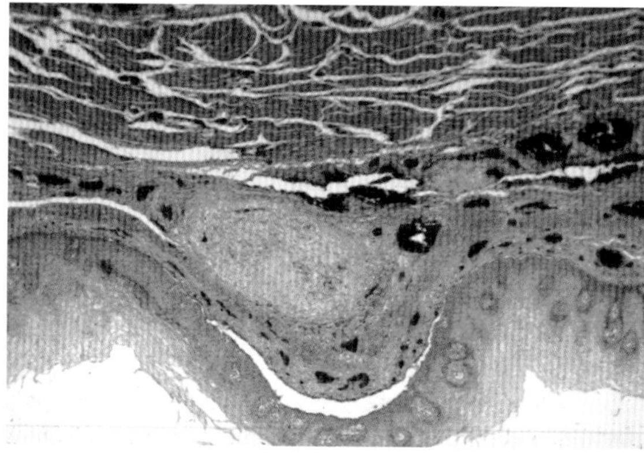

Color Image 33. Sclerosed **esophageal varix.** Overlying esophageal mucosa is generally normal.*

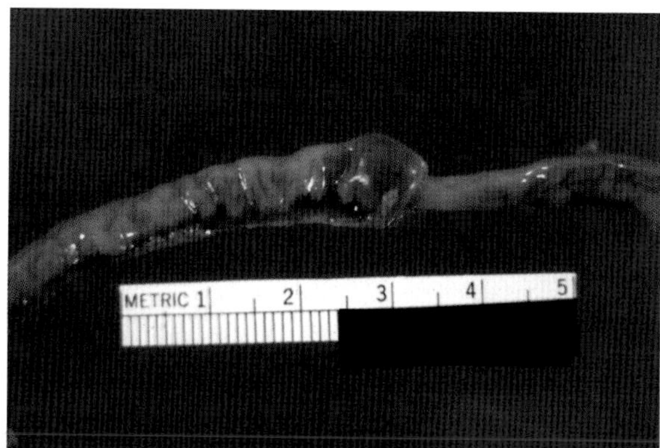

Color Image 34. Intussusception of infant gut, gross.*

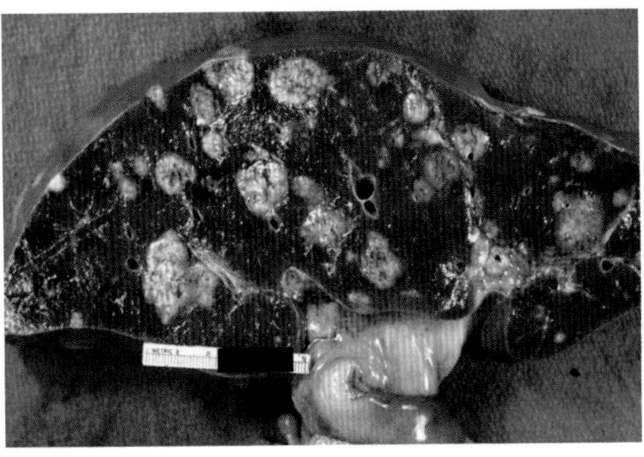

Color Image 27. Metastatic carcinoma to the liver. The most common primary sites are the breast, colon, and lung. Primary tumors of the liver are less common than metastatic disease.*

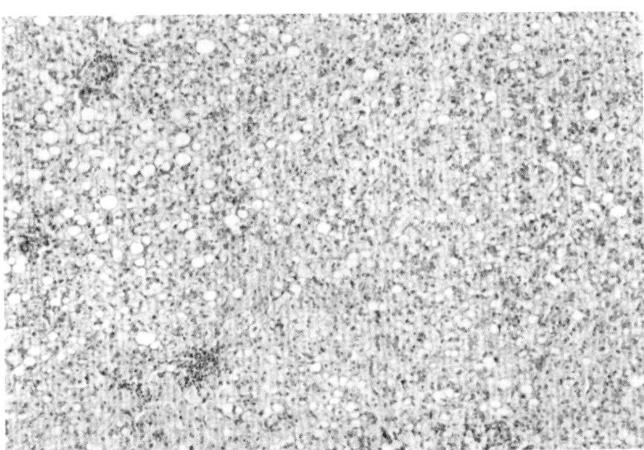

Color Image 28. Fatty metamorphosis (macrovesicular steatosis) of the liver, microscopic. Early reversible change associated with alcohol consumption can be seen; there are abundant fat-filled vacuoles, but as yet there is no inflammation due to fibrosis of more serious alcoholic liver damage.*

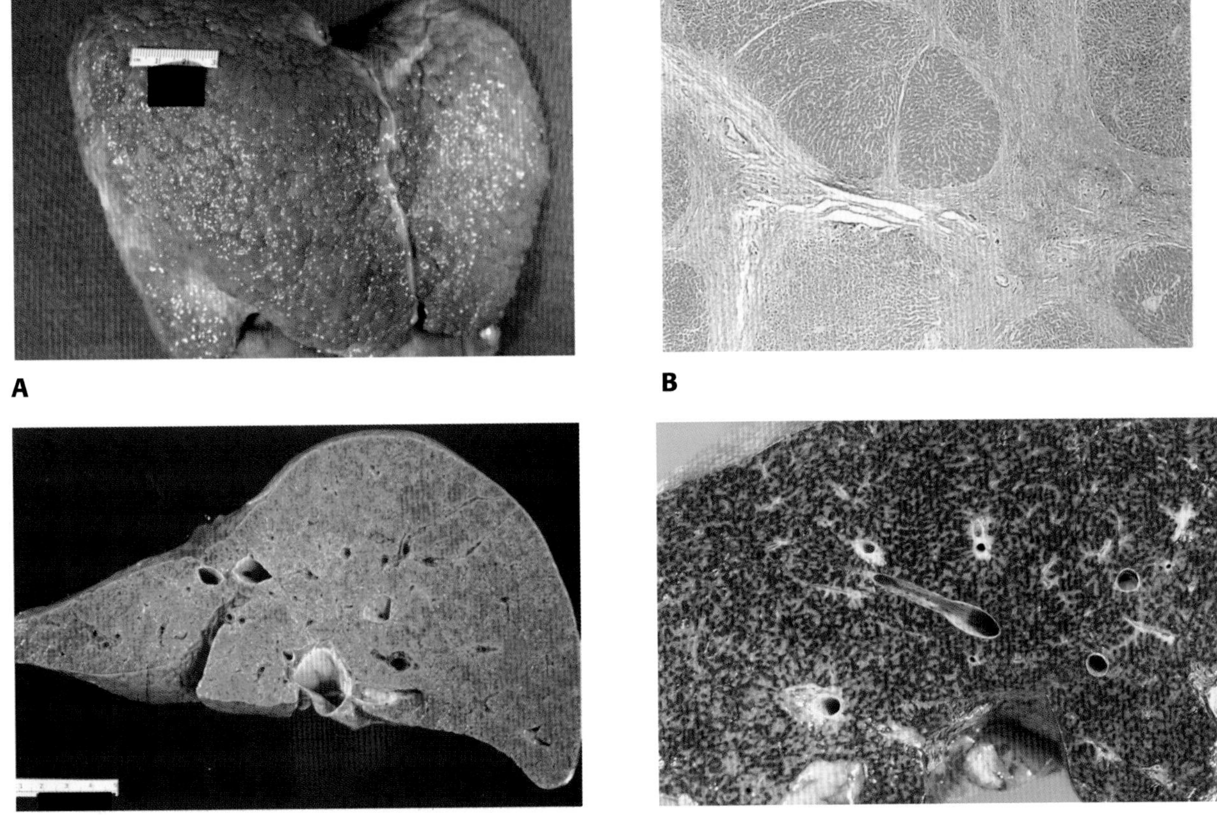

Color Image 29. Cirrhosis. (A) Micronodular cirrhosis of the liver, gross, from an alcoholic patient. The liver is approximately normal in size with a fine, granular appearance. Later stages of disease result in an irregularly shrunken liver with larger nodules, giving it a "hobnail" appearance. **(B) Cirrhosis,** microscopic. Regenerative lesions are surrounded by fibrotic bands of collagen ("bridging fibrosis"), forming the characteristic nodularity. **(C)** Gross natural color with macronodularity that is difficult to see. Hepatitis B surface antigen and core antigen negative. **(D)** Chronic passive biliary congestion gives the liver a "nutmeg" appearance.*

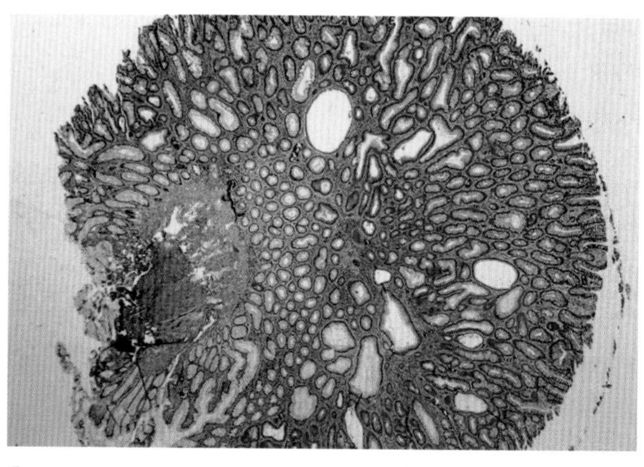

A

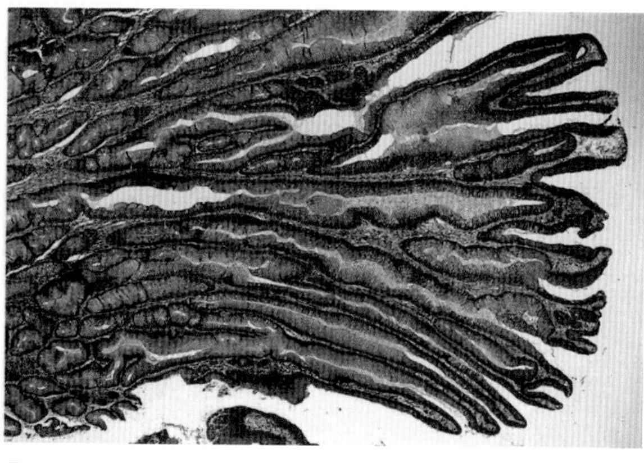

B

Color Image 30. Colonic polyps. Tubular adenomas (A) are smaller and rounded in morphology and have less malignant potential than do **villous adenomas (B),** which are composed of long, fingerlike projections.

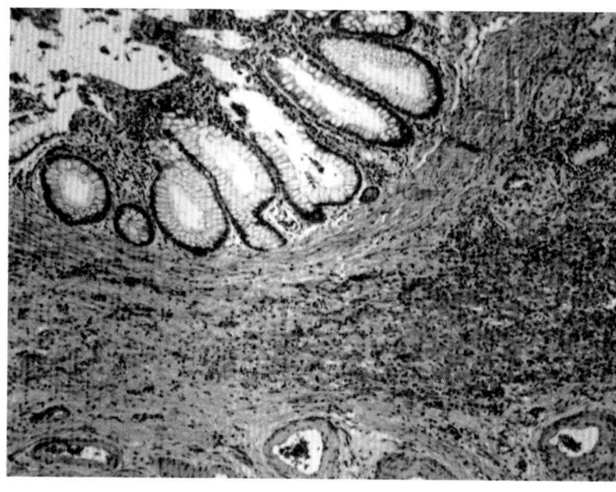

Color Image 31. Diverticulitis. Inflammation of the diverticula typically causes LLQ pain and can progress to perforation, peritonitis, abscess formation, or bowel stenosis. Note the presence of macrophages. Gut lumen is seen at the top of the photo.*

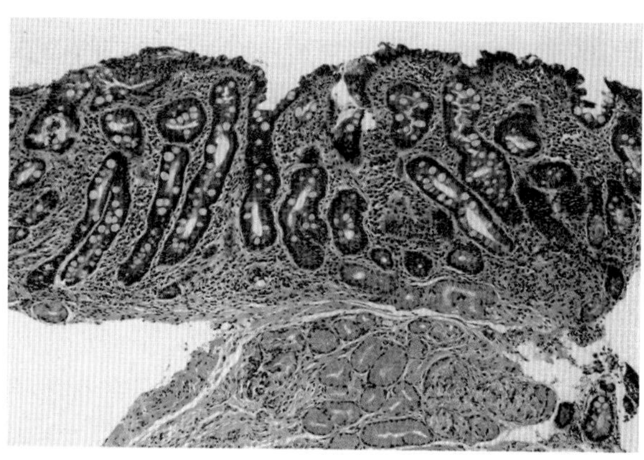

Color Image 32. Celiac sprue (gluten-sensitive enteropathy). Histology shows blunting of villi and crypt hyperplasia.

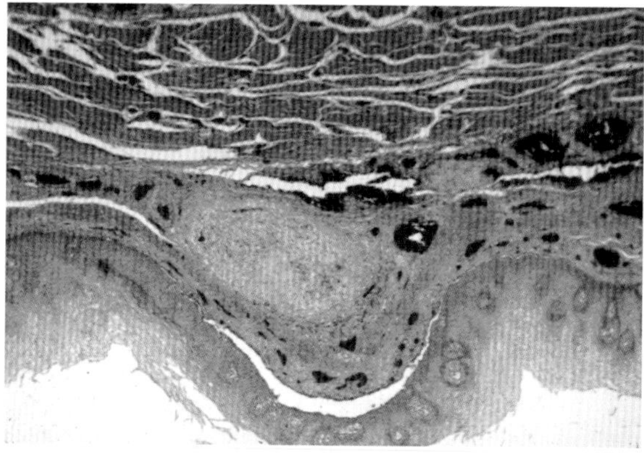

Color Image 33. Sclerosed **esophageal varix.** Overlying esophageal mucosa is generally normal.*

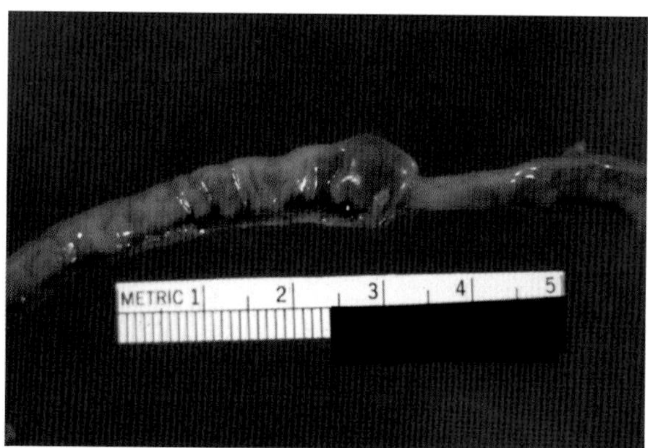

Color Image 34. Intussusception of infant gut, gross.*

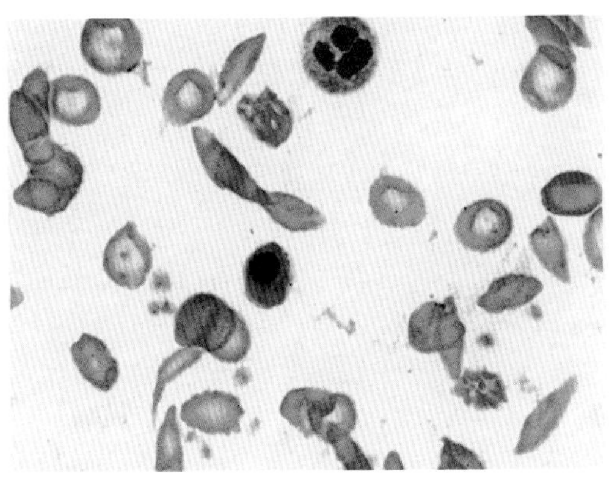

A

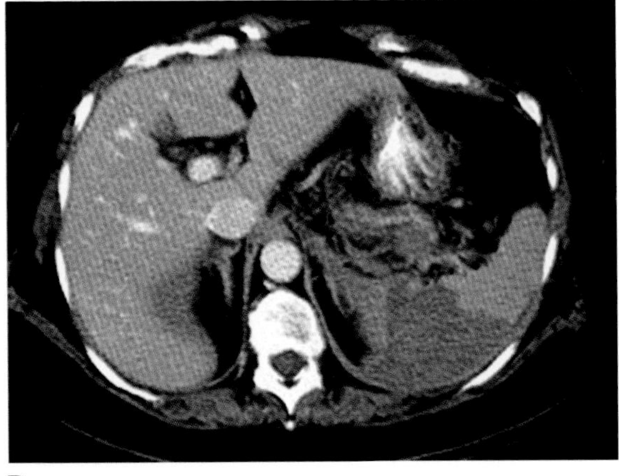

B

Color Image 21. Sickle cell anemia. (A) Sickle cell peripheral blood smear. Note the sickled cells as well as anisocytosis, poikilocytosis, and nucleated RBCs. **(B) Splenic infarction.** The splenic artery lacks collateral supply, making the spleen particularly susceptible to ischemic damage. Coagulative necrosis has occurred in a wedge shape along the pattern of vascular supply. Individual sickle cells cause generalized splenic infarcts that result in autosplenectomy by adolescence.*

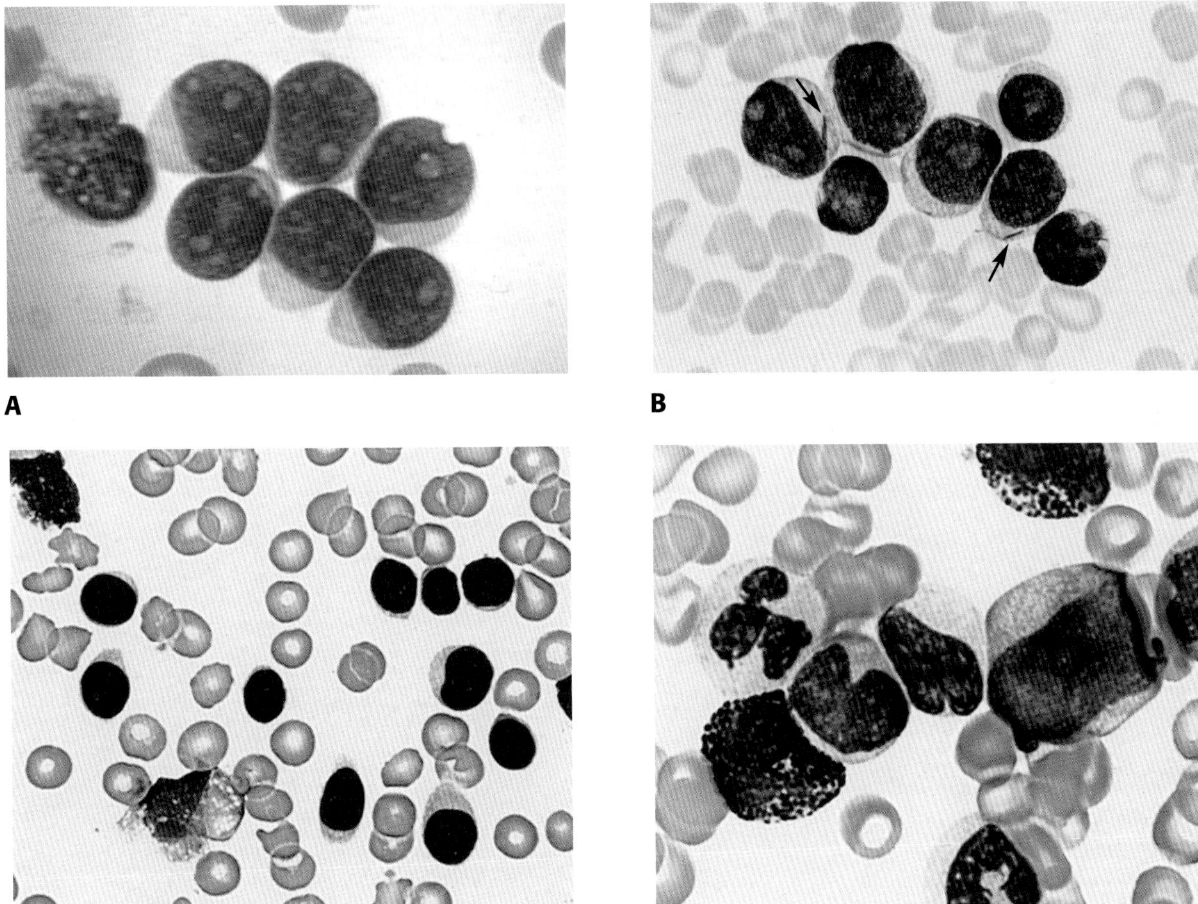

Color Image 22. Leukemia. (A) Acute lymphocytic leukemia, peripheral blood smear. Affects children less than 10 years of age. **(B) Acute myelocytic leukemia** with Auer rods (arrows), peripheral blood smear. Affects adolescents to young adults. **(C) Chronic lymphocytic leukemia,** peripheral blood smear. In CLL, the lymphocytes are excessively fragile. These lymphocytes are easily destroyed during slide preparation, forming "smudge cells." Affects individuals older than 60 years of age. **(D) Chronic myeloid leukemia,** peripheral blood smear. Promyelocytes and myelocytes are seen adjacent to a vascular structure. Affects individuals from 30 to 60 years of age.*

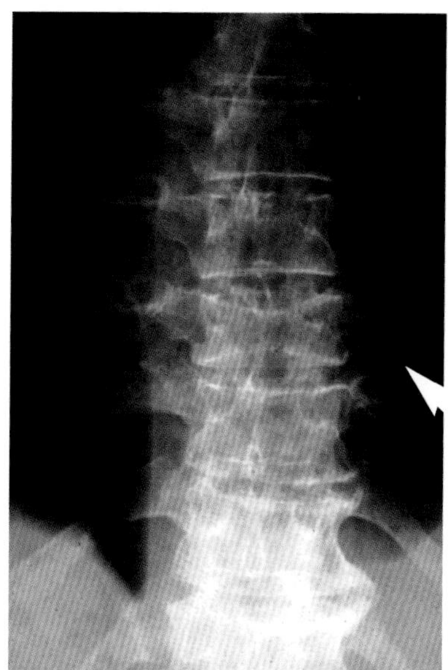

A

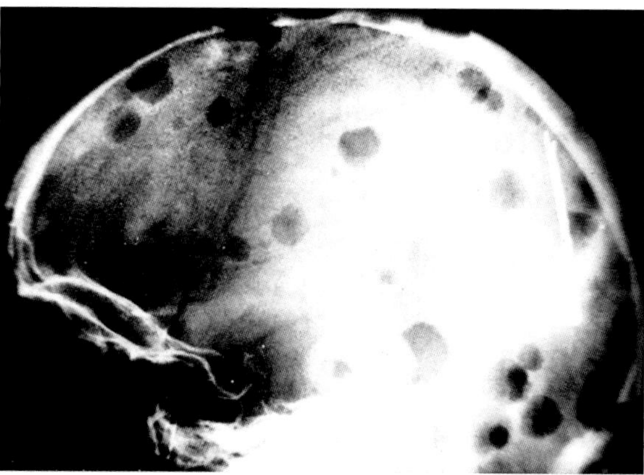

B

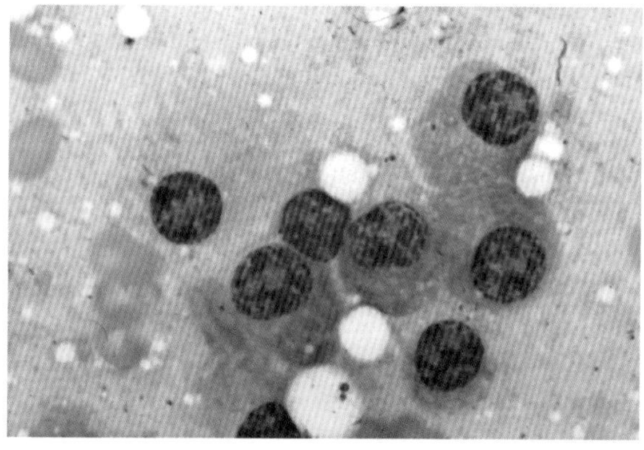

C

Color Image 23. Multiple myeloma. **(A)** X-ray shows numerous punched-out lytic lesions (lucent areas) typical of multiple myeloma. Note the generalized osteopenia and multiple compression fractures (arrow). **(B)** Classic bone lytic lesions seen in multiple myeloma. **(C)** Smears from a patient with multiple myeloma display an abundance of plasma cells. RBCs will often be seen in rouleaux formation, stacked like poker chips. Multiple myeloma is associated with hypercalcemia, lytic bone lesions, and renal insufficiency due to Bence Jones (light-chain) proteinuria.*

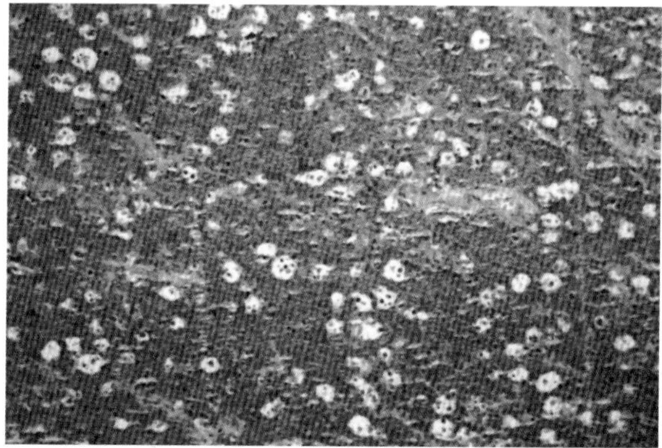

Color Image 24. Burkitt's lymphoma. The classic "starry-sky" appearance from macrophage ingestion of tumor cells can be seen.*

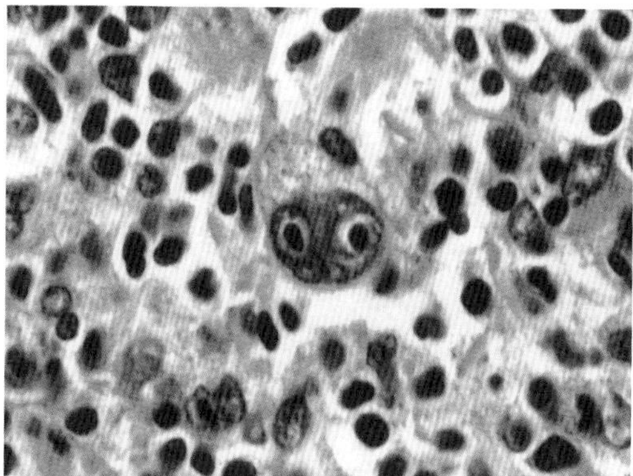

Color Image 25. Hodgkin's disease (Reed-Sternberg cells). Binucleate RS cells displaying prominent inclusion-like nucleoli surrounded by lymphocytes and other reacting inflammatory cells. The RS cell is a necessary but insufficient pathologic finding for the diagnosis of Hodgkin's disease.

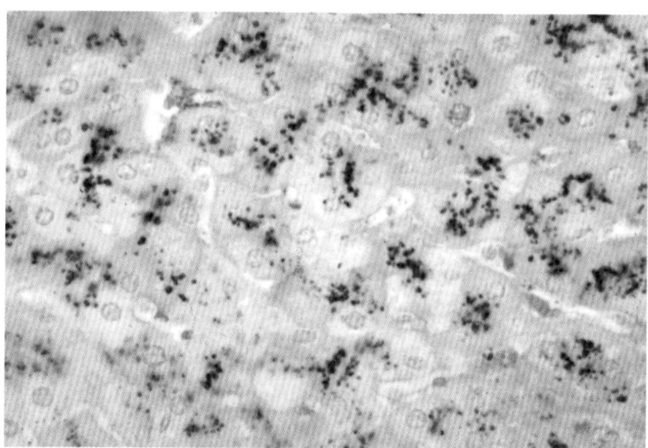

Color Image 26. Hemochromatosis with cirrhosis. Prussian blue iron stain shows hemosiderin in the liver parenchyma. Such deposition occurs throughout the body, causing organ damage and the characteristic darkening of the skin.*

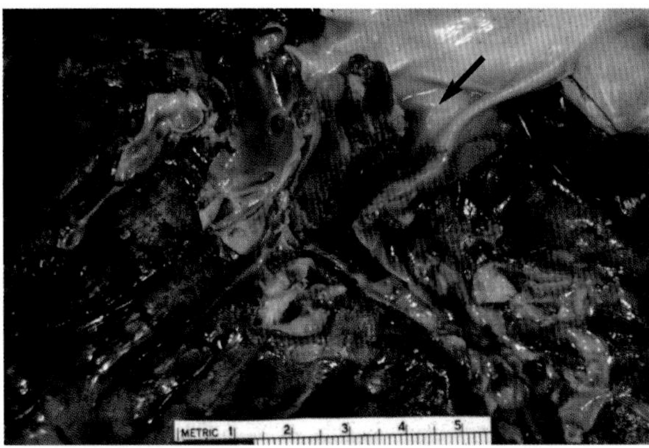

A

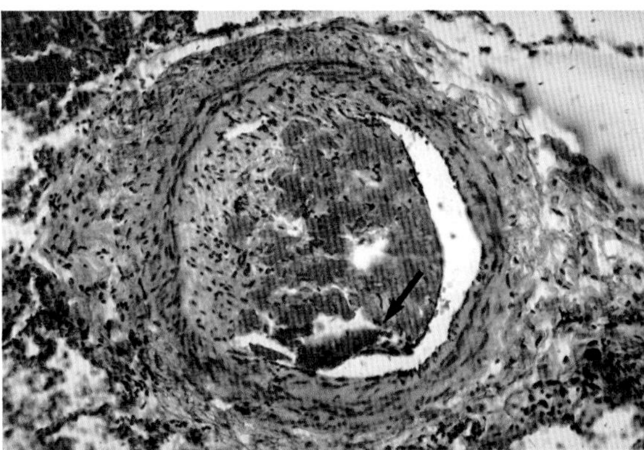

B

Color Image 35. Pulmonary emboli. (A) Pulmonary thromboembolus (arrow), gross. Most often arises from deep venous thrombosis. **(B) Pulmonary thromboembolus** in a small muscular pulmonary artery. The interdigitating areas of pale pink and red within the organizing embolus form the "lines of Zahn" (arrow) characteristic of a thrombus. These lines represent layers of red cells, platelets, and fibrin that are laid down in the vessel as the thrombus forms.*

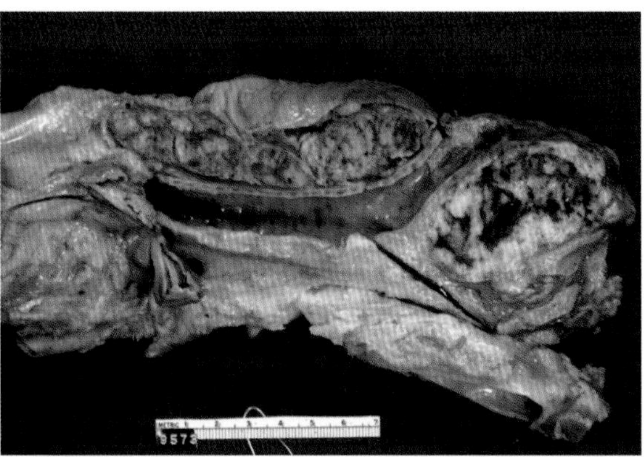

Color Image 36. Squamous cell carcinoma of the lung, gross, from a patient with a long smoking history. This tumor arises from the bronchial epithelium and is centrally located.*

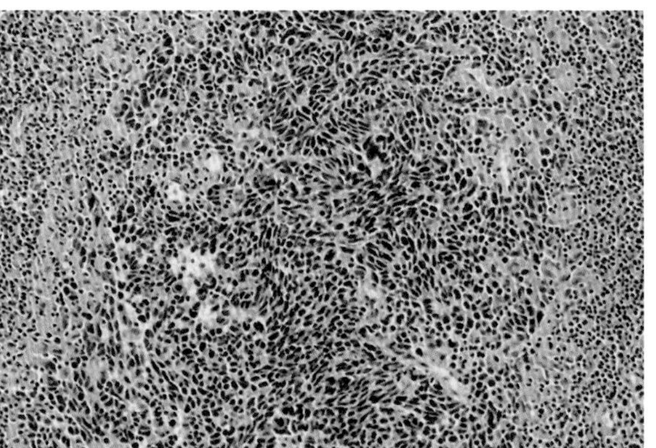

Color Image 37. Small (oat) cell carcinoma in a pulmonary hilar lymph node. Almost all of these tumors are related to tobacco smoking. They can arise anywhere in the lung, most often near the hilum, and quickly spread along the bronchi.*

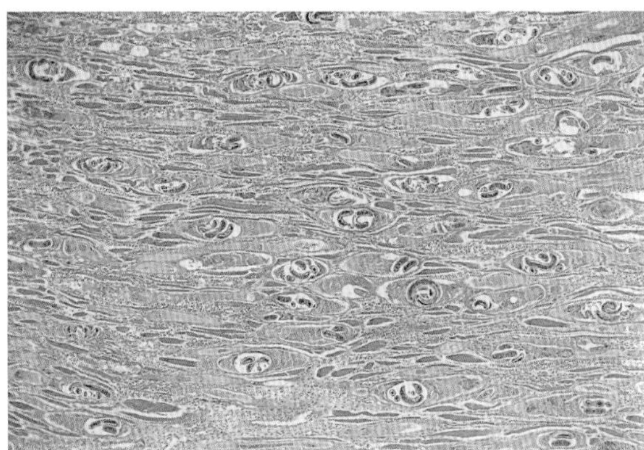

Color Image 38. *Taenia solium*, the pig tapeworm, infesting porcine myocardium. When humans ingest this meat, the larvae attach to the wall of the small intestine and mature to adult worms.

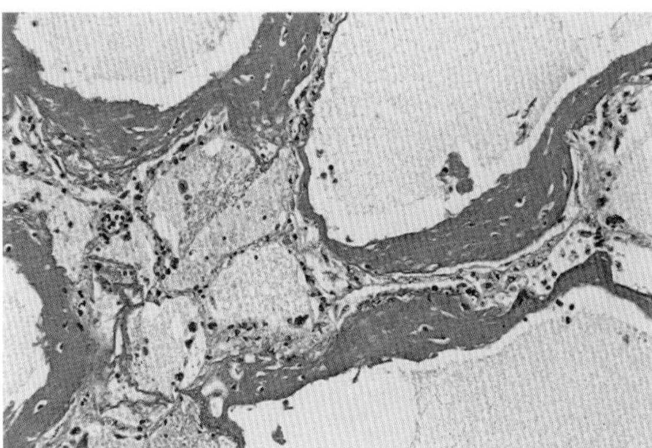

Color Image 39. Acute respiratory distress syndrome (ARDS). Persistent inflammation leads to poor pulmonary compliance and edema; note both alveolar fluid and hyaline membranes.

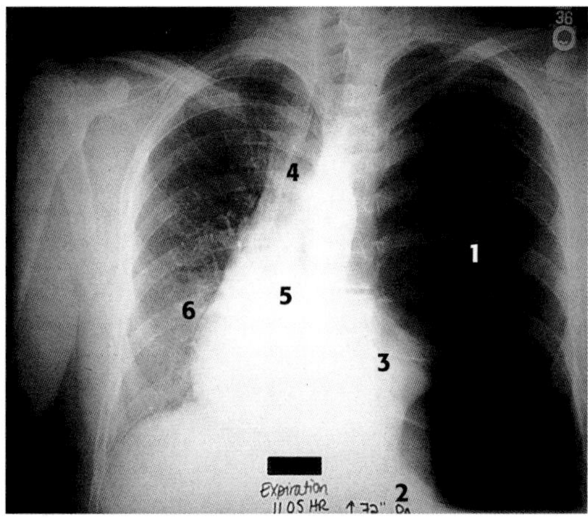

Color Image 40. Tension pneumothorax. Note these features:

1—Hyperlucent lung field
2—Hyperexpansion lowers diaphragm
3—Collapsed lung
4—Deviation of trachea
5—Mediastinal shift
6—Compression of opposite lung

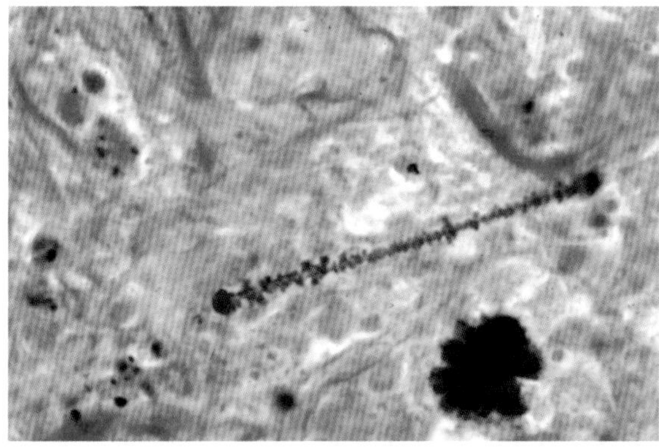

Color Image 42. Asbestosis. Ferruginous bodies (asbestos bodies with Prussian blue iron stain) in the lung, microscopic. Inhaled asbestos fibers are ingested by macrophages.*

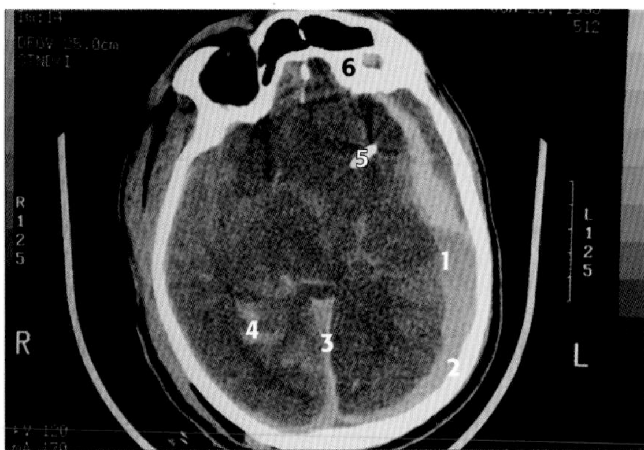

Color Image 43. Subdural hemorrhage. Note the hyperdense extra-axial blood on the left side. Concomitant subarachnoid hemorrhage. 1—subdural blood, layering; 2—skull; 3—falx; 4—subarachnoid blood; 5—shunt catheter; 6—frontal sinus.

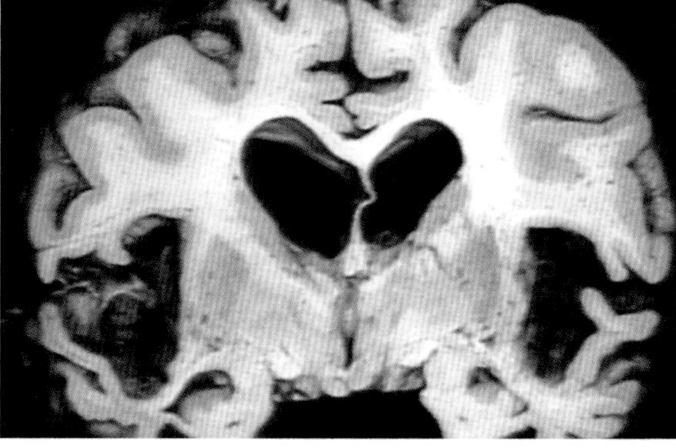

A

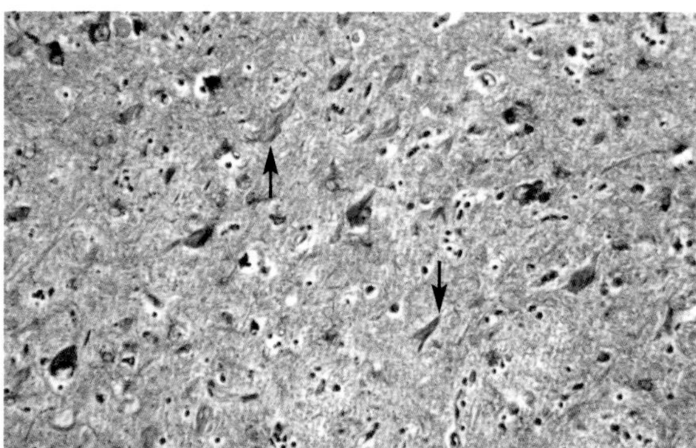

B

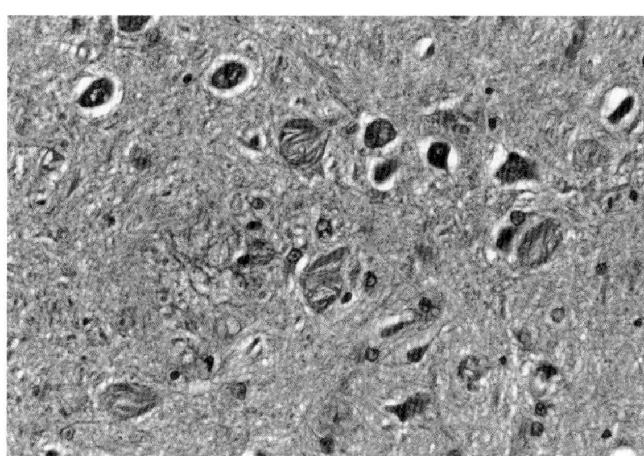

C

Color Image 41. Alzheimer's disease. Key histologic features include "senile plaques" (**A**), a coronal section showing atrophy, especially of the temporal lobes (**B**), and focal masses of interwoven neuronal processes around an amyloid core (neurofibrillary tangles, arrow). The remnants of neuronal degeneration (**C**) are also associated with Alzheimer's disease, the most common cause of dementia in older persons.*

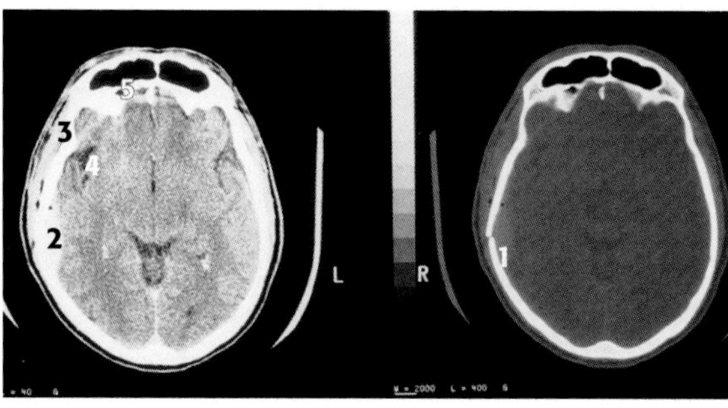

Color Image 44. Epidural hematoma from skull fracture. Note the lens-shaped (biconvex) dense blood next to the fracture. 1—skull fracture; 2—hematoma in epidural space; 3—temporalis muscle; 4—Sylvian fissure; 5—frontal sinus.

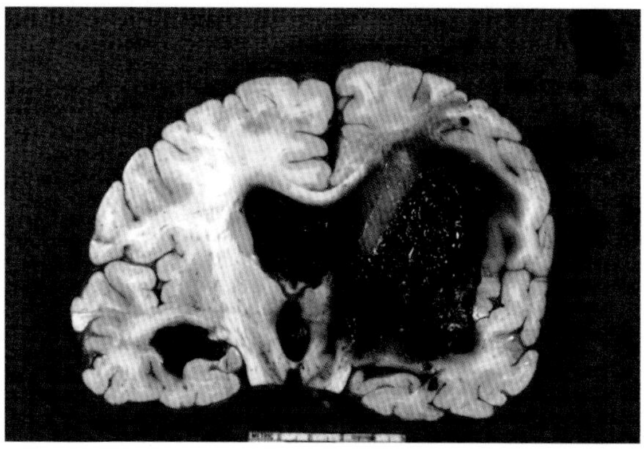

Color Image 45. Brain with **hypertensive hemorrhage** in the region of the basal ganglia, gross.*

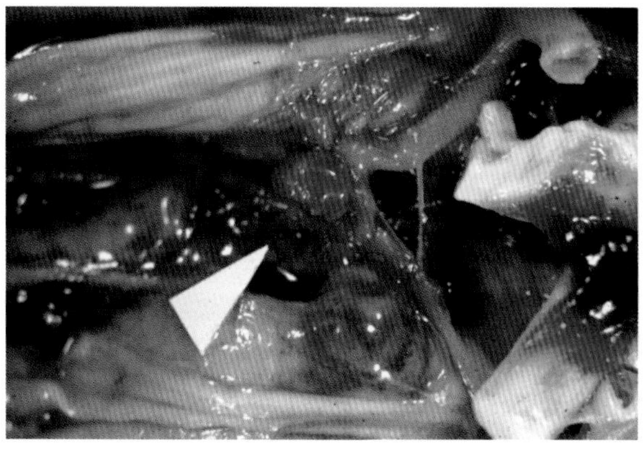

A

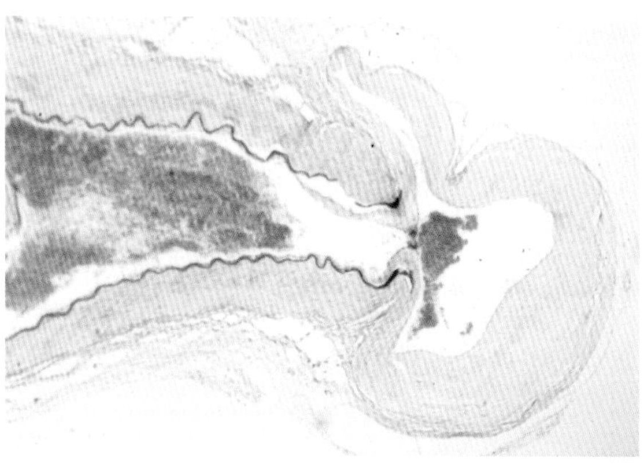

B

Color Image 46. Berry aneurysm (A) located on the anterior cerebral artery. The small, saclike structure can easily rupture during periods of hypertension or stress. The histologic section **(B)** at the origin of the aneurysm shows lack of internal elastic lamina.*

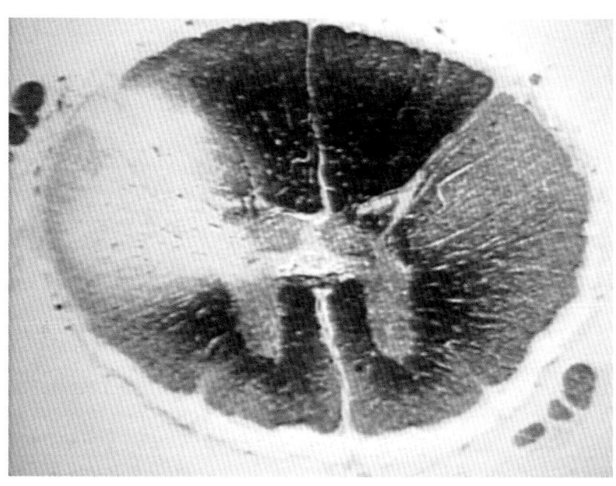

A

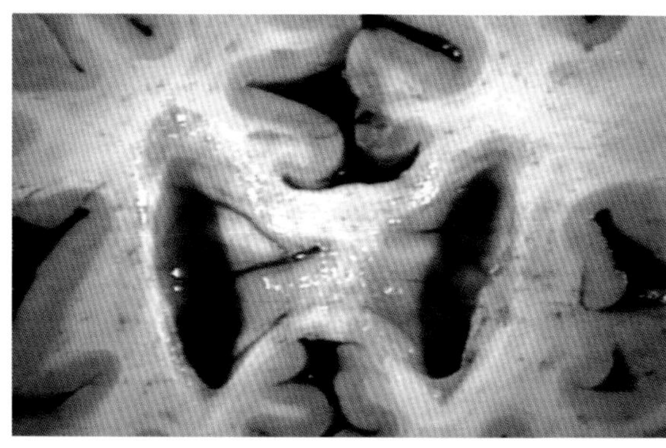

B

Color Image 47. Multiple sclerosis. (A) Lumbar spinal cord with mostly random and asymmetric white-matter lesions. **(B)** Brain with periventricular white-matter plaques of demyelination, gross. Demyelination occurs in a bilateral asymmetric distribution. Classic clinical findings are nystagmus, scanning speech, and intention tremor.*

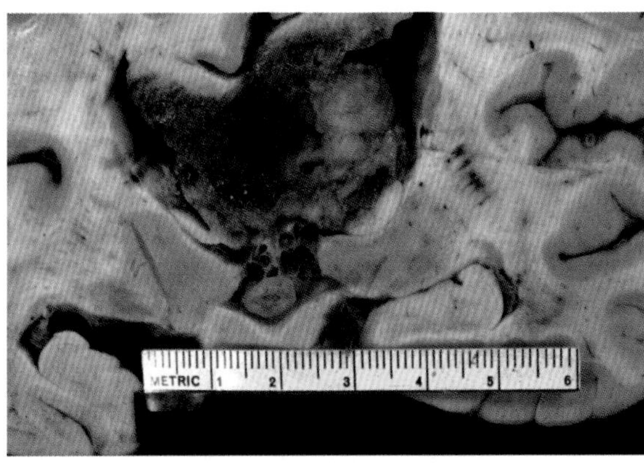

A

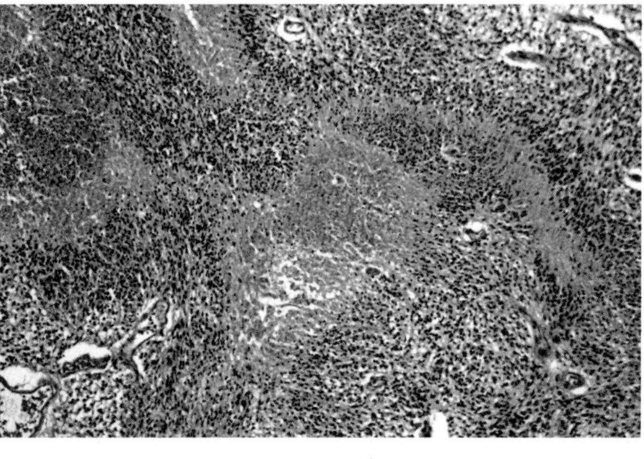

B

Color Image 48. **Glioblastoma multiforme** (**A**) extending across the midline of the cerebral cortex, gross.* (**B**) Histology shows necrosis with surrounding pseudopalisading of malignant tumor cells. (Image B reproduced, with permission, from USMLERx.com.)

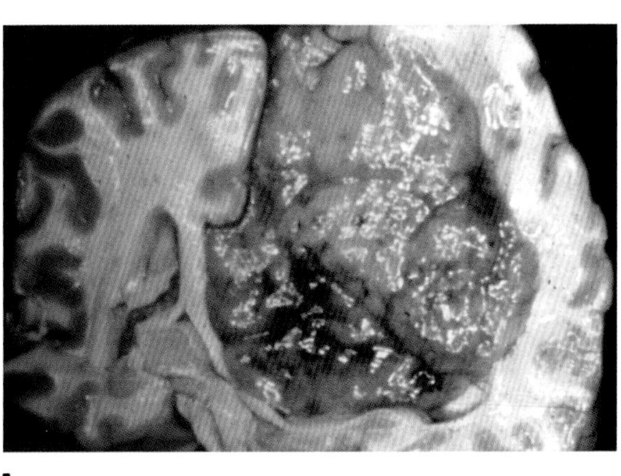

A

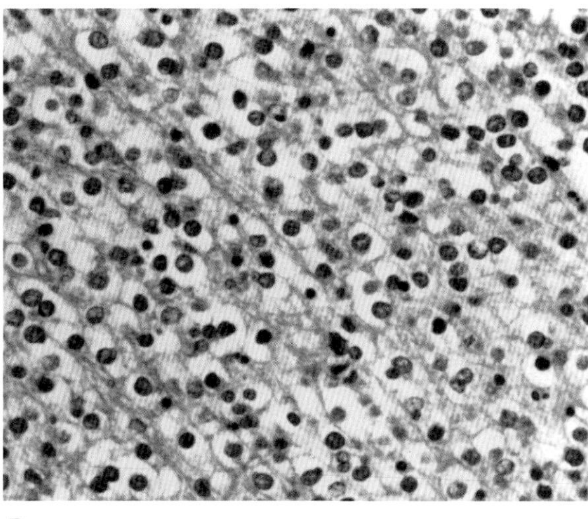

B

Color Image 49. **Oligodendroglioma.** (**A**) Gross natural-color coronal section of cerebral hemisphere with a large lesion of the left parieto-occipital white matter. (**B**) Classic "fried egg" appearance with perinuclear halos and "chicken-wire" capillary pattern.*

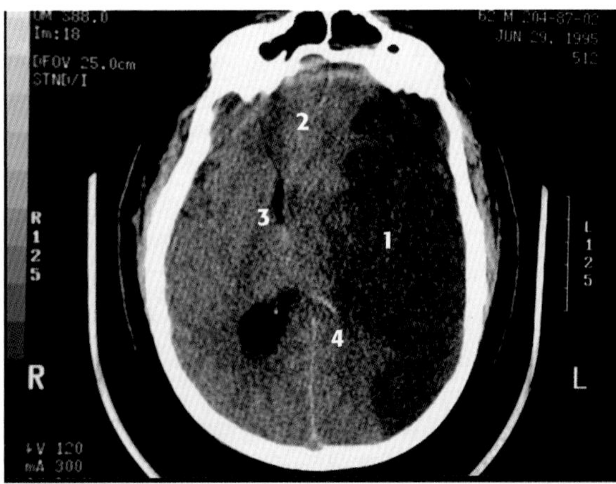

Color Image 50. **Left middle cerebral artery stroke.** Large left MCA territory stroke with edema and mass effect but no visible hemorrhage. The patient experienced deficits in speech and in the right side of the face and upper extremities. 1—ischemic brain parenchyma; 2—subtle midline shift to the right; 3—the right frontal horn of the lateral ventricle; 4—the left lateral ventricles obliterated by edema.

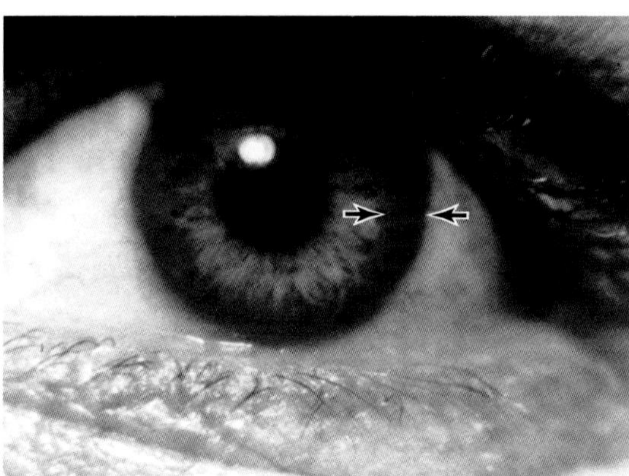

Color Image 51. **Kayser-Fleischer ring** in Wilson's disease. This corneal ring (between arrows) was golden brown and contrasted clearly against a gray-blue iris. Note that the darkness of the ring increases as the outer border (limbus) of the cornea is approached (right arrow). (Photo courtesy of Hoyt, WF.)

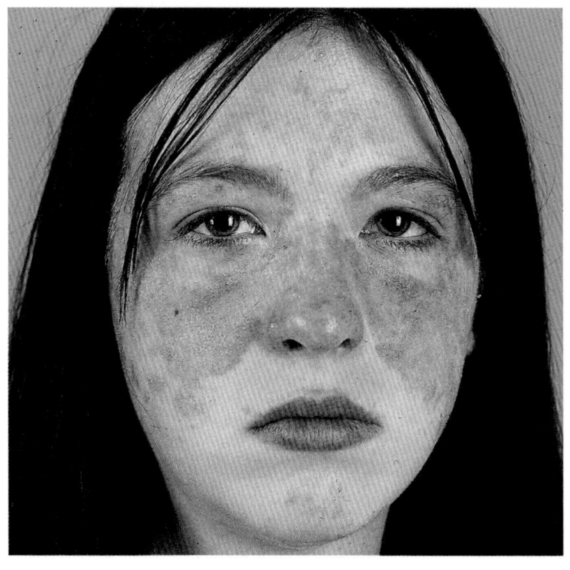

Color Image 52. Acute systemic lupus erythematosus. Bright red, sharply defined erythema is seen with slight edema and minimal scaling in a "butterfly pattern" on the face (the typical "malar rash"). Note also that the patient is female and young. (Reproduced, with permission, from Wolff K et al. *Fitzpatrick's Color Atlas and Synopsis of Clinical Dermatology*, 5th ed. New York: McGraw-Hill, 2005: 385.)

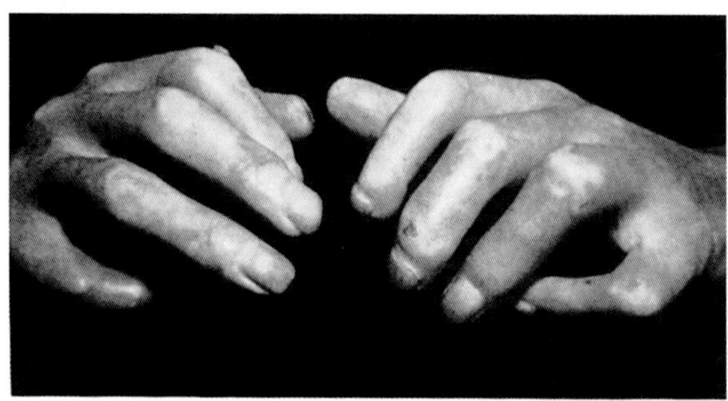

Color Image 53. Scleroderma. The progressive "tightening" of the skin has contracted the fingers and eliminated creases over the knuckles. Fibrosis is widespread and may also involve the esophagus (dysphagia), lung (restrictive disease), and small vessels of the kidney (hypertension).

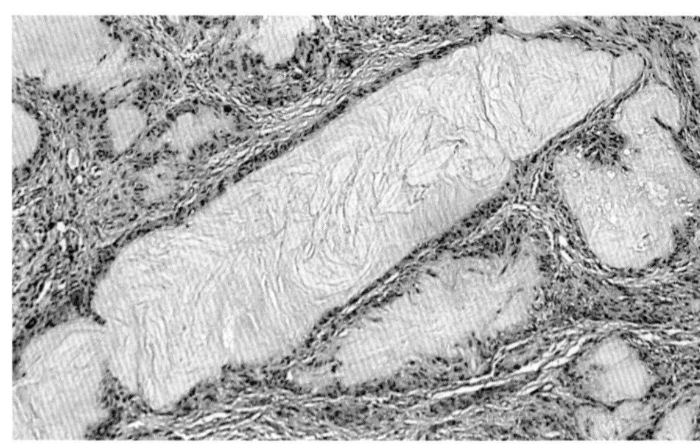

A

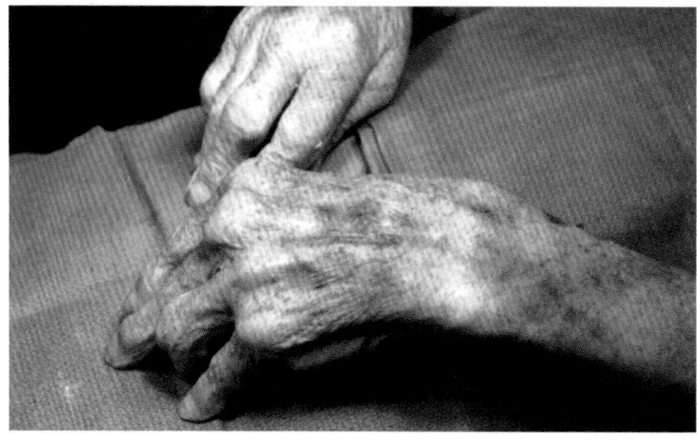

B

Color Image 54. Gout. (**A**) Tophi within joints consist of aggregates of urate crystals surrounded by an inflammatory reaction consisting of macrophages, lymphocytes, and giant cells. (**B**) Tophi affect the proximal interphalangeal (PIP) joints, knees, and elbows, growing like tubers from the bones.* (Image A reproduced, with permission, from USMLERx.com.)

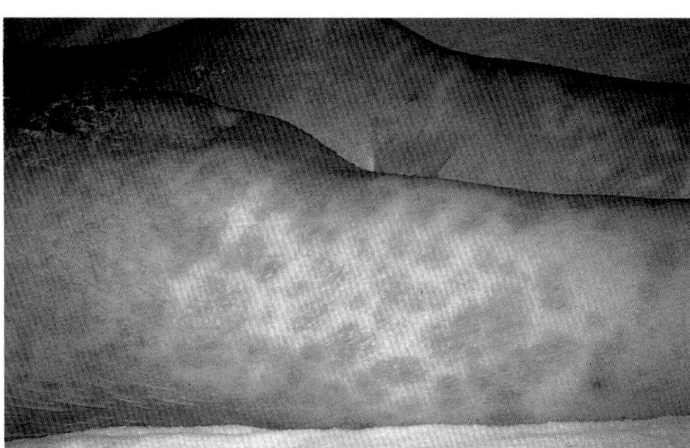

Color Image 55. Erythema multiforme, captopril induced. Erythematous macules, papules, vesicles, bullae, and erosions are seen. (Reproduced, with permission, from Hurwitz RM et al. *Pathology of the Skin: Atlas of Clinical-Pathological Correlation*, 2nd ed. Stamford, CT: Appleton & Lange, 1998.)

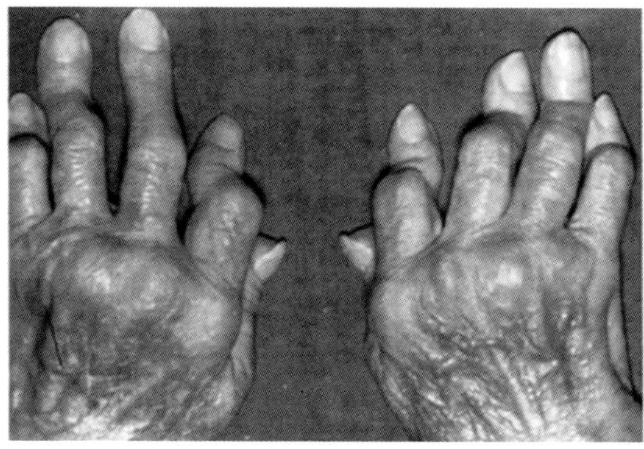

Color Image 56. Rheumatoid arthritis. Note the swan-neck deformities of the digits and severe, symmetric involvement of the PIP joints.

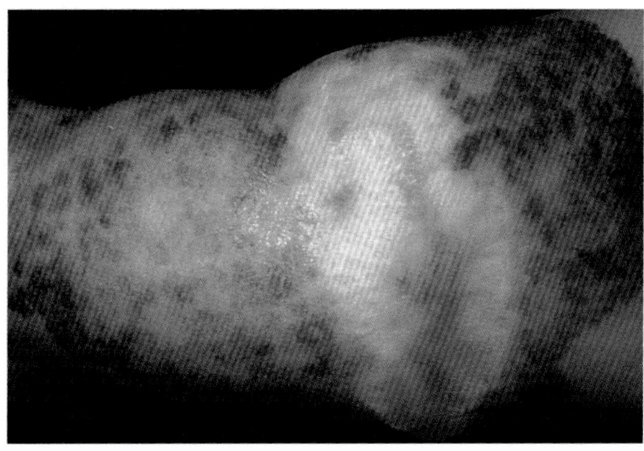

Color Image 57. Arteriovenous malformation. The markedly enlarged and distorted arm of a six-month-old boy with confluent erythematous papules and nodules. (Reproduced, with permission, from Hurwitz RM et al. *Pathology of the Skin: Atlas of Clinical-Pathological Correlation*, 2nd ed. Stamford, CT: Appleton & Lange, 1998.)

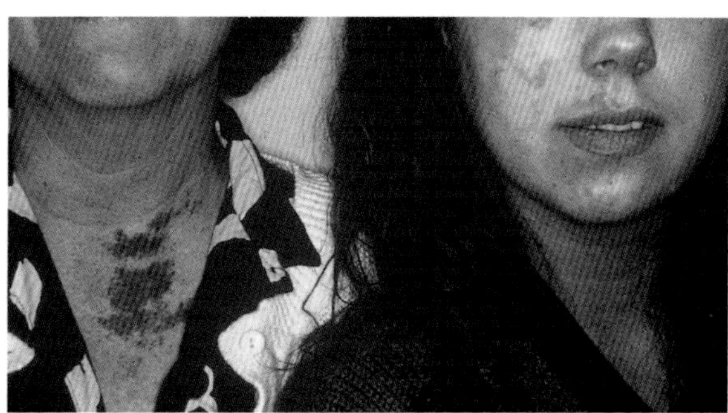

Color Image 58. Capillary malformation, port-wine type. Irregular purple patches and plaques are seen on the neck and chest of the mother, and pink patches are seen on the cheek, lip, chin, neck, and chest of the daughter. Both lesions were present at birth. (Reproduced, with permission, from Hurwitz RM et al. *Pathology of the Skin: Atlas of Clinical-Pathological Correlation*, 2nd ed. Stamford, CT: Appleton & Lange, 1998.)

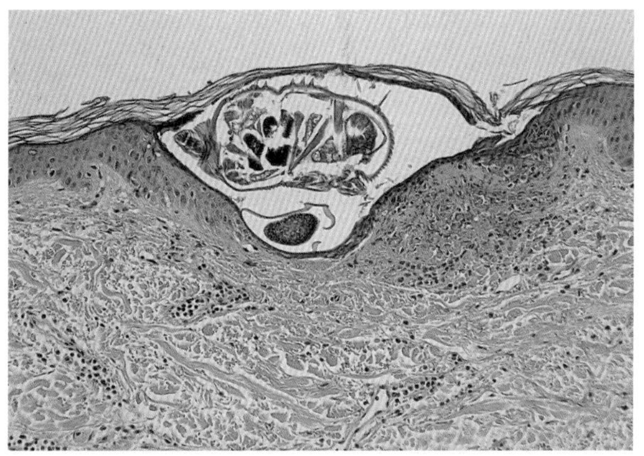

Color Image 59. Scabies. Adult female mite with egg containing embryo within the epidermis. (Reproduced, with permission, from Hurwitz RM et al. *Pathology of the Skin: Atlas of Clinical-Pathological Correlation*, 2nd ed. Stamford, CT: Appleton & Lange, 1998.)

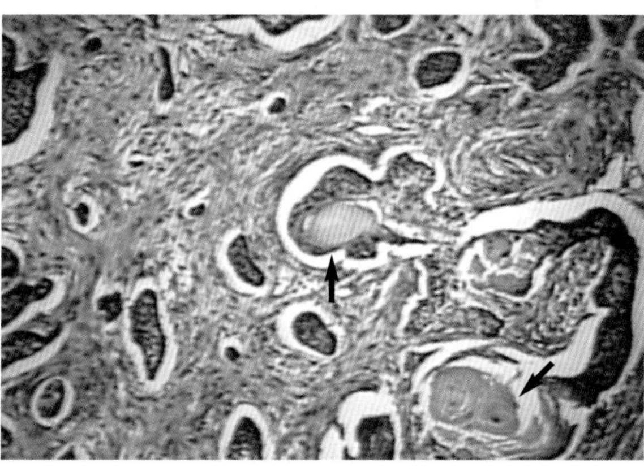

Color Image 60. Squamous cell carcinoma. Malignant skin tumor involving the epidermal skin layer. Note the presence of keratin pearls (arrows).*

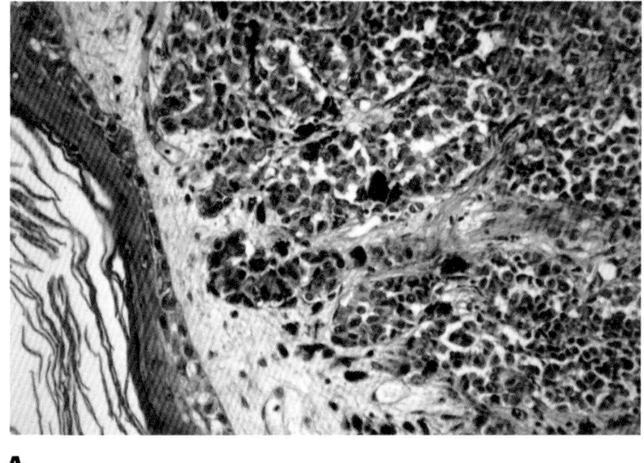

A

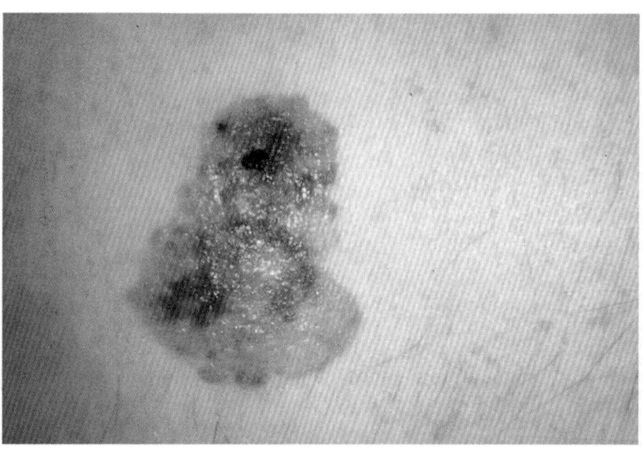

B

Color Image 61. Malignant melanoma. (A) Lesion just beneath the epidermis with pigmented and nonpigmented cells. The tumor cells are usually polyhedral but may be spindle shaped, dendritic, or ballooned or may resemble oat cells. Many but by no means all melanomas make melanin. Large nucleoli are common.* **(B)** A multicolored tan, red, and dark brown irregular plaque on the abdomen. The depth of the lesion is a prognostic indicator. (Image B reproduced, with permission, from Hurwitz RM et al. *Pathology of the Skin: Atlas of Clinical-Pathological Correlation*, 2nd ed. Stamford, CT: Appleton & Lange, 1998.)

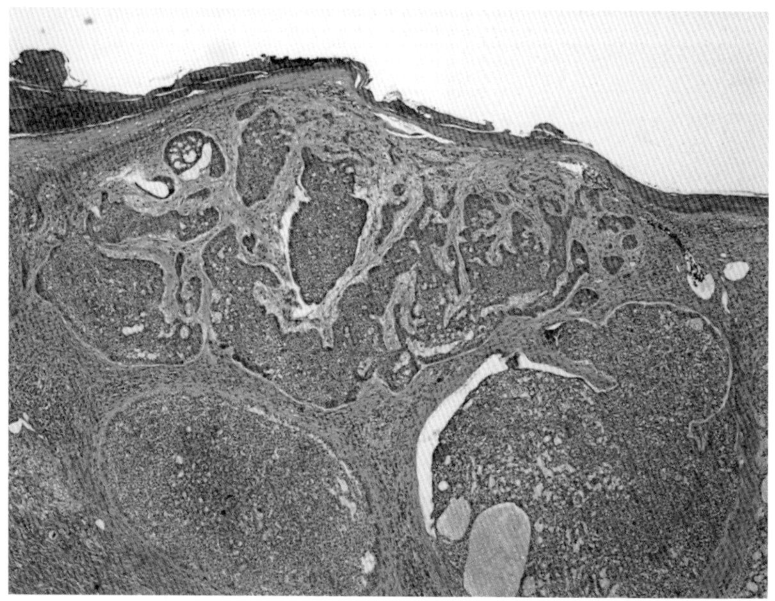

Color Image 62. Basal cell carcinoma. Nests of basaloid cells are present within the dermis with peripheral palisading and prominent retraction artifacts. (Reproduced, with permission, from USMLERx.com.)

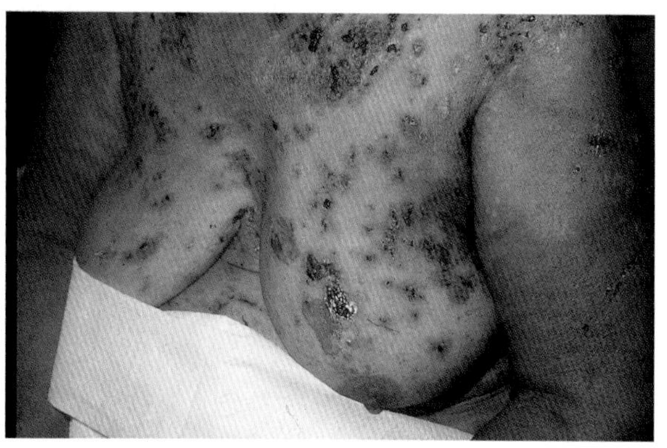

A

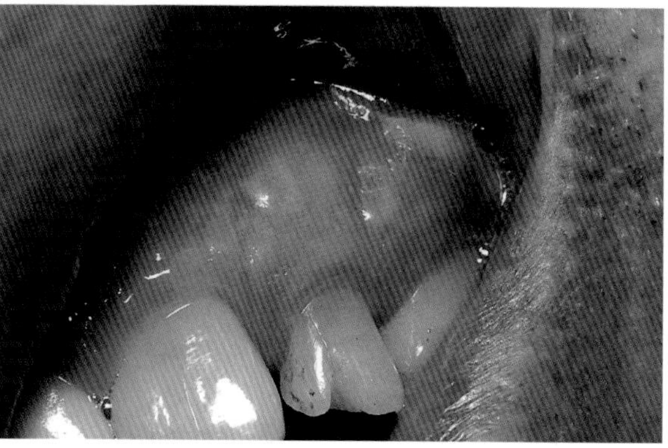

B

Color Image 63. Pemphigus vulgaris. (A) Numerous crusted, denuded, and weepy erythematous plaques are seen on the chest, breast, abdomen, and arms. **(B)** Vesicles on the gingiva. (Reproduced, with permission, from Hurwitz RM et al. *Pathology of the Skin: Atlas of Clinical-Pathological Correlation*, 2nd ed. Stamford, CT: Appleton & Lange, 1998.)

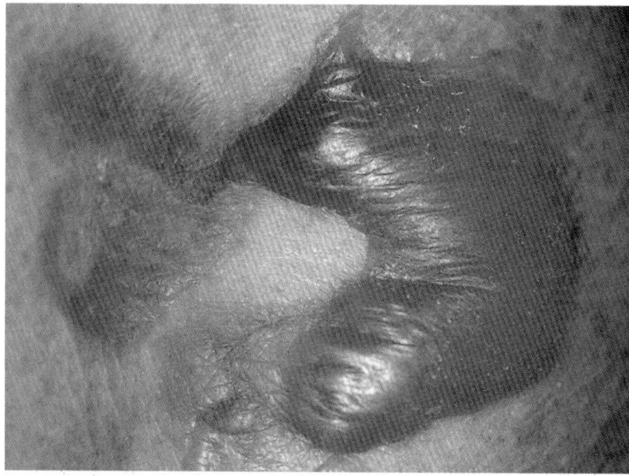

Color Image 64. Bullous pemphigoid. Erythematous plaques contiguous with large bullae. (Reproduced, with permission, from Hurwitz RM et al. *Pathology of the Skin: Atlas of Clinical-Pathological Correlation*, 2nd ed. Stamford, CT: Appleton & Lange, 1998.)

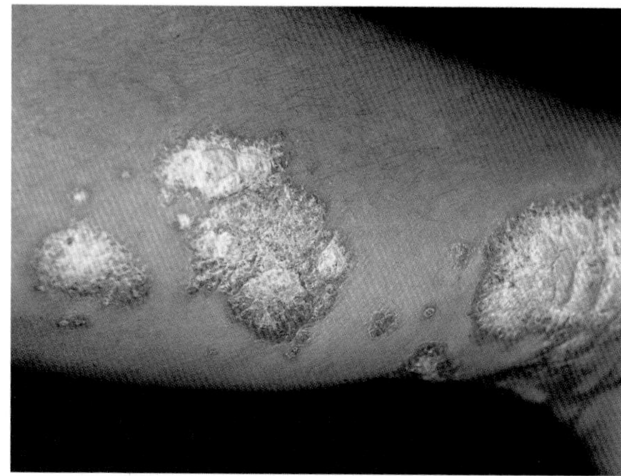

Color Image 65. Psoriasis, fully developed plaque. (Reproduced, with permission, from Hurwitz RM et al. *Pathology of the Skin: Atlas of Clinical-Pathological Correlation*, 2nd ed. Stamford, CT: Appleton & Lange, 1998.)

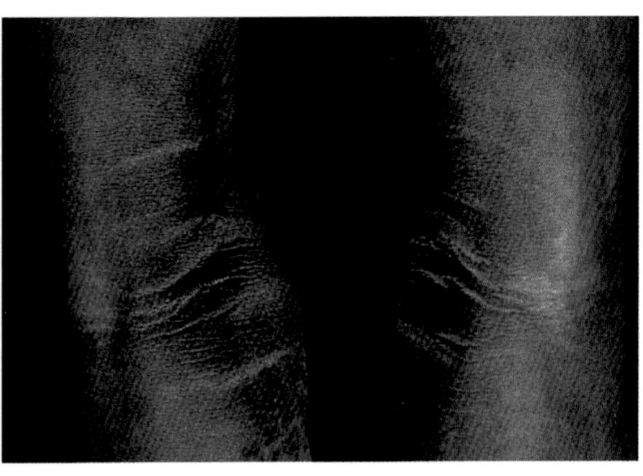

A

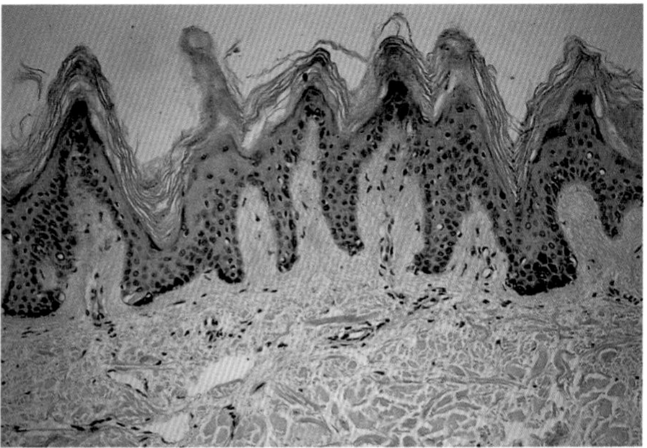

B

Color Image 66. Acanthosis nigricans. (**A**) Extensive hyperpigmented plaques on the arms in a patient with congenital lipodystrophy. This is an unusual distribution for acanthosis nigricans. (**B**) Hyperkeratosis and papillomatosis. (Reproduced, with permission, from Hurwitz RM et al. *Pathology of the Skin: Atlas of Clinical-Pathological Correlation*, 2nd ed. Stamford, CT: Appleton & Lange, 1998.)

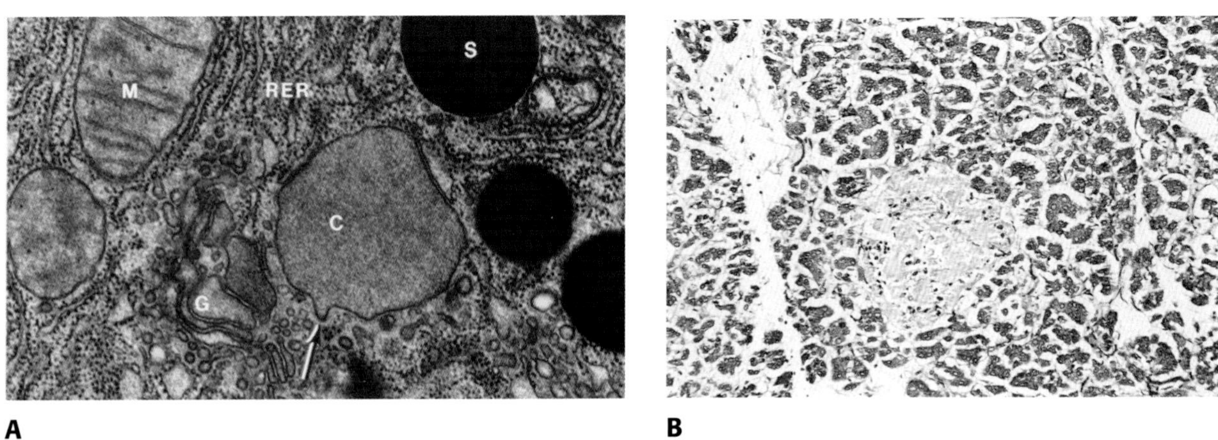

A B

Color Image 67. Pancreas. (A) Pancreatic acinar cell (EM). A condensing vacuole (C) is receiving secretory product (arrow) from the Golgi complex (G). M—mitochondrion; RER—rough endoplasmic reticulum; S—mature condensed secretory zymogen granules. (**B**) Pancreatic islet cells in **diabetes mellitus type 1.** In patients with diabetes mellitus type 1, autoantibodies against β cells cause a chronic inflammation until, over time, islet cells are entirely replaced by amyloid.

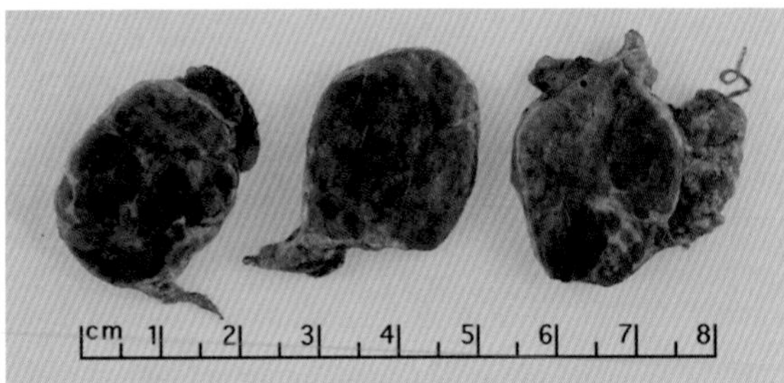

Color Image 68. Adrenocortical adenoma, gross. Cause of hypercortisolism (Cushing's syndrome) or hyperaldosteronism (Conn's syndrome).*

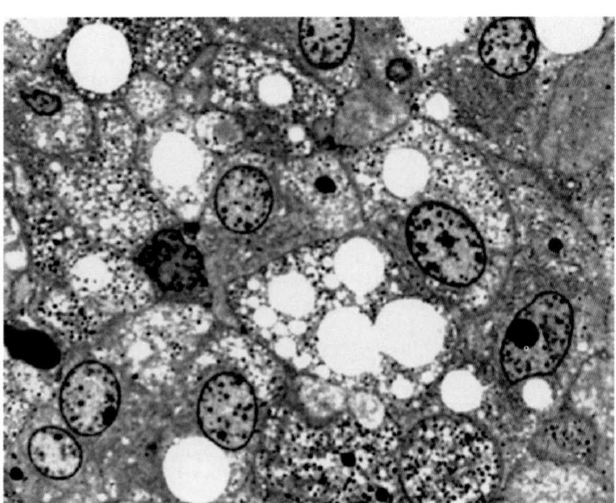

Color Image 69. Pheochromocytoma. The tumor cells have numerous vacuolar spaces within the cytoplasm (pseudoacini). Most of the punctate blue-black granules of variable density are dense-core neurosecretory granules.*

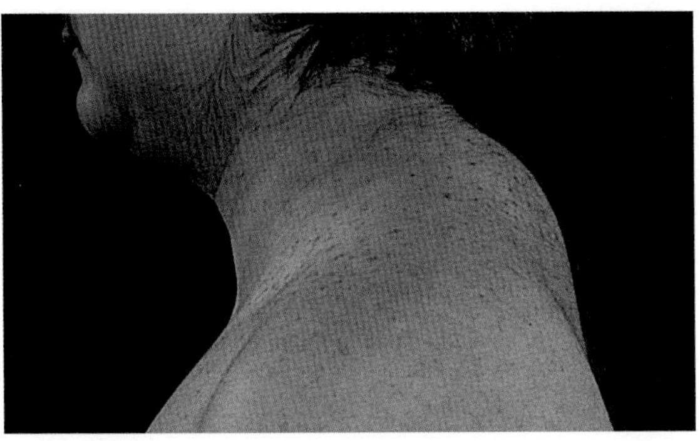

A

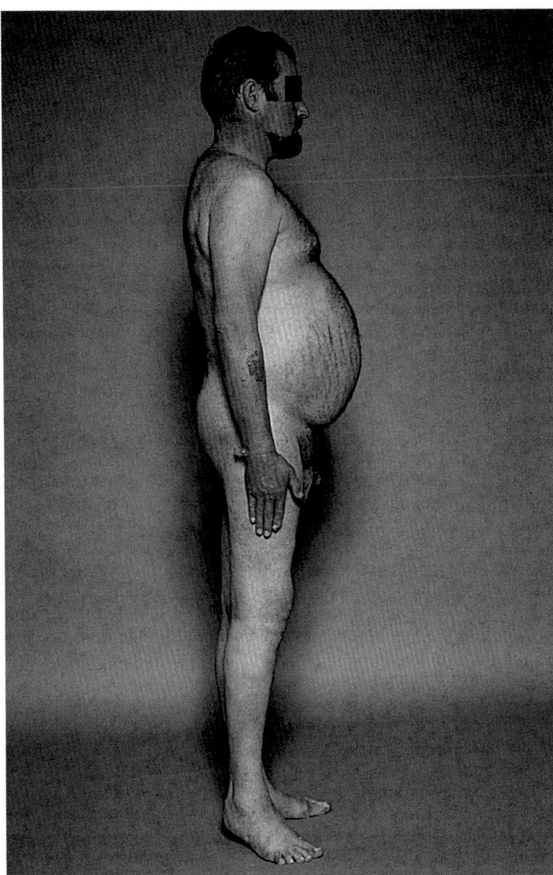

B

Color Image 70. Cushing's disease. The clinical picture includes (**A**) moon facies and buffalo hump and (**B**) truncal obesity and abdominal striae.

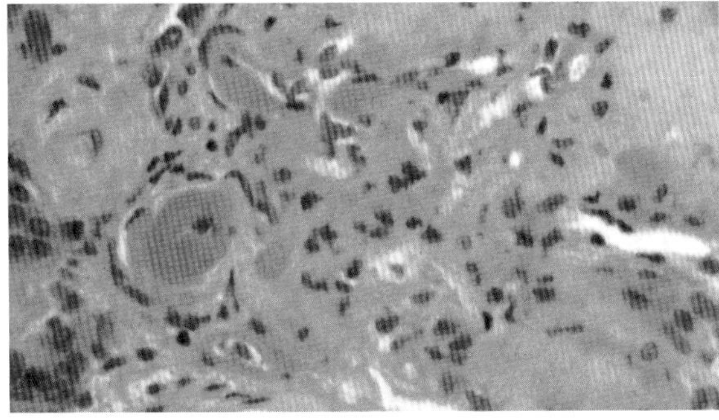

Color Image 72. Arteriolar sclerosis showing masses of hyaline material in glomerular afferent and efferent arterioles and in the glomerulus. From a type 1 diabetic patient.*

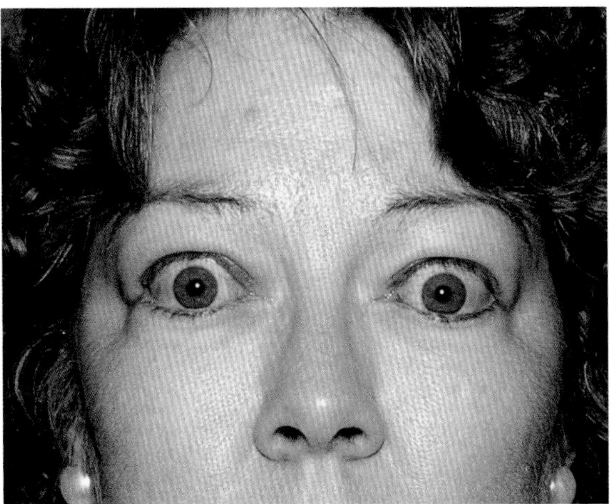

A

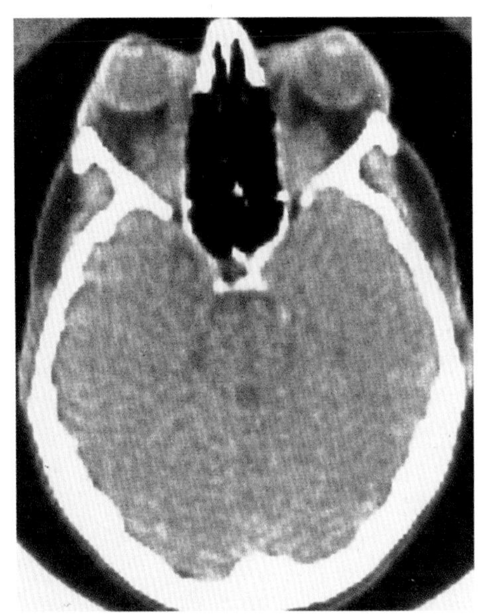

B

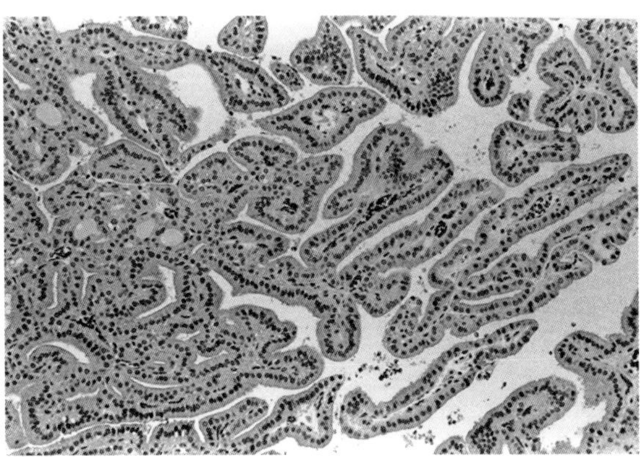

C

Color Image 71. Graves' disease. (**A**) Exophthalmos in a patient with proptosis and periorbital edema. (**B**) CT shows extraocular muscle enlargement at the orbital apex. (**C**) Stimulation of follicular cells by TSH causes the normal uniform architecture to be replaced by hyperplastic papillary, involuted borders, and decreased colloid. Typical medical therapy is propylthiouracil, which inhibits the production of thyroid hormone as well as peripheral conversion of T_4 to T_3.*

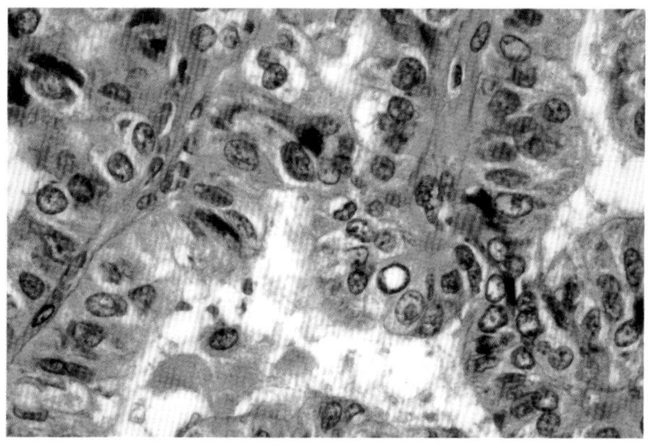

Color Image 73. Papillary carcinoma. The image shows the papillary architecture and classic nuclear features that are key in making the diagnosis, including ground-glass or "Orphan Annie eye" chromatin, nuclear grooves, and intranuclear pseudoinclusions. Psammoma bodies are not seen here but are often present. (Reproduced, with permission, from USMLERx.com.)

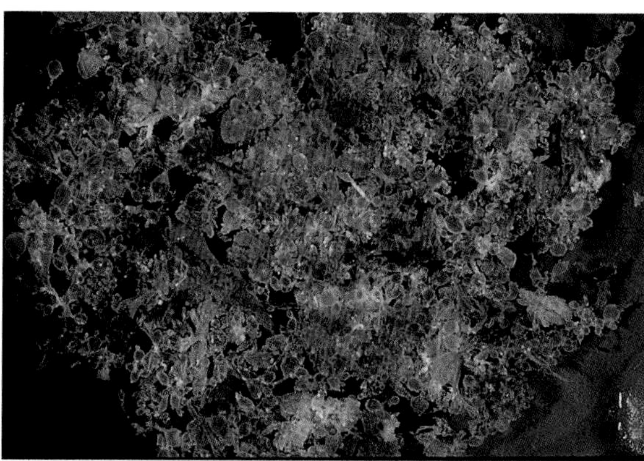

Color Image 74. Hydatidiform mole. The characteristic gross appearance is a "bunch of grapes." Hydatidiform moles are the most common precursors of choriocarcinoma. Complete moles usually display a 46,XX diploid pattern with all the chromosomes derived from the sperm. In partial moles, the karyotype is triploid or tetraploid, and fetal parts may be present.

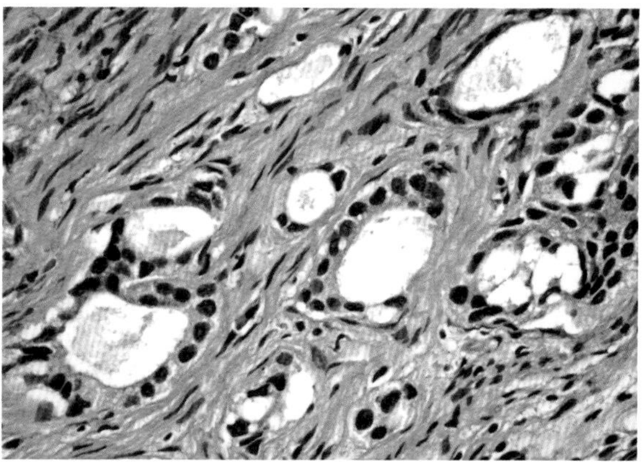

Color Image 75. Prostatic adenocarcinoma. Histology shows infiltrating glands lined by a single layer of cuboidal epithelium with enlarged nuclei and visible nucleoli. Note the absence of the outer basal layer that is usually present in normal glands. (Reproduced, with permission, from USMLERx.com.)

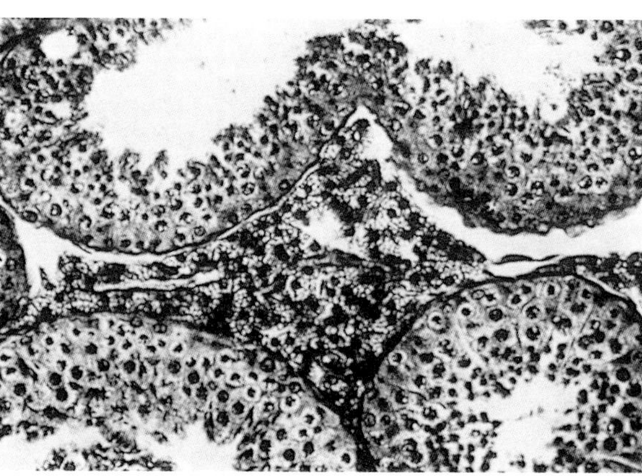

Color Image 76. Seminiferous tubules. Sertoli cells play a supportive and protective role in spermatogenesis. Note cells in various stages of differentiation, with spermatogonia near the basal lamina and more mature forms near the lumen.

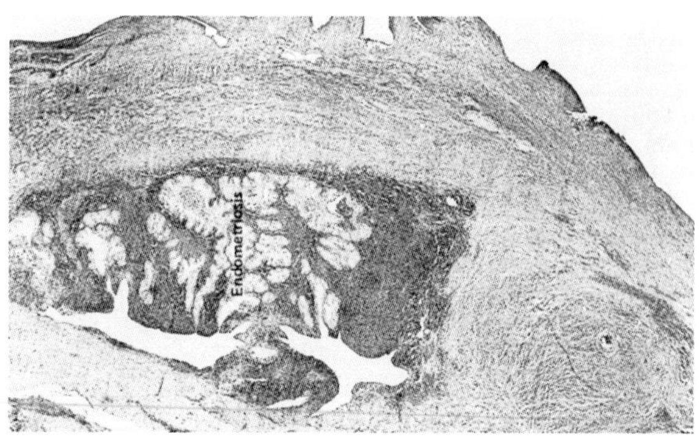

A

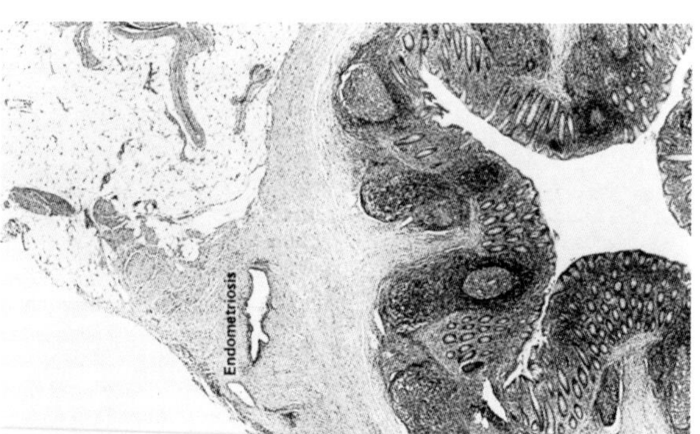

B

Color Image 77. Histologic appearance of endometriosis. **(A)** Endometriosis of the ovary. **(B)** Endometriosis of the cervix. (Reproduced, with permission, from DeCherney AH. *Current Obstetric and Gynecologic Diagnosis and Treatment*, 9th ed. New York: McGraw-Hill, 2003.)

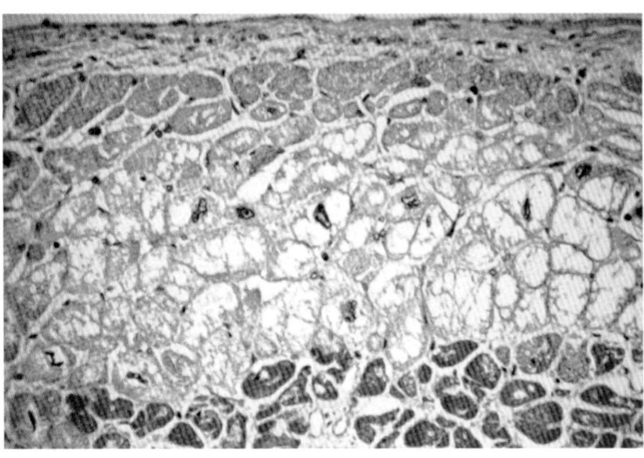

Color Image 78. Endocardial chronic ischemia. Microscopic example of myocytolysis and coagulation necrosis beneath the endocardium.*

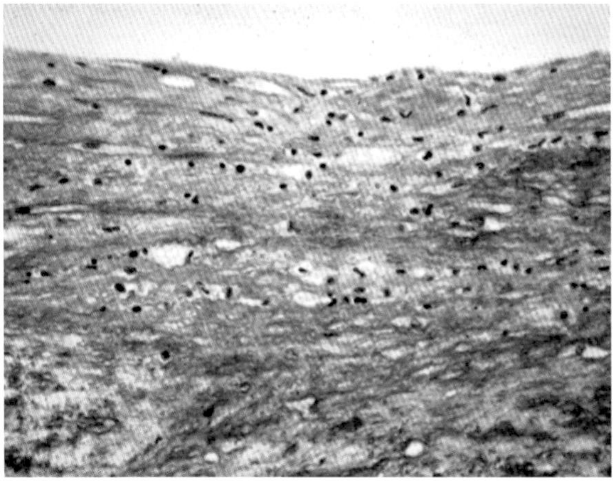

Color Image 79. Atherosclerosis. Aorta with fibrous intimal thickening and foam cells dispersed throughout smooth muscle cells, micro.*

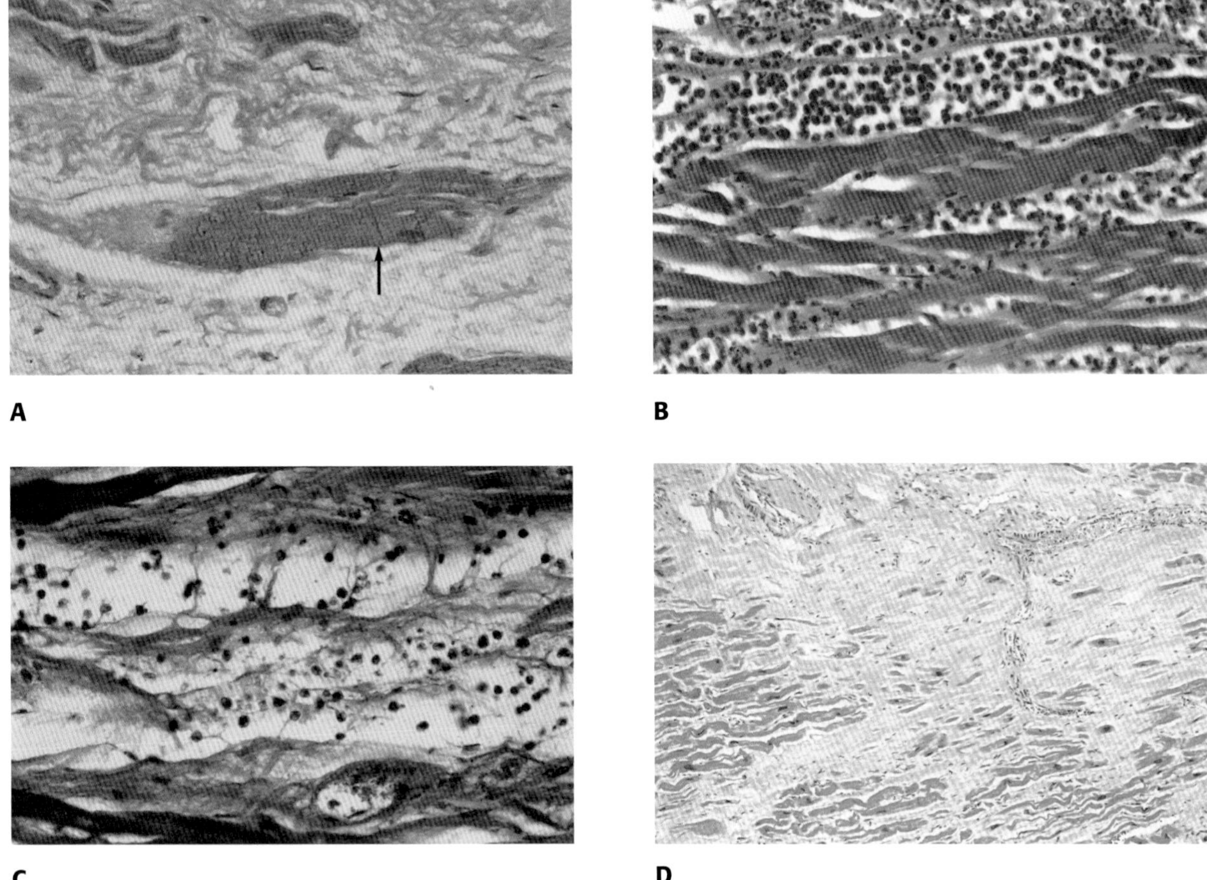

Color Image 80. Evolution of a myocardial infarction. Contraction band necrosis (arrow) is the first visible change, occurring in one to two hours (**A**). In the first three days, neutrophilic infiltration and coagulation necrosis occur (**B**). By three to seven days, neutrophils have been replaced by macrophages, and clearing of myocyte debris has begun (**C**). Within weeks, granulation and scarring occur (**D**).

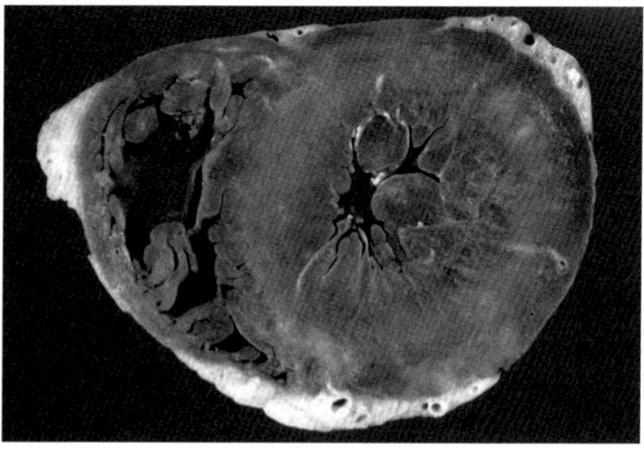

Color Image 81. Heart with marked concentric **left ventricular hypertrophy** from hypertension, gross.*

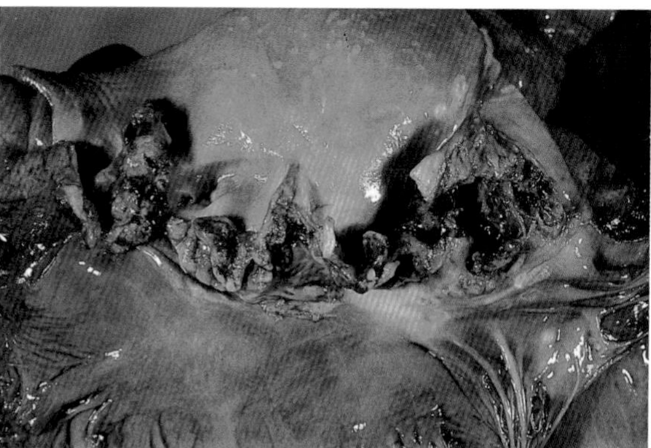

Color Image 82. **Acute bacterial endocarditis.** Virulent organisms (e.g., *Staphylococcus aureus*) infect previously normal valves, causing marked damage (here, in the aortic valve) and potentially giving rise to septic emboli.

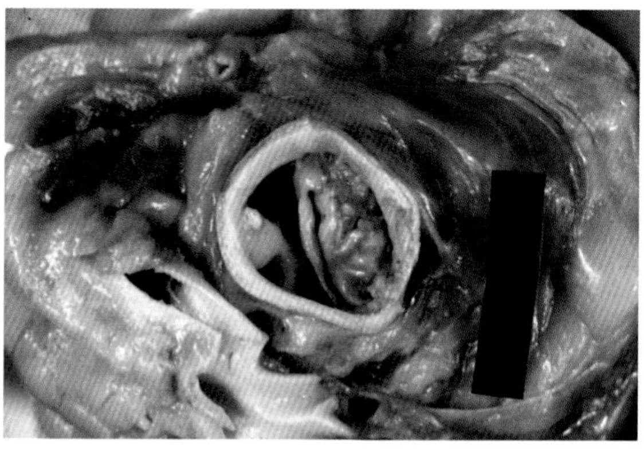

Color Image 83. Calcified **bicuspid aortic valve** showing false raphe. The abnormal architecture of the valve makes its leaflets susceptible to otherwise ordinary hemodynamic stresses, which ultimately leads to valvular thickening, calcification, increased rigidity, and stenosis.*

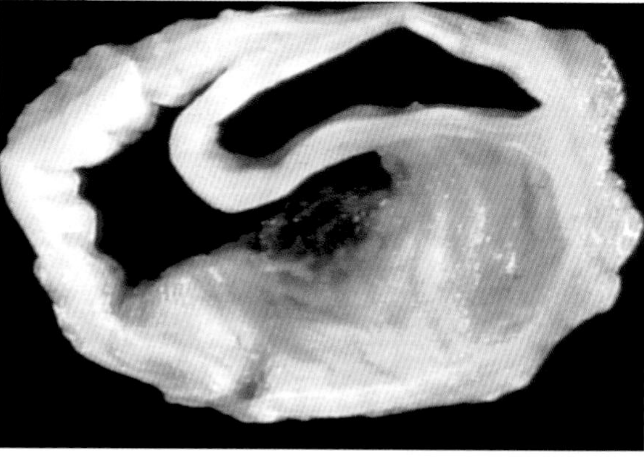

Color Image 84. **Aortic dissection** with a blood clot compressing the aortic lumen. A tear in the intima allowed blood to surge through the muscular layer to the adventitia (may lead to sudden death from hemothorax). Risk factors are hypertension, Marfan's syndrome, pregnancy, Ehlers-Danlos syndrome, and trauma.*

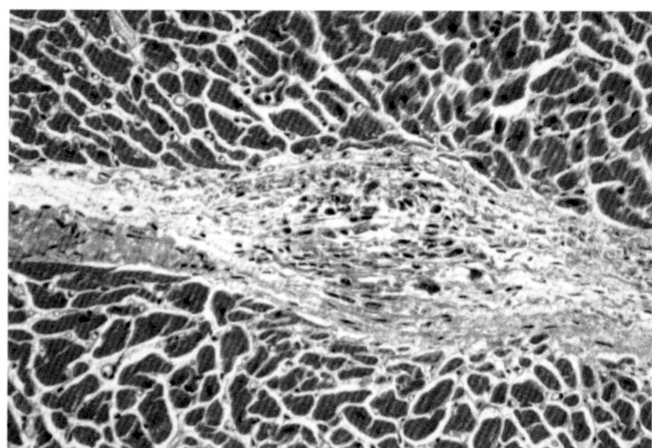

Color Image 85. The **Aschoff body**, an area of fibrinoid necrosis surrounded by mononuclear and multinucleated giant cells, is pathognomonic for **rheumatic heart disease.** The mitral valve is most commonly affected.*

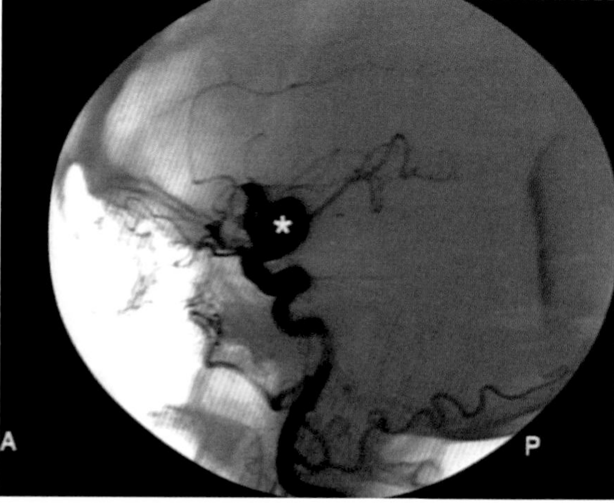

Color Image 86. **Carotid angiogram showing aneurysm.** Note the path of the internal carotid artery through the neck and its major branches (ophthalmic artery, anterior cerebral artery, middle cerebral artery). The aneurysm is inferior to the terminal branches in this angiogram.*

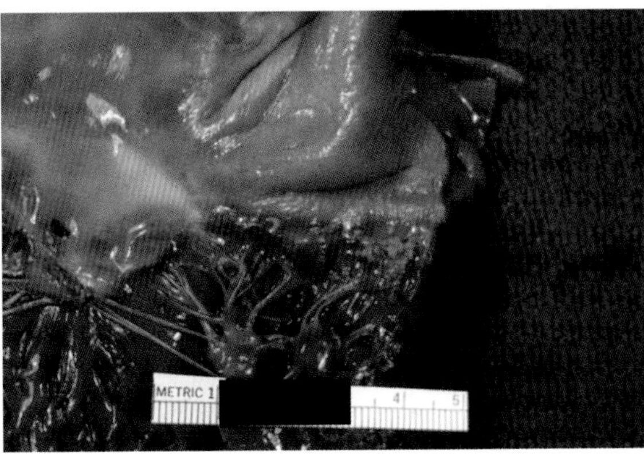

Color Image 87. Bacterial endocarditis of the mitral valve. Vegetations can embolize and infect distant organ systems.*

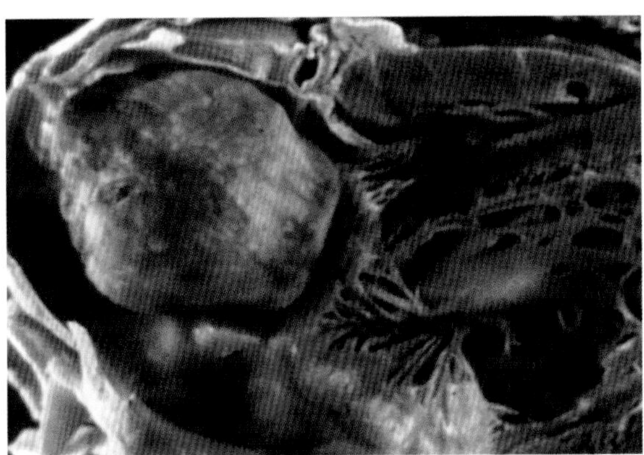

Color Image 88. Left atrial myxoma. The most common primary cardiac tumor; known to produce VEGF (vascular endothelial growth factor).*

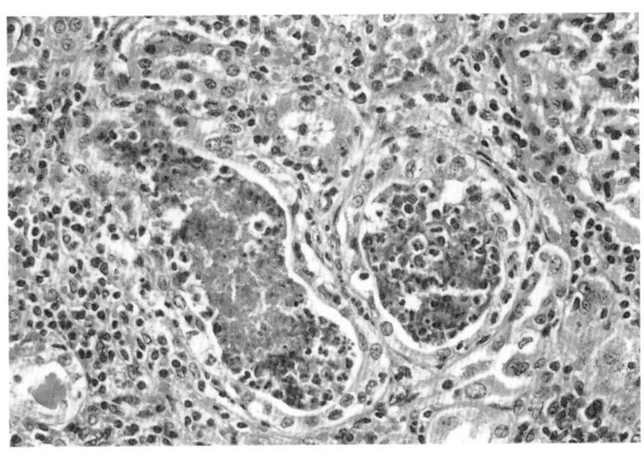

A

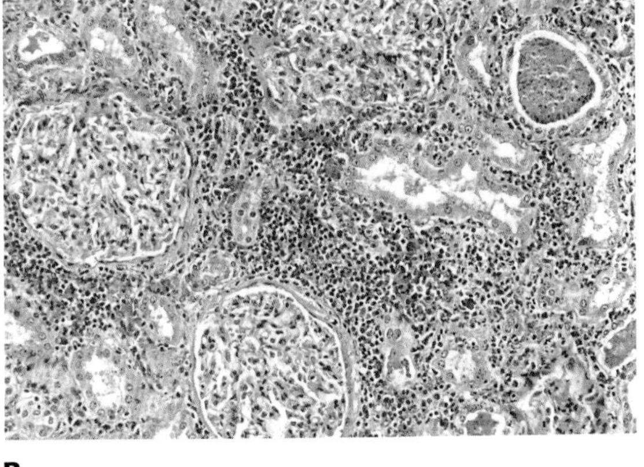

B

Color Image 89. Acute pyelonephritis (A) is characterized by neutrophilic infiltration and abscess formation within the renal interstitium. Abscesses may rupture, introducing collections of white cells to the tubular lumen. In contrast, **chronic pyelonephritis (B)** has a lymphocytic invasion with fibrosis.

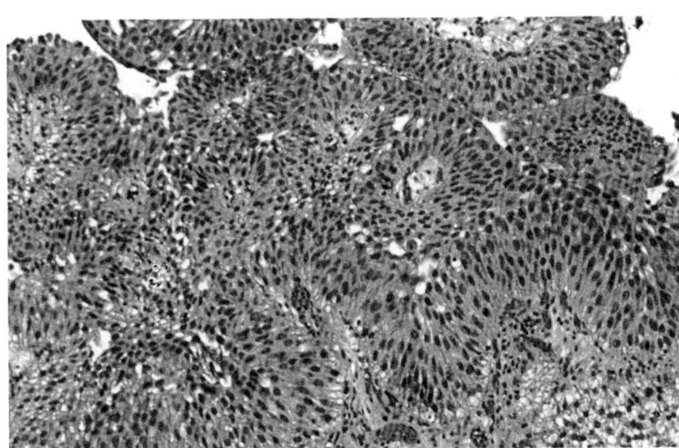

Color Image 90. Transitional cell carcinoma. The image shows a papillary growth lined by transitional epithelium with mild nuclear atypia and pleomorphism. (Reproduced, with permission, from USMLERx.com.)

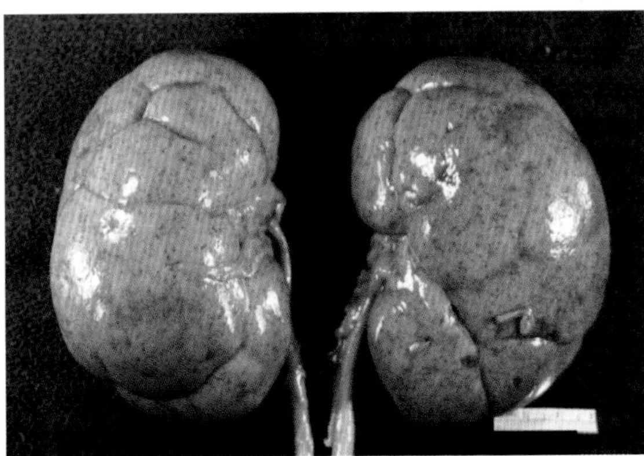

Color Image 91. Lupus erythematosus, kidneys. Enlarged, very pale kidneys with "flea bite" or ectasia from a patient with nephrotic syndrome or subacute glomerulonephritis as a result of lupus erythematosus.*

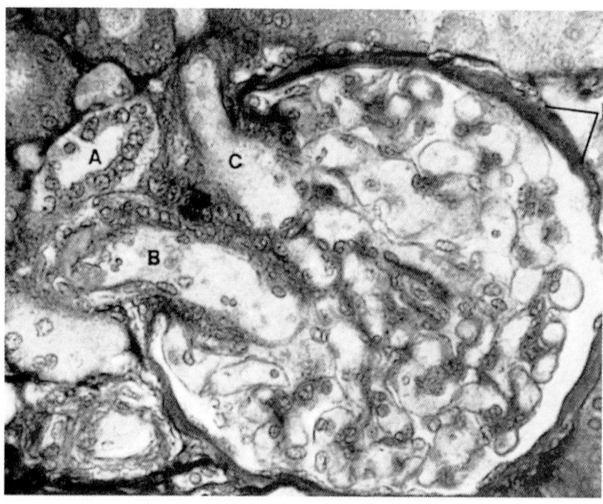

Color Image 92. Normal glomerulus, microscopic, with (**A**) macula densa and (**B**) afferent and (**C**) efferent arterioles.

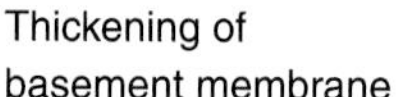

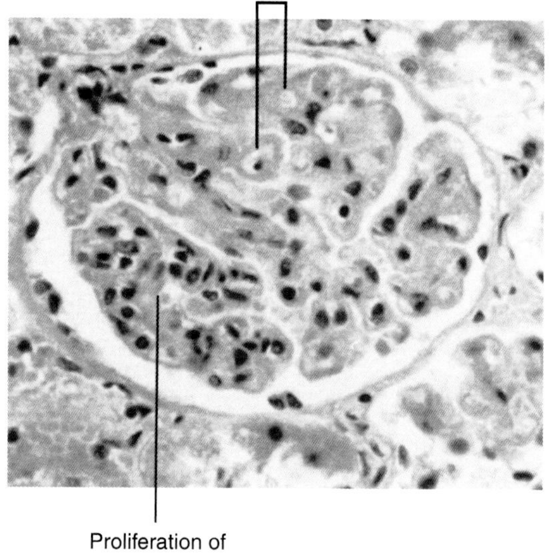

Color Image 94. Systemic lupus erythematosus, kidney pathology. In the membranous glomerulonephritic pattern, "wire-loop" thickening occurs as a result of subendothelial immune complex deposition.

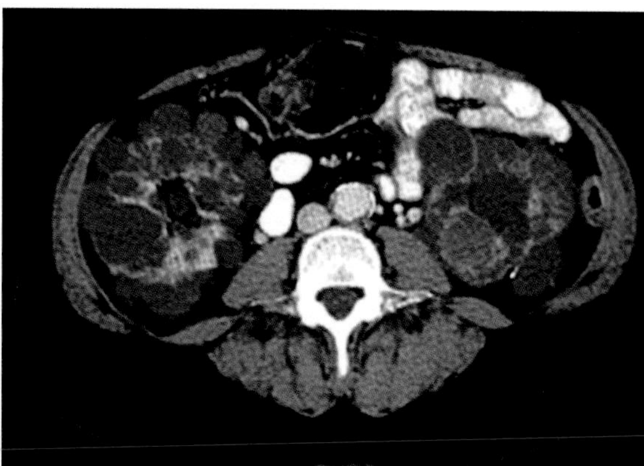

Color Image 96. Polycystic kidney disease. Abdominal CT shows multiple cysts in both kidneys. PKD is an autosomal-dominant disease and is often associated with aneurysm formation in the brain. The disease occurs bilaterally and presents with flank pain and hematuria.*

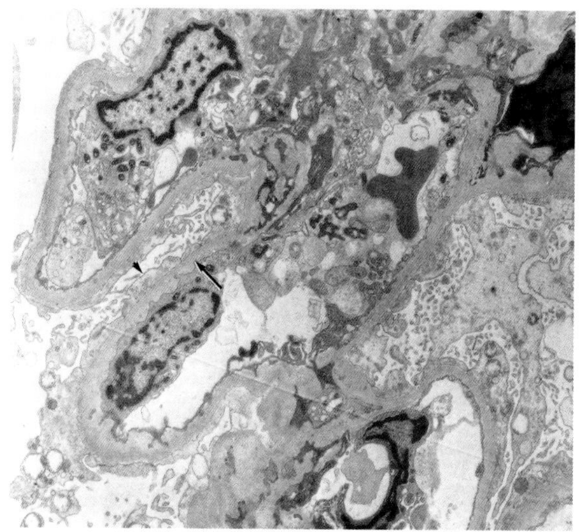

Color Image 93. Minimal change disease (lipoid nephrosis) shows normal glomeruli on light microscopy but effacement of foot processes on EM (arrowhead). The full arrow points to a normal foot process. Treatment consists of corticosteroids.

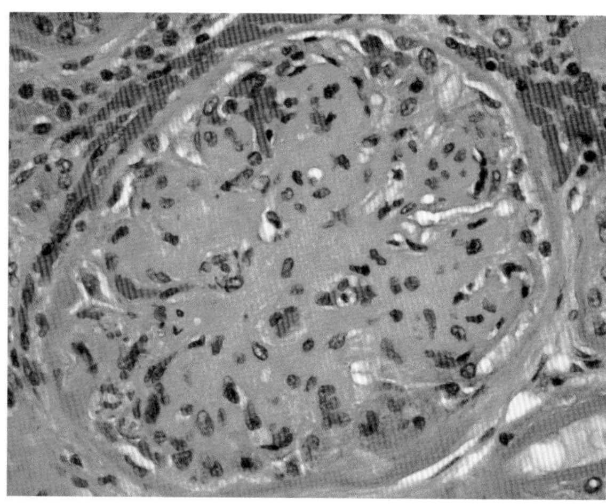

Color Image 95. Diabetic glomerulosclerosis. Nodular diabetic glomerulosclerosis is also known as Kimmelstiel-Wilson syndrome and is characterized by acellular ovoid nodules in the periphery of the glomerulus. (Reproduced, with permission, from USMLERx.com.)

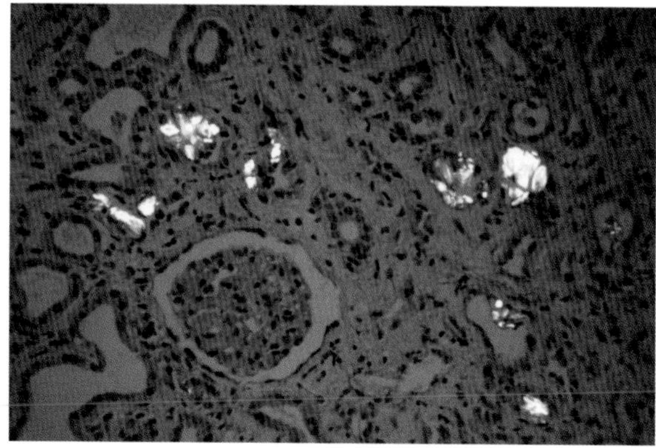

Color Image 97. Calcium oxalate crystals in the kidney, viewed with partially crossed polarizers. Tubular failure in oxalate nephropathy can result from vitamin C or antifreeze abuse.*

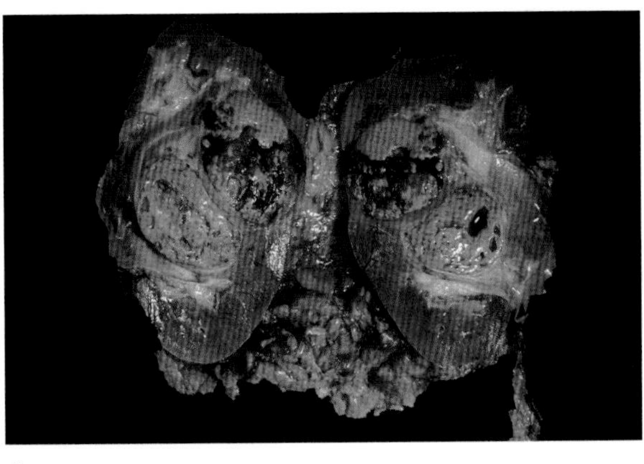

A

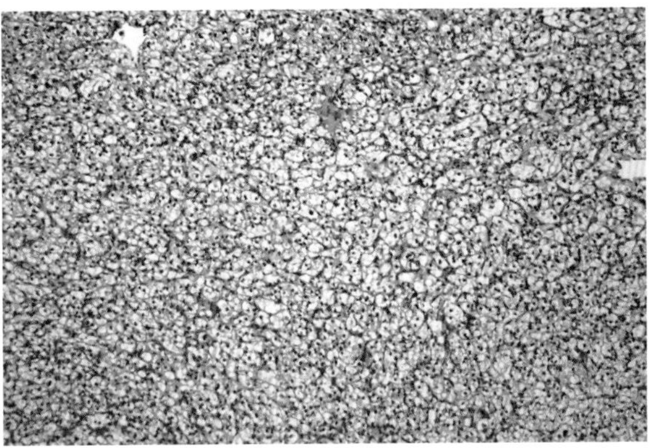

B

Color Image 98. Renal cell carcinoma. (**A**) Gross. The kidney has been bivalved, revealing a nodular, golden-yellow tumor in the midkidney with areas of hemorrhage and necrosis. (**B**) Histology shows polygonal cells with small nuclei and abundant clear cytoplasm with a rich, delicate branching vasculature. (Reproduced, with permission, from USMLERx.com.)

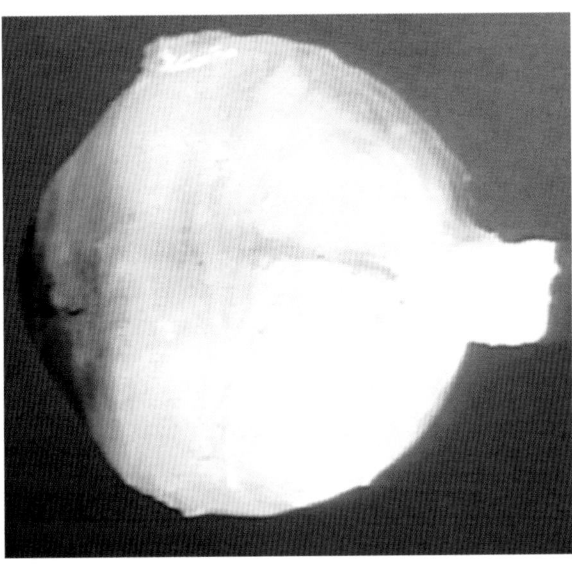

A

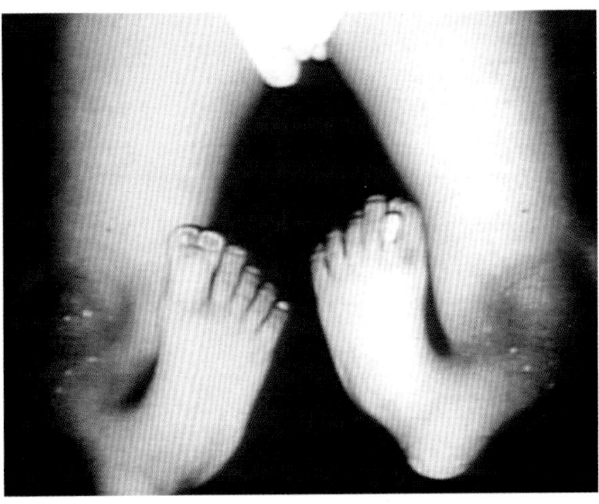

B

Color Image 99. Osteogenesis imperfecta. (**A**) Blue sclera caused by translucency of connective tissue over the choroid. The optic nerve is on the right side of the image. (**B**) Abnormal collagen synthesis results from a variety of gene mutations and causes brittle bones and connective tissue malformations.*

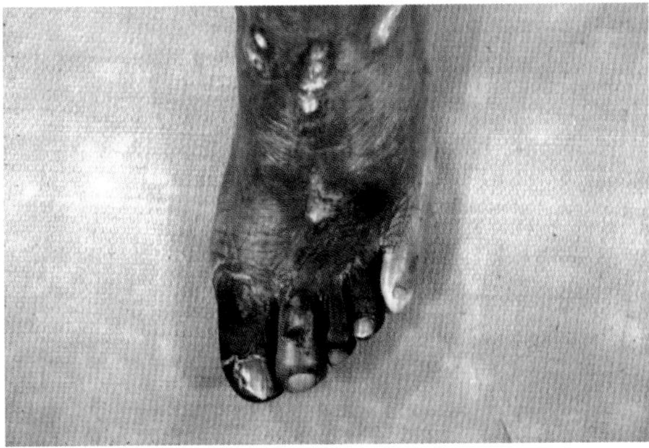

Color Image 100. Foot gangrene. The first four toes and adjacent skin are dry, shrunken, and blackened with superficial necrosis and peeling of the skin. A well-defined line of demarcation separates the black region from the viable skin.*

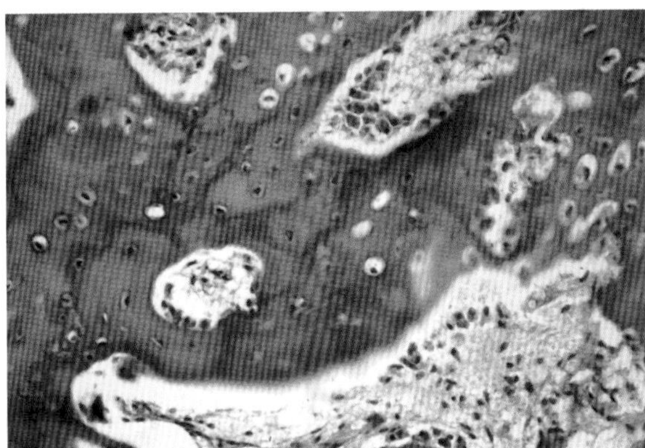

Color Image 101. Bone fracture. New bone formation with osteoblasts.*

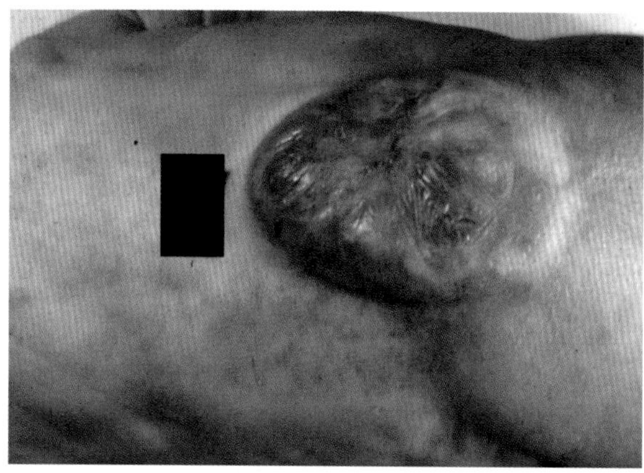

Color Image 102. Meningomyelocele. A neural tube defect in which the meninges and spinal cord herniate through the spinal canal; gross image of infant's lower back.*

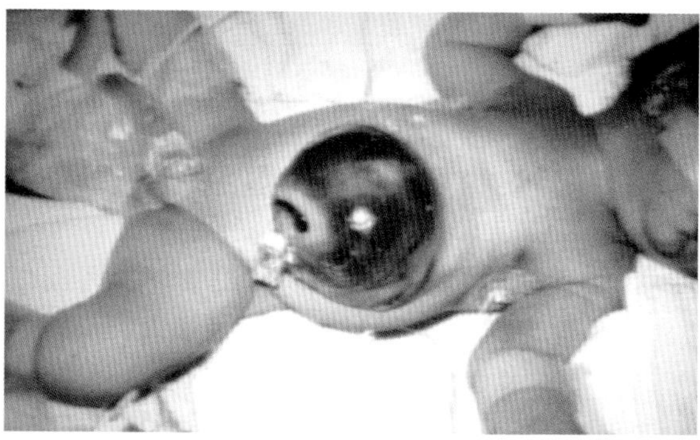

Color Image 103. Omphalocele in a newborn. Note that the defect is midline and is covered by peritoneum, as opposed to gastroschisis, which is not covered by peritoneum and is often not midline.*

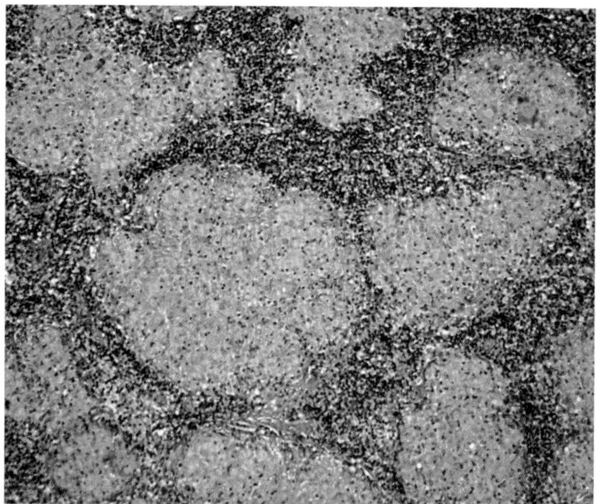

Color Image 104. Sarcoidosis. Numerous tightly formed granulomas are seen on histology of a lymph node in a patient with sarcoidosis. (Reproduced, with permission, from USMLERx.com.)

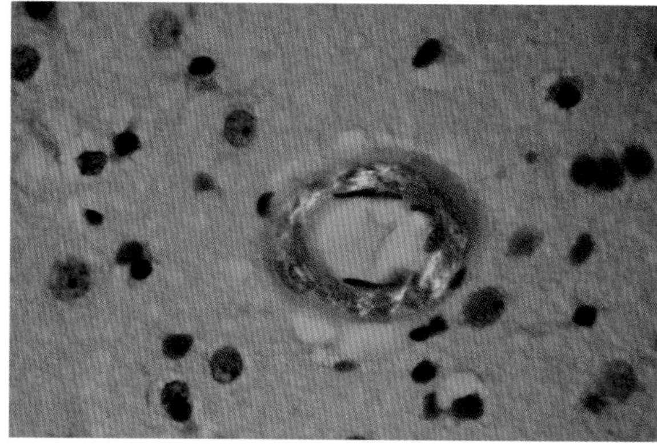

Color Image 105. Amyloidosis. Congo red stain demonstrates amyloid deposits in the artery wall that show apple-green birefringence under polarized light. (Reproduced, with permission, from USMLERx.com.)

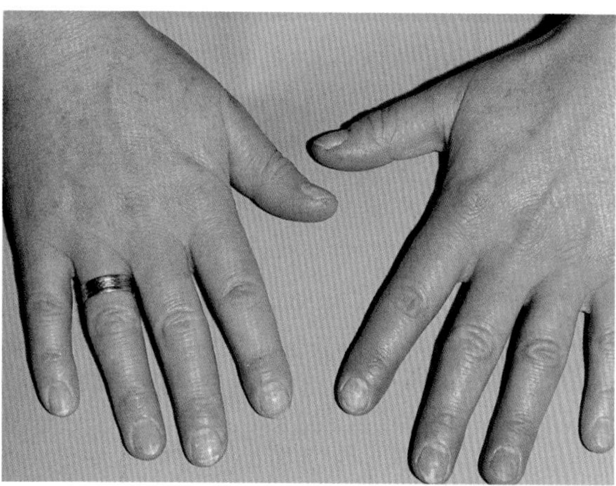

Color Image 106. Raynaud's disease. The left hand exhibits a distal cyanosis compared to the right hand; it is seen especially well in the nail beds. Unilateral episodes such as this one may occur after contact with a cold object. (Reproduced, with permission, from Wolff K et al. *Fitzpatrick's Color Atlas and Synopsis of Clinical Dermatology*, 5th ed. New York: McGraw-Hill, 2005: 403.)

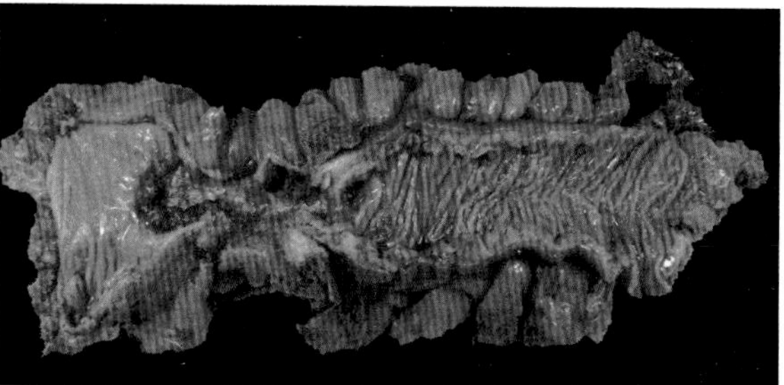

Color Image 107. Colon cancer. Note the circumferential tumor with heaped-up edges and central ulceration. (Reproduced, with permission, from USMLERx.com.)

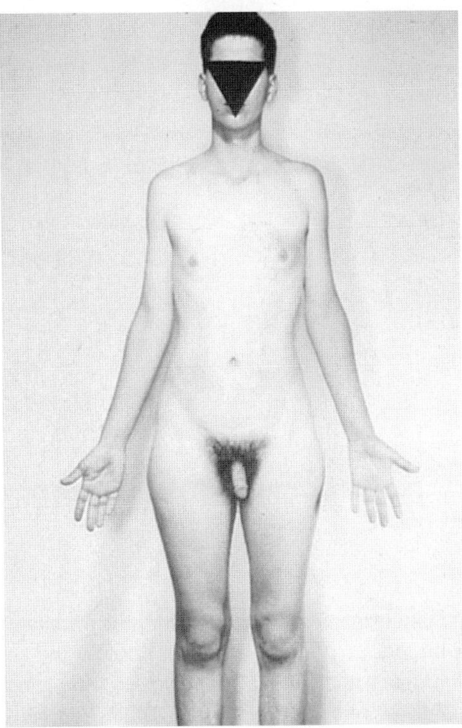

Image 108. Klinefelter's syndrome (XXY). Phenotype includes a female fat distribution with male external genitalia.

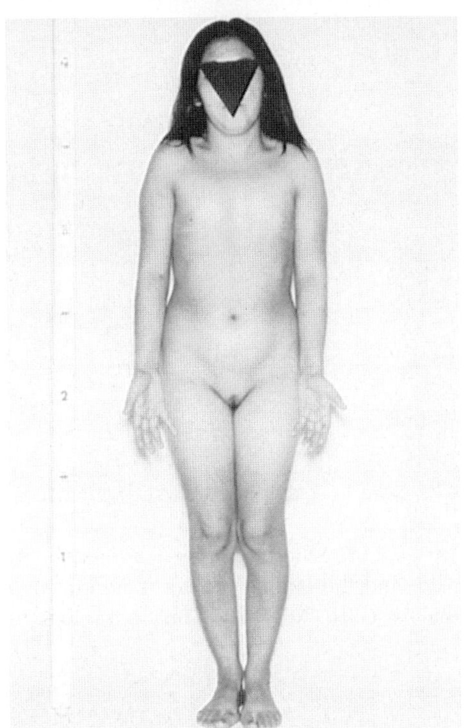

Image 109. Turner's syndrome (XO). Phenotype includes short stature, webbing of the neck, and poorly developed secondary sex characteristics.

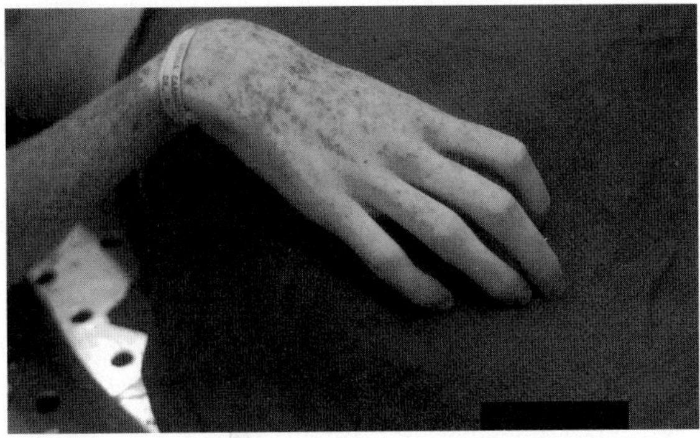

Image 110. Marfan's syndrome. Patients are tall with very long extremities. The joints are hyperextensible, with slim bone structure and wiry muscles.*

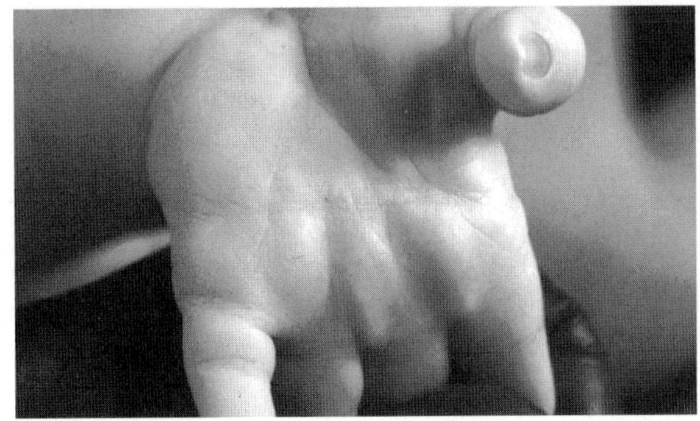

Image 111. Simian crease. A characteristic feature of Down syndrome (trisomy 21). The palm has a single transverse crease instead of the normal two creases.*

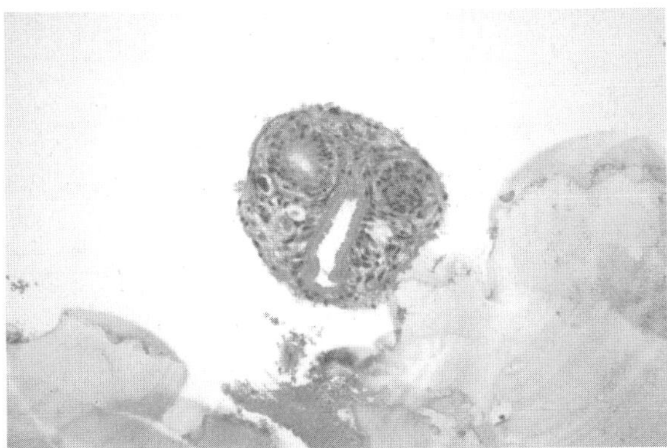

Image 112. Hydatid cyst. Echinococcus eggs develop into larvae in the intestine, penetrate the intestinal wall, and disseminate throughout the body. The larvae form hydatid cysts in the liver and, less commonly, in the lungs, kidney, and brain. (Reproduced, with permission, from USMLERx.com.)

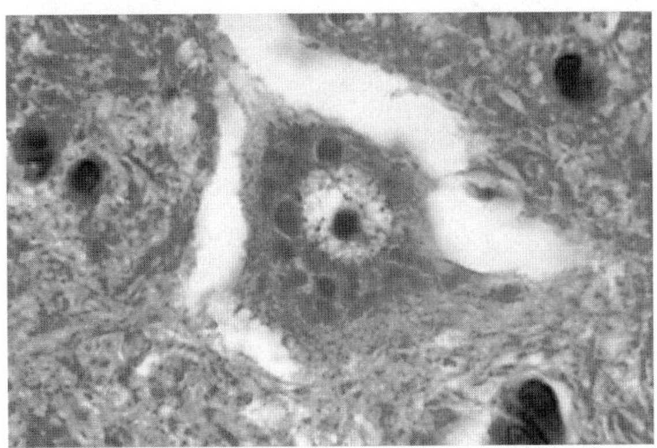

Image 113. Negri bodies are pathognomonic inclusions in the cytoplasm of neurons infected by the rabies virus. (Reproduced, with permission, from the Centers for Disease Control and Prevention, Atlanta, GA.)

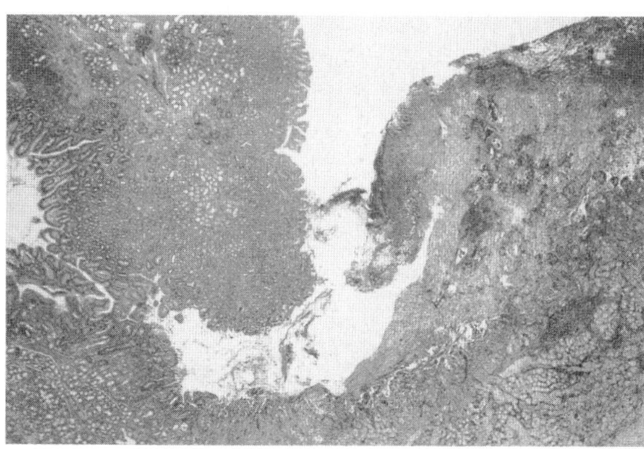

Image 114. Duodenal ulcer. The epithelium is ulcerated, and the lamina propria is infiltrated with inflammatory cells. Necrotic debris is present in the ulcer crater.

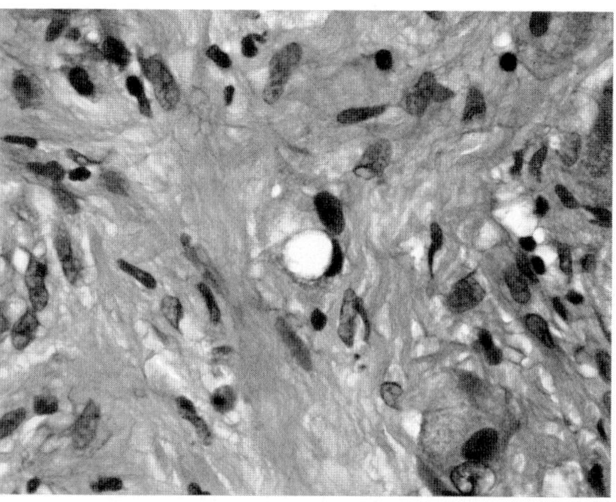

Image 115. Signet ring cell. Mucin expands the cytoplasm and pushes the nucleus to the periphery, creating the appearance of a signet ring. The diffuse type of gastric carcinoma is composed of widely infiltrative signet ring cells. (Reproduced, with permission, from USMLERx.com.)

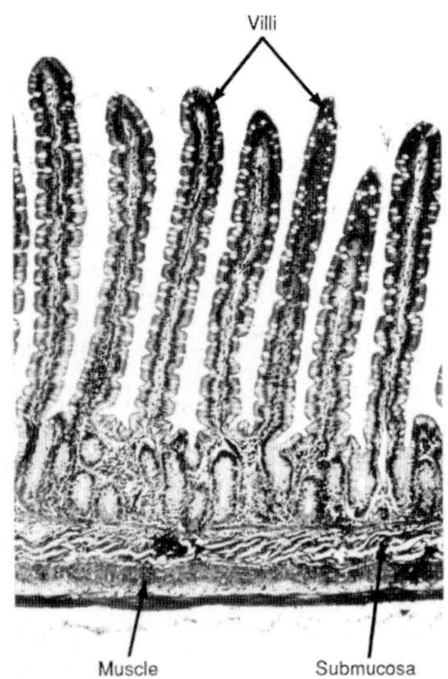

Image 116. Photomicrograph of the **small intestine.**

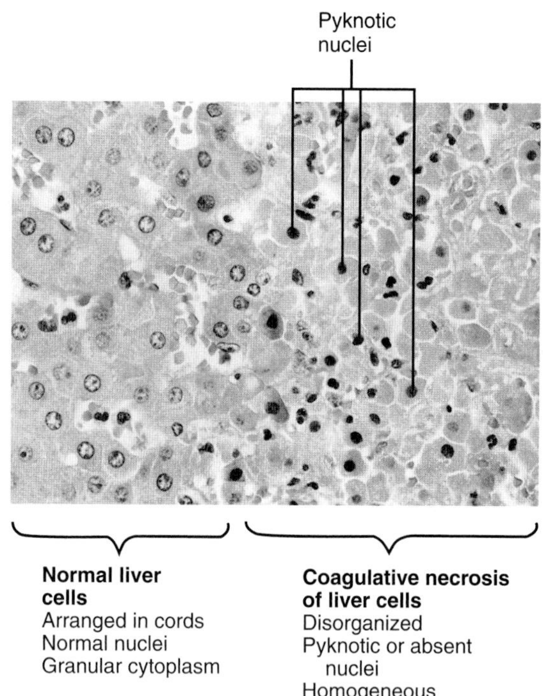

Image 117. Coagulative necrosis of hepatocytes.

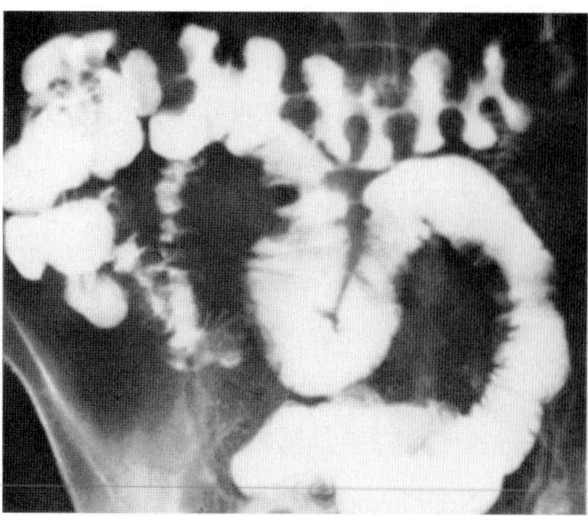

Image 118. Crohn's disease. Barium x-ray showing spicules, edema, and ulcers. (Reproduced, with permission, from Le T et al. *First Aid for the Wards*, 3rd ed. New York: McGraw-Hill, 2006: 399.)

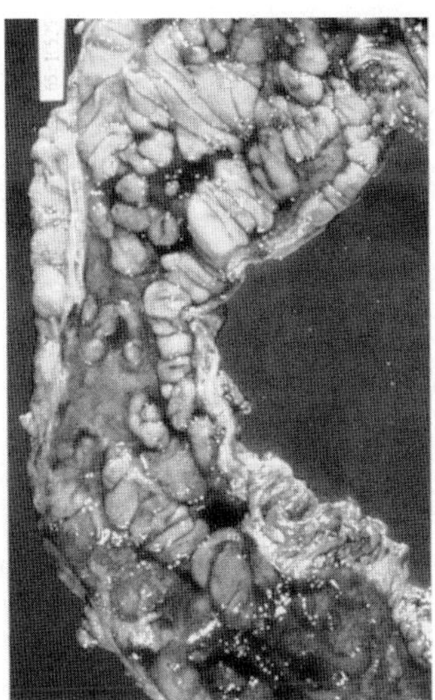
A

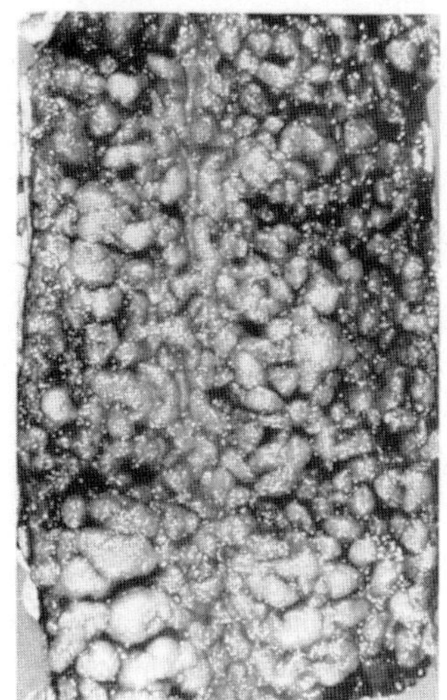
B

Image 119. Inflammatory bowel disease. In **Crohn's disease** (**A**), the juxtaposition of ulcerated and normal mucosa gives a "cobblestone" appearance. In acute **ulcerative colitis** (**B**), the intestinal mucosa is inflamed and edematous and has a pseudopolypoid appearance. Chronically, ulcerative colitis has a more atrophic appearance.

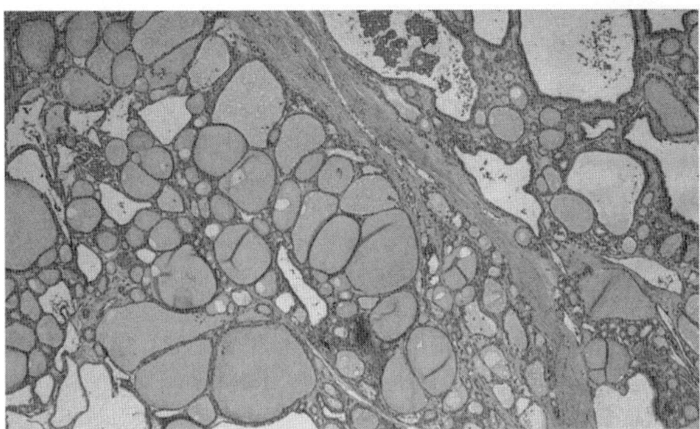

Image 120. Multinodular goiter with hyperplasia and subsequent involution of the thyroid gland. The image shows follicles distended with colloid and lined by a flattened epithelium with areas of fibrosis and hemorrhage. (Reproduced, with permission, from USMLERx.com.)

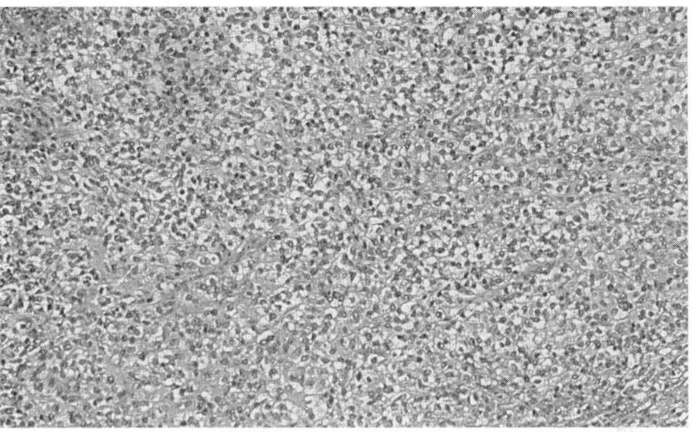

Image 121. Ewing's sarcoma. This malignant tumor of bone occurs in children and is characterized by the (11;22) translocation that results in the fusion gene EWS-FLI1. The tumor is composed of sheets of uniform small, round cells. (Reproduced, with permission, from USMLERx.com.)

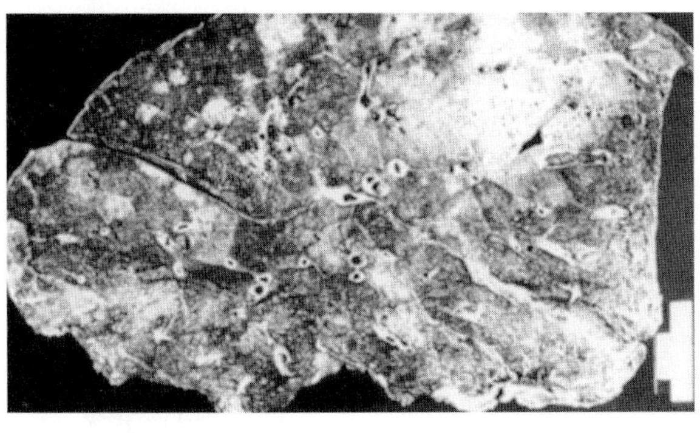
A

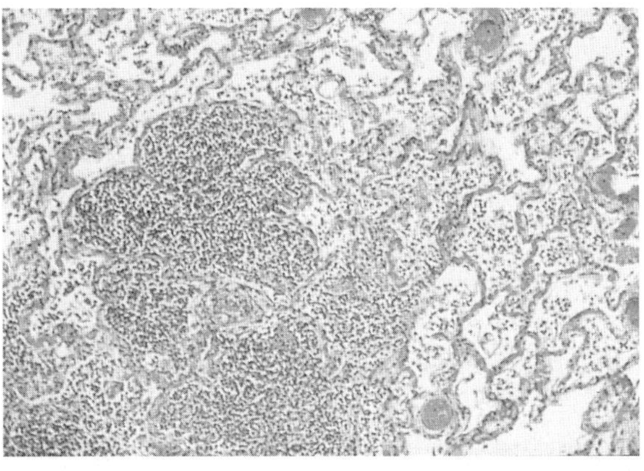
B

Image 122. Bronchopneumonia. (**A**) Gross. Note the large area of consolidation at the base plus multiple small areas of consolidation (pale) involving bronchioles and surrounding alveolar sacs throughout the lung. (**B**) Bronchopneumonia with neutrophils in alveolar spaces, microscopic.

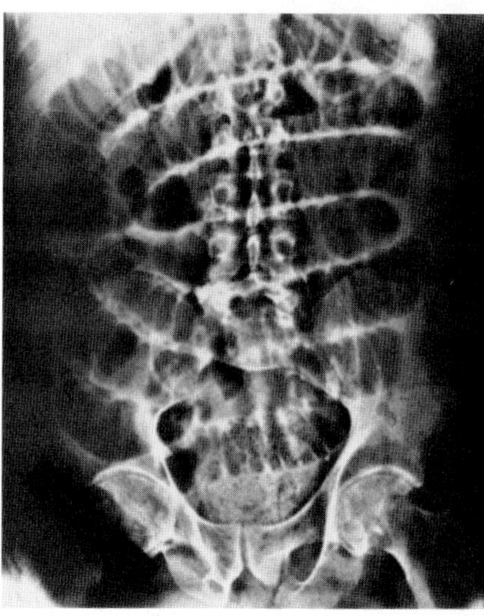

Image 123. Small bowel obstruction on supine abdominal x-ray. Note dilated loops of small bowel in a ladder-like pattern. Air-fluid levels may be seen if an upright x-ray is done. (Reproduced, with permission, from Le T et al. *First Aid for the Wards*, 3rd ed. New York: McGraw-Hill, 2006: 392.)

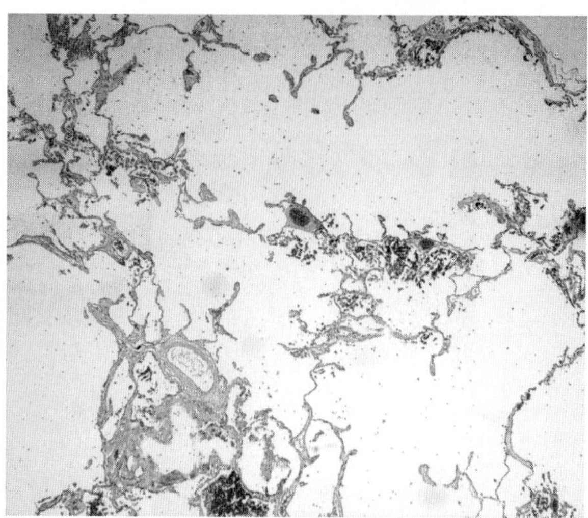

Image 124. Emphysema. Note the abnormal permanent enlargement of the airspaces distal to the terminal bronchiole. On microscopy, enlarged alveoli are seen separated by thin septa, some of which appear to float within the alveolar spaces. (Reproduced, with permission, from USMLERx.com.)

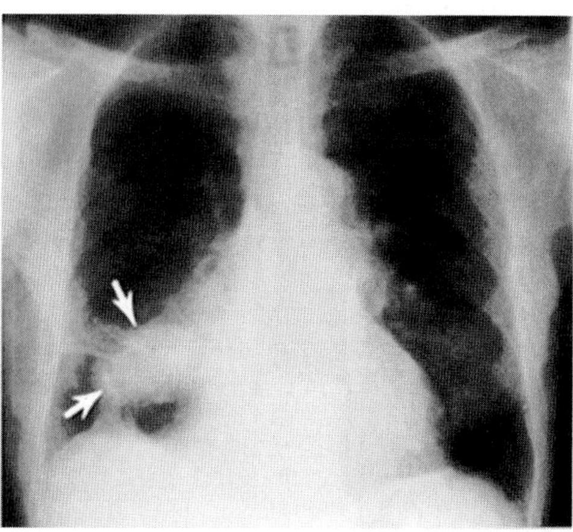

Image 125. Squamous cell carcinoma in the right lower lobe. (Reproduced, with permission, from Le T et al. *First Aid for the Wards*, 3rd ed. New York: McGraw-Hill, 2006: 133.)

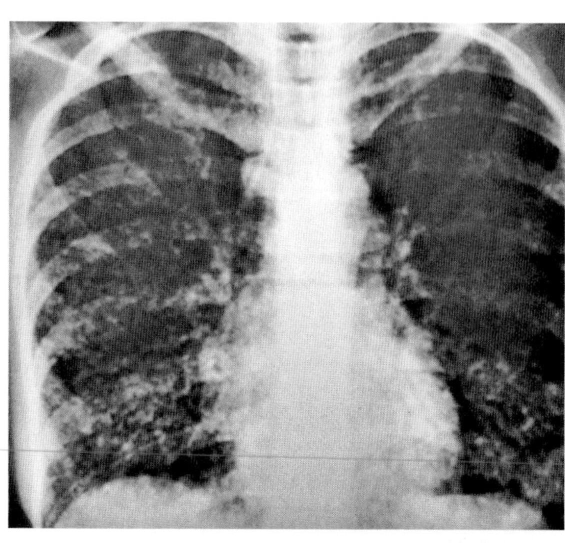

A

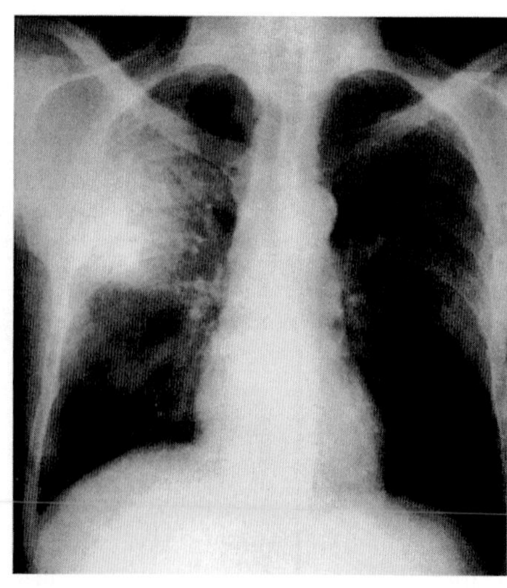

B

Image 126. Compare the diffuse, patchy bilateral infiltrates of "atypical" **interstitial pneumonia (A)** with the localized, dense lesion of **lobar pneumonia (B)**.

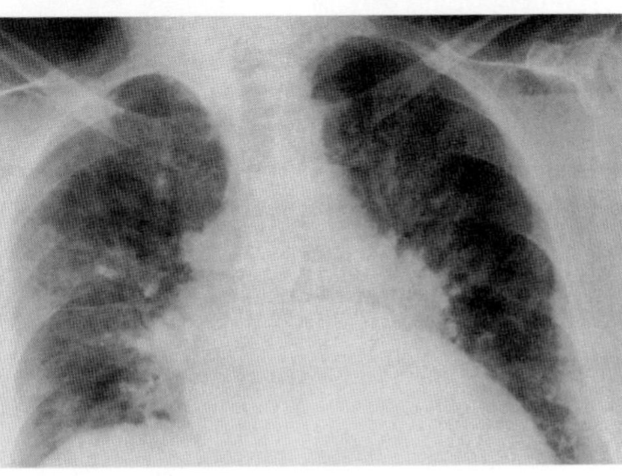

Image 127. Pulmonary edema. Posteroanterior chest x-ray in a man with acute pulmonary edema due to left ventricular failure. Note the bat's-wing density, cardiac enlargement, increased size of upper lobe vessels, and pulmonary venous congestion. (Reproduced, with permission, from McPhee SJ et al. *Pathophysiology of Disease: An Introduction to Clinical Medicine*, 4th ed. New York: McGraw-Hill, 2002.)

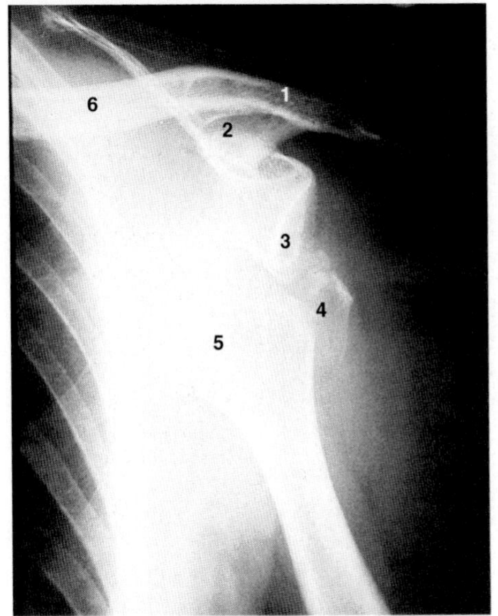

Image 128. Anterior shoulder dislocation. Note the humeral head inferior and medial to the glenoid fossa and fracture fragments from the greater tuberosity.

1—Acromion
2—Coracoid
3—Glenoid fossa
4—Fracture fragments
5—Humeral head
6—Clavicle

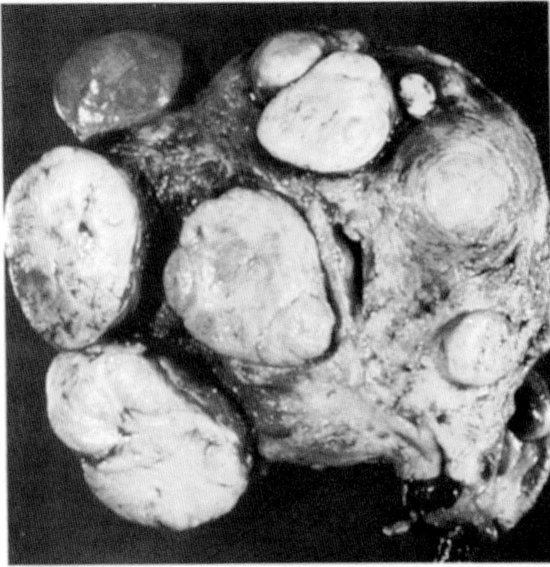

Image 129. Multiple **leiomyomas** (fibroids) of the uterus. A common benign uterine tumor. Fibroids beneath the endometrium may present with vaginal bleeding; they also develop subserosally or within the myometrium.

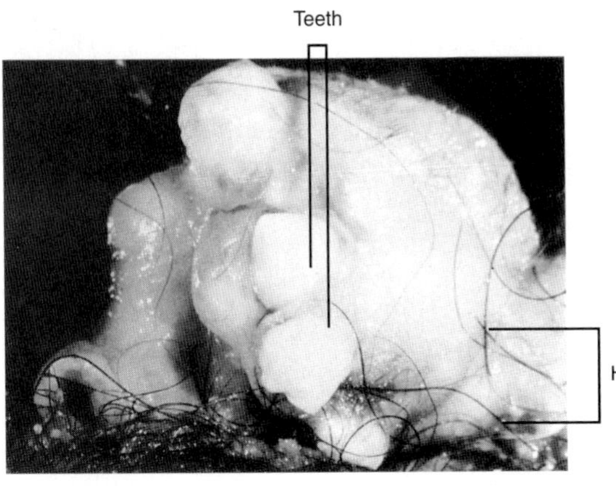

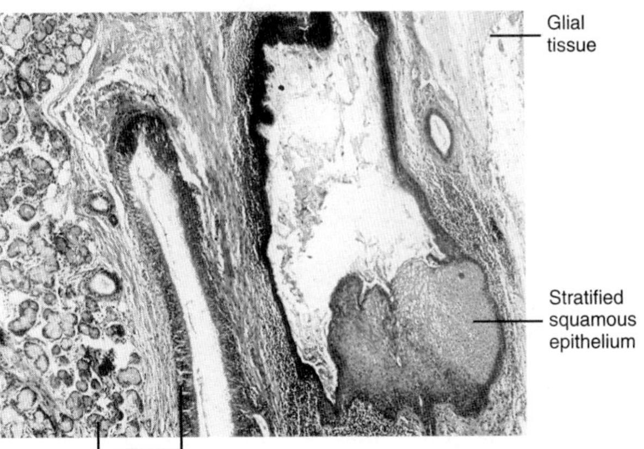

Images 130 and 131. Teratoma (benign) of the ovary containing teeth and hair—an incidental finding during abdominal surgery. In females, teratomas are generally benign, whereas in males they account for roughly 30% of testicular tumors.

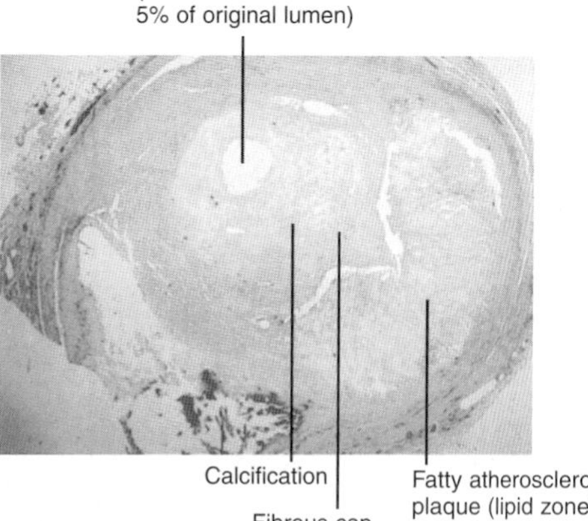

Image 132. Atherosclerosis in a coronary vessel. Calcified plaques have narrowed the lumen of the artery, increasing the risk for occlusion—i.e., myocardial infarction.

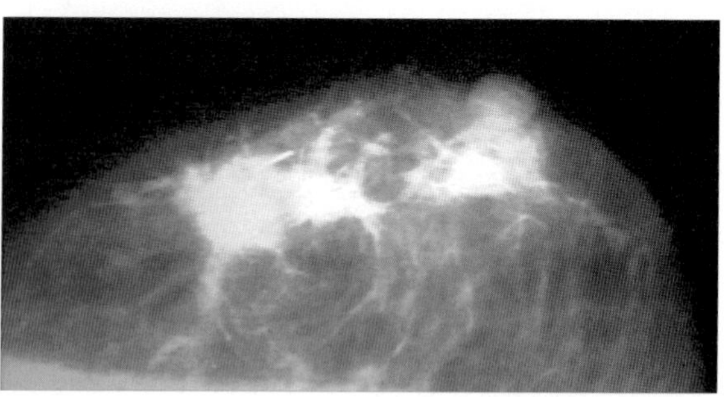

Image 133. Breast mammogram diagnostic of breast cancer. The upper half of the breast shows a dense, irregularly shaped mass with long, branching tentacles extending toward the nipple. Numerous tiny calcium deposits looking like grains of sand (microcalcifications) are seen both in the mass and in the surrounding tissue.*

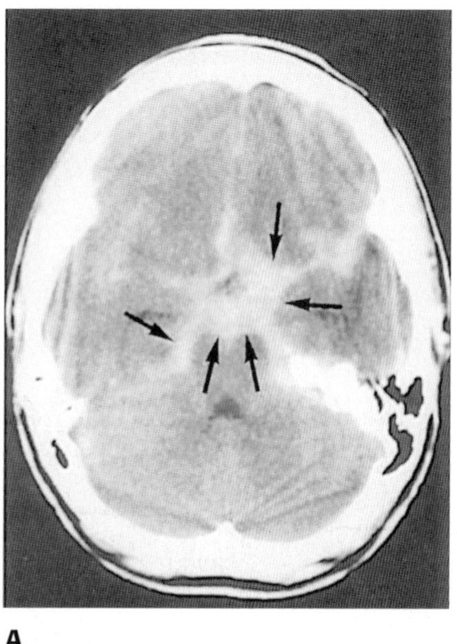

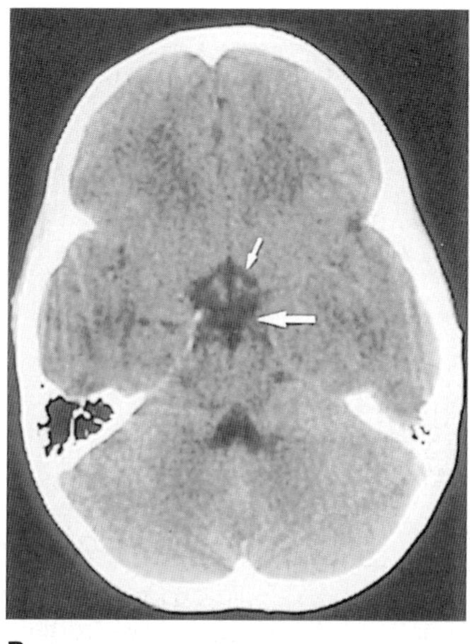

Image 134. Subarachnoid hemorrhage. CT scan with contrast reveals blood in the subarachnoid space at the base of the brain.

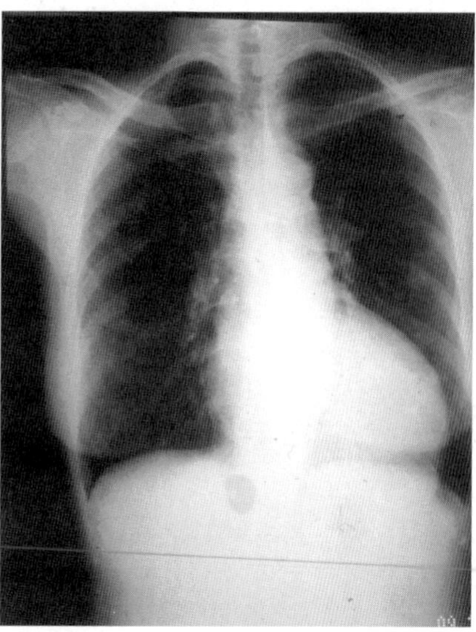

Image 135. Left ventricular hypertrophy (mediastinum wider than 50% of the width of the chest) from aortic valve stenosis.*

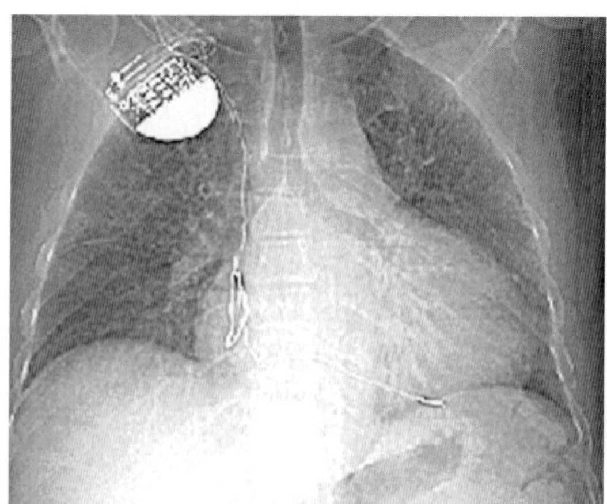

Image 136. Amiodarone toxicity. Diffuse interstitial bilateral pulmonary markings in a reticular nodular pattern, most prominent in the lung bases and posteriorly, are evidence of pulmonary fibrosis.*

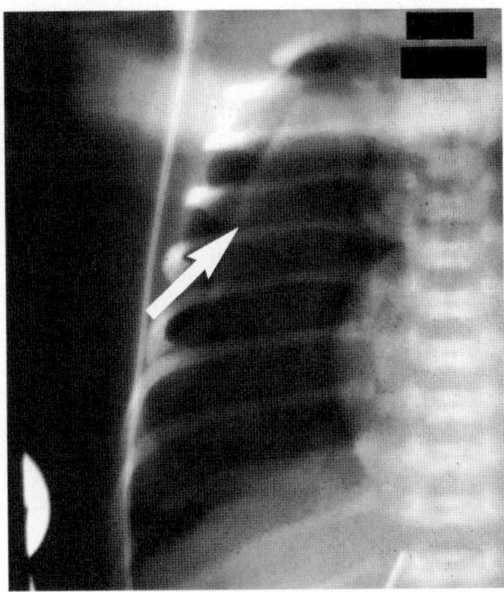

Image 137. Pneumothorax. The right lung is collapsed; the apparent straight line off the rightmost edge of the pleural space indicated by the arrow shows the edge of the collapsed lung.*

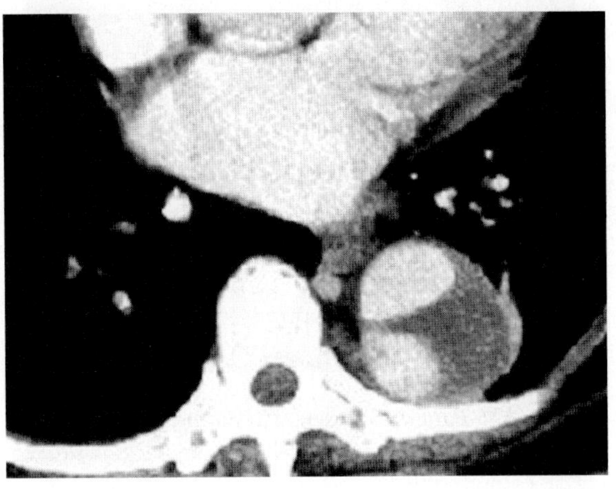

Image 138. Descending aortic dissection. Presents with severe chest pain. Type A is proximal to the subclavian artery and type B distal to the subclavian.*

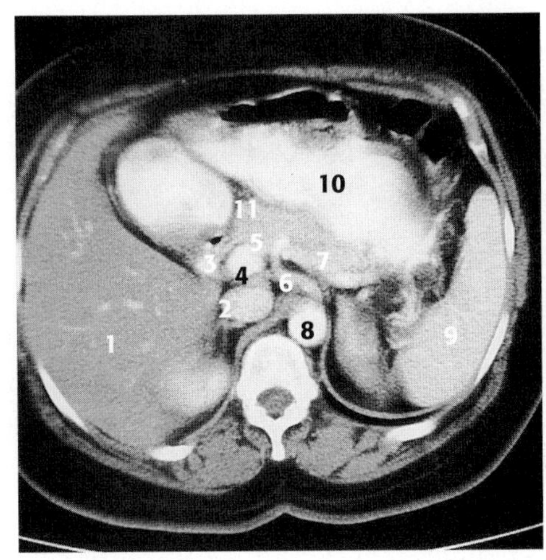

Image 139. CT of the abdomen with contrast—normal anatomy.

1—Liver
2—IVC
3—Portal vein
4—Hepatic artery
5—Gastroduodenal artery
6—Celiac trunk
7—Splenic vein
8—Aorta
9—Spleen
10—Stomach
11—Pancreas

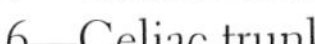

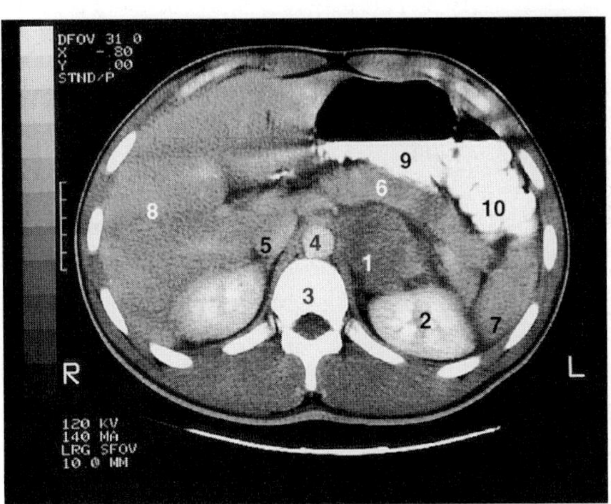

Image 140. Left adrenal mass.

1—Large left adrenal mass
2—Kidney
3—Vertebral body
4—Aorta
5—IVC
6—Pancreas
7—Spleen
8—Liver
9—Stomach with air and contrast
10—Colon–splenic flexure

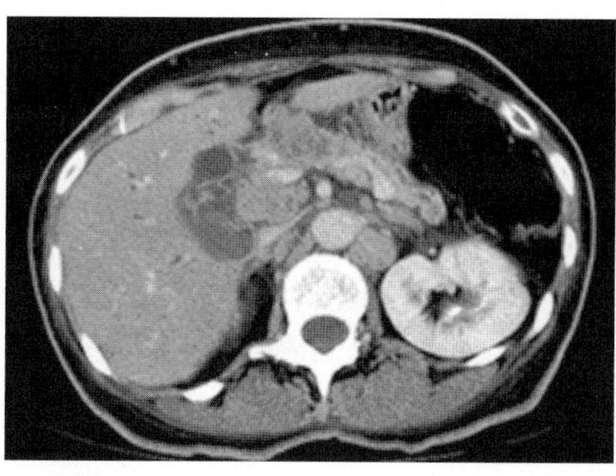

Image 141. Pancreatic adenocarcinoma. A large, heterogeneously enhancing mass is visible at the neck of the pancreas, compressing the common bile duct, portal vein, splenic vein, superior mesenteric vein, and IVC. No liver metastases are apparent.*

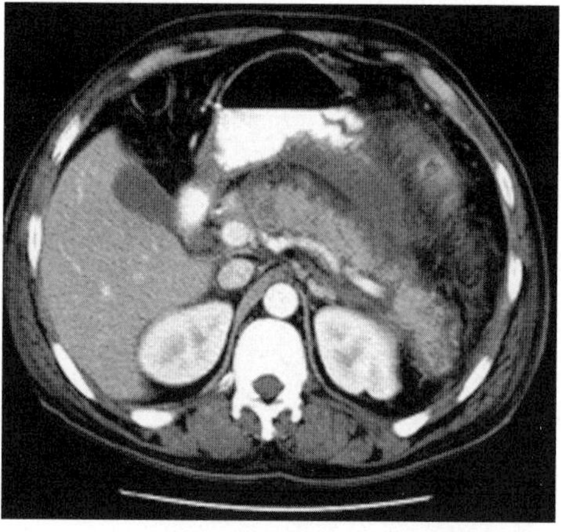

Image 142. Acute pancreatitis, typically from alcohol abuse or gallstone obstruction of the pancreatic duct. No evidence of necrosis or fluid collection is seen.*

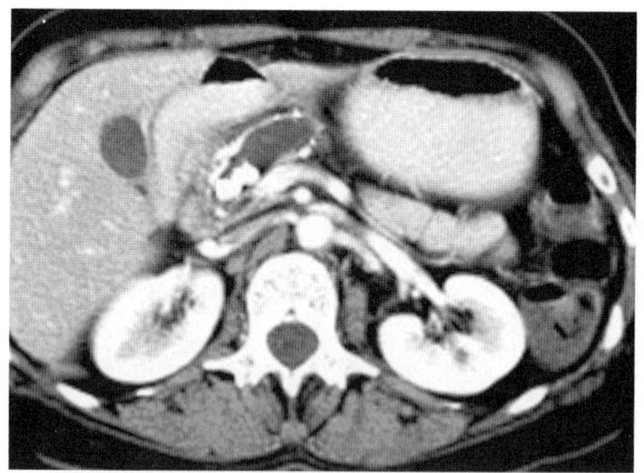

Image 143. Chronic pancreatitis precipitated by large duct stones. A small fatty infiltrate is visible to the left of the liver. Mild central biliary dilatation and a prominent common bile duct are also seen.*

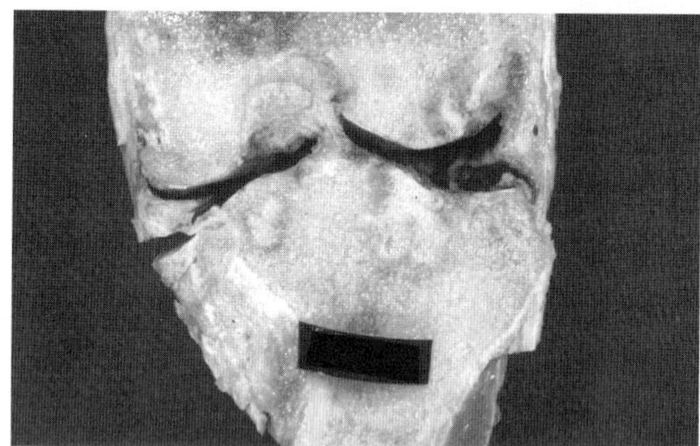

Image 144. Osteoarthritis. Increased fibrosis of the joint and a decreased amount of cartilage are apparent.*

CO_2 transport

Carbon dioxide is transported from tissues to the lungs in 3 forms:

1. **Bicarbonate (90%)**

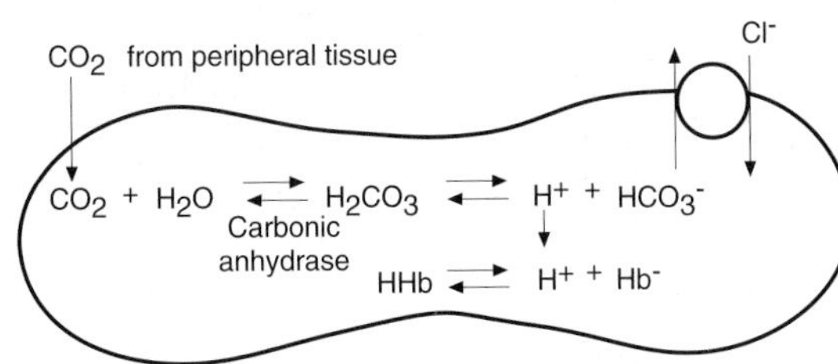

2. Bound to hemoglobin as carbaminohemoglobin (5%)
3. Dissolved CO_2 (5%)

(Adapted, with permission, from Ganong WF. *Review of Medical Physiology,* 22nd ed. New York: McGraw-Hill, 2005: 670.)

In lungs, oxygenation of Hb promotes dissociation of H^+ from Hb. This shifts equilibrium toward CO_2 formation; therefore, CO_2 is released from RBCs (Haldane effect).

In peripheral tissue, ↑ H^+ from tissue metabolism shifts curve to right, unloading O_2 (Bohr effect).

Response to high altitude

1. Acute ↑ in ventilation
2. Chronic ↑ in ventilation
3. ↑ erythropoietin → ↑ hematocrit and hemoglobin (chronic hypoxia)
4. ↑ 2,3-DPG (binds to hemoglobin so that hemoglobin releases more O_2)
5. Cellular changes (↑ mitochondria)
6. ↑ renal excretion of bicarbonate (e.g., can augment by use of acetazolamide) to compensate for the respiratory alkalosis
7. Chronic hypoxic pulmonary vasoconstriction results in RVH

Obstructive lung disease (COPD)

Obstruction of air flow resulting in air trapping in the lungs. Airways close prematurely at high lung volumes, resulting in ↑ RV and ↓ FVC. PFTs: ↓↓ FEV_1, ↓ FVC → ↓ FEV_1/FVC ratio (hallmark), V/Q mismatch.

Type	Pathology	Other
Chronic Bronchitis ("Blue Bloater")	Hypertrophy of mucus-secreting glands in the bronchioles → Reid index = gland depth / total thickness of bronchial wall; in COPD, Reid index > 50%.	Productive cough for > 3 consecutive months in ≥ 2 years. Disease of small airways. Findings—wheezing, crackles, cyanosis.
Emphysema ("pink puffer," barrel-shaped chest)	Enlargement of air spaces and ↓ recoil resulting from destruction of alveolar walls. Centriacinar—caused by smoking. Panacinar—α_1-antitrypsin deficiency (also liver cirrhosis). Paraseptal emphysema—associated with bullae → can rupture → spontaneous pneumothorax; often in young, otherwise healthy males.	↑ elastase activity. ↑ lung compliance due to loss of elastic fibers. Exhale through pursed lips to ↑ airway pressure and prevent airway collapse during exhalation. Findings—dyspnea, ↓ breath sounds, tachycardia, ↓ I/E ratio.
Asthma	Bronchial hyperresponsiveness causes reversible bronchoconstriction. Smooth muscle hypertrophy and Curschmann's spirals (shed epithelium from mucous plugs).	Can be triggered by viral URIs, allergens, and stress. Findings: cough, wheezing, dyspnea, tachypnea, hypoxemia, ↓ I/E ratio, pulsus paradoxus, mucus plugging.
Bronchiectasis	Chronic necrotizing infection of bronchi → permanently dilated airways, purulent sputum, recurrent infections, hemoptysis.	Associated with bronchial obstruction, CF, poor ciliary motility, Kartagener's syndrome. Can develop aspergillosis.

Restrictive lung disease

Restricted lung expansion causes ↓ lung volumes (↓ FVC and TLC). PFTs—FEV_1/FVC ratio > 80%.

Types:

1. Poor breathing mechanics (extrapulmonary, peripheral hypoventilation):
   a. Poor muscular effort—polio, myasthenia gravis
   b. Poor structural apparatus—scoliosis, morbid obesity
2. Interstitial lung diseases (pulmonary, lowered diffusing capacity):
   a. Adult respiratory distress syndrome (ARDS)
   b. Neonatal respiratory distress syndrome (hyaline membrane disease)
   c. Pneumoconioses (coal miner's silicosis, asbestosis)
   d. Sarcoidosis
   e. Idiopathic pulmonary fibrosis (repeated cycles of lung injury and wound healing with ↑ collagen)
   f. Goodpasture's syndrome
   g. Wegener's granulomatosis
   h. Eosinophilic granuloma (histiocytosis X)
   i. Drug toxicity (bleomycin, busulfan, amiodarone)

Neonatal respiratory distress syndrome	Surfactant deficiency leading to ↑ surface tension, resulting in alveolar collapse. Surfactant is made by type II pneumocytes most abundantly after 35th week of gestation. The lecithin-to-sphingomyelin ratio in the amniotic fluid, a measure of lung maturity, is usually < 1.5 in neonatal respiratory distress syndrome. Surfactant—dipalmitoyl phosphatidylcholine. Treatment: maternal steroids before birth; artificial surfactant for infant.
Adult respiratory distress syndrome (ARDS)	May be caused by trauma, sepsis, shock, gastric aspiration, uremia, acute pancreatitis, or amniotic fluid embolism. Diffuse alveolar damage → ↑ alveolar capillary permeability → protein-rich leakage into alveoli. Results in formation of intra-alveolar hyaline membrane. Initial damage due to neutrophilic substances toxic to alveolar wall, activation of coagulation cascade, or oxygen-derived free radicals (see Color Image 39).

Obstructive vs. restrictive lung disease

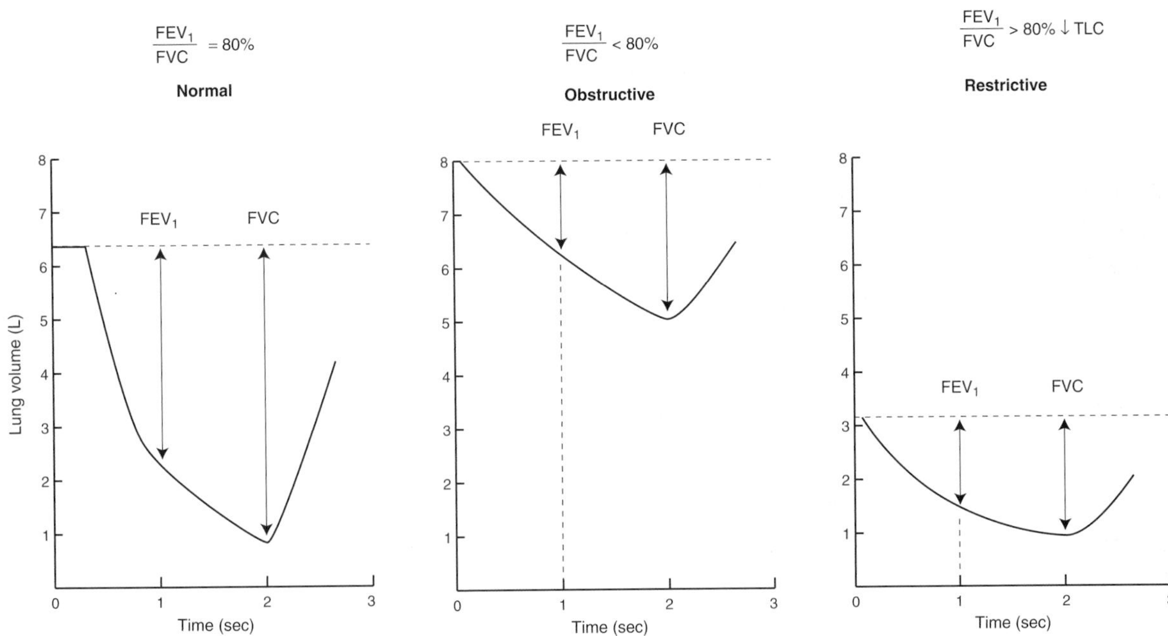

Note: Obstructive lung volumes > normal (↑ TLC, ↑ FRC, ↑ RV); restrictive lung volumes < normal. In both obstructive and restrictive, FEV_1 and FVC are reduced, but in obstructive, FEV_1 is more dramatically reduced, resulting in a ↓ FEV_1/FVC ratio.

Sleep apnea	Person stops breathing for at least 10 seconds repeatedly during sleep. **Central sleep apnea**—no respiratory effort. **Obstructive sleep apnea**—respiratory effort against airway obstruction. Associated with obesity, loud snoring, systemic/pulmonary hypertension, arrhythmias, and possibly sudden death. Individuals may become chronically tired.	Treatment: weight loss, CPAP, surgery.

Asbestosis

Diffuse pulmonary interstitial fibrosis caused by inhaled asbestos fibers. ↑ risk of pleural mesothelioma and bronchogenic carcinoma. Long latency. Ferruginous bodies in lung (asbestos fibers coated with hemosiderin). Ivory-white pleural plaques (see Color Image 42).

Mainly affects lower lobes. Other pneumoconioses affect upper lobes (e.g., coal worker's lung).

Asbestosis and smoking greatly ↑ risk of bronchogenic cancer (smoking not additive with mesothelioma).

Seen in shipbuilders, roofers, and plumbers.

Lung—physical findings

Abnormality	Breath Sounds	Resonance	Fremitus	Tracheal Deviation
Bronchial obstruction	Absent/↓ over affected area	↓	↓	Toward side of lesion
Pleural effusion	↓ over effusion	Dullness	↓	—
Pneumonia (lobar)	May have bronchial breath sounds over lesion	Dullness	↑	—
Pneumothorax	↓	Hyperresonant	Absent	Away from side of lesion (see Color Image 40)

Lung cancer

Lung cancer is the leading cause of cancer death. Presentation: cough, hemoptysis, bronchial obstruction, wheezing, pneumonic "coin" lesion on x-ray film.

SPHERE of complications:
- Superior vena cava syndrome
- Pancoast's tumor
- Horner's syndrome
- Endocrine (paraneoplastic)
- Recurrent laryngeal symptoms (hoarseness)
- Effusions (pleural or pericardial)

Type	Location	Characteristics	Histology
Squamous cell carcinoma (Squamous Sentral Smoking)	Central	Hilar mass arising from bronchus; Cavitation; Clearly linked to Smoking; parathyroid-like activity → PTHrP (see Color Image 36, Image 125).	Keratin pearls and intercellular bridges.
Adenocarcinoma: Bronchial Bronchioloalveolar	Peripheral	Develops in site of prior pulmonary inflammation or injury (most common lung cancer in nonsmokers and females). Not linked to smoking.	Both types: Clara cells → type II pneumocytes; multiple densities on x-ray of chest.
Small cell (oat cell) carcinoma	Central	Undifferentiated → very aggressive; often associated with ectopic production of ACTH or ADH; may lead to Lambert-Eaton syndrome (autoantibodies against calcium channels). Responsive to chemotherapy.	Neoplasm of neuroendocrine Kulchitsky cells → small dark blue cells (see Color Image 37).
Large cell carcinoma	Peripheral	Highly anaplastic undifferentiated tumor; poor prognosis; less tendency to metastasize and less responsive to chemotherapy. Removed surgically.	Pleomorphic giant cells with leukocyte fragments in cytoplasm.
Carcinoid tumor	—	Secretes serotonin, can cause carcinoid syndrome (flushing, diarrhea, wheezing, salivation).	—
Metastases	—	Very common. Brain (epilepsy), bone (pathologic fracture), and liver (jaundice, hepatomegaly).	—

Pancoast's tumor

Carcinoma that occurs in apex of lung and may affect cervical sympathetic plexus, causing Horner's syndrome.

Horner's syndrome—ptosis, miosis, anhidrosis.

Pneumonia

Type	Organism(s)	Characteristics
Lobar	Pneumococcus most frequently	Intra-alveolar exudate → consolidation; may involve entire lung
Bronchopneumonia	*S. aureus, H. flu, Klebsiella, S. pyogenes*	Acute inflammatory infiltrates from bronchioles into adjacent alveoli; patchy distribution involving ≥ 1 lobes (see Image 122).
Interstitial (atypical) pneumonia	Viruses (RSV, adenoviruses), *Mycoplasma, Legionella, Chlamydia*	Diffuse patchy inflammation localized to interstitial areas at alveolar walls; distribution involving ≥ 1 lobes (see Image 126).

Lung abscess — Localized collection of pus within parenchyma, usually resulting from bronchial obstruction (e.g., cancer) or aspiration of gastric contents (especially in patients predisposed to loss of consciousness, e.g., alcoholics or epileptics). Often due to *S. aureus* or anaerobes.

Pleural effusions

Transudate	↓ protein content. Due to CHF, nephrotic syndrome, or hepatic cirrhosis.
Exudate	↑ protein content, cloudy. Due to malignancy, pneumonia, collagen vascular disease, trauma.
Lymphatic	Milky fluid; ↑ triglycerides.

► RESPIRATORY–PHARMACOLOGY

H_1 blockers	Reversible inhibitors of H_1 histamine receptors.
1st generation	Diphenhydramine, dimenhydrinate, chlorpheniramine.
Clinical uses	Allergy, motion sickness, sleep aid.
Toxicity	Sedation, antimuscarinic, anti-α-adrenergic.
2nd generation	Loratadine, fexofenadine, desloratadine, cetirizine.
Clinical uses	Allergy.
Toxicity	Far less sedating than 1st generation because of ↓ entry into CNS.

Asthma drugs

Nonspecific β-agonists	**Isoproterenol**—relaxes bronchial smooth muscle (β_2). Adverse effect is tachycardia (β_1).
β_2-agonists	**Albuterol**—relaxes bronchial smooth muscle (β_2). Use during acute exacerbation. **Salmeterol**—long-acting agent for prophylaxis. Adverse effects are tremor and arrhythmia.
Methylxanthines	**Theophylline**—likely causes bronchodilation by inhibiting phosphodiesterase, thereby ↓ cAMP hydrolysis. Usage is limited because of narrow therapeutic index (cardiotoxicity, neurotoxicity); metabolized by P-450.
Muscarinic antagonists	**Ipratropium**—competitive block of muscarinic receptors, preventing bronchoconstriction. Also used for COPD.
Cromolyn	Prevents release of mediators from mast cells. Effective only for the prophylaxis of asthma. Not effective during an acute asthmatic attack. Toxicity is rare.
Corticosteroids	**Beclomethasone, prednisone**—inhibit the synthesis of virtually all cytokines. Inactivate NF-κB, the transcription factor that induces the production of TNF-α, among other inflammatory agents. 1st-line therapy for chronic asthma.
Antileukotrienes	**Zileuton**—A 5-lipoxygenase pathway inhibitor. Blocks conversion of arachidonic acid to leukotrienes. **Zafirlukast, montelukast**—block leukotriene receptors. Especially good for aspirin-induced asthma.

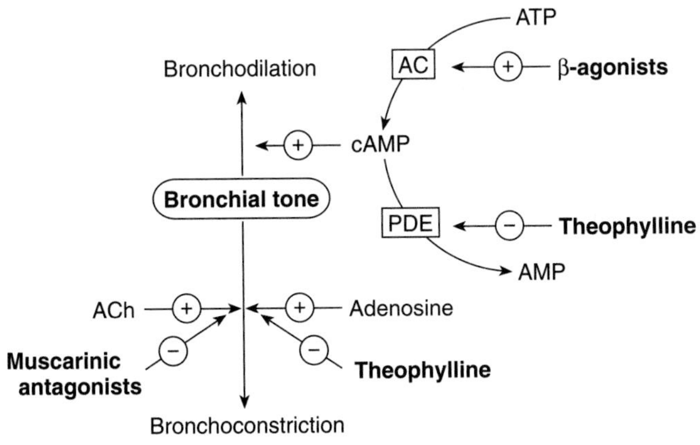

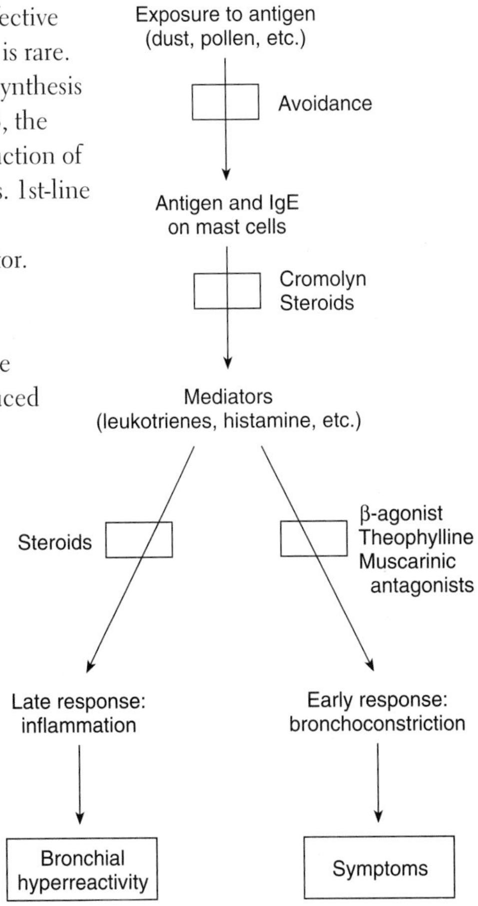

Exposure to antigen (dust, pollen, etc.)
Avoidance
Antigen and IgE on mast cells
Cromolyn
Steroids
Mediators (leukotrienes, histamine, etc.)
Steroids
β-agonist
Theophylline
Muscarinic antagonists
Late response: inflammation
Early response: bronchoconstriction
Bronchial hyperreactivity
Symptoms

Treatment strategies in asthma

ATP
Bronchodilation
AC
β-agonists
cAMP
Bronchial tone
PDE
Theophylline
AMP
ACh
Adenosine
Muscarinic antagonists
Theophylline
Bronchoconstriction

(Adapted, with permission, from Katzung BG, Trevor AJ. *Pharmacology: Examination & Board Review,* 5th ed. Stamford, CT: Appleton & Lange, 1998: 159 and 161.)

Expectorants

Guaifenesin (Robitussin)	Removes excess sputum but large doses necessary; does not suppress cough reflex.
N-acetylcysteine	Mucolytic → can loosen mucous plugs in CF patients. Also used as an antidote for acetaminophen overdose.

Rapid Review

The following tables represent a collection of high-yield associations of diseases, "buzzwords," findings, and associated pathologies that may be useful for quick review right before the exam.

Disease/Finding	Association
Actinic keratosis	Often precedes squamous cell carcinoma
Addison's disease	1° adrenocortical deficiency
Albright's syndrome	Polyostotic fibrous dysplasia, precocious puberty, café-au-lait spots, short stature, young girls
Albuminocytologic dissociation	Guillain-Barré (↑ protein in CSF with only modest ↑ in cell count)
Alport's syndrome	Hereditary nephritis with nerve deafness
Anti–basement membrane antibodies	Goodpasture's syndrome
Anticentromere antibodies	Scleroderma (CREST)
Anti-double-stranded DNA antibodies (ANA antibodies)	SLE (type III hypersensitivity)
Anti–epithelial cell antibodies	Pemphigus vulgaris
Antigliadin antibodies	Celiac disease
Antihistone antibodies	Drug-induced SLE
Anti-IgG antibodies	Rheumatoid arthritis
Antimitochondrial antibodies	1° biliary cirrhosis
Antineutrophil antibodies	Vasculitis
Antiplatelet antibodies	Idiopathic thrombocytopenic purpura
Arachnodactyly	Marfan's syndrome
Argyll Robertson pupil	Neurosyphilis
Arnold-Chiari malformation	Cerebellar tonsillar herniation
Aschoff bodies	Rheumatic fever
Atrophy of the mammillary bodies	Wernicke's encephalopathy
Auer rods	Acute myelogenous leukemia (especially the promyelocytic type)
Autosplenectomy	Sickle cell anemia
Babinski's sign	UMN lesion
Baker's cyst in popliteal fossa	Rheumatoid arthritis
"Bamboo spine" on x-ray	Ankylosing spondylitis
Bartter's syndrome	Hyperreninemia
Basophilic stippling of RBCs	Lead poisoning
Becker's muscular dystrophy	Defective dystrophin; less severe than Duchenne's
Bell's palsy	LMN CN VII palsy
Bence Jones proteins	Multiple myeloma (kappa or lambda Ig light chains in urine), Waldenström's macroglobulinemia (IgM)

Berger's disease	IgA nephropathy
Bernard-Soulier disease	Defect in platelet adhesion
Bilateral hilar adenopathy, uveitis	Sarcoidosis
Birbeck granules on EM	Histiocytosis X (eosinophilic granuloma)
Bloody tap on LP	Subarachnoid hemorrhage
"Blue bloater"	Chronic bronchitis
Blue-domed cysts	Fibrocystic change of the breast
Blue sclera	Osteogenesis imperfecta
Boot-shaped heart on x-ray	Tetralogy of Fallot; RVH
Bouchard's nodes	Osteoarthritis (PIP swelling 2° to osteophytes)
Boutonnière deformity	Rheumatoid arthritis
Branching rods in oral infection	*Actinomyces israelii*
"Brown tumor" of bone	Hemorrhage causes brown color of osteolytic cysts: 1. Hyperparathyroidism 2. Osteitis fibrosa cystica (von Recklinghausen's disease)
Bruton's disease	X-linked agammaglobulinemia
Budd-Chiari syndrome	Posthepatic venous thrombosis
Buerger's disease	Small/medium-artery vasculitis
Burkitt's lymphoma	8:14 translocation; associated with EBV; "starry sky" appearance on histology
Burton's lines	Lead poisoning
c-ANCA, p-ANCA	Wegener's granulomatosis, microscopic polyangiitis
Café-au-lait spots on skin	Neurofibromatosis
Caisson disease	Gas emboli
Calf pseudohypertrophy	Duchenne's muscular dystrophy
Call-Exner bodies	Granulosa-theca cell tumor of the ovary
Cardiomegaly with apical atrophy	Chagas' disease
Cerebriform nuclei	Mycosis fungoides (cutaneous T-cell lymphoma)
Chagas' disease	Trypanosome infection
Chancre	1° syphilis (not painful)
Chancroid	*Haemophilus ducreyi* (painful)
Charcot's triad	Multiple sclerosis (nystagmus, intention tremor, scanning speech), cholangitis (jaundice, RUQ pain, fever)
Charcot-Leyden crystals	Bronchial asthma (eosinophil membranes)
Chédiak-Higashi disease	Phagocyte deficiency

Cherry-red spot on macula	Tay-Sachs, Niemann-Pick disease, central retinal artery occlusion
Cheyne-Stokes respirations	Central apnea in CHF and ↑ intracranial pressure
"Chocolate cysts"	Endometriosis (frequently involves both ovaries)
Chronic atrophic gastritis	Predisposition to gastric carcinoma
Chvostek's sign	Hypocalcemia (facial muscle spasm upon tapping)
Clear cell adenocarcinoma of the vagina	DES exposure in utero
Clue cells	*Gardnerella* vaginitis
Codman's triangle on x-ray	Osteosarcoma
Cold agglutinins	*Mycoplasma pneumoniae,* infectious mononucleosis
Cold intolerance	Hypothyroidism
Condylomata lata	2° syphilis
Continuous machinery murmur	Patent ductus arteriosus
Cori's disease	Debranching enzyme deficiency
Cotton-wool spots	Chronic hypertension
Cough, conjunctivitis, coryza + fever	Measles
Councilman bodies	Toxic or viral hepatitis
Cowdry type A bodies	Herpesvirus
Crescents in Bowman's capsule	Rapidly progressive crescentic glomerulonephritis
Crigler-Najjar syndrome	Congenital unconjugated hyperbilirubinemia
Curling's ulcer	Acute gastric ulcer associated with severe burns
Currant-jelly sputum	*Klebsiella*
Curschmann's spirals	Bronchial asthma (whorled mucous plugs)
Cushing's ulcer	Acute gastric ulcer associated with CNS injury
D-dimers	DIC
Depigmentation of neurons in substantia nigra	Parkinson's disease (basal ganglia disorder—rigidity, resting tremor, bradykinesia)
Dermatitis, dementia, diarrhea	Pellagra (niacin, vitamin B_3 deficiency)
Diabetes insipidus + exophthalmos + lesions of skull	Hand-Schüller-Christian disease
Dog or cat bite	*Pasteurella multocida*
Donovan bodies	Granuloma inguinale
Dressler's syndrome	Post-MI fibrinous pericarditis

Dubin-Johnson syndrome	Congenital conjugated hyperbilirubinemia (black liver)
Duchenne's muscular dystrophy	Deleted dystrophin gene (X-linked recessive)
Eburnation	Osteoarthritis (polished, ivory-like appearance of bone)
Edwards' syndrome	Trisomy 18 associated with rocker-bottom feet, low-set ears, heart disease
Eisenmenger's complex	Late cyanosis shunt (uncorrected L $\rightarrow$ R shunt becomes R $\rightarrow$ L shunt)
Elastic skin	Ehlers-Danlos syndrome
Erb-Duchenne palsy	Superior trunk (C5–C6) brachial plexus injury ("waiter's tip")
Erythema chronicum migrans	Lyme disease
Fanconi's syndrome	Proximal tubular reabsorption defect
"Fat, female, forty, and fertile"	Acute cholecystitis
Fatty liver	Alcoholism
Ferruginous bodies	Asbestosis
Gardner's syndrome	Colon polyps with osteomas and soft tissue tumors
Gaucher's disease	Glucocerebrosidase deficiency
Ghon focus	1° TB
Gilbert's syndrome	Benign congenital unconjugated hyperbilirubinemia
Glanzmann's thrombasthenia	Defect in platelet aggregation
Goodpasture's syndrome	Autoantibodies against alveolar and glomerular basement membrane proteins
Gowers' maneuver	Duchenne's (use of patient's arms to help legs pick self off the floor)
Guillain-Barré syndrome	Idiopathic polyneuritis
"Hair-on-end" (crew-cut) appearance on x-ray	β-thalassemia, sickle cell anemia (extramedullary hematopoiesis)
Hand-Schüller-Christian disease	Chronic progressive histiocytosis
HbF	Thalassemia major
HbS	Sickle cell anemia
hCG elevated	Choriocarcinoma, hydatidiform mole (occurs with and without embryo)
Heberden's nodes	Osteoarthritis (DIP swelling 2° to osteophytes)
Heinz bodies	G6PD deficiency
Henoch-Schönlein purpura	Hypersensitivity vasculitis associated with hemorrhagic urticaria and URIs
Heterophil antibodies	Infectious mononucleosis (EBV)
High-output cardiac failure (dilated cardiomyopathy)	Wet beriberi (thiamine, vitamin B_1 deficiency)
HLA-B27	Reiter's syndrome, ankylosing spondylitis
HLA-DR3 or -DR4	Diabetes mellitus type 1 (caused by autoimmune destruction of β cells)
Homer Wright rosettes	Neuroblastoma
Honeycomb lung on x-ray	Interstitial fibrosis

Horner's syndrome	Ptosis, miosis, and anhidrosis
Howell-Jolly bodies	Splenectomy (or nonfunctional spleen)
Huntington's disease	Caudate degeneration (autosomal dominant)
Hyperphagia + hypersexuality + hyperorality + hyperdocility	Klüver-Bucy syndrome (amygdala)
Hyperpigmentation of skin	1° adrenal insufficiency (Addison's disease)
Hypersegmented neutrophils	Macrocytic anemia
Hypertension + hypokalemia	Conn's syndrome
Hypochromic microcytosis	Iron deficiency anemia, lead poisoning
Increased α-fetoprotein in amniotic fluid/maternal serum	Anencephaly, spina bifida (neural tube defects)
Increased uric acid levels	Gout, Lesch-Nyhan syndrome, myeloproliferative disorders, loop and thiazide diuretics
Intussusception	Adenovirus (causes hyperplasia of Peyer's patches)
Janeway lesions	Endocarditis
Jarisch-Herxheimer reaction	Syphilis––overaggressive treatment of an asymptomatic patient that causes symptoms due to rapid lysis
Job's syndrome	Neutrophil chemotaxis abnormality
Kaposi's sarcoma	AIDS in MSM (men who have sex with men)
Kartagener's syndrome	Dynein defect
Kayser-Fleischer rings	Wilson's disease
Keratin pearls	Squamous cell carcinoma
Kimmelstiel-Wilson nodules	Diabetic nephropathy
Klüver-Bucy syndrome	Bilateral amygdala lesions
Koilocytes	HPV
Koplik spots	Measles
Krukenberg tumor	Gastric adenocarcinoma with ovarian metastases
Kussmaul hyperpnea	Diabetic ketoacidosis
Lens dislocation + aortic dissection + joint hyperflexibility	Marfan's syndrome (fibrillin deficit)
Lesch-Nyhan syndrome	HGPRT deficiency
Lewy bodies	Parkinson's disease
Libman-Sacks disease	Endocarditis associated with SLE
Lines of Zahn	Arterial thrombus
Lisch nodules	Neurofibromatosis (von Recklinghausen's disease)

Low serum ceruloplasmin	Wilson's disease
Lucid interval	Epidural hematoma
"Lumpy-bumpy" appearance of glomeruli on immunofluorescence	Poststreptococcal glomerulonephritis
Lytic bone lesions on x-ray	Multiple myeloma
Mallory bodies	Alcoholic liver disease
Mallory-Weiss syndrome	Esophagogastric lacerations
McArdle's disease	Muscle phosphorylase deficiency
McBurney's sign	Appendicitis
MLF syndrome (INO)	Multiple sclerosis
Monoclonal antibody spike	Multiple myeloma (called the M protein; usually IgG or IgA), MGUS (monoclonal gammopathy of undetermined significance), Waldenström's (M protein = IgM) macroglobulinemia
Myxedema	Hypothyroidism
Necrotizing vasculitis (lungs) and necrotizing glomerulonephritis	Wegener's and Goodpasture's (hemoptysis and glomerular disease)
Needle-shaped, negatively birefringent crystals	Gout
Negri bodies	Rabies
Nephritis + cataracts + hearing loss	Alport's syndrome
Neurofibrillary tangles	Alzheimer's disease
Niemann-Pick disease	Sphingomyelinase deficiency
No lactation postpartum	Sheehan's syndrome (pituitary infarction)
Nutmeg liver	CHF
Occupational exposure to asbestos	Malignant mesothelioma
"Orphan Annie" nuclei	Papillary carcinoma of the thyroid
Osler's nodes	Endocarditis
Owl's eye	CMV
Painless jaundice	Pancreatic cancer (head)
Palpable purpura on legs and buttocks	Henoch-Schönlein purpura
Pancoast's tumor	Bronchogenic apical tumor associated with Horner's syndrome
Pannus	Rheumatoid arthritis
Parkinson's disease	Nigrostriatal dopamine depletion
Periosteal elevation on x-ray	Pyogenic osteomyelitis
Peutz-Jeghers syndrome	Benign polyposis
Peyronie's disease	Penile fibrosis

Philadelphia chromosome (*bcr-abl*)	CML (may sometimes be associated with AML)
Pick bodies	Pick's disease
Pick's disease	Progressive dementia, similar to Alzheimer's
"Pink puffer"	Emphysema (centroacinar [smoking], panacinar [α_1-antitrypsin deficiency])
Plummer-Vinson syndrome	Esophageal webs with iron deficiency anemia
Podagra	Gout (MP joint of hallux)
Podocyte fusion	Minimal change disease
Polyneuropathy, cardiac pathology, and edema	Dry beriberi (thiamine, vitamin B_1 deficiency)
Polyneuropathy preceded by GI or respiratory infection	Guillain-Barré syndrome
Pompe's disease	Lysosomal glucosidase deficiency associated with cardiomegaly
Port-wine stain	Hemangioma
Positive anterior "drawer sign"	Anterior cruciate ligament injury
Pott's disease	Vertebral tuberculosis
Pseudopalisade tumor cell arrangement	Glioblastoma multiforme
Pseudorosettes	Ewing's sarcoma
Ptosis, miosis, anhidrosis	Horner's syndrome (Pancoast's tumor)
Rash on palms and soles	2° syphilis, Rocky Mountain spotted fever
Raynaud's syndrome	Recurrent vasospasm in extremities
RBC casts in urine	Acute glomerulonephritis
Recurrent pulmonary *Pseudomonas* and *S. aureus* infections	Cystic fibrosis
Red urine in the morning	Paroxysmal nocturnal hemoglobinuria
Reed-Sternberg cells	Hodgkin's lymphoma
Reid index (increased)	Chronic bronchitis
Reinke crystals	Leydig cell tumor
Reiter's syndrome	Urethritis, conjunctivitis, arthritis
Renal cell carcinoma + cavernous hemangiomas + adenomas	von Hippel–Lindau disease
Renal epithelial casts in urine	Acute toxic/viral nephrosis
Rhomboid crystals, positively birefringent	Pseudogout

Rib notching	Coarctation of aorta
Roth's spots in retina	Endocarditis
Rotor's syndrome	Congenital conjugated hyperbilirubinemia
Rouleaux formation (RBCs)	Multiple myeloma
S3	Left-to-right shunt (VSD, PDA, ASD), mitral regurgitation, LV failure (CHF)
S4	Aortic stenosis, hypertrophic subaortic stenosis
Schiller-Duval bodies	Yolk sac tumor
Senile plaques	Alzheimer's disease
Sézary syndrome	Cutaneous T-cell lymphoma
Sheehan's syndrome	Postpartum pituitary necrosis
Shwartzman reaction	*Neisseria meningitidis*
Signet-ring cells	Gastric carcinoma
Simian crease	Down syndrome
Sipple's syndrome	MEN type IIa
Sjögren's syndrome	Dry eyes, dry mouth, arthritis
Skip lesions	Crohn's
Slapped cheeks	Erythema infectiosum (fifth disease)
Smith antigen	SLE
"Smudge cell"	CLL
Soap bubble on x-ray	Giant cell tumor of bone
Spike and dome on EM	Membranous glomerulonephritis
Spitz nevus	Benign juvenile melanoma
Splinter hemorrhages in fingernails	Endocarditis
Starry-sky pattern	Burkitt's lymphoma
"Strawberry tongue"	Scarlet fever
Streaky ovaries	Turner's syndrome
String sign on x-ray	Crohn's disease
Subepithelial humps on EM	Poststreptococcal glomerulonephritis
Suboccipital lymphadenopathy	Rubella
Sulfur granules	*Actinomyces israelii*
Swollen gums, bruising, poor wound healing, anemia	Scurvy (ascorbic acid, vitamin C deficiency)––vitamin C is necessary for hydroxylation of proline and lysine in collagen synthesis
Systolic ejection murmur (crescendo-decrescendo)	Aortic valve stenosis

t(8;14)	Burkitt's lymphoma (c-*myc* activation)
t(9;22)	Philadelphia chromosome, CML (*bcr-abl* hybrid)
t(14;18)	Follicular lymphomas (*bcl*-2 activation)
Tabes dorsalis	3° syphilis
Tendon xanthomas (classically Achilles)	Familial hypercholesterolemia
Thumb sign on lateral x-ray	Epiglottitis (*Haemophilus influenzae*)
Thyroidization of kidney	Chronic bacterial pyelonephritis
Tophi	Gout
"Tram-track" appearance on LM	Membranoproliferative glomerulonephritis
Trousseau's sign	Visceral cancer, pancreatic adenocarcinoma (migratory thrombophlebitis), hypocalcemia (carpal spasm)
Virchow's node	Left supraclavicular node enlargement from metastatic carcinoma of the stomach
Virchow's triad	Pulmonary embolism (triad = blood stasis, endothelial damage, hypercoagulation)
von Recklinghausen's disease	Neurofibromatosis with café-au-lait spots
von Recklinghausen's disease of bone	Osteitis fibrosa cystica ("brown tumor")
Wallenberg's syndrome	PICA thrombosis
Waterhouse-Friderichsen syndrome	Adrenal hemorrhage associated with meningococcemia
Waxy casts	Chronic end-stage renal disease
WBC casts in urine	Acute pyelonephritis
WBCs in urine	Acute cystitis
Wermer's syndrome	MEN type I
Whipple's disease	Malabsorption syndrome caused by *Tropheryma whippelii*
Wilson's disease	Hepatolenticular degeneration
"Wire loop" appearance on LM	Lupus nephropathy
"Worst headache of my life"	Berry aneurysm—associated with adult polycystic kidney disease
Xanthochromia (CSF)	Subarachnoid hemorrhage
Xerostomia + arthritis + keratoconjunctivitis sicca	Sjögren's syndrome
Zenker's diverticulum	Upper GI diverticulum
Zollinger-Ellison syndrome	Gastrin-secreting tumor associated with ulcers

Most Common ...	
Bacteremia/pneumonia (IVDA)	*S. aureus*
Bacteria associated with cancer	*H. pylori*
Bacteria found in GI tract	*Bacteroides* (2nd most common is *E. coli*)
Brain tumor (adults)	Mets > astrocytoma (including glioblastoma multiforme) > meningioma > schwannoma
Brain tumor (kids)	Medulloblastoma (cerebellum)
Brain tumor--supratentorial (kids)	Craniopharyngioma
Breast cancer	Infiltrating ductal carcinoma (in the United States, 1 in 9 women will develop breast cancer)
Breast mass	Fibrocystic change (in postmenopausal women, carcinoma is the most common)
Breast tumor (benign)	Fibroadenoma
Bug in debilitated, hospitalized pneumonia patient	*Klebsiella*
Cardiac 1° tumor (adults)	Myxoma (4:1 left to right atrium; "ball and valve")
Cardiac 1° tumor (kids)	Rhabdomyoma
Cardiac tumor (adults)	Mets
Cardiomyopathy	Dilated cardiomyopathy
Chromosomal disorder	Down syndrome (associated with ALL, Alzheimer's dementia, and endocardial cushion defects)
Chronic arrhythmia	Atrial fibrillation (associated with high risk of emboli)
Congenital cardiac anomaly	VSD
Constrictive pericarditis	Tuberculosis
Coronary artery involved in thrombosis	LAD > RCA > LCA
Cyanosis (early; less common)	Tetralogy of Fallot, transposition of great vessels, truncus arteriosus
Cyanosis (late; more common)	VSD, ASD, PDA (close with indomethacin; open with misoprostol)
Demyelinating disease	Multiple sclerosis
Dietary deficit	Iron
Epiglottitis	*Haemophilus influenzae* type B
Esophageal cancer	Squamous cell carcinoma
Gene involved in cancer	p53 tumor suppressor gene
Group affected by cystic fibrosis	Caucasians (fat-soluble vitamin deficiencies, mucous plugs/lung infections)
Gynecologic malignancy	Endometrial carcinoma
Heart murmur	Mitral valve prolapse

Heart valve in bacterial endocarditis	Mitral
Heart valve in bacterial endocarditis in IVDA	Tricuspid
Heart valve (rheumatic fever)	Mitral valve (aortic is 2nd)
Helminth infection (U.S.)	*Enterobius vermicularis* (*Ascaris lumbricoides* is 2nd most common)
Hereditary bleeding disorder	von Willebrand's
Kidney stones	Calcium = radiopaque (2nd most common is ammonium = radiopaque; formed by urease-positive organisms such as *Proteus vulgaris* or *Staphylococcus*)
Liver disease	Alcoholic liver disease
Location of brain tumors (adults)	Supratentorial
Location of brain tumors (kids)	Infratentorial
Lysosomal storage disease	Gaucher's disease
Male cancer	Prostatic carcinoma
Malignancy associated with noninfectious fever	Hodgkin's disease
Malignant skin tumor	Basal cell carcinoma (rarely metastasizes)
Mets to bone	Breast, lung, thyroid, testes, prostate, kidney
Mets to brain	Lung, breast, skin (melanoma), kidney (renal cell carcinoma), GI
Mets to liver	Colon, gastric, pancreatic, breast, and lung carcinomas
Motor neuron disease	ALS
Neoplasm (kids)	ALL (2nd most common is cerebellar medulloblastoma)
Nephrotic syndrome	Membranous glomerulonephritis
Obstruction of male urinary tract	BPH
Opportunistic infection in AIDS	*Pneumocystis carinii* pneumonia
Organ receiving mets	Adrenal glands (due to rich blood supply)
Organ sending mets	Lung > breast, stomach
Ovarian tumor (benign)	Serous cystadenoma
Ovarian tumor (malignant)	Serous cystadenocarcinoma
Pancreatic tumor	Adenocarcinoma (head of pancreas)
Patient with ALL/CLL/AML/CML	ALL–child, CLL–adult > 60, AML–adult > 60, CML–adult 35–50
Patient with Hodgkin's	Young male (except nodular sclerosis type—female)
Patient with minimal change disease	Young child
Patient with Reiter's	Male
Pituitary tumor	Prolactinoma (2nd--somatotropic "acidophilic" adenoma)

Preventable cancer	Lung cancer
Primary bone tumor (adults)	Multiple myeloma
Primary hyperparathyroidism	Adenomas (followed by hyperplasia, then carcinoma)
Primary liver tumor	Hepatoma
Renal tumor	Renal cell carcinoma––associated with von Hippel–Lindau and acquired polycystic kidney disease; paraneoplastic syndromes (erythropoietin, renin, PTH, ACTH)
Secondary hyperparathyroidism	Hypocalcemia of chronic renal failure
Sexually transmitted disease	*Chlamydia*
Site of diverticula	Sigmoid colon
Site of metastasis	Regional lymph nodes
Site of metastasis (2nd most common)	Liver
Sites of atherosclerosis	Abdominal aorta > coronary > popliteal > carotid
Skin cancer	Basal cell carcinoma
Stomach cancer	Adenocarcinoma
Testicular tumor	Seminoma
Thyroid cancer	Papillary carcinoma
Tracheoesophageal fistula	Lower esophagus joins trachea/upper esophagus––blind pouch
Tumor in men	Prostate carcinoma
Tumor in women	Leiomyoma (estrogen dependent)
Tumor of infancy	Hemangioma
Tumor of the adrenal medulla (adults)	Pheochromocytoma (benign)
Tumor of the adrenal medulla (kids)	Neuroblastoma (malignant)
Type of Hodgkin's	Nodular sclerosis (vs. mixed cellularity, lymphocytic predominance, lymphocytic depletion)
Type of non-Hodgkin's	Follicular, small cleaved
Type of pituitary adenoma	Prolactinoma
Vasculitis	Temporal arteritis (risk of ipsilateral blindness due to thrombosis of ophthalmic artery)
Viral encephalitis	HSV
Vitamin deficiency (U.S.)	Folic acid (pregnant women are at high risk; body stores only 3- to 4-month supply)

Most Frequent Cause of ...	
Addison's	Autoimmune (infection is the 2nd most common cause)
Aneurysm, dissecting	Hypertension
Aortic aneurysm, abdominal and descending aorta	Atherosclerosis
Aortic aneurysm, ascending	3° syphilis
Bacterial meningitis (adults)	*Streptococcus pneumoniae*
Bacterial meningitis (elderly)	*S. pneumoniae*
Bacterial meningitis (kids)	*S. pneumoniae* or *Neisseria meningitidis*
Bacterial meningitis (newborns)	Group B streptococcus
Cancer associated with AIDS	Kaposi's sarcoma
Congenital adrenal hyperplasia	21-hydroxylase deficiency
Cretinism	Iodine deficit/hypothyroidism
Cushing's syndrome	Corticosteroid therapy (2nd most common cause is excess ACTH secretion by pituitary)
Death in CML	Blast crisis
Death in SLE	Lupus nephropathy
Dementia	Alzheimer's (2nd most common is multi-infarct)
DIC	Gram-negative sepsis, obstetric complications, cancer, burn trauma
Ejection click	Aortic/pulmonic stenosis
Food poisoning	*S. aureus*
Glomerulonephritis (adults)	IgA nephropathy (Berger's disease)
Hematoma--epidural	Rupture of middle meningeal artery (arterial bleeding is fast)
Hematoma--subdural	Rupture of bridging veins (trauma; venous bleeding is slow)
Hemochromatosis	Multiple blood transfusions (can result in CHF and ↑ risk of hepatocellular carcinoma)
Hepatic cirrhosis	EtOH
Hepatocellular carcinoma	Cirrhotic liver (often associated with hepatitis B and C)
Holosystolic murmur	VSD, tricuspid regurgitation, mitral regurgitation
Hypertension, 2°	Renal disease
Hypoparathyroidism	Thyroidectomy
Hypopituitarism	Adenoma
Infection in blood transfusion	Hepatitis C
Infection in burn victims	*Pseudomonas*

Leukemia (adults)	AML
"Machine-like" murmur	PDA
Mental retardation	Down syndrome (fragile X is the 2nd most common cause)
MI	Atherosclerosis
Mitral valve stenosis	Rheumatic heart disease
Myocarditis	Coxsackie B
Nephrotic syndrome (adults)	Membranous glomerulonephritis
Nephrotic syndrome (kids)	Minimal change disease (associated with infections/vaccinations; treat with corticosteroids)
Opening snap	Mitral stenosis
Osteomyelitis	*S. aureus*
Osteomyelitis in patients with sickle cell disease	*Salmonella*
Osteomyelitis with IVDA	*Pseudomonas*
Pancreatitis (acute)	EtOH and gallstones
Pancreatitis (chronic)	EtOH (adults), cystic fibrosis (kids)
Peau d'orange	Carcinoma of the breast
PID	*Neisseria gonorrhoeae* (monoarticular arthritis)
Pneumonia, hospital-acquired	*Klebsiella*
Pneumonia in cystic fibrosis, burn infection	*Pseudomonas aeruginosa*
Preventable blindness	*Chlamydia*
Primary amenorrhea	Turner's (XO)
Primary hyperaldosteronism	Adenoma of adrenal cortex
Primary hyperparathyroidism	Adenoma
Pulmonary hypertension	COPD
Right heart failure due to a pulmonary cause	Cor pulmonale
Right-sided heart failure	Left-sided heart failure
Sheehan's syndrome	Postpartum pituitary infarction 2° to hemorrhage
SIADH	Small cell carcinoma of the lung
UTI	*E. coli*
UTI (young women)	*E. coli* and *Staphylococcus saprophyticus*

▶ EQUATION REVIEW

Topic	Equation	Page
Sensitivity	$\text{Sensitivity} = \frac{a}{a+c}$	65
Specificity	$\text{Specificity} = \frac{d}{b+d}$	65
Positive predictive value	$\text{PPV} = \frac{a}{a+b}$	65
Negative predictive value	$\text{NPV} = \frac{d}{c+d}$	65
Relative risk	$\text{RR} = \frac{\left[\frac{a}{a+b}\right]}{\left[\frac{c}{c+d}\right]}$	66
Attributable risk	$\text{AR} = \left[\frac{a}{a+b}\right] - \left[\frac{c}{c+d}\right]$	66
Hardy-Weinberg equilibrium	$p^2 + 2pq + q^2 = 1$ $p + q = 1$	115
Henderson-Hasselbalch equation	$\text{pH} = \text{pKa} + \log \frac{[HCO_3^-]}{0.03\ P_{CO_2}}$	427
Volume of distribution	$V_d = \frac{\text{amount of drug in the body}}{\text{plasma drug concentration}}$	221
Clearance	$\text{CL} = \frac{\text{rate of elimination of drug}}{\text{plasma drug concentration}}$	221
Half-life	$t_{1/2} = \frac{0.7 \times V_d}{\text{CL}}$	221
Loading dose	$\text{LD} = C_p \times \frac{V_d}{F}$	222
Maintenance dose	$\text{MD} = C_p \times \frac{\text{CL}}{F}$	222
Cardiac output	$\text{CO} = \frac{\text{rate of } O_2 \text{ consumption}}{\text{arterial } O_2 \text{ content} - \text{venous } O_2 \text{ content}}$	244
Cardiac output	$\text{CO} = \text{stroke volume} \times \text{heart rate}$	244
Mean arterial pressure	$\text{MAP} = \text{cardiac output} \times \text{total peripheral resistance}$	244
Mean arterial pressure	$\text{MAP} = \frac{1}{3}\text{ systolic} + \frac{2}{3}\text{ diastolic}$	244
Stroke volume	$\text{SV} = \text{end diastolic volume} - \text{end systolic volume}$	244
Ejection fraction	$\text{EF} = \frac{\text{stroke volume}}{\text{end diastolic volume}} \times 100$	245
Resistance	$R = \frac{\text{driving pressure}}{\text{flow}} = \frac{8\eta\ (\text{viscosity}) \times \text{length}}{\pi r^4}$	246
Net filtration pressure	$P_{net} = \left[(P_c - P_i) - (\pi_c - \pi_i)\right]$	255

Glomerular filtration rate	$GFR = U_{inulin} \times \frac{V}{P_{inulin}} = C_{inulin}$	422
Glomerular filtration rate	$GFR = K_f [(P_{GC} - P_{BS}) - (\pi_{GC} - \pi_{BS})]$	422
Effective renal plasma flow	$ERPF = U_{PAH} \times \frac{V}{P_{PAH}} = C_{PAH}$	422
Renal blood flow	$RBF = \frac{RPF}{1 - Hct}$	422
Filtration fraction	$FF = \frac{GFR}{RPF}$	423
Free water clearance	$C_{H_2O} = V - C_{osm}$	423
Physiologic dead space	$V_D = V_T \times \frac{(Paco_2 - Peco_2)}{Paco_2}$	459

NOTES

SECTION IV

Top-Rated Review Resources

- How to Use the Database
- Internet Sites
- Comprehensive
- Anatomy and Embryology
- Behavioral Science
- Biochemistry
- Cell Biology and Histology
- Microbiology and Immunology
- Pathology
- Pharmacology
- Physiology
- Commercial Review Courses
- Publisher Contacts

▶ HOW TO USE THE DATABASE

This section is a database of top-rated basic science review books, sample examination books, software, Web sites, and commercial review courses that have been marketed to medical students studying for the USMLE Step 1. At the end of the section is a list of publishers and independent bookstores with addresses and phone numbers. For each recommended resource, we list the **Title** of the book, the **First Author** (or editor), the **Series Name** (where applicable), the **Current Publisher**, the **Copyright Year**, the **Number of Pages**, the **ISBN Code**, the **Approximate List Price**, the **Format** of the resource, and the **Number of Test Questions**. The entries for most books also include **Summary Comments** that describe their style and overall utility for studying. Finally, each recommended resource receives a **Rating**. Recommended resources are sorted into a comprehensive section as well as into sections corresponding to eight traditional basic medical science disciplines (anatomy and embryology, behavioral science, biochemistry, cell biology and histology, microbiology and immunology, pathology, pharmacology, and physiology). Within each section, books are arranged first by Rating and then alphabetically by First Author within each Rating group.

For the 2008 edition of *First Aid for the® USMLE Step 1,* the database of rated review books has been reorganized and updated with the addition of many new books and software and with the removal of some older, outdated items. A letter rating scale with six different grades reflects the detailed student evaluations for **Rated Resources.** Each rated resource receives a rating as follows:

A+	Excellent for boards review.
A A–	Very good for boards review; choose among the group.
B+ B	Good, but use only after exhausting better sources.
B–	Fair, but there are many better books in the discipline; or low-yield subject material.

The Rating is meant to reflect the overall usefulness of the resource in helping medical students prepare for the USMLE Step 1 examination. This is based on a number of factors, including:

- The cost
- The readability of the text
- The appropriateness and accuracy of the material
- The quality and number of sample questions
- The quality of written answers to sample questions
- The quality and appropriateness of the illustrations (e.g., graphs, diagrams, photographs)
- The length of the text (longer is not necessarily better)
- The quality and number of other resources available in the same discipline
- The importance of the discipline for the USMLE Step 1 examination

Please note that ratings do not reflect the quality of the resources for purposes other than reviewing for the USMLE Step 1 examination. Many books with lower ratings are well written and informative but are not ideal for boards preparation. We have not listed or commented on general textbooks available in the basic sciences.

Evaluations are based on the cumulative results of formal and informal surveys of thousands of medical students at many medical schools across the country. The summary comments and overall ratings represent a consensus opinion, but there may have been a broad range of opinion or limited student feedback on any particular resource.

Please note that the data listed are subject to change in that:

- Publishers' prices change frequently.
- Bookstores often charge an additional markup.
- New editions come out frequently, and the quality of updating varies.
- The same book may be reissued through another publisher.

We actively encourage medical students and faculty to submit their opinions and ratings of these basic science review materials so that we may update our database. (See p. xv, How to Contribute.) In addition, we ask that publishers and authors submit for evaluation review copies of basic science review books, including new editions and books not included in our database. We also solicit reviews of new books or suggestions for alternate modes of study that may be useful in preparing for the examination, such as flash cards, computer-based tutorials, commercial review courses, and World Wide Web sites.

Disclaimer/Conflict of Interest Statement

No material in this book, including the ratings, reflects the opinion or influence of the publisher. All errors and omissions will gladly be corrected if brought to the attention of the authors through the publisher. Please note that *USMLERx* and the *First Aid for the USMLE* series are publications by the senior authors of this book; their ratings are based solely on recommendations from the student authors of this book as well as data from the student survey and feedback forms.

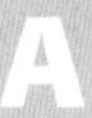

WebPath: The Internet Pathology Laboratory | ***Free*** | Review/1000 q

KLATT

http://library.med.utah.edu/WebPath/webpath.html

Features a wealth of outstanding gross and microscopic illustrations, clinical vignette questions, and case studies. Contains many classic, high-quality illustrations. Includes 8 general pathology exams and 11 system-based exams with approximately 1000 questions. Also includes 170 questions associated with images. Questions reflect current boards format and difficulty level but are typically shorter. A WebPath CD-ROM is available for $60.00 and features the online Web site plan supplemented with additional illustrations, topics, tutorials, and radiology.

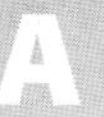

USMLEWorld Qbank | ***$90 for 1 month; $175 for 3 months*** | Test/2000 q

USMLEWORLD

www.usmleworld.com

A new high-quality USMLE question bank. Very well constructed questions. Excellent, detailed explanations with figures and tables. Questions tend to be more difficult than those on the actual exam. Features a number of test customization and analysis options. Web program does not allow other application windows to be open for studying. Reasonably priced. Compare closely to Kaplan and USMLERx.

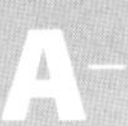

Kaplan Qbank | ***$199 for 1 month; $279 for 3 months*** | Test/2350 q

KAPLAN

www.kaplanmedical.com

A high-quality but expensive question bank providing tailored boards-format exams. Test content and performance feedback are organized by organ system and discipline. Questions are similar in style and content to those on the actual exam but are somewhat reliant on buzzwords. Includes well-written, detailed explanations. Additional Qbanks for physiology and clinical vignettes are available. Compare closely to USMLERx and USMLEWorld.

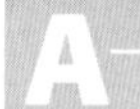

USMLERx Step 1 Qmax | ***$69 for 1 month; $129 for 3 months*** | Test/2600+ q

MEDIQ LEARNING

LE

www.usmlerx.com

A well-priced question bank that closely simulates the USMLE. Question length and level of difficulty are similar to those of the actual exam. Explanations are to the point and feature high-yield facts from *First Aid for the USMLE Step 1*. Provides many helpful test selection options and detailed performance analyses. Overall, an excellent resource for high-yield questions with useful test analysis options.

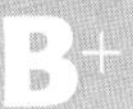

USMLE Steps 123 Step 1 Question Bank | **_$99 for 1 month; $199 for 3 months_** | Test/2500+ q

ELSEVIER

www.studentconsult.com/usmle

A solid question bank that can be divided according to discipline and subject area. Includes both practice and test modes. Question length, difficulty, and test interface (FRED) are similar to those of the actual exam. Offers concise explanations with links to StudentConsult and FirstConsult content. Users can see cumulative results over time and compared to other test takers. Overall, a good source of practice questions, with a number of subscription periods available. Limited student feedback.

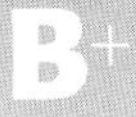

The Pathology Guy | 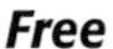 **_Free_** | Review

FRIEDLANDER

www.pathguy.com

A free Web site containing extensive but poorly organized information on a variety of fundamental concepts in pathology. An excellent collection of high-yield facts can be found in "Ed's Pathology Review for USMLE," which is buried at the end of each pathology topic page. Philosophical and religious digressions can impede a rapid review of the site.

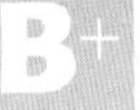

Digital Anatomist Interactive Atlases | **_Free_** | Review

UNIVERSITY OF WASHINGTON

www9.biostr.washington.edu/da.html

A good site containing an interactive neuroanatomy course along with a three-dimensional atlas of the brain, thorax, and knee. Atlases have computer-generated images along with cadaver dissections. Each atlas also has a useful quiz in which users identify structures in the slide images. An excellent source for reviewing neuro images.

B

The Whole Brain Atlas | **_Free_** | Review

JOHNSON

www.med.harvard.edu/AANLIB/home.html

A collection of high-quality brain MR and CT images with views of normal, aging, and diseased brains (CVA, degenerative, neoplastic, and inflammatory diseases). The interface is technologically impressive but complex. Guided tours and image correlations to cases are especially useful. Although not all of the images are particularly high yield for the boards, this is an excellent introduction to neuroimaging.

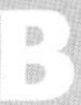

Lippincott's 350-Question Practice Test for USMLE Step 1 ***Free*** Test/350 q

LIPPINCOTT WILLIAMS & WILKINS

www.lww.com/medstudent/usmle

Previously Blackwell's Step 1 Online Q&A. A full-length, seven-block, 350-question practice exam in a format similar to that of the real exam. Questions come with explanations related to the selected answer only. Users can bookmark questions and can take the test all at once or by section.

USMLEasy ***$99 for 1 month; $199 for 3 months*** Test/2800 q

MCGRAW-HILL

www.usmleasy.com

An Internet-based question bank based on the PreTest series. Requires an online subscription. Some questions are more obscure than those appearing on the actual exam. Users can track questions completed as well as customize tests. Presented in boards format. Useful as a supplemental review after other resources have been exhausted.

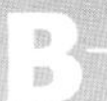

Active Learning Centre ***Free*** Test/100 q

TURCHIN

www.med.jhu.edu/medcenter/quiz/home.cgi

A quiz engine site based on a large database with an extensive list of bugs, drugs, and vaccines. Questions test the basic characteristics of each element in the database in a multiple-choice, matching, or essay format that the user selects. Questions are not boards style but are useful for learning the memory-intensive subjects of microbiology and pharmacology.

A

First Aid Cases for the USMLE Step 1 ***$39.95*** Review

LE

McGraw-Hill, 2006, 334 pages, ISBN 0071464107

A series of cases organized into the same sections as *First Aid for the USMLE Step 1*. Provides 9–45 cases per general principle or organ system. Each case includes a paragraph-long clinical vignette followed by questions and detailed explanations. Many cases include images that are highly relevant to boards review. Overall, a good supplemental USMLE review resource that provides just the right amount of depth.

A–

Kaplan's USMLE Step 1 Home Study Program ***$499.00*** Review

Kaplan, 2006, 1900 pages, ISBN 0X63410105

Includes two general-principle review books along with two organ system–based review books, all of which are lengthy and comprehensive. Useful only if started early, possibly with coursework. Excellent as a reference for studying. Expensive for the amount of material. Books can be purchased by calling 1-800-KAP-ITEM or by visiting www.kaptest.com.

A–

USMLE Q&A for the USMLE Step 1 ***$39.95*** Test/1000 q

LE

McGraw-Hill, 2006, 416 pages, ISBN 0071481729

A great resource for review questions drawn from the USMLE Step 1 Qmax. Offers 1000 questions organized according to subject along with one full-length examination consisting of 350 questions. Questions are similar to those of the actual exam in both complexity and length. Explanations are brief but adequate.

A–

medEssentials ***6 months for $129; 12 months for $189; 25 months for $279*** Review

MANLEY

Kaplan, 2006, 500 pages, ISBN BK5023A

A comprehensive review book with great tables and figures. Divided into general principles and organ systems. Contains some high-yield color images in the back. Too detailed in some parts. Comes with a monthly subscription to online interactive exercises that are of limited value. Limited student feedback.

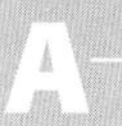

Step-Up: A High-Yield, Systems-Based Review for the USMLE Step 1 **_$39.95_** Review

MEHTA

Lippincott Williams & Wilkins, 2006, 448 pages, ISBN 078178090X

An organ system–based review text that is useful for integrating the basic sciences covered in Step 1. Composed primarily of outlines, charts, tables, and diagrams. The appendix includes 38 clinical cases and an alphabetical section on pharmacology. The previous edition contained some errors. The organ system format appeals to many students and serves as a good contrast to other review sources. Includes useful "quick hit" facts. Limited feedback on the new edition.

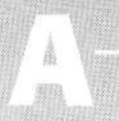

Deja Review: USMLE Step 1 **_$22.95_** Review

NAHEEDY

McGraw-Hill, 2006, 192 pages, ISBN 0071447903

A review book featuring questions and answers in a two-column, quiz-yourself format, divided according to discipline. Includes a section at the end with high-yield clinical vignettes. Has a few mistakes throughout, but still a great last-second review before the exam. Compare with the Recall series. Limited student feedback.

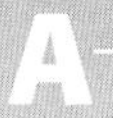

USMLE Step 1 Recall Audio **_$37.95_** Audio—MP3

REINHEIMER

Lippincott Williams & Wilkins, 2007, ISBN 0781765544

Downloads accessed at http://thepoint.lww.com/audio. Offers the same content as that of the corresponding text. The use of two different voices allows listeners to distinguish questions from answers. Content contains some errors, but overall a useful review resource that can be used during downtime.

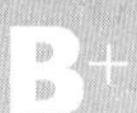

USMLE Step 1 Secrets **_$39.95_** Review

BROWN

Elsevier, 2004, 324 pages, ISBN 1560535709

Clarifies difficult concepts in a concise, easy-to-read manner. Complements other boards study material, with a focus on understanding preclinical fundamentals rather than on rote memorization. Easy-to-read style allows for rapid review during downtime. Good integration of information.

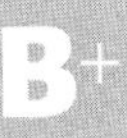

Medical Boards—Step 1 Made Ridiculously Simple **$29.95** Review

CARL

MedMaster, 2007, 351 pages, ISBN 0940780712

Quick and easy reading. The table and chart format is organized by subject, but some charts are poorly labeled. Reviews are mixed. Consider as an adjunct. Compare with *Crashing the Boards: USMLE Step 1*. Limited feedback on the recent edition.

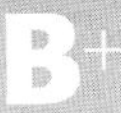

Blueprints Step 1 Q&A **$34.95** Test/350 q

CLEMENT

Lippincott Williams & Wilkins, 2003, 184 pages, ISBN 140510323X

Contains one full-length exam of 350 questions written by students. Good for practicing the multistep questions common on the actual exam. Questions are at times easier than those on the actual test. A good supplemental source for practice questions on high-yield facts.

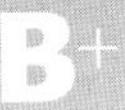

Lange Outline Review: USMLE Step 1 **$39.95** Review

GOLDBERG

McGraw-Hill, 2006, 364 pages, ISBN 0071451919

A comprehensive outline review of basic science topics. Includes essential facts, diseases, and disorders. Also offers a bulleted treatment of major abnormal processes by system. Includes black-and-white images of pathology and histology throughout.

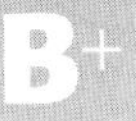

Lange Practice Tests USMLE Step 1 **$42.95** Review/650 q

GOLDBERG

McGraw-Hill, 2005, 240 pages, ISBN 007144615X

A good resource for review questions consisting of 13 blocks of 50 questions with explanations. Less lengthy and challenging than the actual USMLE questions.

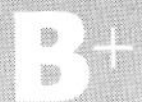

Rapid Review for USMLE Step 1 **$34.95** Review/1400 q

GOLJAN

Elsevier, 2002, 314 pages + CD-ROM, ISBN 0323008410

Outline format with high-yield marginal notes, figures, and tables that highlight key content. Narrative clinical boxes illustrate clinical relevance. Practice exams provide USMLE-style questions of mixed quality. The CD-ROM includes the questions from the book, but the user cannot omit previously used questions from practice sessions.

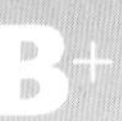

Lange Q&A: USMLE Step 1 **$41.95** Review/1100+ q

KING

McGraw-Hill, 2005, 528 pages, ISBN 0071445781

A large source of review questions. Offers more than 1100 questions organized according to subject along with three sections of comprehensive practice exams. Slightly less challenging than the actual USMLE questions.

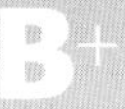

PreTest Clinical Vignettes for the USMLE Step 1 **$29.95** Test/400 q

MCGRAW-HILL

McGraw-Hill, 2007, 416 pages, ISBN 0071471847

Clinical vignette–style questions with detailed explanations, organized as eight blocks of 50 questions covering basic sciences. Serves as a good self-evaluation tool, but questions may not mirror those on the actual exam.

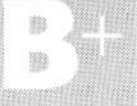

USMLE Step 1 Recall: Buzzwords for the Boards **$40.95** Review

REINHEIMER

Lippincott Williams & Wilkins, 2007, 467 pages, ISBN 0781778735

Quizzes on main topics and key points presented in a two-column question-and-answer format. Good for self-testing, group study, and quick review. Useful as a change of pace. Covers many important clinical features, but not comprehensive or tightly organized. Sometimes focuses on obscure details and memorization rather than on the comprehension and integration that the USMLE emphasizes. Compare with the Deja Review series.

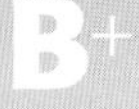

Underground Clinical Vignettes: Step 1 Bundle **$159.95** Review

SWANSON

Lippincott Williams & Wilkins, 2007, 9 volumes, ISBN 0781763622

Bundle includes nine books. Designed for easy quizzing with a group. Case-based vignettes provide a good review supplement. Best when started early with coursework or when used in conjunction with another primary review source.

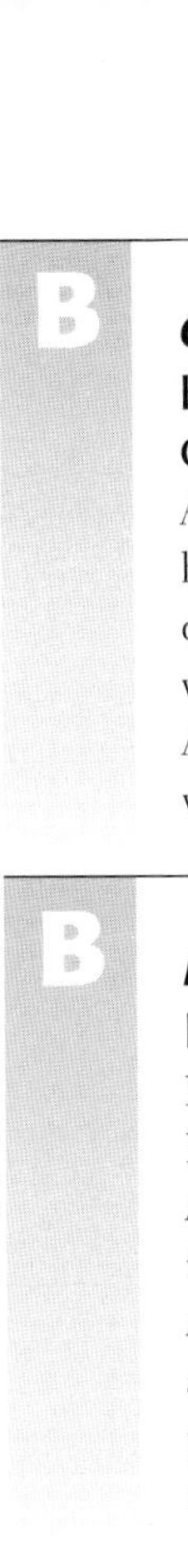

B

Gold Standard Prep Set for USMLE Step 1 **$309.00** Review

KNOUSE

Gold Standard, 2004

A set of 55 CDs covering USMLE Step 1 material in more than 70 hours. Limited but positive feedback on an updated and expanded set of CDs. Used by some students as a way to review while driving, while working out, and during downtime. Contains some inaccuracies. Available only by mail order through the company's Web site, www.boardprep.net.

B

NMS Review for USMLE Step 1 **$44.95** Test/850 q

LAZO

Lippincott Williams & Wilkins, 2005, 480 pages + CD-ROM, ISBN 0781779219

A text that includes a CD-ROM and serves as a good source of practice questions and answers. Some questions are too picky or difficult. Annotated explanations are well written but are sometimes unnecessarily detailed. Organized as 17 practice exams. The six pages of color plates are helpful. The CD-ROM attempts to simulate the CBT format but is disorganized.

B

Kaplan's USMLE Step 1 Qbook **$44.95** Test/850 q

MANLEY

Kaplan, 2006, 464 pages, ISBN 1419551493

Consists of seventeen 50-question exams organized by the traditional basic science disciplines. Offers good USMLE-style questions with clear, detailed explanations, but lacks the classic images typically seen on the exam. Also includes a guide on test-taking strategies. Comparable to the First Aid and NMS question reviews.

B

USMLE Step 1 Recall PDA: Buzzwords for the Boards **$37.95** PDA

REINHEIMER

Lippincott Williams & Wilkins, 2004, ISBN 0781754216

The PDA version of the book of the same name. Useful for quick review.

B

PreTest Physical Diagnosis **$25.95** Test/500 q

RETEGUIZ

McGraw-Hill, 2006, 434 pages, ISBN 0071455515

A collection of clinical vignettes organized by body system, presented in a style similar to that of other books in the PreTest series. May be beyond the scope of Step 1, but could also be used in the clinical years of medical school. Limited student feedback.

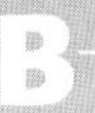

Exam Master Step 1 — ***$149.00*** — Test/8000 q

EXAM MASTER

Exam Master Corporation, 2004, ISBN 158129087X

Windows/Mac-based testing software with access to up to 8000 Step 1 questions. Interface and exam setup can be difficult. Questions are of mixed quality and can be relatively simple or very obscure. Offers the ability to hide multiple-choice options.

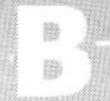

Cracking the Boards: USMLE Step 1 — ***$34.95*** — Review/400 q

STEIN

Random House, 2000, 832 pages, ISBN 0375761632

A comprehensive text review based on the USMLE content outline, written by past and present medical students. The style is wordy and broad but offers few details. The organ-based format appeals to some students. Includes many labeled illustrations, charts, and photos.

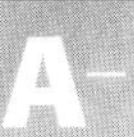

High-Yield Embryology | **$25.95** | Review

DUDEK

Lippincott Williams & Wilkins, 2006, 208 pages, ISBN 0781768721

A very good, concise review of embryology for the USMLE. Offers excellent organization with clinical correlations. Includes a high-yield list of embryologic origins of tissues. No index or questions.

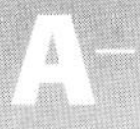

High-Yield Neuroanatomy | **$25.95** | Review

FIX

Lippincott Williams & Wilkins, 2005, 178 pages, ISBN 0781758998

A clean, easy-to-read outline format. Offers straightforward text with excellent diagrams and illustrations. The first several chapters are particularly good. Compare with *Clinical Neuroanatomy Made Ridiculously Simple*. No index.

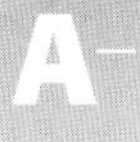

Case Files: Gross Anatomy | **$29.95** | Review

TOY

McGraw-Hill, 2005, 345 pages, ISBN 0071437797

A resource that offers both gross anatomy basics and clinical cases covering several high-yield anatomy topics. Also features a concise discussion of anatomy essentials. Diagrams are sparse but high yield.

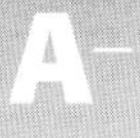

USMLE Road Map: Gross Anatomy | **$25.95** | Review/100 q

WHITE

McGraw-Hill, 2005, 240 pages, ISBN 0071445161

An outline treatment of gross anatomy with clinical correlations throughout. Also features high-yield facts in boldface along with numerous high-yield charts and figures. Clinical problems with explanations are given at the end of each chapter. An especially effective chart format is used throughout, with clearly labeled illustrations of basic anatomy. Good integration of facts.

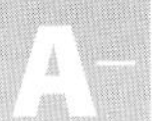

USMLE Road Map: Neuroscience | **$24.95** | Review/80 q

WHITE

McGraw-Hill, 2004, 208 pages, ISBN 0071422870

An outline review of basic anatomy and physiology with clinical correlations throughout. Also features high-yield facts in boldface along with numerous high-yield charts and figures. Clinical problems with explanations are given at the end of each chapter.

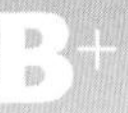

Elsevier's Integrated Anatomy and Embryology — **$34.95** — Book

BOGART

Elsevier, 2007, 378 pages, ISBN 1416031650

Part of the new Integrated series that focuses on core knowledge in a specific basic science discipline while linking that information to related concepts from other disciplines. Case-based and USMLE-style questions at the end of each chapter allow readers to gauge their comprehension of the material. Includes online access. Best if used during coursework. Limited student feedback.

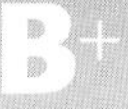

High-Yield Gross Anatomy — **$26.95** — Review

DUDEK

Lippincott Williams & Wilkins, 2007, 190 pages, ISBN 0781770157

An excellent, concise review with clinical correlations. Contains well-labeled, high-yield radiologic images. May be useful to supplement with an atlas. No index.

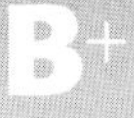

Clinical Neuroanatomy Made Ridiculously Simple — **$19.95** — Review/Few q

GOLDBERG

MedMaster, 2007, 96 pages + CD-ROM, ISBN 0940780577

An easy-to-read, memorable, and simplified format with clever hand-drawn diagrams. Offers a quick, high-yield review of clinical neuroanatomy. Good emphasis on clinically relevant pathways, cranial nerves, and neurologic diseases. Includes a CD-ROM that offers CT and MRI images as well as a tutorial on neurologic localization. Compare with *High-Yield Neuroanatomy*.

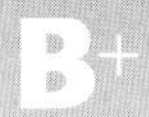

Crash Course: Anatomy — **$29.95** — Review

GRANGER

Elsevier, 2006, 225 pages, ISBN 0323043194

Part of the Crash Course review series for basic sciences, integrating clinical topics. Offers two-color illustrations, handy study tools, and USMLE review questions. Includes online access. Provides a solid review of anatomy for Step 1. Best if started early.

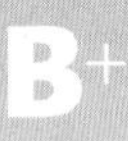

Rapid Review: Gross and Developmental Anatomy — **$34.95** — Review/350 q

MOORE

Elsevier, 2006, 400 pages, ISBN 0323045510

A detailed treatment of basic anatomy and embryology, presented in an outline format similar to that of other books in the series. At times more detailed than necessary for boards review. Contains high-yield charts and figures throughout. Two 50-question tests with extensive explanations are included, with 250 additional questions online.

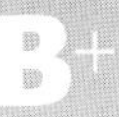

Underground Clinical Vignettes: Anatomy **$22.95** Review/20 q

SWANSON

Lippincott Williams & Wilkins, 2007, 224 pages, ISBN 0781764750

Concise clinical cases illustrating approximately 100 frequently tested diseases with an anatomic basis. Also includes 20 additional boards-style questions. Cardinal signs, symptoms, and buzzwords are highlighted. A useful source for isolating important anatomy concepts to concentrate on for Step 1.

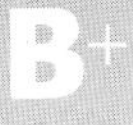

Deja Review: Neuroscience **$22.95** Review

TREMBLAY

McGraw-Hill, 2006, 250 pages, ISBN 0071474625

A review book featuring questions and answers in a two-column, quiz-yourself format similar to that of the Recall series. Provides a sound review in a format that differs from straight text. A perfect length for USMLE neurophysiology and anatomy review.

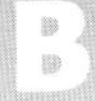

Neuroscience at a Glance **$34.95** Review

BARKER

Blackwell Science, 2003, 132 pages, ISBN 1405111240

A high-yield treatment of basic principles in neuroscience using figures only, with one topic presented on each page. Includes a highly effective appendix of pathways. Most useful when used in conjunction with a neuroscience course. Limited student feedback.

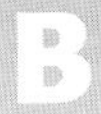

Platinum Vignettes: Anatomy & Embryology **$26.95** Review

BROCHERT

Elsevier, 2003, 110 pages, ISBN 1560535814

Fifty clinical case scenarios presented in a user-friendly format, with questions appearing on the front of each page and answers printed on the back. Similar in style to other books in the Platinum Vignettes series; may be of benefit for students who wish to self-quiz. Relatively few cases are presented considering that both anatomy and embryology are covered. Expensive for the amount of material covered.

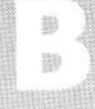

Gray's Anatomy Flash Cards **$34.95** Flash cards

DRAKE

Elsevier, 2005, 320 pages, ISBN 0443069107

The front of each card offers detailed anatomical illustrations, while the back of each card identifies the structures in each illustration along with systemically and clinically relevant information. Includes some radiology review cards and clinical question cards that are good for boards review. Overall, may be too detailed for USMLE preparation. Includes online access.

B

BRS Embryology **$36.95** Review/500 q

DUDEK

Lippincott Williams & Wilkins, 2007, 304 pages,
ISBN 0781771161

An outline-based review of embryology that is typical of the BRS series. Offers a good but overly detailed review of important embryology. A discussion of congenital malformations is included at the end of each chapter along with relevant questions. The comprehensive exam at the end of the book is high yield.

B

BRS Neuroanatomy **$36.95** Review/500 q

FIX

Lippincott Williams & Wilkins, 2007, 480 pages,
ISBN 0781772451

An updated text that covers the anatomy and embryology of the nervous system. Complete but too lengthy for USMLE review; requires time commitment. Compare with *High-Yield Neuroanatomy* by the same author.

B

Clemente's Anatomy Flash Cards **$36.95** Review

GEST

Lippincott Williams & Wilkins, 2007, 700 pages,
ISBN 0781765269

Organized by region, with 350 full-color illustrations. Based on Clemente's *Anatomy: A Regional Atlas of the Human Body*, 5th edition. Labels are designed for self-testing, with numbers on the front of each card and answers on the back. Tables on the back of the cards provide additional information about bones, muscles, nerves, arteries, veins, ligaments, topographic features, lymphatics, and organs. Great for use during coursework, but too detailed for boards review.

B

Clinical Anatomy Made Ridiculously Simple **$29.95** Review

GOLDBERG

MedMaster, 2007, 187 pages, ISBN 0940780798

An easy-to-read text offering simple diagrams along with numerous mnemonics and amusing associations. Incomplete. The humorous style has variable appeal to students, so browse before buying. Offers good coverage of selected topics. Best if used during coursework.

B

Clinical Anatomy Flash Cards **$36.95** Review

GOULD

Lippincott Williams & Wilkins, 2007, 696 pages,
ISBN 0781765099

Based on Moore and Dalley's *Clinically Oriented Anatomy,* 5th edition, and Agur and Dalley's *Grant's Atlas of Anatomy,* 11th edition. Organized by region, with 450 full-color illustrations offering realistic anatomic renderings from Grant's Atlas. Cards feature clinically relevant descriptions of structures, concise versions of the text's clinical "Blue Boxes," and correlating images. Great for use during coursework, but too detailed for boards review.

B

Netter's Anatomy Flash Cards **$34.95** Flash cards

HANSEN

Elsevier, 2006, 324 cards, ISBN 1416039740

A series of 324 flash cards featuring illustrations from Netter's *Atlas of Human Anatomy,* 4th edition. Cards are hole-punched and include a metal ring for easy portability. Includes access to www.netteranatomy.com, where cards can be viewed online. Great for use during coursework, but too detailed for boards review.

B

Netter's Clinical Anatomy **$48.95** Review

HANSEN

Elsevier, 2005, 600 pages, ISBN 192900771X

A review book that includes many of the famous Netter's anatomy and embryology images along with short descriptions. It also offers helpful clinical correlation pages for many of the common diseases. Definitely a wonderful anatomy reference text during boards studying, but too long and detailed to be used as a primary review source.

B

Crash Course: Nervous System **$29.95** Review

MIHAILOFF

Elsevier, 2005, 272 pages, ISBN 0323034438

Part of the Crash Course review series for basic sciences, integrating clinical topics. Offers two-color illustrations, handy study tools, and USMLE review questions. Includes online access. A good overall review of neuroscience with integration of multiple areas.

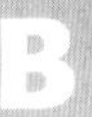

Elsevier's Integrated Neuroscience — **_$34.95_** — Book

NOLTE

Elsevier, 2007, 336 pages, ISBN 0323034098

Part of the new Integrated series that focuses on core knowledge in a specific basic science discipline while linking that information to related concepts from other disciplines. Case-based and USMLE-style questions at the end of each chapter allow readers to gauge their comprehension of the material. Includes online access. Best if used during coursework. Limited student feedback.

B

PreTest Neuroscience — **_$25.95_** — Test/500 q

SIEGEL

McGraw-Hill, 2007, 384 pages, ISBN 0071471804

Similar to other books in the PreTest series. Features a question-and-answer format that is not necessarily in USMLE style. Black-and-white images are referenced to questions throughout. Includes a brief high-yield section. Improved 2007 edition.

B

BRS Gross Anatomy Flash Cards — **_$31.99_** — Flash cards

SWANSON

Lippincott Williams & Wilkins, 2005, 254 pages, ISBN 0781756545

High-yield anatomy clinical cases presented in flash-card format. Anatomy basics are generally excluded. A useful, boards-relevant resource for students who like to study with flash cards and are reasonably well versed in anatomy.

B

Blueprints Notes & Cases: Neuroscience — **_$28.95_** — Review

WECHSLER

Lippincott Williams & Wilkins, 2003, 240 pages, ISBN 1405103493

High-yield cases followed by a discussion and tables, presented in a format similar to that of other books in the Blueprints series. Offers important gross neuroanatomy and neurophysiology facts, but diagrams must be improved if the book is to be considered sufficiently comprehensive for boards review.

B

Rapid Review: Neuroscience — **_$34.95_** — Book

WEYHENMEYER & GALLMAN

Elsevier, 2006, 304 pages, ISBN 0323022618

A detailed treatment of neuroscience, presented in an outline format similar to that of other books in the series. Should be started early given its extensive treatment of a relatively narrow topic. Contains high-yield charts and figures throughout. Two 50-question tests with extensive explanations are included, with 250 additional questions online.

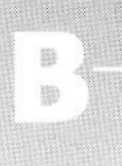

Anatomy Recall | **_$34.95_** | Review

ANTEVIL

Lippincott Williams & Wilkins, 2005, 384 pages,
ISBN 078179885X

Presented in question-and-answer format. Good for quick review, but too detailed for boards review.

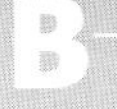

BRS Gross Anatomy | **_$36.95_** | Review/500 q

CHUNG

Lippincott Williams & Wilkins, 2007, 544 pages,
ISBN 0781771749

A detailed, lengthy text in outline format with illustrations and tables. Better for coursework than for quick boards review, especially for a lower-yield subject. Features a good clinical correlation section.

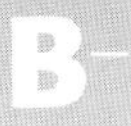

Netter's Neuroscience Flash Cards | **_$34.95_** | Flash cards

FELTEN

Elsevier, 2005, 235 cards, ISBN 1929007647

Color codes identify corresponding sections from the atlas for easy cross-referencing and review. Explanatory comments are given on the back of each card along with integrative clinical points. Great for coursework, but too detailed for boards review.

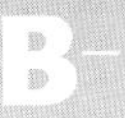

Manter and Gatz's Essentials of Clinical Neuroanatomy and Neurophysiology | **_$33.95_** | Review

GILMAN

F. A. Davis, 2002, 281 pages, ISBN 0803607725

A well-organized discussion of neuroanatomy, neurophysiology, and neuropharmacology presented with illustrations and images. Too dense for boards review.

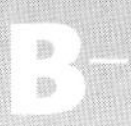

Biotest Study Aids: Histology and Neural Anatomy | **_$25.95_** | Review/2000 q

PAPKA

Biotest, Inc., 2004, 427 pages, ISBN 1893720136

A comprehensive outline review. Lacks illustrations and includes a large number of low-quality questions with no explanations, but answers are cross-referenced to the text. Consider using with coursework. Limited student feedback.

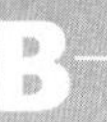

Clinical Anatomy: An Illustrated Review — ***$39.95*** — Review/500 q

SNELL

Lippincott Williams & Wilkins, 2003, 294 pages, ISBN 0781743168

A well-organized summary of Snell's major book. Includes excellent diagrams and tables. Questions incorporate radiographs, CT scans, and MRIs. Does not cover neuroanatomy or embryology. Neither the text nor the questions are as clinical as the title implies. Only some answers have explanations, and most are too short.

B-

Imaging Atlas of Human Anatomy — ***$49.95*** — Text

WEIR

Elsevier, 2003, 224 pages, ISBN 0723432112

An atlas of diagnostic images for all major systems, including MRIs, CT scans, and brief explanations of diagnostic methods. Useful primarily as an imaging reference for boards review.

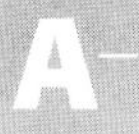

A

High-Yield Behavioral Science **$26.95** Review

FADEM

Lippincott Williams & Wilkins, 2001, 144 pages, ISBN 0781730848

A clear, concise, quick review of behavioral science. Offers a logical presentation with crammable charts, graphs, and tables. Features a short but adequate statistics chapter. No index.

A–

BRS Behavioral Science **$36.95** Review/500 q

FADEM

Lippincott Williams & Wilkins, 2004, 296 pages, ISBN 0781757274

An easy-to-read outline format with boldfacing of key terms. Offers good, detailed coverage of high-yield topics. The text is lengthy and gives more information than may be needed for the USMLE. Includes excellent tables and charts as well as a short but complete statistics chapter. Offers great coverage of ethics and patient communication topics. Also features good review questions, including a 100-question comprehensive exam at the end of the book.

A–

Deja Review: Behavioral Science **$22.95** Review

STANFORD

McGraw-Hill, 2007, 200 pages, ISBN 0071468684

A review book featuring questions and answers in a two-column, quiz-yourself format similar to that of the Recall series. Provides a sound review in a format that differs from straight text. Allows a more interactive review of some hard-to-memorize details needed for USMLE behavioral science questions.

A–

Rapid Review: Behavioral Science **$34.95** Review/350 q

STEVENS

Elsevier, 2006, 352 pages, ISBN 0323045715

A quick outline format covering basic topics in behavioral science, human development, and biostatistics, presented in a format similar to that of other books in the Rapid Review series. Two 50-question multiple-choice tests are included with explanations. Somewhat more detailed on specific disorders, but not sufficient as a sole biostatistics review. The CD-ROM contains additional questions. Compare with *High-Yield Behavioral Science.* Limited student feedback.

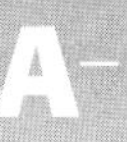

Underground Clinical Vignettes: Behavioral Science ***$22.95*** Review/20 q

SWANSON

Lippincott Williams & Wilkins, 2007, 224 pages,
ISBN 0781764645

Concise clinical cases illustrating commonly tested diseases in behavioral science. Cardinal signs, symptoms, and buzzwords are highlighted. Useful for picking out important points in this very broad subject. Use as a supplement to other review sources. Also includes 20 additional boards-style questions.

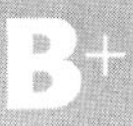

Behavioral Sciences and Outpatient Medicine for the Boards and Wards ***$19.95*** Review

AYALA

Lippincott Williams & Wilkins, 2001, 112 pages,
ISBN 0632045787

Presented in a clear and informative format similar to that of other books in the Boards and Wards series. Covers some low-yield topics.

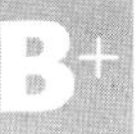

Platinum Vignettes: Behavioral Science & Biostatistics ***$26.95*** Review

BROCHERT

Elsevier, 2003, 100 pages, ISBN 1560535768

A series of cases followed by explanations and discussions on the subsequent page, presented in a format similar to that of other books in the Platinum Vignettes series. In contrast to *Underground Clinical Vignettes: Behavioral Science,* the Platinum Vignettes series includes vignettes for biostatistics; however, there are only half as many cases. Expensive for the amount of material.

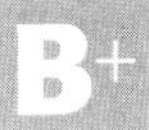

High-Yield Brain and Behavior ***$29.95*** Review

FADEM

Lippincott Williams & Wilkins, 2007, 256 pages,
ISBN 0781792282

Part of the new High-Yield Systems series that covers embryology, gross anatomy, radiology, histology, physiology, microbiology, and pharmacology as they relate to the nervous system. Written by the same author as the High-Yield and BRS Behavioral Science texts. Overall, provides a good review of neuroscience and behavioral science.

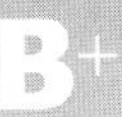

High-Yield Biostatistics **$26.95** Review

GLASER

Lippincott Williams & Wilkins, 2004, 128 pages,
ISBN 078179644X

A well-written text, but some explanations are confusing. Offers extensive coverage for a low-yield topic. Includes good review questions and tables. For the motivated student; not for last-minute cramming. Suitable as a course companion. Best used in conjunction with a behavioral science resource.

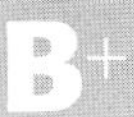

Blueprints Notes & Cases: Behavioral Science and Epidemiology **$29.95** Review/184 q

NEUGROSCHL

Lippincott Williams & Wilkins, 2003, 224 pages,
ISBN 1405103558

A case-oriented approach to behavioral science, presented as part of the Blueprints Notes & Cases series. Includes the HPI, a basic science review and discussion, key points, and questions. The 8.5″ × 11″ layout may feel overwhelming to some, but the font size is conducive to easy review. A good way to master the intangibles of behavioral science, but slightly more detailed than warranted for boards review.

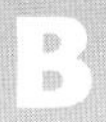

PreTest Behavioral Science **$24.95** Test/500 q

EBERT

McGraw-Hill, 2001, 300 pages, ISBN 0071374701

Contains detailed answers cross-referenced with other resources along with good test questions. Requires time commitment. Includes a brief high-yield section. Need updating.

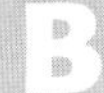

Kaplan USMLE Medical Ethics **$39.00** Review

FISCHER

Kaplan, 2007, 208 pages, ISBN 1419542091

Includes 100 cases, each followed by a single multiple-choice question with detailed explanations. The first part of the book is primarily in text format. Also offers guidelines on how the USMLE requires test takers to think about ethics and medicolegal questions. Too long for review of a low-yield subject area, but its 100 cases could be a useful resource.

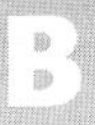

Behavioral Science Made Ridiculously Simple — ***$16.95*** — Review

SIERLES

MedMaster, 1998, 171 pages, ISBN 0940780348

Easy reading, and reasonably high yield for the amount of material. Includes medical sociology along with strong coverage of psychopathology with illustrative examples. No biostatistics. Sometimes offers too much detail on low-yield topics.

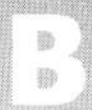

Rapid Review: Behavioral Science — ***$34.95*** — Review/350 q

STEVENS

Elsevier, 2006, 320 pages, ISBN 0323045715

Similar in style to other books in the Rapid Review series, providing a good review of a broad subject. Includes 100 questions and explanations along with an additional 250 questions online. Limited student feedback.

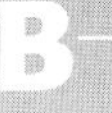

Epidemiology & Biostatistics Secrets — ***$39.95*** — Review

NORDNESS

Elsevier, 2005, 288 pages, ISBN 0323034063

Presents information in a format similar to that of other Secrets books. A useful resource for a notably hard-to-study topic, with case questions and discussions. Comes with Student Consult online access and extras. Too long and detailed for boards review, but a useful reference for biostatistics.

A–

Lippincott's Illustrated Reviews: Biochemistry | **_$52.95_** | Review/250 q

CHAMPE

Lippincott Williams & Wilkins, 2007, 528 pages, ISBN 0781769604

An excellent book that offers good clinical correlations as well as highly effective color diagrams. Offers a comprehensive review of biochemistry, including some low-yield topics. The new edition also features high-yield chapter summaries and a "big picture" chapter at the end of the book that highlights the most important concepts. Requires time commitment; skim high-yield diagrams to maximize USMLE review. Best used with coursework.

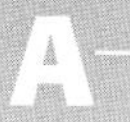

Deja Review: Biochemistry | **_$22.95_** | Review

MANZOUL

McGraw-Hill, 2007, 200 pages, ISBN 0071474633

A review book featuring questions and answers in a two-column, quiz-yourself format similar to that of the Recall series. Provides a sound review in a format that differs from straight text. Includes a helpful chapter on molecular biology. Limited student feedback.

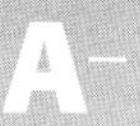

Rapid Review: Biochemistry | **_$34.95_** | Review/350 q

PELLEY

Elsevier, 2006, 320 pages, ISBN 0323044379

A quick outline format covering basic topics in biochemistry, presented in a format similar to that of other books in the Rapid Review series. High-yield disease correlation boxes are useful for review. Excellent tables and high-yield figures are featured throughout. Also includes two 50-question multiple-choice tests with explanations plus 250 questions online.

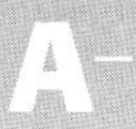

BRS Biochemistry and Molecular Biology Flash Cards | **_$29.95_** | Review

SWANSON

Lippincott Williams & Wilkins, 2006, 512 pages, ISBN 0781779022

Flash cards covering a range of topics in biochemistry and molecular biology. Although not comprehensive, they provide a good source of review for these topics.

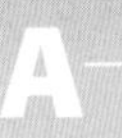

Underground Clinical Vignettes: Biochemistry ***$22.95*** Review/20 q

SWANSON

Lippincott Williams & Wilkins, 2007, 256 pages, ISBN 0781764726

Concise clinical cases illustrating approximately 100 frequently tested diseases with a biochemical basis. Cardinal signs, symptoms, and buzzwords are highlighted. Also includes 20 additional boards-style questions. A nice review of "take-home" points for biochemistry, and a useful supplement to other sources of review.

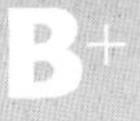

Crash Course: Metabolism and Nutrition ***$29.95*** Book

CLARK

Elsevier, 2005, 256 pages, ISBN 1416031170

Part of the Crash Course review series for basic sciences, integrating clinical topics. Offers two-color illustrations, handy study tools, and USMLE review questions. Includes online access. Although lengthy, it provides a clear and concise review of biochemistry for Step 1. Best if started early.

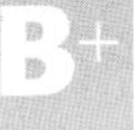

Elsevier's Integrated Biochemistry ***$34.95*** Book

PELLEY

Elsevier, 2006, 300 pages, ISBN 0323034101

Part of the new Integrated series that focuses on core knowledge in a specific basic science discipline while linking that information to related concepts from other disciplines. Case-based and USMLE-style questions at the end of each chapter allow readers to gauge their comprehension of the material. Includes online access. Best if used during coursework. Limited student feedback.

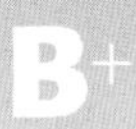

High-Yield Biochemistry ***$26.95*** Review

WILCOX

Lippincott Williams & Wilkins, 2003, 107 pages, ISBN 0781743141

A concise and crammable text in outline format with good clinical correlations at the end of each chapter. Features many diagrams and tables. Good as a study supplement.

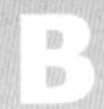

Clinical Biochemistry ***$51.95*** Review

GAW

Churchill Livingstone, 2004, 180 pages, ISBN 0443072698

Biochemistry and physiology presented in a clinical framework. Visually pleasing. Focuses on adult medicine; skimpy on inherited disorders, genetics, and molecular biochemistry. Case studies are included throughout, but no standard question-and-answer exercises are given. Best if used during a biochemistry course.

B

Clinical Biochemistry Made Ridiculously Simple — ***$22.95*** — Review

GOLDBERG

MedMaster, 2004, 93 pages + foldout, ISBN 0940780305

A conceptual approach to clinical biochemistry, presented with humor. The casual style does not appeal to all students. Mnemonics tend to be somewhat complicated. Offers a good overview and integration of all metabolic pathways. Includes a 23-page clinical review that is very high yield and crammable. Also contains a unique foldout "road map" of metabolism. For students with a firm biochemistry background.

B

PreTest Biochemistry & Genetics — ***$25.95*** — Test/500 q

INGRAM-SMITH

McGraw-Hill, 2007, 432 pages, ISBN 0071471839

Difficult questions with detailed, referenced explanations. Best for motivated students who use it along with a review book. Contains some questions on biochemical disorders and metabolism but no clinical vignettes. Features a useful high-yield-facts section at the front of the book.

B

Case Files: Biochemistry — ***$29.95*** — Review

TOY

McGraw-Hill, 2005, 450 pages, ISBN 0071437819

A text that is divided into clinical cases followed by clinical correlations, a discussion, and take-home pearls, presented in a format similar to others in the Case Files series. A few questions accompany each case. The black-and-white figures are sometimes too small to read, but the clinical correlations make biochemistry concepts easier to remember. Too lengthy for rapid review; best for students who enjoy problem-based learning.

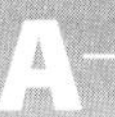

High-Yield Cell and Molecular Biology | ***$26.95*** | Review

DUDEK

Lippincott Williams & Wilkins, 2006, 254 pages,
ISBN 078176887X

Cellular and molecular biology presented in an outline format, with good diagrams and clinical correlations. The new, recently published edition is brief but complete. Includes descriptions of laboratory techniques and genetic disorders. No questions or vignettes.

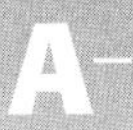

Deja Review: Histology & Medical Cell Biology | ***$22.95*** | Review

GRISSON

McGraw-Hill, 2006, 200 pages, ISBN 0323034101

Features questions and answers in a two-column, quiz-yourself format similar to that of the Recall series. Provides a sound review in a format that differs from straight text.

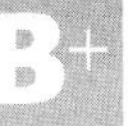

Crash Course: Cell Biology and Genetics | ***$29.95*** | Review

LAMB

Elsevier, 2006, 250 pages, ISBN 0323044948

Part of the Crash Course review series for basic sciences, integrating clinical topics. Offers two-color illustrations, handy study tools, and USMLE review questions. Includes online access. Too much coverage for a limited subject.

B

Elsevier's Integrated Genetics | ***$34.95*** | Book

ADLISON

Elsevier, 2007, 336 pages, ISBN 0323043291

Part of the new Integrated series that focuses on core knowledge in a specific basic science discipline while linking that information to related concepts from other disciplines. Case-based and USMLE-style questions at the end of each chapter allow readers to gauge their comprehension of the material. Includes online access. Best if used during coursework. Limited student feedback.

B

Rapid Review: Histology and Cell Biology | ***$34.95*** | Review/350 q

BURNS

Elsevier, 2006, 336 pages, ISBN 0323044255

Similar to other books in the Rapid Review series. Features an outline of basic concepts with numerous charts, but histology images are very limited. Two 50-question multiple-choice tests are presented with explanations, along with 250 questions online.

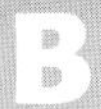

High-Yield Histology **$26.95** Review

DUDEK

Lippincott Williams & Wilkins, 2004, 288 pages,
ISBN 0781747635

A quick and easy review of a relatively low-yield subject. Tables include some high-yield information. Contains good pictures. The appendix features classic electron micrographs. Too lengthy for USMLE review.

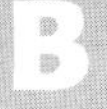

BRS Cell Biology and Histology **$37.95** Review/500 q

GARTNER

Lippincott Williams & Wilkins, 2006, 384 pages + CD-ROM,
ISBN 0781785774

An outline format that is useful for looking up cell biology and histology information, presented in a style that is typical of the BRS series. Can be used alone for cell biology review, but does not include enough histology images to be considered comprehensive. Includes a CD-ROM with questions.

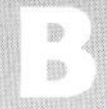

PreTest Anatomy, Histology, & Cell Biology **$25.95** Test/500 q

KLEIN

McGraw-Hill, 2007, 576 pages, ISBN 0071471855

Difficult questions with detailed answers as well as some illustrations. Requires extensive time commitment. Includes a high-yield section that highlights clinically relevant relationships and lessons.

B

Wheater's Functional Histology **$72.95** Text

YOUNG

Elsevier, 2006, 448 pages, ISBN 044306850X

A color atlas with illustrations of normal histology and accompanying text. Useful as a text for coursework. Skim through the photomicrographs for USMLE review. Image captions provide an excellent source for the review of basic cell biology.

B-

Elsevier's Integrated Histology **$34.95** Book

TELSER

Elsevier, 2007, 336 pages, ISBN 0323033881

Part of the new Integrated series that focuses on core knowledge in a specific basic science discipline while linking that information to related concepts from other disciplines. Case-based and USMLE-style questions at the end of each chapter allow readers to gauge their comprehension of the material. Includes online access. Best if used during coursework. Limited student feedback.

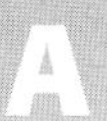

Clinical Microbiology Made Ridiculously Simple ***$32.95*** Review

GLADWIN

MedMaster, 2007, 392 pages, ISBN 094078081X

A very good chart-based review of microbiology that includes clever and humorous mnemonics. The best of this series. The text is easy to read, and an excellent antibiotic review is useful for pharmacology as well. The style of the series does not appeal to everyone. Requires a supplemental source for immunology. Excellent if you have limited time or are "burning out."

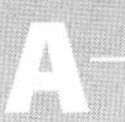

Basic Immunology ***$61.95*** Review

ABBAS

Elsevier, 2006, 336 pages, ISBN 1416029745

A text that includes colorful diagrams, images, and tables that students will find useful for quick review. Also offers abundant text as well as a lengthy glossary for those who wish to delve into the topic further. Features online access.

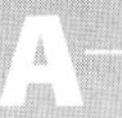

Deja Review: Microbiology & Immunology ***$22.95*** Review

CHEN

McGraw-Hill, 2006, 250 pages, ISBN 0071468668

Features questions and answers in a two-column, quiz-yourself format similar to that of the Recall series. Provides a sound review in a format that differs from straight text. A great resource once a primary review of microbiology has already been done. Limited student feedback.

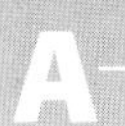

Microcards ***$34.95*** Flash cards

HARPAVAT

Lippincott Williams & Wilkins, 2007, 300 pages, ISBN 0781769248

A highly useful resource for students who like to use flash cards for review. Some cards include excellent flow charts of important classes of bacteria or viruses. Most of the other cards include the bacterium or virus, clinical presentation, pathobiology, diagnosis, treatment, and important quick facts. Recommended for initial use with coursework.

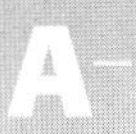

High-Yield Immunology | **$26.95** | Review

JOHNSON

Lippincott Williams & Wilkins, 2005, 112 pages, ISBN 0781774691

A review book presented in a format typical of the High-Yield series. Accurately covers high-yield details within the topic in proportion to the boards' coverage of immunology. Good for quick review. The new edition includes many improvements.

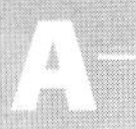

Review of Medical Microbiology and Immunology | **$41.95** | Review/654 q

LEVINSON

McGraw-Hill, 2006, 580 pages, ISBN 0071460314

A clear, concise text with excellent diagrams and tables. Includes an excellent immunology section. The "Summary of Medically Important Organisms" is highly crammable. Requires time commitment. Can be detailed and dense; best if started early with the course. Covers all topics, including some that are low yield. Includes good practice questions and a comprehensive exam, but questions have letter answers only. Compare with *Lippincott's Illustrated Reviews: Microbiology*.

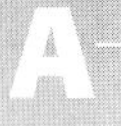

Review of Medical Microbiology | **$36.95** | Test/550 q

MURRAY

Elsevier, 2005, 176 pages, ISBN 0323033253

USMLE-style questions divided into bacteriology, virology, mycology, and parasitology. Contains high-quality color images for many questions and detailed answer explanations for each. Questions are similar to those on the boards and provide a nice review. Supplements Murray's *Medical Microbiology* textbook.

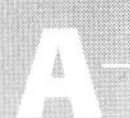

Crash Course: Immunology | **$29.95** | Review

NOVAK

Elsevier, 2006, 144 pages, ISBN 1416030077

Part of the Crash Course review series for basic sciences, integrating clinical topics. Offers two-color illustrations, handy study tools, and USMLE review questions. Includes online access. Good length and detail for boards review.

B

Appleton & Lange Outline Review: Microbiology and Immunology
Yotis
McGraw-Hill, 2003, 200 pages, ISBN 0071405666
A well-organized approach to the microbiology section of the boards, addressing all areas included in the exam. Lacks detailed treatment of autoimmune disorders, but an excellent resource to use in addition to class notes. A good resource for organization of the material. Its sparse use of images could be a drawback.

$30.95 Review

B−

Platinum Vignettes: Microbiology
Brochert
Elsevier, 2003, 114 pages, ISBN 1560535741
Fifty clinical case scenarios presented in a unique format, with the case question appearing on the front of the page and the answer printed on the back. May be useful for students who wish to self-quiz. Expensive for the amount of material.

$26.95 Review

B−

BRS Microbiology and Immunology
Johnson
Lippincott Williams & Wilkins, 2001, 302 pages, ISBN 0781727707
A concise outline format with good questions and illustrations. The immunology section is especially useful. For the motivated student.

$36.95 Review/500 q

B−

PreTest Microbiology
Kettering
McGraw-Hill, 2007, 352 pages, ISBN 0071471790
Mixed-quality questions with detailed, sometimes verbose explanations. Useful for additional question-based review in bacteriology and virology, but not high yield. Includes a useful high-yield-facts section.

$25.95 Test/500 q

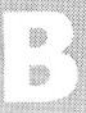

Instant Notes in Immunology

$35.95 Review/125 q

LYDYARD

Garland Science, 2004, 336 pages, ISBN 1859960391

A comprehensive review of immunology with effective figures throughout. Well organized, but too detailed for boards review. Best used during the course. Questions are not in current USMLE format and do not include explanations. High-yield tables of principal cytokines and selected molecules are included. Limited student feedback.

B

How the Immune System Works

$29.95 Review

SOMPAYRAC

Blackwell Science, 2002, 144 pages, ISBN 063204702X

A concise overview of immunology that attempts to simplify complicated concepts. Offers a good general overview for coursework, but lacks many of the details that are needed for boards review. Best used as a companion to other, more detailed resources, although many students find it useful as an initial refresher to get the "big picture." Weak in clinical immunology for the USMLE.

B

BRS Micro Flash Cards

$29.95 Flash cards

SWANSON

Lippincott Williams & Wilkins, 2003, 250 pages, ISBN 078174427X

A series of flash cards featuring questions with answers on the reverse side. Useful for students who enjoy an active style of review. A good last-second microbiology review.

B

Clinical Microbiology Review

$36.95 Review

WARINNER

Wysteria, 2001, 150 pages, ISBN 0967783933

A concise yet comprehensive review in chart format with some clinical correlations. Each page covers a single organism with ample space for adding notes during class. Contains no immunology. Spatial organization, color coding, and bulleting of facts facilitate review. A great cross-reference section groups organisms by general characteristics. Includes color plates of significant microbes. Limited student feedback.

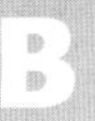

Appleton & Lange Outline Review: Microbiology and Immunology — ***$30.95*** — Review

YOTIS

McGraw-Hill, 2003, 200 pages, ISBN 0071405666

A well-organized approach to the microbiology section of the boards, addressing all areas included in the exam. Lacks detailed treatment of autoimmune disorders, but an excellent resource to use in addition to class notes. A good resource for organization of the material. Its sparse use of images could be a drawback.

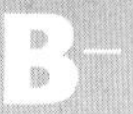

Platinum Vignettes: Microbiology — ***$26.95*** — Review

BROCHERT

Elsevier, 2003, 114 pages, ISBN 1560535741

Fifty clinical case scenarios presented in a unique format, with the case question appearing on the front of the page and the answer printed on the back. May be useful for students who wish to self-quiz. Expensive for the amount of material.

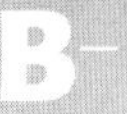

BRS Microbiology and Immunology — ***$36.95*** — Review/500 q

JOHNSON

Lippincott Williams & Wilkins, 2001, 302 pages, ISBN 0781727707

A concise outline format with good questions and illustrations. The immunology section is especially useful. For the motivated student.

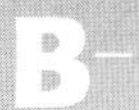

PreTest Microbiology — ***$25.95*** — Test/500 q

KETTERING

McGraw-Hill, 2007, 352 pages, ISBN 0071471790

Mixed-quality questions with detailed, sometimes verbose explanations. Useful for additional question-based review in bacteriology and virology, but not high yield. Includes a useful high-yield-facts section.

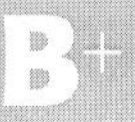

Case Files: Microbiology ***$29.95*** Review
TOY
McGraw-Hill, 2005, 430 pages, ISBN 0071445749
Fifty clinical microbiology cases reviewed in an interactive learning format. Each case is followed by a clinical correlation, a discussion with boldfaced buzzwords, and questions. Cases are useful for boards review, since key ideas can be readily associated with the appropriate clinical scenario.

B

Microbiology and Immunology for the Boards and Wards ***$24.95*** Review/100 q
AYALA
Lippincott Williams & Wilkins, 2005, 256 pages, ISBN 1405104686
Similar in style to other books in the Boards and Wards series. Includes many high-yield tables and buzzwords. Some parts are too detailed for USMLE review. Limited student feedback.

B

Blueprints Notes & Cases: Microbiology and Immunology ***$29.95*** Review
GANDHI
Lippincott Williams & Wilkins, 2003, 224 pages, ISBN 1405103477
Fifty-eight succinct clinical cases covering boards-relevant microbiology and immunology facts. Charts, tables, illustrations, and useful "thumbnails" are included in the discussion section to facilitate rapid synthesis of key concepts. Best used during microbiology coursework. For students proficient in immunology.

B

Lippincott's Illustrated Reviews: Microbiology ***$37.95*** Review/Few q
HARVEY
Lippincott Williams & Wilkins, 2006, 432 pages, ISBN 0781782155
A comprehensive, highly illustrated review of microbiology similar in style to Champe's *Lippincott's Illustrated Reviews: Biochemistry*. Includes a 50-page color section with more than 150 clinical and laboratory photographs. Compare with Levinson's *Review of Medical Microbiology and Immunology*.

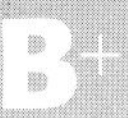

Concise Medical Immunology **$39.95** Review

DOAN

Lippincott Williams & Wilkins, 2005, 256 pages, ISBN 078175741X

A concise text with useful diagrams, illustrations, and tables. Good for students who need extra immunology review or wish to study the subject thoroughly for the boards. End-of-chapter multiple-choice questions help reinforce key concepts.

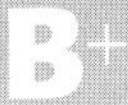

Bugcards: The Complete Microbiology Review Flash Cards for Class, the Boards, and the Wards **$26.50** Flash cards

LEVINE

BL Publishing, 2004, 150 pages, ISBN 0967165539

High-quality flash cards designed for rapid class and USMLE microbiology review. Cards cover all medically relevant bacteria, viruses, fungi, and parasites and include important buzzwords, mnemonics, and clinical vignettes to aid in recall. Unique "disease process cards" summarize all organisms for a particular disease (e.g., UTI, pneumonia).

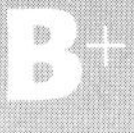

Review of Immunology **$32.95** Test/500 q

LICHTMAN

Elsevier, 2005, 192 pages, ISBN 0721603432

Complements Abbas's *Cellular and Molecular Immunology* and *Basic Immunology* textbooks. Contains 500 USMLE-style questions with full-color illustrations along with explanations of all answers. A good resource for questions in a lower-yield area. Limited student feedback.

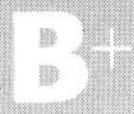

Case Studies in Immunology: Clinical Companion **$49.95** Review

ROSEN

Garland Science, 2007, 328 pages, ISBN 0815341458

Originally designed as a clinical companion to Janeway's *Immunobiology*, this text provides an excellent synopsis of the major disorders of immunity in a clinical vignette format. Integrates basic and clinical sciences. Excellent images, illustrations, questions, and discussion.

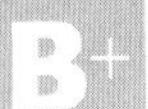

Rapid Review: Microbiology and Immunology **$34.95** Review/350 q

ROSENTHAL

Elsevier, 2006, 368 pages, ISBN 0323044263

Similar to other books in the Rapid Review series. Contains a significant number of excellent tables and figures. Two 50-question tests with extensive explanations complement the topics covered in the review, along with 250 questions online. Limited student feedback.

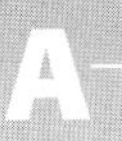

High-Yield Immunology **$26.95** Review

JOHNSON

Lippincott Williams & Wilkins, 2005, 112 pages, ISBN 0781774691

A review book presented in a format typical of the High-Yield series. Accurately covers high-yield details within the topic in proportion to the boards' coverage of immunology. Good for quick review. The new edition includes many improvements.

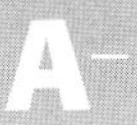

Review of Medical Microbiology and Immunology **$41.95** Review/654 q

LEVINSON

McGraw-Hill, 2006, 580 pages, ISBN 0071460314

A clear, concise text with excellent diagrams and tables. Includes an excellent immunology section. The "Summary of Medically Important Organisms" is highly crammable. Requires time commitment. Can be detailed and dense; best if started early with the course. Covers all topics, including some that are low yield. Includes good practice questions and a comprehensive exam, but questions have letter answers only. Compare with *Lippincott's Illustrated Reviews: Microbiology*.

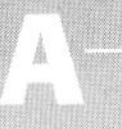

Review of Medical Microbiology **$36.95** Test/550 q

MURRAY

Elsevier, 2005, 176 pages, ISBN 0323033253

USMLE-style questions divided into bacteriology, virology, mycology, and parasitology. Contains high-quality color images for many questions and detailed answer explanations for each. Questions are similar to those on the boards and provide a nice review. Supplements Murray's *Medical Microbiology* textbook.

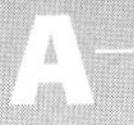

Crash Course: Immunology **$29.95** Review

NOVAK

Elsevier, 2006, 144 pages, ISBN 1416030077

Part of the Crash Course review series for basic sciences, integrating clinical topics. Offers two-color illustrations, handy study tools, and USMLE review questions. Includes online access. Good length and detail for boards review.

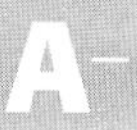

Medical Microbiology and Immunology Flashcards ***$34.95*** Flash cards

ROSENTHAL

Elsevier, 2005, 414 pages, ISBN 032303392X

Flash cards covering the most commonly asked-about bugs. Features full-color images of a microscopic view of each bug and its clinical presentation on one side, with the other side offering relevant bug information in conjunction with a short case. Well-organized information, and comes in a nice carrying case. Also comes with StudentConsult online access and extras. A little too much emphasis is placed on "trigger words" relating to each bug.

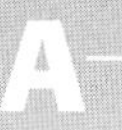

Underground Clinical Vignettes: Microbiology Vol. I: Virology, Immunology, Parasitology, Mycology ***$22.95*** Review/20 q

SWANSON

Lippincott Williams & Wilkins, 2007, 224 pages, ISBN 078176470X

Concise clinical cases illustrating frequently tested diseases in microbiology and immunology (100 cases in each volume). Cardinal signs, symptoms, and buzzwords are highlighted. Also includes 20 additional boards-style questions. Use as a supplement to other sources of review.

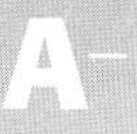

Underground Clinical Vignettes: Microbiology Vol. II: Bacteriology ***$22.95*** Review/20 q

SWANSON

Lippincott Williams & Wilkins, 2007, 224 pages, ISBN 0781764718

Concise clinical cases illustrating frequently tested diseases in bacteriology (100 cases in each volume). Cardinal signs, symptoms, and buzzwords are highlighted. Also includes 20 additional boards-style questions. Use as a supplement to other sources of review.

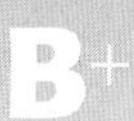

Elsevier's Integrated Immunology and Microbiology ***$34.95*** Book

ACTOR

Elsevier, 2006, 336 pages, ISBN 032303389X

Part of the new Integrated series that focuses on core knowledge in a specific basic science discipline while linking that information to related concepts from other disciplines. Case-based and USMLE-style questions at the end of each chapter allow users to gauge their comprehension of the material. Includes online access. Best if used during coursework. Limited student feedback.

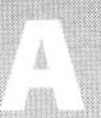

Rapid Review: Pathology **$34.95** Review/350 q

GOLJAN

Elsevier, 2006, 768 pages, ISBN 032304414X

The best of the Rapid Review series. Addresses key concepts in pathology in a bulleted outline format with many tables and figures. Focuses on key facts with a strong clinical orientation. Much longer than other books in this series, but very high yield.

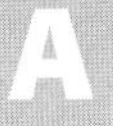

BRS Pathology **$36.95** Review/500 q

SCHNEIDER

Lippincott Williams & Wilkins, 2005, 412 pages, ISBN 0781760224

An excellent, concise review with appropriate content emphasis. Features outline-format chapters with boldfacing of key facts. Includes good questions with explanations at the end of each chapter along with a comprehensive exam at the end of the book. Offers well-organized tables and diagrams as well as some good black-and-white photographs representative of classic pathology that can be correlated with color photographs from an atlas. Also contains a chapter on laboratory testing and "key associations" with each disease. Short on clinical details for vignette questions, but worth the time investment. Most effective if started early and then reviewed during study periods.

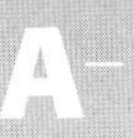

Pathophysiology for the Boards and Wards: Diagnosis and Therapy **$36.95** Review/75 q

AYALA

Lippincott Williams & Wilkins, 2003, 352 pages, ISBN 1405103426

A system-based outline with a focus on pathology. Well organized with glossy color plates of relevant pathology and excellent, concise tables. The appendix includes a helpful overview of neurology, immunology, "zebras," syndromes, and pearls. Good integration of USMLE-relevant material from various subject areas.

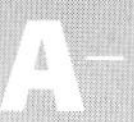

Lange Flash Cards: Pathology | ***$31.95*** | Flash cards

BARON

McGraw-Hill, 2004, 280 pages, ISBN 0071436901

Pathology flash cards with information on one disease per card. Includes pathophysiology, clinical manifestations, treatment, and clinical vignette. Most effective when used at the beginning of the second year through Step 1 preparation. A useful resource with which to organize the breadth of pathology topics covered on the USMLE. Limited student feedback.

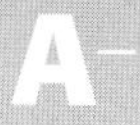

Lippincott's Review of Pathology: Illustrated, Interactive Q & A | ***$39.95*** | Review/1100+ q

FENDERSON

Lippincott, Williams & Wilkins, 2007, 352 pages, ISBN 078179580X

A review book featuring more than 1100 multiple-choice questions that follow the USMLE template. Questions frequently involve "two-step" logic, a strategy that probes the student's ability to integrate basic science knowledge into a clinical situation. Detailed rationales are linked to clinical vignettes and address incorrect answer choices. More than 300 full-color images link clinical and pathologic findings, with normal lab values provided for reference. Questions are presented both online and in print. Students can work through the online questions either in "quiz mode," which provides instant feedback, or in "test mode," which simulates the USMLE experience. Overall, a resource that is similar in quality to Robbins' question book.

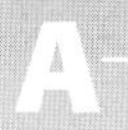

Deja Review: Pathology | ***$22.95*** | Review

GALFIONE

McGraw-Hill, 2007, 275 pages, ISBN 0071474951

Features questions and answers in a two-column, quiz-yourself format similar to that of the Recall series. Provides a sound review in a format that differs from straight text. Includes many pathophysiology relationships as opposed to just pathology. Limited student feedback.

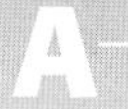

Robbins and Cotran Review of Pathology | ***$44.95*** | Review/1000 q

KLATT

Elsevier, 2004, 432 pages, ISBN 0721601944

A review question book that follows the main Robbins textbooks. Questions are often more detailed than those of the actual test, but the text offers a great review of pathology. Thorough answer explanations reinforce key points.

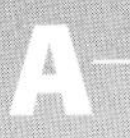

Underground Clinical Vignettes: Pathophysiology, Vol. I ***$22.95*** Review/20 q

SWANSON

Lippincott Williams & Wilkins, 2007, 224 pages,

ISBN 0781764653

Concise clinical cases illustrating 100 frequently tested pathology and physiology cases. Cardinal signs, symptoms, and buzzwords are highlighted. Also includes 20 additional boards-style questions. Use as a supplement to other sources of review.

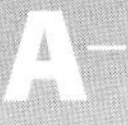

Underground Clinical Vignettes: Pathophysiology, Vol. II ***$22.95*** Review/20 q

SWANSON

Lippincott Williams & Wilkins, 2007, 224 pages,

ISBN 0781764661

Concise clinical cases illustrating 100 frequently tested pathology and physiology cases. Cardinal signs, symptoms, and buzzwords are highlighted. Also includes 20 additional boards-style questions. Use as a supplement to other sources of review.

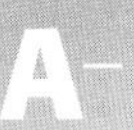

Underground Clinical Vignettes: Pathophysiology, Vol. III ***$22.95*** Review/20 q

SWANSON

Lippincott Williams & Wilkins, 2007, 224 pages,

ISBN 0781764688

Concise clinical cases illustrating 100 frequently tested pathology and physiology cases. Cardinal signs, symptoms, and buzzwords are highlighted. Also includes 20 additional boards-style questions. Use as a supplement to other sources of review.

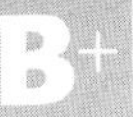

MedMaps for Pathophysiology ***$29.95*** Review

AGOSTI

Lippincott Williams & Wilkins, 2007, 240 pages,

ISBN 0781777550

A rapid review that contains 102 concept maps of disease processes and mechanisms, organized by organ system, as well as classic diseases. Useful both for course exams and for Step 1 preparation. Ample room is provided for notes. Provides a good resource for looking up specific mechanisms, especially when used in conjunction with other primary review sources.

B+

High-Yield Heart **$29.95** Review

DUDEK

Lippincott Williams & Wilkins, 2007, 192 pages,

ISBN 0781755689

Part of the new High-Yield Systems series that covers embryology, gross anatomy, radiology, histology, physiology, microbiology, and pharmacology as they relate to the cardiovascular system. Appropriate length and detail for boards review. Limited student feedback.

B+

High-Yield Kidney **$29.95** Review

DUDEK

Lippincott Williams & Wilkins, 2007, 224 pages,

ISBN 0781755697

Part of the new High-Yield Systems series that covers embryology, gross anatomy, radiology, histology, physiology, microbiology, and pharmacology as they relate to the kidneys. Appropriate length and detail for boards review. Limited student feedback.

B+

High-Yield Lung **$29.95** Review

DUDEK

Lippincott Williams & Wilkins, 2007, 162 pages,

ISBN 0781755700

Part of the new High-Yield Systems series that covers embryology, gross anatomy, radiology, histology, physiology, microbiology, and pharmacology as they relate to the respiratory system. Appropriate length and detail for boards review. Limited student feedback.

B+

Pocket Companion to Robbins Pathologic Basis of Disease **$38.95** Review

MITCHELL

Elsevier, 2006, 816 pages, ISBN 0721602657

A review book that is good for reviewing associations between keywords and specific diseases. Presented in a format that is highly condensed, complete, and easy to understand. Explains most important diseases and pathologic processes. Contains no photographs or illustrations. Useful as a quick reference.

B+

PreTest Pathophysiology **$25.95** Test/500 q

MUFSON

McGraw-Hill, 2004, 480 pages, ISBN 0071434925

Includes 500 questions and answers with detailed explanations. Questions may be more difficult than those on the boards. Features a brief section of high-yield topics.

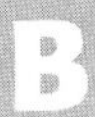

Platinum Vignettes: Pathology I — ***$26.95*** — Review

BROCHERT

Elsevier, 2003, 118 pages, ISBN 1560535695

A text consisting of vignettes that are very similar in style to those of the *Underground Clinical Vignettes* series. However, each volume contains 50 cases for a total of 100, whereas the UCVs offer 300 cases split over three volumes. Overall, offers less "bang for the buck" than the UCVs.

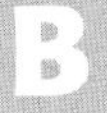

Platinum Vignettes: Pathology II — ***$26.95*** — Review

BROCHERT

Elsevier, 2003, 104 pages, ISBN 1560535725

A text consisting of vignettes that are very similar in style to those of the *Underground Clinical Vignettes* series. However, each volume contains 50 cases for a total of 100, whereas the UCVs offer 300 cases split over three volumes. Overall, offers less "bang for the buck" than the UCVs.

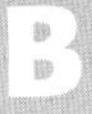

PreTest Pathology — ***$25.95*** — Test/500 q

BROWN

McGraw-Hill, 2007, 592 pages., ISBN 0071471820

Picky, difficult questions with detailed, complete answers. Questions are often obscure or esoteric. Features high-quality black-and-white photographs but no color illustrations. Can be used as a supplement to other review books. For the motivated student. Thirty-nine pages of high-yield facts are useful for concept summaries.

B

Appleton & Lange's Review of Pathology — ***$36.95*** — Test/850 q

CATALANO

McGraw-Hill, 2002, 344 pages, ISBN 0071389954

Short text sections followed by numerous questions with answers. Some useful high-yield tables are included at the beginning of each section. Features good photomicrographs. Covers both general and organ-based pathology. Can be used as a supplement to more detailed texts. A good review when time is short.

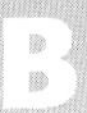

Blueprints Notes & Cases–Pathophysiology: Renal, Hematology, and Oncology **$29.95** Review

CAUGHEY

Lippincott Williams & Wilkins, 2003, 208 pages, ISBN 1405103523

This book follows the format of the Blueprints series, in which each case takes the form of a discussion followed by key points and a series of questions. The pathophysiology volumes would be a good companion to organ-based teaching modules, but the material is neither comprehensive enough nor sufficiently concise to be high yield for intensive boards preparation.

B

Pathology Recall **$34.95** Review

CHABRA

Lippincott Williams & Wilkins, 2002, 552 pages, ISBN 0781734061

A quiz-based text featuring thousands of brief questions. Not in USMLE format. Similar to others in the Recall series. Beyond the scope of Step 1, but an entertaining break from other reviews. Contains numerous errors throughout the book.

B

Colour Atlas of Anatomical Pathology **$91.95** Review

COOKE

Elsevier, 2003, 300 pages, ISBN 0443073600

An impressive photographic atlas of gross pathology. Offers easy-to-read, clinically relevant content. Limited student feedback.

B

Pathology: Review for USMLE, Step 1 **$49.95** Review/524 q

DEPALMA

J&S Publishing, 2007, 302 pages, ISBN 1888308192

A pathology review book with questions and well-discussed answer explanations. Organization is similar to that of other pathology texts (general pathology and specific areas). Includes color and black-and-white illustrations. A solid review book, but lacking in detail. Limited student feedback.

B

High-Yield Histopathology **$26.95** Review

DUDEK

Lippincott Williams & Wilkins, 2005, 336 pages, ISBN 0781769590

A new book that reviews the relationship of basic histology to the pathology, physiology, and pharmacology of clinical conditions that are tested on the USMLE Step 1 and seen in clinical practice. Includes case studies, numerous light and electron micrographs, and pathology photographs. Given its considerable length, should be started with coursework. Limited feedback.

B

Blueprints Notes & Cases—Pathophysiology: Pulmonary, Gastrointestinal, and Rheumatology **$29.95** Review

FILBIN

Lippincott Williams & Wilkins, 2003, 192 pages, ISBN 1405103515

A review book that follows the format of the Blueprints series, in which each case takes the form of a discussion followed by key points and a series of questions. The pathophysiology volumes would be a good companion to organ-based teaching modules, but the material is neither comprehensive enough nor sufficiently concise to be high yield for intensive boards preparation.

B

Crash Course: Pathology **$29.95** Review

FISHBACK

Elsevier, 2005, 368 pages, ISBN 0323033083

Part of the Crash Course review series for basic sciences, integrating clinical topics. Offers two-color illustrations, handy study tools, and USMLE review questions. Includes online access. Best if started early during coursework.

B

Elsevier's Integrated Pathology **$34.95** Review

KING

Elsevier, 2006, 336 pages, ISBN 0323043283

Part of the new Integrated series that links various disciplines. A good text for initial coursework, but too long for Step 1 review. Case-based and USMLE-style questions are included at the end of each chapter. Limited student feedback.

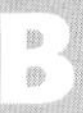

Blueprints Notes & Cases–Pathophysiology: Cardiovascular, Endocrine, and Reproduction **$29.95** Review

LEUNG

Lippincott Williams & Wilkins, 2003, 208 pages,
ISBN 1405103507

A review book that follows the format of the Blueprints series, in which each case takes the form of a discussion followed by key points and a series of questions. The pathophysiology volumes would be a good companion to organ-based teaching modules, but the material is neither comprehensive enough nor sufficiently concise to be high yield for intensive boards preparation.

Pathophysiology of Heart Disease **$39.95** Text

LILLY

Lippincott Williams & Wilkins, 2006, 464 pages,
ISBN 0781763215

A collaborative project by medical students and faculty at Harvard. Well organized, easy to read, and concise; offers comprehensive coverage of cardiovascular pathophysiology from the medical student's perspective. Serves as an excellent bridge between the basic and clinical sciences. Very good for review of this subject, but does not cover other areas of pathology tested on the boards. May be too detailed for boards review.

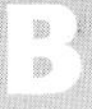

Pathcards **$34.95** Flash cards

MARCUCCI

Lippincott Williams & Wilkins, 2003, 553 pages,
ISBN 0781743990

Presents comprehensive and detailed information in flash-card format rather than attempting to condense boards-relevant material into just one fact per disease state. Appropriate to the level of depth with which pathology is tested on the USMLE.

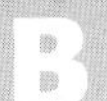

Pathophysiology of Disease: Introduction to Clinical Medicine **$57.95** Review/Few q

MCPHEE

McGraw-Hill, 2005, 784 pages, ISBN 007144159X

An interdisciplinary course text useful for understanding the pathophysiology of clinical symptoms. Effectively integrates the basic sciences with mechanisms of disease. Features great graphs, diagrams, and tables. Most helpful if used during coursework owing to its length. Includes a few non-boards-style questions. The text's clinical emphasis nicely complements *BRS Pathology*.

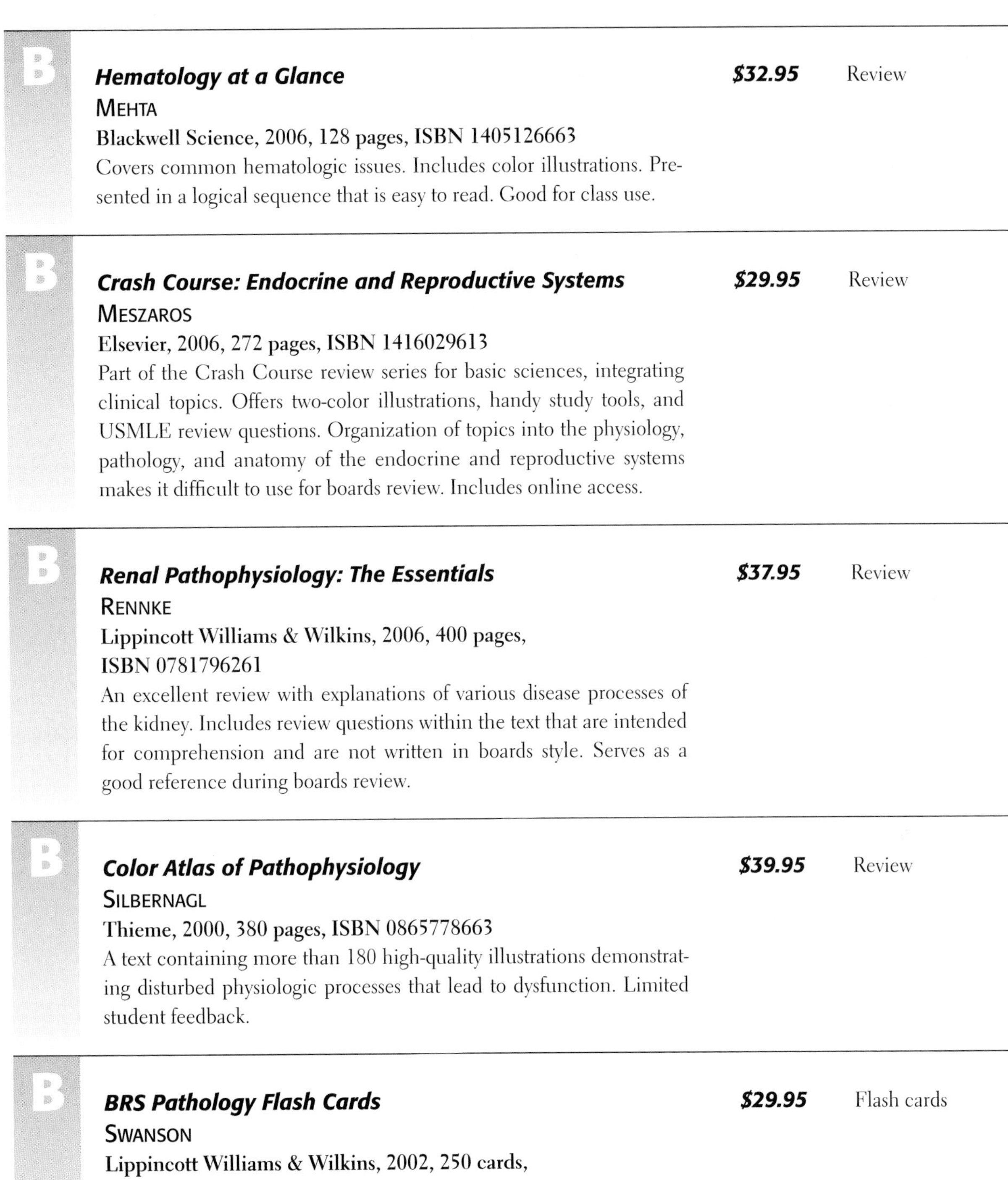

B

Hematology at a Glance — ***$32.95*** — Review

MEHTA

Blackwell Science, 2006, 128 pages, ISBN 1405126663

Covers common hematologic issues. Includes color illustrations. Presented in a logical sequence that is easy to read. Good for class use.

B

Crash Course: Endocrine and Reproductive Systems — ***$29.95*** — Review

MESZAROS

Elsevier, 2006, 272 pages, ISBN 1416029613

Part of the Crash Course review series for basic sciences, integrating clinical topics. Offers two-color illustrations, handy study tools, and USMLE review questions. Organization of topics into the physiology, pathology, and anatomy of the endocrine and reproductive systems makes it difficult to use for boards review. Includes online access.

B

Renal Pathophysiology: The Essentials — ***$37.95*** — Review

RENNKE

Lippincott Williams & Wilkins, 2006, 400 pages, ISBN 0781796261

An excellent review with explanations of various disease processes of the kidney. Includes review questions within the text that are intended for comprehension and are not written in boards style. Serves as a good reference during boards review.

B

Color Atlas of Pathophysiology — ***$39.95*** — Review

SILBERNAGL

Thieme, 2000, 380 pages, ISBN 0865778663

A text containing more than 180 high-quality illustrations demonstrating disturbed physiologic processes that lead to dysfunction. Limited student feedback.

B

BRS Pathology Flash Cards — ***$29.95*** — Flash cards

SWANSON

Lippincott Williams & Wilkins, 2002, 250 cards, ISBN 0781737109

A series of 250 pathology flash cards categorized by organ system. Effective when used with the *BRS Pathology* textbook, but not comprehensive enough when used alone. Most cards have only one high-yield fact.

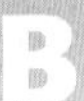

B

Case Files: Pathology **$29.95** Review

Toy

McGraw-Hill, 2006, 414 pages, ISBN 0071437800

A clinical case review book consisting of 49 cases along with useful tables. Uses a problem-based learning approach that provides a good alternative to learning an extensive subject. Limited student feedback.

B

Crash Course: Musculoskeletal System **$29.95** Review

Walji

Elsevier, 2006, 248 pages, ISBN 1416030085

Part of the Crash Course review series for basic sciences, integrating clinical topics. Offers two-color illustrations, handy study tools, and USMLE review questions. Organization of topics into the physiology, pathology, and anatomy of the musculoskeletal system makes it difficult to use for boards review. Includes online access.

A–

Pharmacology Flash Cards | **_$34.95_** | Flash cards

Brenner

Elsevier, 2006, 576 pages, ISBN 1416031863

Flash cards for more than 200 of the most commonly tested drugs. Cards include the name of the drug (both generic and brand) on the front and basic drug information on the back. Divided and color-coded by class. Comes with a useful compact carrying case. Limited student feedback.

A–

Lippincott's Illustrated Reviews: Pharmacology | **_$52.95_** | Review/125 q

Howland

Lippincott Williams & Wilkins, 2005, 559 pages, ISBN 0781741181

An outline format with practice questions and many excellent illustrations and tables. Text is cross-referenced to other books in Lippincott's Illustrated Reviews series. Good for the "big picture," and takes an effective pathophysiologic approach. Highly detailed, so use with coursework and review for the USMLE. For the motivated student.

A–

Katzung and Trevor's Pharmacology: Examination and Board Review | **_$45.95_** | Review/1000 q

Trevor

McGraw-Hill, 2004, 640 pages, ISBN 0071422900

A well-organized text in narrative format with concise explanations. Features good charts and tables. Good for drug interactions and toxicities. Offers two practice exams with questions and detailed answers. Includes some low-yield/obscure drugs. The crammable list of "top boards drugs" is especially high yield. Compare with *Lippincott's Illustrated Reviews: Pharmacology*.

A–

Deja Review: Pharmacology | **_$22.95_** | Review

Young

McGraw-Hill, 2007, 186 pages, ISBN 0071474617

Features questions and answers in a two-column, quiz-yourself format similar to that of the Recall series. Provides a sound review in a format that differs from straight text. Allows for a more interactive review of some hard-to-memorize details needed for USMLE pharmacology questions.

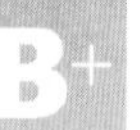

Pharmacology for the Boards and Wards **$34.95** Review/150 q

AYALA

Blackwell Science, 2006, 256 pages, ISBN 1405105119

Like other books in the Boards and Wards series, the pharmacology volume is presented primarily in tabular format with bulleted key points. Review questions are in USMLE style. At times can be too dense, but does a great job at focusing on the clinical aspects of drugs.

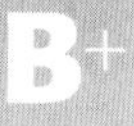

Crash Course: Pharmacology **$29.95** Book

BARNES

Elsevier, 2006, 248 pages, ISBN 1416029591

Part of the Crash Course review series for basic sciences, integrating clinical topics. Offers two-color illustrations, handy study tools, and USMLE review questions. Includes online access. Gives a solid, easy-to-follow overview of pharmacology for Step 1. Limited student feedback.

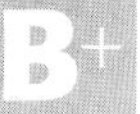

Pharm Cards: A Review for Medical Students **$36.95** Flash cards

JOHANNSEN

Lippincott Williams & Wilkins, 2002, 228 pages, ISBN 0781734010

Cards highlight important features of major drugs and drug classes. Good for class review; also offers a quick, focused review for the USMLE. Lacks pharmacokinetics, but features good charts and diagrams. Well liked by students who enjoy flash card–based review. Bulky to carry around.

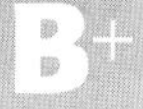

Elsevier's Integrated Pharmacology **$34.95** Review

KESTER

Elsevier, 2006, 336 pages, ISBN 032303408X

Part of the new Integrated series that focuses on core knowledge in a specific basic science discipline while linking that information to related concepts from other disciplines. Case-based and USMLE-style questions at the end of each chapter allow readers to gauge their comprehension of the material. Includes online access. Best if used during coursework. Limited student feedback.

B+

BRS Pharmacology Flash Cards **$29.95** Flash cards

KIM

Lippincott Williams & Wilkins, 2004, 640 pages, ISBN 0781747961

Cards focus on facilitating the recall of drugs used for particular diseases rather than describing these drugs in detail. May be useful for those who find Pharm Cards overwhelming. Considered by many to be an excellent resource for quick review before the boards.

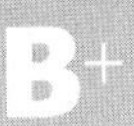

Rapid Review: Pharmacology **$34.95** Review

PAZDERNIK & KERECSEN

Elsevier, 2006, 352 pages, ISBN 0323045502

A detailed treatment of pharmacology, presented in an outline format similar to that of other books in the series. At times more detailed than necessary for boards review. Contains high-yield charts and figures throughout. Two 50-question tests with extensive explanations are included, with 250 additional questions online.

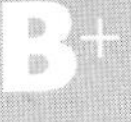

Lange Smart Charts: Pharmacology **$38.95** Review

PELLETIER

McGraw-Hill, 2003, 386 pages, ISBN 0071388788

Pharmacology concepts organized into a tabular format. Most useful when used as a secondary source for organization when reviewing material. Limited student feedback.

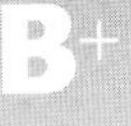

Pharmacology Recall **$34.95** Review

RAMACHANDRAN

Lippincott Williams & Wilkins, 2006, 544 pages, ISBN 078175562X

An approach to pharmacology review presented in a question-and-answer Recall format. Includes a high-yield drug summary. Good for cramming and memorization.

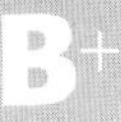

Underground Clinical Vignettes: Pharmacology **$22.95** Review/20 q

SWANSON

Lippincott Williams & Wilkins, 2007, 224 pages, ISBN 0781764858

Concise clinical cases illustrating approximately 100 frequently tested pharmacology concepts. Cardinal signs, symptoms, and buzzwords are highlighted. The clinical vignette style can help readers learn important drug connections for Step 1. Also includes 20 additional boards-style questions. Use as a supplement to other sources of review.

B

Clinical Pharmacology Made Ridiculously Simple **$22.95** Review

OLSON

MedMaster, 2006, 163 pages, ISBN 0940780763

A review text that includes general principles as well as many drug summary charts. Particularly strong in cardiovascular drugs and antimicrobials; incomplete in other areas. Consists primarily of tables; lacks the humorous illustrations and mnemonics typical of this series. Well organized, but occasionally too detailed. Effective as a chart-based review book but not as a sole study source. Must be supplemented with a more detailed text.

B

BRS Pharmacology **$36.95** Review

ROSENFELD

Lippincott Williams & Wilkins, 2006, 464 pages, ISBN 0781780748

A text that includes end-of-chapter review tests featuring updated USMLE-style questions. Two-color tables and figures summarize essential information for quick recall. Also features drug lists for each chapter. This updated edition includes additional USMLE-style comprehensive examination questions and explanations. An additional question bank is available online.

B

PreTest Pharmacology **$25.95** Test/500 q

SHLAFER

McGraw-Hill, 2007, 430 pages, ISBN 0071471812

This new edition represents a significant improvement over previous editions of the book. A good resource to use after other sources of questions have been exhausted.

B

Case Files: Pharmacology **$29.95** Review

TOY

McGraw-Hill, 2005, 456 pages, ISBN 0071445730

A clinical case review book consisting of 52 cases along with useful tables. The text may appeal to students who prefer problem-based learning, but some may find it difficult to review pharmacology using a clinical vignette format.

B–

High-Yield Pharmacology **$26.95** Review

CHRIST

Lippincott Williams & Wilkins, 2003, 138 pages, ISBN 0781745128

A pharmacology review presented in an easy-to-follow outline format. Contains no questions or index. Offers a good summary. Best used with a more extensive text.

B–

Appleton & Lange's Review of Pharmacology ***$36.95*** Test/800 q

KRZANOWSKI

McGraw-Hill, 2002, 155 pages, ISBN 0071377433

A text that contains plenty of questions along with a 50-question practice test. Answers have no accompanying text or explanations. Use when better resources are exhausted.

REVIEW RESOURCES

PHARMACOLOGY

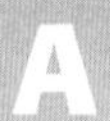

BRS Physiology — ***$37.95*** — Review/400 q

COSTANZO

Lippincott Williams & Wilkins, 2006, 352 pages,
ISBN 0781773113

A clear, concise review of physiology that is both comprehensive and efficient, making for fast, easy reading. Includes great charts and tables. Good practice questions are given along with explanations and a clinically oriented final exam. An excellent review book, but may not be enough for in-depth coursework. Respiratory and acid-base sections are comparatively weak.

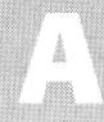

Physiology — ***$54.95*** — Text

COSTANZO

Elsevier, 2006, 512 pages, ISBN 1416023208

Comprehensive coverage of concepts outlined in *BRS Physiology*. Offers excellent diagrams and charts. Each systems-based chapter includes a detailed summary of objectives and a boards-relevant clinical case. Includes access to online interactive extras. Requires time commitment.

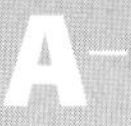

BRS Physiology Cases and Problems — ***$36.95*** — Review/Many q

COSTANZO

Lippincott Williams & Wilkins, 2006, 384 pages,
ISBN 078176078X

Roughly 50 cases in vignette format with several questions per case. Includes detailed answers with explanations. For the motivated student.

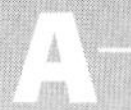

Deja Review: Physiology — ***$22.95*** — Review

LIN

McGraw-Hill, 2007, 216 pages, ISBN 0071475109

Features questions and answers in a two-column, quiz-yourself format similar to that of the Recall series. Provides a sound review in a format that differs from straight text. Includes helpful graphics and tables. Limited student feedback.

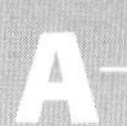

USMLE Road Map: Physiology — ***$26.95*** — Review/50 q

PASLEY

McGraw-Hill, 2006, 208 pages, ISBN 0071400761

A text in outline format incorporating high-yield illustrations. Provides a concise approach to physiology. Clinical correlations are referenced to the text. Questions build on basic concepts and include detailed explanations. Limited student feedback.

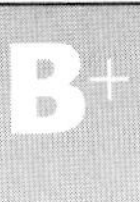

Rapid Review: Physiology **$34.95** Review

BROWN

Elsevier, 2007, 272 pages, ISBN 0323019919

Part of the Rapid Review series. Provides a good review of physiology for Step 1 with an easy-to-follow format. Includes 100 questions with explanations in the book along with an additional 250 questions online with other extra features. Limited student feedback.

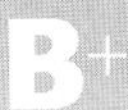

High-Yield Acid Base **$26.95** Review

LONGENECKER

Lippincott Williams & Wilkins, 2006, 128 pages, ISBN 0781796555

A concise and well-written description of acid-base disorders. Includes chapters discussing differential diagnoses and 12 clinical cases. Introduces a multistep approach to the material. A bookmark with useful factoids is included with the text. No index or questions.

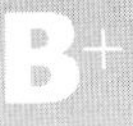

Appleton & Lange's Review of Physiology **$34.95** Test/700 q

PENNEY

McGraw-Hill, 2003, 278 pages, ISBN 0071377263

Boards-style questions divided into subcategories under physiology. Good if subject-specific questions are desired, but may be too detailed for many students. Some diagrams are used to explain answers. A good way to test your knowledge after coursework.

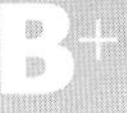

Respiratory Physiology: The Essentials **$37.95** Review/100 q

WEST

Lippincott Williams & Wilkins, 2004, 208 pages, ISBN 0781751527

Comprehensive coverage of respiratory physiology. Clearly organized with useful charts and diagrams. The new edition includes appendices with more than 100 questions and answers with explanations. Best used as a course supplement.

B

Elsevier's Integrated Physiology **$34.95** Review

CARROLLI

Elsevier, 2006, 336 pages, ISBN 0323043186

Part of the new Integrated series that links various disciplines. A good text for initial coursework, but too long for Step 1 review. Case-based and USMLE-style questions are included at the end of each chapter. Limited student feedback.

B

Color Atlas of Physiology | ***$39.95*** | Review

DESPOPOULOS

Thieme, 2003, 448 pages, ISBN 1588900614

A compact text with more than 150 colorful but complicated diagrams on the right and dense explanatory text on the left. Suffers from some translation problems. Overall, a unique, highly visual approach that is worthy of consideration. Useful as an adjunct to other review books.

B

Clinical Physiology Made Ridiculously Simple | ***$19.95*** | Review

GOLDBERG

MedMaster, 2007, 160 pages, ISBN 0940780216

Easy reading with many amusing associations. The style does not work for everyone. Not as well illustrated as the rest of the series. Use as a supplement to other review books.

B

Guyton and Hall Physiology Review | ***$30.95*** | Test/1000 q

HALL

Elsevier, 2005, 260 pages, ISBN 072168307X

More than 1000 questions that provide a good review of physiology. Questions are much shorter than those on the boards and are not as complex. Best if used as a review resource for areas of weakness in physiology. Limited student feedback.

B

Lange Smart Charts: Physiology | ***$34.95*** | Review

LYN

McGraw-Hill, 2004, 400 pages, ISBN 0071395075

Major topics in physiology organized into chart form according to body system. Includes mnemonics and definitions of key terms, but lacks detail at times. Suitable as an adjunct to another source. Limited student feedback.

B

Acid-Base, Fluids, and Electrolytes Made Ridiculously Simple | ***$18.95*** | Review

PRESTON

MedMaster, 2002, 156 pages, ISBN 0940780313

Covers major electrolyte disturbances and fluid management issues with which medical students should be familiar. A great reference for the internal medicine clerkship. Provides information beyond the scope of the USMLE, but remains a useful companion for understanding physiology, kidney function, and fluids. Includes scattered diagrams and questions at the end of each chapter that test comprehension more than facts. Some questions involve calculations.

B	***PreTest Physiology*** RYAN **McGraw-Hill, 2007, 400 pages, ISBN 0071476636** Questions with detailed, well-written explanations. The new edition offers more USMLE-oriented questions as well as more focused explanations. One of the best of the PreTest series. May be useful for the motivated student following extensive review of other sources. Includes a useful high-yield-facts section.	***$25.95***	Test/500 q
B	***Metabolism at a Glance*** SALWAY **Blackwell Science, 2004, 128 pages, ISBN 1405107162** A concise and impressive review of the biochemical pathways involved in metabolism. Intricate figures depict the interplay between the various reactions. Beyond the scope of the USMLE, but a unique resource for coursework.	***$36.95***	Review
B	***Case Files: Physiology*** TOY **McGraw-Hill, 2005, 455 pages, ISBN 0071445757** A review text divided into 51 clinical cases followed by clinical correlations, a discussion, and take-home pearls, presented in a format similar to that of other texts in the Case Files series. A few questions accompany each case. Too lengthy for rapid review; best for students who enjoy problem-based learning.	***$29.95***	Review

NOTES

SECTION IV

Commercial Review Courses

- Falcon Physician Reviews
- Kaplan Medical
- Northwestern Medical Review
- Postgraduate Medical Review Education (PMRE)
- The Princeton Review
- Doctor Youel's Prep, Inc.

Commercial preparation courses can be helpful for some students, but such courses are expensive and require significant time commitment. They are usually an effective tool for students who feel overwhelmed by the volume of material they must review in preparation for the boards. Note, too, that the multiweek review courses may be quite intense and may thus leave limited time for independent study. Also note that while some commercial courses are designed for first-time test takers, others focus on students who are repeating the examination. Still other courses focus on IMGs who want to take all three Steps in a limited amount of time. Finally, student experience and satisfaction with review courses are highly variable, and course content and structure can evolve rapidly. We thus suggest that you discuss options with recent graduates of review courses you are considering. Some student opinions can be found in discussion groups on the World Wide Web.

Falcon Physician Reviews

Established in 2002, Falcon Physician Reviews provides intensive and comprehensive live reviews for students preparing for the USMLE and COMLEX. The seven-week Step 1 reviews are held throughout the year with small class sizes in order to increase student involvement and instructor accessibility. Falcon Physician Reviews uses an active learning system that focuses on comprehension, retention, and application of concepts. Program components include:

- Application-based lecture materials
- Free tutoring
- More than 12,000 USMLE-type sample questions
- Clinical vignettes
- USMLE questions integrated into each lecture
- Case histories
- Sample tests

Programs are currently offered in Dallas, Texas, and Miami, Florida. The fee is $3950. The all-inclusive program tuition fee includes:

- Books and study materials
- More than 325 contact hours
- Hotel accommodations
- Daily full breakfast and lunch
- Ground transportation to and from the airport
- Shuttle service to shopping, movies, and other areas of interest

For more information, contact:

Falcon Physician Reviews
1431 Greenway Drive #800
Irving, TX 75038
Phone: (214) 632-5466
Fax: (214) 292-8568
info@falconreviews.com
URL: www.falconreviews.com

Kaplan Medical

Kaplan Medical offers a wide range of options for USMLE preparation, including live lectures, center-based study, and online products. All of its courses and products focus on providing the most exam-relevant information available.

Live Lectures. Kaplan's IntensePrep offers a highly structured, interactive live review led by expert faculty. Designed for medical students with little time to prepare, it includes approximately 15 days of live lectures during which faculty members cover the material students need to know to master the Step 1 exam. IntensePrep students also receive six months of access to Kaplan's online lectures, which includes more than 80 hours of high-yield, audio-streamed lectures. This course features seven volumes of lecture notes and a question book that includes 850 practice questions.

Kaplan also offers live-lecture courses ranging from 6 to 14 weeks with all-inclusive options to stay and study in high-end hotel accommodations, all of which are aimed at students who are repeating the exam as well as students and physicians who seek more time to prepare.

Center Study. CenterPrep 30 Visits, Kaplan's center-based lecture course, is designed for medical students seeking flexibility. It is offered at more than 160 Kaplan Centers across the United States and includes 30 visits to one Kaplan Center, where students are given access to over 160 hours of video lecture review. This course also features seven volumes of lecture notes; a question book that includes 850 practice questions; and a full-length simulated exam with a complete performance analysis and detailed explanations. For those who would like more access to study resources, Kaplan offers CenterPrep, which includes a personalized learning system (PLS) and three months of access to any Kaplan Center of your choice.

Online Resources. Kaplan Medical provides online content- and question-based review. WebPrep offers 80 hours of audio-streamed lectures, seven volumes of lecture notes, a full online Step 1 simulated exam, and access to Kaplan Medical's popular online question bank, Qbank, which contains more than 2150 USMLE-style practice questions with detailed explanations. WebPrep is designed to provide students with the most flexible content- and question-based review available.

Kaplan's popular Qbank allows students to create practice tests by discipline and organ system, receive instant on-screen feedback, and track their cumulative performance. Kaplan also offers Integrated Vignettes Qbank (IV Qbank), an online clinical-case question bank that allows users to practice answering case-based, USMLE-style vignettes that are organized by symptom. Each vignette contains multidisciplinary questions covering different ways the underlying basic science concepts could be tested.

Kaplan's most comprehensive question practice option is Qreview, which contains more than 3750 questions and provides six months of simultaneous access to both Step 1 Qbank and IV Qbank. Qreview provides students with collective reporting of their results across both Qbanks and also includes an online simulated exam for further USMLE practice. Qbank demos are available at www.kaplanmedical.com.

More information on all of Kaplan's review options can be obtained at (800) 533-8850 or by visiting www.kaplanmedical.com.

Northwestern Medical Review

Northwestern Medical Review offers live-lecture review courses for both the COMLEX Level I and USMLE Step 1 examinations. Four review plans are available for each exam: NBI 100, a three-day course; NBI 150, a four-day course; NBI 200, a five-day course; and NBI 300, a 10- or 15-day course. All courses are in live-lecture format, and most are taught by the authors of the Northwestern Review Books. In addition to organized lecture notes and books for each subject, courses include Web-based question bank access, audio CDs, and a large pool of practice questions and simulated exams. All plans are available in a customized, onsite format for groups of second-year students from individual U.S. medical schools. Additionally, public sites are frequently offered in East Lansing and Detroit, Michigan; Philadelphia, Pennsylvania; St. Louis, Missouri; San Antonio, Texas; Los Angeles, California; Baltimore, Maryland; and Long Island, New York. International sites may also be offered at the request of groups of students and international educational organizations.

Tuition ranges from $390 for the 3-day to $1380 for the 15-day course. Tuition includes all study materials and Web usage services, and it is based on group size, program duration, and early-enrollment discounts. Home-study materials, CBT question-bank access, and DVD materials are also available for purchase independent of the live-lecture plans. Northwestern offers a retake option as well as a liberal cancellation policy.

For more information, contact:

Northwestern Medical Review
P.O. Box 22174
Lansing, MI 48909-2174
Phone: (866) MedPass
Fax: (517) 347-7005
E-mail: registrar@northwesternmedicalreview.com
URL: www.northwesternmedicalreview.com

Postgraduate Medical Review Education (PMRE)

Established in 1976, PMRE offers complete home-study courses for the USMLE Step 1 in the form of audio cassettes, CDs, DVDs, and books. Home Study Package A offers live classes on audiotapes and a transcript book with a compilation of handout notes for $998. For an additional $85, a DVD of 11 hours of Pathology will be included in Package A. Package C offers 15 hours of audiotapes and a transcript book containing 3500 keywords, 400 exam strategies, and 150 acronyms for the seven basic sciences (Biochemistry, Microbiology, Physiology, Pharmacology, Pathology, Anatomy, and Behavioral Science) for $295. Package E features 9000 questions and answers on 20 hours of audiotape for $250. There is also a workshop book with 4200 questions and answers with explanations and 10 hours of audiotapes for $229. PMRE offers a book of about 350 mnemonics for $85. PMRE uses professors who write questions for USMLE exams in conjunction with professionally recorded materials. Books are being sold at the UCLA medical book store and McGill Medical University book store, Montreal, Canada.

For more information, contact:

PMRE
1909 Tyler Street, Suite 305
Hollywood, FL 33020
Phone: (800) 323-6430
Fax: (954) 926-3333
E-mail: sales@pmre.com
URL: www.PMRE.com

The Princeton Review

The Princeton Review offers three flexible preparation options for the USMLE Step 1: the USMLE Online Course, the USMLE Classroom Course, and the USMLE Online Workout. In selected cities, The Princeton Review also offers a more intensive preparation course for IMGs.

USMLE Step 1 Classroom Courses for Medical Students. The USMLE Classroom Courses offer comprehensive preparation that includes the following:

- Seventy-five hours of online review, including lessons, vignettes, and drills
- Three full-length diagnostic tests with detailed score reports
- Seven comprehensive review manuals consisting of more than 1500 pages
- Seven minitests to gauge students' knowledge in each subject
- Twenty-four-hour e-mail support from Princeton Review Online instructors
- Three months of online access

USMLE Online Workout. The USMLE Online Workout offers the following:

- Two thousand USMLE-style questions presented in the CBT format
- Three full-length diagnostic exams
- Seven minitests covering Anatomy, Behavioral Science, Biochemistry, Microbiology and Immunology, Pathology, Pharmacology, and Physiology
- More than 40 subject-specific drills
- A high-yield slide review for Anatomy and Pathology
- Complete explanations of all questions and answers
- Three months of access

USMLE Online Courses. The USMLE Online Courses offer the following:

- Seventy-five hours of online review, including lessons, vignettes, and drills
- Complete review of all USMLE Step 1 subjects
- Three full-length CBTs
- Seven one-hour subject-based tests
- Complete set of print materials
- E-mail support from expert instructors
- 24/7 real-time support from the Princeton Review Online Coach
- Three months of access to tests, drills, and lessons

More information can be found on The Princeton Review's Web site at www.princetonreview.com.

Doctor Youel's Prep, Inc.

Doctor Youel's Prep, Inc., has specialized in medical board preparation for 30 years. The company provides DVDs, audiotapes, videotapes, a CD (Pre-Prep™, Quick Start™), a book (*Seven Steps to Board Success*), live lectures, and tutorials for small groups as well as for individuals (TutorialPrep™). All DVDs, videotapes, audiotapes, live lectures, and tutorials are correlated with a three-book set of Prep Notes© consisting of two textbooks, *Youel's Jewels I*© and *Youel's Jewels II*© (984 pages), and *Case Studies*©, a question-and-answer book (1854 questions, answers, and explanations).

The Comprehensive DVD program consists of 56 hours of lectures by the systems with a three-book set: *Youel's Jewels I and II* and *Case Studies.* Integrated with these programs are pre-tests and post-tests.

All Doctor Youel's Prep courses are taught and written by physicians, reflecting the clinical slant of the boards. All programs are systems based. In addition, all programs are updated continuously. Accordingly, books are not printed until the order is received.

Delivery in the United States or overseas is usually within one week. Optional express delivery is also available. Doctor Youel's Prep Home Study Program™ allows students to own their materials and to use them for repetitive study in the convenience of their homes. Purchasers of any of Doctor Youel's Prep materials, programs, or services are enrolled as members of the Doctor Youel's Prep Family of Students™, which affords them access to free telephone tutoring at (800) 645-3985. Students may call 24/7. Doctor Youel's Prep live lectures are held at select medical schools at the invitation of the school and students.

Programs are custom-designed for content, number of hours, and scheduling to fit students' needs. First-year students are urged to call early to arrange live-lecture programs at their schools for next year.

For more information, contact:

Doctor Youel's Prep
P.O. Box 31479
Palm Beach Gardens, FL 33420
Phone: (800) 645-3985
Fax: (561) 622-4858
E-mail: info@youelsprep.com
www.youelsprep.com

Publisher Contacts

ASM Press
P.O. Box 605
Herndon, VA 20172
(800) 546-2416
Fax: (703) 661-1501
asmmail@presswarehouse.com
www.asmpress.org

Biotest Publishing Company, Inc.
5850 Thille Street, Suite 103
Ventura, CA 93003
SkeletonDude@BiotestOnline.com
www.biotestonline.com

Churchill Livingstone
(see Elsevier Science)

Elsevier Science
Order Fulfillment
11830 Westline Industrial Drive
St. Louis, MO 63146
(800) 545-2522
Fax: (800) 535-9935
www.us.elsevierhealth.com

Exam Master
500 Ethel Court
Middletown, DE 19709-9410
(800) 572-3627
Fax: (302) 378-1153
customer_service@exammaster.com
www.exammaster.com

Garland Science Publishing
Taylor & Francis Group Ltd
2 Park Square
Milton Park, Abingdon
Oxford
OX14 4RN
UK
Tel: +44 (0) 20 7017 6000
Fax: +44 (0) 20 7017 6699
www.garlandscience.co.uk

Gold Standard Board Prep
2619 West Loughlin Drive
Chandler, AZ 85224
Fax: (480) 219-9070
www.boardprep.net

Icon Learning Systems
(see Elsevier Science)
www.netterart.com

John Wiley & Sons
10475 Crosspoint Blvd.
Indianapolis, IN 46256
(877) 762-2974
Fax: (800) 597-3299
consumers@wiley.com
www.wiley.com

Kaplan, Inc.
888 7th Avenue
New York, NY 10106
(212) 492-5800
www.kaplan.com

Lippincott Williams & Wilkins
P.O. Box 1600
Hagerstown, MD 21740
(800) 638-3030
Fax: (301) 223-2400
orders@lww.com
www.lww.com

MedMaster, Inc.
P.O. Box 640028
Miami, FL 33164
(800) 335-3480
Fax: (954) 962-4508
mmbks@aol.com
www.medmaster.net

McGraw-Hill Companies
Order Services
P.O. Box 182604
Columbus, OH 43272-3031
(877) 833-5524
Fax: (614) 759-3749
customer.service@mcgraw-hill.com
www.mhprofessional.com

Mosby-Year Book
(see Elsevier Science)

Parthenon Publishing/CRC Press
Taylor & Francis Group
6000 Broken Sound Parkway, NW, Suite 300
Boca Raton, FL 33487
(800) 272-7737
Fax: (800) 374-3401
orders@crcpress.com
www.crcpress.com

Princeton Review
2315 Broadway
New York, NY 10024
(212) 874-8282
Fax: (212) 874-0775
www.princetonreview.com

Thieme New York
333 Seventh Avenue
New York, NY 10001
(800) 782-3488
Fax: (212) 947-1112
www.thieme.com
customerservice@thieme.com

W. B. Saunders
(see Elsevier Science)

Wysteria Publishing
(888) 997-8300
www.wysteria.com

NOTES

APPENDIX

Abbreviations and Symbols

Abbreviation	Meaning
1°	primary
2°	secondary
3°	tertiary
AA	amino acid
AAMC	Association of American Medical Colleges
aa-tRNA	aminoacyl-tRNA
Ab	antibody
ABP	androgen-binding protein
ACC	acetyl-CoA carboxylase
Ac-CoA	acetylcoenzyme A
ACD	anemia of chronic disease
ACE	angiotensin-converting enzyme
ACh	acetylcholine
AChE	acetylcholinesterase
AChR	acetylcholine receptor
ACL	anterior cruciate ligament
ACTH	adrenocorticotropic hormone
ADA	adenosine deaminase, Americans with Disabilities Act
ADH	antidiuretic hormone
ADHD	attention-deficit hyperactivity disorder
ADP	adenosine diphosphate
AFP	α-fetoprotein
Ag	antigen
AICA	anterior inferior cerebellar artery
AIDS	acquired immunodeficiency syndrome
AL	amyloidosis
ALA	aminolevulinic acid
ALL	acute lymphocytic leukemia
ALP	alkaline phosphatase
ALS	amyotrophic lateral sclerosis
ALT	alanine transaminase
AML	acute myelocytic leukemia
AMP	adenosine monophosphate
ANA	antinuclear antibody
ANCA	antineutrophil cytoplasmic antibody
ANOVA	analysis of variance
ANP	atrial natriuretic peptide
ANS	autonomic nervous system
AOA	American Osteopathic Association
AP	action potential
APC	antigen-presenting cell
APKD	adult polycystic kidney disease

Abbreviation	Meaning
APRT	adenine phosphoribosyltransferase
APSAC	anistreplase
aPTT	activated partial thromboplastin time
AR	attributable risk, autosomal recessive
ARC	Appalachian Regional Commission
ARDS	adult respiratory distress syndrome
Arg	arginine
ASA	acetylsalicylic acid
ASD	atrial septal defect
ASO	antistreptolysin O
Asp	aspartic acid
AST	aspartate transaminase
AT	angiotensin
ATCase	aspartate transcarbamoylase
ATP	adenosine triphosphate
ATPase	adenosine triphosphatase
AV	atrioventricular, azygous vein
AVM	arteriovenous malformation
AZT	azidothymidine
BAL	British anti-Lewisite [dimercaprol]
BM	basement membrane
BMI	body-mass index
BMR	basal metabolic rate
BP	bisphosphate, blood pressure
BPG	bisphosphoglycerate
BPH	benign prostatic hyperplasia
BUN	blood urea nitrogen
CAD	coronary artery disease
cAMP	cyclic adenosine monophosphate
c-ANCA	cytoplasmic antineutrophil cytoplasmic antibody
CBG	corticosteroid-binding globulin
Cbl	cobalamin
CBSSA	Comprehensive Basic Science Self-Assessment
CBT	computer-based testing
CCK	cholecystokinin
CCl_4	carbon tetrachloride
CCS	computer-based case simulation
CCT	cortical collecting tubule
CD	cluster of differentiation
CDK	cyclin-dependent kinase
CE	cholesterol ester
CEA	carcinoembryonic antigen

Abbreviation	Meaning
CETP	cholesterol-ester transfer protein
CF	cystic fibrosis
CFTR	cystic fibrosis transmembrane conductance regulator
CFX	circumflex [artery]
cGMP	cyclic guanosine monophosphate
CGN	*cis*-Golgi network
ChAT	choline acetyltransferase
CHF	congestive heart failure
CI	confidence interval
CIN	candidate identification number, cervical intraepithelial neoplasia
CJD	Creutzfeldt-Jakob disease
CK	clinical knowledge
CK-MB	creatine kinase, MB fraction
CL	clearance
CLL	chronic lymphocytic leukemia
CML	chronic myeloid leukemia
CMV	cytomegalovirus
CN	cranial nerve, cyanide
CNS	central nervous system
CO	cardiac output
CoA	coenzyme A
COGME	Council on Graduate Medical Education
COMLEX	Comprehensive Osteopathic Medical Licensing Examination
COMT	catechol-O-methyltransferase
COP	coat protein
COPD	chronic obstructive pulmonary disease
CoQ	coenzyme Q
COX	cyclooxygenase
C_p	plasma concentration
CPAP	continuous positive airway pressure
CPK	creatine phosphokinase
CRC	colorectal cancer
CRF	chronic renal failure
CRH	corticotropin-releasing hormone
CS	clinical skills
CSF	cerebrospinal fluid, colony-stimulating factor
CT	computed tomography
CVA	cerebrovascular accident, costovertebral angle
Cx	complication
CXR	chest x-ray
Cys	cysteine
d4T	didehydrodeoxythymidine [stavudine]
DAF	decay-accelerating factor
DAG	diacylglycerol
dATP	deoxyadenosine triphosphate
DCIS	ductal carcinoma in situ
ddC	dideoxycytidine
ddI	didanosine
DES	diethylstilbestrol
DHAP	dihydroxyacetone phosphate
DHB	dihydrobiopterin
DHEA	dehydroepiandrosterone

Abbreviation	Meaning
DHF	dihydrofolic acid
DHS	Department of Homeland Security
DHT	dihydrotestosterone
DI	diabetes insipidus
DIC	disseminated intravascular coagulation
DIP	distal interphalangeal [joint]
DIT	diiodotyrosine
DKA	diabetic ketoacidosis
DNA	deoxyribonucleic acid
2,4-DNP	2,4-dinitrophenol
DO	doctor of osteopathy
2,3-DPG	2,3-diphosphoglycerate
DPM	doctor of podiatric medicine
DPPC	dipalmitoyl phosphatidylcholine
DS	double stranded
dsDNA	double-stranded deoxyribonucleic acid
dsRNA	double-stranded ribonucleic acid
dTMP	deoxythymidine monophosphate
DTR	deep tendon reflex
DTs	delirium tremens
dTTP	deoxythymidine triphosphate
dUMP	deoxyuridine monophosphate
DVT	deep venous thrombosis
EBV	Epstein-Barr virus
EC_{50}	median effective concentration
ECF	extracellular fluid
ECFMG	Educational Commission for Foreign Medical Graduates
ECG	electrocardiogram
ECL	enterochromaffin-like [cell]
ECT	electroconvulsive therapy
ED_{50}	median effective dose
EDRF	endothelium-derived relaxing factor
EDTA	ethylenediamine tetra-acetic acid
EDV	end-diastolic volume
EEG	electroencephalogram
EF	ejection fraction, elongation factor
EGF	epidermal growth factor
eIF	eukaryotic initiation factor
ELISA	enzyme-linked immunosorbent assay
EM	electron micrograph, electron microscopic, electron microscopy
EOM	extraocular muscle
epi	epinephrine
EPO	erythropoietin
EPS	extrapyramidal system
ER	endoplasmic reticulum, estrogen receptor
ERAS	Electronic Residency Application Service
ERCP	endoscopic retrograde cholangiopancreatography
ERP	effective refractory period
ERPF	effective renal plasma flow
ERT	estrogen replacement therapy
ERV	expiratory reserve volume
ESR	erythrocyte sedimentation rate
ESV	end-systolic volume

Abbreviation	Meaning
EtOH	ethyl alcohol
EV	esophageal vein
F6P	fructose-6-phosphate
FAD	oxidized flavin adenine dinucleotide
$FADH_2$	reduced flavin adenine dinucleotide
FAP	familial adenomatous polyposis
FBPase	fructose bisphosphatase
FcR	Fc receptor
5f-dUMP	5-fluorodeoxyuridine monophosphate
Fe_{Na}	excreted fraction of filtered sodium
FEV_1	forced expiratory volume in 1 second
FF	filtration fraction
FFA	free fatty acid
FGF	fibroblast growth factor
FISH	fluorescence in situ hybridization
FLEX	Federation Licensing Examination
f-met	formylmethionine
FMG	foreign medical graduate
FMN	flavin mononucleotide
FRC	functional residual capacity
FSH	follicle-stimulating hormone
FSMB	Federation of State Medical Boards
FTA-ABS	fluorescent treponemal antibody—absorbed
5-FU	5-fluorouracil
FVC	forced vital capacity
G3P	glucose-3-phosphate
G6P	glucose-6-phosphate
G6PD	glucose-6-phospate dehydrogenase
GABA	γ-aminobutyric acid
GBM	glomerular basement membrane
G-CSF	granulocyte colony-stimulating factor
GDP	guanosine diphosphate
GE	gastroesophageal
GERD	gastroesophageal reflux disease
GFAP	glial fibrillary acid protein
GFR	glomerular filtration rate
GGT	γ-glutamyl transpeptidase
GH	growth hormone
GHRH	growth hormone–releasing hormone
GI	gastrointestinal
GIP	gastric inhibitory peptide
GIST	gastrointestinal stromal tumor
Glu	glutamic acid
GLUT	glucose transporter
GM-CSF	granulocyte-macrophage colony-stimulating factor
GMP	guanosine monophosphate
GN	glomerulonephritis
GnRH	gonadotropin-releasing hormone
GP	glycogen phosphorylase, glycoprotein
GPe	globus pallidus externa
GPi	globus pallidus interna
GPI	glycosyl phosphatidylinositol
GPP	glycogen phosphorylase phosphatase
GS	glycogen synthase
GSH	reduced glutathione
GS-P	glycogen synthase phosphatase
GSSG	oxidized glutathione

Abbreviation	Meaning
GTP	guanosine triphosphate
GU	genitourinary
HAART	highly active antiretroviral therapy
HAV	hepatitis A virus
HAVAb	hepatitis A antibody
Hb	hemoglobin
HBcAb	hepatitis B core antibody
HBcAg	hepatitis B core antigen
HBeAb	hepatitis B early antibody
HBeAg	hepatitis B early antigen
HBsAb	hepatitis B surface antibody
HBsAg	hepatitis B surface antigen
HBV	hepatitis B virus
hCG	human chorionic gonadotropin
Hct	hematocrit
HCV	hepatitis C virus
HDL	high-density lipoprotein
HDV	hepatitis D virus
H&E	hematoxylin and eosin
HEV	hepatitis E virus
HGPRT	hypoxanthine-guanine phosphoribosyltransferase
HHS	[Department of] Health and Human Services
HHV	human herpesvirus
5-HIAA	5-hydroxyindoleacetic acid
His	histidine
HIT	heparin-induced thrombocytopenia
HIV	human immunodeficiency virus
HL	hepatic lipase
HLA	human leukocyte antigen
HMG-CoA	hydroxymethylglutaryl-coenzyme A
HMP	hexose monophosphate
HMWK	high-molecular-weight kininogen
HNPCC	hereditary nonpolyposis colorectal cancer
hnRNA	heterogeneous nuclear ribonucleic acid
HPA	hypothalamic-pituitary-adrenal [axis]
HPSA	Health Professional Shortage Area
HPV	human papillomavirus
HR	heart rate
HRT	hormone replacement therapy
HSV	herpes simplex virus
HSV-1	herpes simplex virus 1
HSV-2	herpes simplex virus 2
5-HT	5-hydroxytryptamine (serotonin)
HTLV	human T-cell leukemia virus
HUS	hemolytic-uremic syndrome
HVA	homovanillic acid
IBD	inflammatory bowel disease
IC	inspiratory capacity
ICA	internal carotid artery
ICAM	intracellular adhesion molecule
ICF	intracellular fluid
ICP	intracranial pressure
ID_{50}	median infectious dose
IDDM	insulin-dependent diabetes mellitus
IDL	intermediate-density lipoprotein

Abbreviation	Meaning
I/E	inspiratory/expiratory [ratio]
IEV	inferior epigastric vein
IF	immunofluorescence
IFN	interferon
Ig	immunoglobulin
IGF	insulin-like growth factor
IL	interleukin
Ile	isoleucine
IMA	inferior mesenteric artery
IMED	International Medical Education Directory
IMG	international medical graduate
IMP	inosine monophosphate
IMV	inferior mesenteric vein
INH	isonicotine hydrazine [isoniazid]
INR	International Normalized Ratio
IO	inferior oblique [muscle]
IP_3	inositol triphosphate
IPV	inactivated polio vaccine
IR	inferior rectus [muscle]
IRV	inferior rectal vein, inspiratory reserve volume
ITP	idiopathic thrombocytopenic purpura
IV	intravenous
IVC	inferior vena cava
JG	juxtaglomerular [cells]
JGA	juxtaglomerular apparatus
JVD	jugular venous distention
K_f	filtration constant
KOH	potassium hydroxide
KSHV	Kaposi's sarcoma–associated herpesvirus
LA	left atrial, left atrium
LAD	left anterior descending [artery]
LAF	left anterior fascicle
LCA	left coronary artery
LCAT	lecithin-cholesterol acyltransferase
LCFA	long-chain fatty acid
LCL	lateral collateral ligament
LCME	Liaison Committee on Medical Education
LCV	lymphocytic choriomeningitis virus
LD_{50}	median toxic dose
LDH	lactate dehydrogenase
LDL	low-density lipoprotein
LES	lower esophageal sphincter
Leu	leucine
LFA-1	leukocyte function–associated antigen 1
LFT	liver function test
LGN	lateral geniculate nucleus
LGV	left gastric vein
LH	luteinizing hormone
LLQ	left lower quadrant
LM	light microscopy
LMN	lower motor neuron
LOR	letter of recommendation
LPL	lipoprotein lipase
LPS	lipopolysaccharide

Abbreviation	Meaning
LR	lateral rectus [muscle]
LSE	Libman-Sacks endocarditis
LT	leukotriene
LV	left ventricle, left ventricular
Lys	lysine
MAC	membrane attack complex, minimal alveolar concentration
MALT	mucosa-associated lymphoid tissue
MAO	monoamine oxidase
MAOI	monoamine oxidase inhibitor
MAP	mean arterial pressure
MCA	middle cerebral artery
MCHC	mean corpuscular hemoglobin concentration
MCL	medial collateral ligament
MCP	metacarpophalangeal [joint]
MCV	mean corpuscular volume
MEN	multiple endocrine neoplasia
MEOS	microsomal ethanol oxidizing system
Met	methionine
MGN	medial geniculate nucleus
MGUS	monoclonal gammopathy of undetermined significance
MHC	major histocompatibility complex
MHPSA	Mental Health Professional Shortage Area
MI	myocardial infarction
MIT	monoiodotyrosine
MLCK	myosin light-chain kinase
MLF	medial longitudinal fasciculus
MMR	measles, mumps, rubella [vaccine]
6-MP	6-mercaptopurine
MPO	myeloperoxidase
MPTP	1-methyl-4-phenyl-1,2,3,6-tetrahydropyridine
MR	medial rectus [muscle], mental retardation, mitral regurgitation
MRI	magnetic resonance imaging
mRNA	messenger ribonucleic acid
MRSA	methicillin-resistant S. *aureus*
MS	multiple sclerosis
MSH	melanocyte-stimulating hormone
mTOR	mammalian target of rapamycin
MTP	metatarsophalangeal [joint]
MTX	methotrexate
MUA/P	Medically Underserved Area and Population
MVO_2	myocardial oxygen consumption
NAD^+	oxidized nicotinamide adenine dinucleotide
NADH	reduced nicotinamide adenine dinucleotide
$NADP^+$	oxidized nicotinamide adenine dinucleotide phosphate
NADPH	reduced nicotinamide adenine dinucleotide phosphate
NBME	National Board of Medical Examiners
NBOME	National Board of Osteopathic Medical Examiners

Abbreviation	Meaning
NBPME	National Board of Podiatric Medical Examiners
NE	norepinephrine
NF	neurofibromatosis
NH_3	ammonia
NIDDM	non-insulin-dependent diabetes mellitus
NK	natural killer [cells]
NMJ	neuromuscular junction
NO	nitric oxide
NPV	negative predictive value
NSAID	nonsteroidal anti-inflammatory drug
OAA	oxaloacetic acid
OCD	obsessive-compulsive disorder
OCP	oral contraceptive pill
OMT	osteopathic manipulative technique
OPV	oral polio vaccine
OR	odds ratio
PA	posteroanterior
PABA	para-aminobenzoic acid
PAH	para-aminohippuric acid
PALS	periarterial lymphatic sheath
p-ANCA	perinuclear antineutrophil cytoplasmic antibody
PAS	periodic acid Schiff
PBP	penicillin-binding protein
P_c	capillary pressure
PC	pyruvate carboxylase
PCL	posterior cruciate ligament
P_{CO_2}	partial pressure of carbon dioxide
PCOS	polycystic ovarian syndrome
PCP	phencyclidine hydrochloride, *Pneumocystis carinii* (now *jiroveci*) pneumonia
PCR	polymerase chain reaction
PCWP	pulmonary capillary wedge pressure
PD	posterior descending [artery]
PDA	patent ductus arteriosus
PDE	phosphodiesterase
PDH	pyruvate dehydrogenase
PE	pulmonary embolism
PEP	phosphoenolpyruvate
PFK	phosphofructokinase
PFT	pulmonary function test
PG	phosphoglycerate, prostaglandin
Phe	phenylalanine
P_i	interstitial fluid pressure
PICA	posterior inferior cerebellar artery
PID	pelvic inflammatory disease
PIP	proximal interphalangeal [joint]
PIP_2	phosphatidylinositol 4,5-bisphosphate
PK	pyruvate kinase
PKA	protein kinase A
PKD	polycystic kidney disease
PKU	phenylketonuria
PLP	pyridoxal phosphate
PML	progressive multifocal leukoencephalopathy
PMN	polymorphonuclear [leukocyte]

Abbreviation	Meaning
P_{net}	net filtration pressure
PNET	primitive neuroectodermal tumor
PNH	paroxysmal nocturnal hemoglobinuria
PNS	peripheral nervous system
P_{O_2}	partial pressure of oxygen
POMC	pro-opiomelanocortin
PPD	purified protein derivative
PPI	proton pump inhibitor
PPRF	paramedian pontine reticular formation
PPV	positive predictive value
PR	progesterone receptor
PRPP	phosphoribosylpyrophosphate
PSA	prostate-specific antigen
PSS	progressive systemic sclerosis
PT	prothrombin time
PTH	parathyroid hormone
PTHrP	parathyroid hormone–related protein
PTSD	post-traumatic stress disorder
PTT	partial thromboplastin time
PUV	paraumbilical vein
PV	plasma volume, portal vein
RA	rheumatoid arthritis, right atrium
RBC	red blood cell
RBF	renal blood flow
RCA	right coronary artery
RDS	respiratory distress syndrome
RDW	red-cell distribution width
REM	rapid eye movement
RER	rough endoplasmic reticulum
RNA	ribonucleic acid
RNP	ribonucleoprotein
RPF	renal plasma flow
RPR	rapid plasma reagin
RR	relative risk, respiratory rate
rRNA	ribosomal ribonucleic acid
RS	Reed-Sternberg [cells]
RSV	respiratory syncytial virus
RUQ	right upper quadrant
RV	renal vein, residual volume, right ventricle, right ventricular
RVH	right ventricular hypertrophy
SA	sinoatrial, subarachnoid
SAA	serum amyloid–associated [protein]
SAM	S-adenosylmethionine
SARS	severe acute respiratory syndrome
SC	subcutaneous
SCC	squamous cell carcinoma
SCID	severe combined immunodeficiency disease
SCJ	squamocolumnar junction
SD	standard deviation, subdural
SEM	standard error of the mean
SER	smooth endoplasmic reticulum
SEV	superior epigastric vein
SEVIS	Student and Exchange Visitor Information System
SEVP	Student and Exchange Visitor Program

Abbreviation	Meaning
SGOT	serum glutamic oxaloacetic transaminase
SGPT	serum glutamic pyruvate transaminase
SHBG	sex hormone–binding globulin
SIADH	syndrome of inappropriate antidiuretic hormone
SLE	systemic lupus erythematosus
SLL	small lymphocytic lymphoma
SMA	superior mesenteric artery
SMV	superior mesenteric vein
SMX	sulfamethoxazole
SNc	substantia nigra compacta
snRMP	small nuclear ribonucleoprotein
SO	superior oblique [muscle]
SOD	superoxide dismutase
SR	sarcoplasmic reticulum, superior rectus [muscle]
SRP	sponsoring residency program
SRV	superior rectal vein
SS	single stranded
SSB	single-stranded binding
ssDNA	single-stranded deoxyribonucleic acid
SSPE	subacute sclerosing panencephalitis
SSRI	selective serotonin reuptake inhibitor
ssRNA	single-stranded ribonucleic acid
SSSS	staphylococcal scalded-skin syndrome
STD	sexually transmitted disease
STN	subthalamic nucleus
SV	sinus venosus, splenic vein, stroke volume
SVC	superior vena cava
SVT	supraventricular tachycardia
$t_{1/2}$	half-life
T_3	triiodothyronine
T_4	thyroxine
TA	truncus arteriosus
TB	tuberculosis
TBG	thyroxine-binding globulin
TBW	total body weight
3TC	dideoxythiacytidine [lamivudine]
TCA	tricarboxylic acid [cycle], tricyclic antidepressant
Tc cell	cytotoxic T cell
TCR	T-cell receptor
TFT	thyroid function test
TG	triglyceride
TGA	trans-Golgi apparatus
TGF	transforming growth factor
THB	tetrahydrobiopterin
Th cell	helper T cell
THF	tetrahydrofolate
Thr	threonine
TI	therapeutic index
TIBC	total iron-binding capacity
TLC	total lung capacity
TMP-SMX	trimethoprim-sulfamethoxazole

Abbreviation	Meaning
TNF	tumor necrosis factor
TNM	tumor, node, metastases [staging]
TOEFL	Test of English as a Foreign Language
tPA	tissue plasminogen activator
TPP	thiamine pyrophosphate
TPR	total peripheral resistance
TRAP	tartrate-resistant acid phosphatase
TRH	thyrotropin-releasing hormone
tRNA	transfer ribonucleic acid
Trp	tryptophan
TSH	thyroid-stimulating hormone
TSI	thyroid-stimulating immunoglobulin
TSS	toxic shock syndrome
TSST	toxic shock syndrome toxin
TTP	thrombotic thrombocytopenic purpura
TV	tidal volume
TXA	thromboxane
UA	urinalysis
UCV	Underground Clinical Vignettes
UDP	uridine diphosphate
UMN	upper motor neuron
URI	upper respiratory infection
USDA	United States Department of Agriculture
USIA	United States Information Agency
USMLE	United States Medical Licensing Examination
UTI	urinary tract infection
UV	ultraviolet
VA	ventral anterior [nucleus], Veterans Administration
Val	valine
VC	vital capacity
V_d	volume of distribution
VDRL	Venereal Disease Research Laboratory
VF	ventricular fibrillation
VHL	von Hippel–Lindau [disease]
VIP	vasoactive intestinal peptide
VIPoma	vasoactive intestinal polypeptide-secreting tumor
VL	ventral lateral [nucleus]
VLDL	very low density lipoprotein
VMA	vanillylmandelic acid
VPL	ventral posterior nucleus, lateral
VPM	ventral posterior nucleus, medial
VPN	ventral posterior nucleus
V/Q	ventilation/perfusion [ratio]
VRE	vancomycin-resistant enterococcus
VSD	ventricular septal defect
vWF	von Willebrand factor
VZV	varicella-zoster virus
WBC	white blood cell
XR	X-linked recessive
ZDV	zidovudine [formerly AZT]

Index

Note: boldface indicates a First Aid fact title.

P

U

V

W

X

Y

Z

NOTES

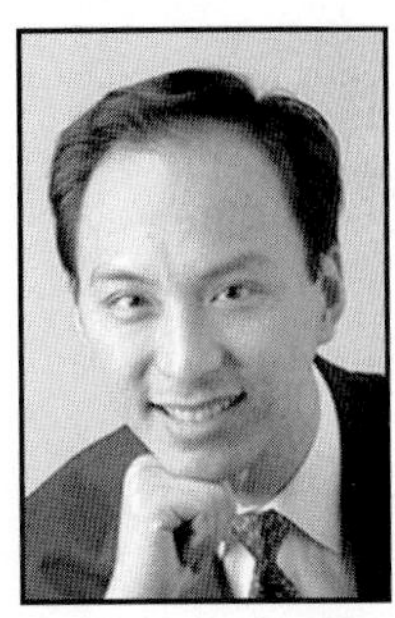

Tao Le, MD, MHS

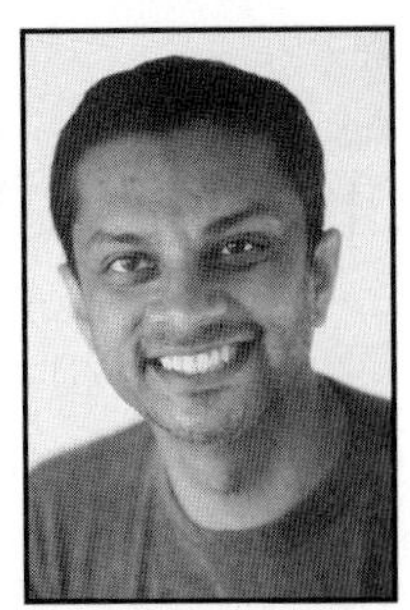

Vikas Bhushan, MD

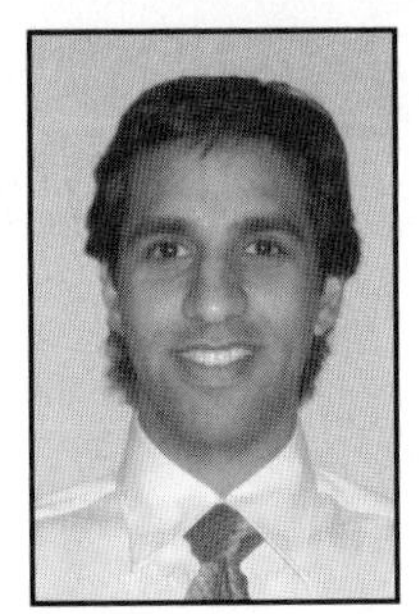

Deepak A. Rao, MS, MPhil

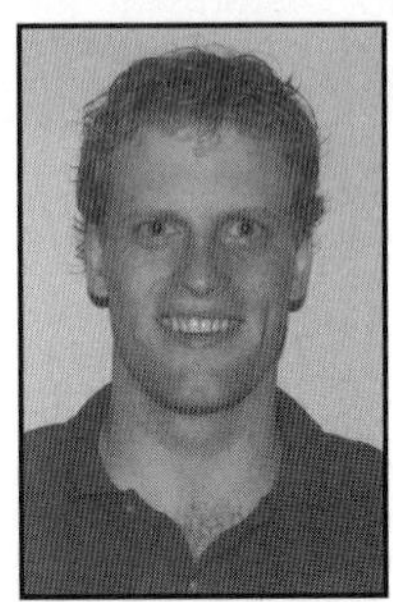

Lars Grimm

Tao Le, MD, MHS

Tao has been a well-recognized figure in medical education for the past 15 years. As senior editor, he has led the expansion of *First Aid* into a global educational series. In addition, he is the founder of the *USMLERx* online test bank series as well as a cofounder of the *Underground Clinical Vignettes* series. As a medical student, he was editor-in-chief of the University of California, San Francisco *Synapse,* a university newspaper with a weekly circulation of 9000. Tao earned his medical degree from the University of California, San Francisco in 1996 and completed his residency training in internal medicine at Yale University and allergy and immunology fellowship training at Johns Hopkins University. At Yale, he was a regular guest lecturer on the USMLE review courses and an adviser to the Yale University School of Medicine curriculum committee. Tao subsequently went on to cofound Medsn and served as its chief medical officer. He is currently pursuing research in asthma education at the University of Louisville.

Vikas Bhushan, MD

Vikas is an author, editor, entrepreneur, and roaming teleradiologist who divides his days between Los Angeles, Maui, and balmy remote locales with abundant bandwidth. In 1992 he conceived and authored the original *First Aid for the USMLE Step 1*, and in 1998 he originated and coauthored the *Underground Clinical Vignettes* series. His entrepreneurial adventures include a successful software company; a medical publishing enterprise (S2S); an e-learning company (Medsn); and, most recently, an ER teleradiology venture (24/7 Radiology). His eclectic interests include medical informatics, independent film, humanism, Urdu poetry, world music, South Asian diasporic culture, and avoiding a day job. He has also coproduced a music documentary on qawwali; coproduced and edited *Shabash 2.0: The Hip Guide to All Things South Asian in North America* (available at www.artwallah.org/shabash); and is now completing a CD/book project on Sufi poetry translated into four languages. Vikas completed a bachelor's degree in biochemistry from the University of California, Berkeley; an MD with thesis from the University of California, San Francisco; and a radiology residency from the University of California, Los Angeles.

Deepak A. Rao, MS, MPhil

Deepak is currently a sixth-year MD-PhD student at the Yale University School of Medicine, and this is his fourth year on the *First Aid* team. Born and raised in Philadelphia, Deepak developed an interest in basic science research as an undergraduate at Harvard University, where he received an AB degree in 2001. He participated in a one-year pre-IRTA training fellowship at the NIH studying muscular dystrophy before enrolling in the Medical Scientist Training Program at Yale. He has worked as a private tutor for several years and has also participated on the education and curriculum committee at Yale. Deepak is currently working toward a PhD in immunology, studying immune responses generated against the vasculature of solid organ transplants. He looks forward to returning to medical school after completing his PhD.

Lars Grimm

Lars is a fourth-year medical student at the Yale School of Medicine. Raised predominantly in Naples, Florida, he graduated from Stanford University in 2004 and received a BS degree in geological and environmental sciences. He is currently pursuing a master's degree in health science, focusing his research on qualitative assessments of trauma resuscitation. Lars has been involved in a variety of extracurricular charity and social activities at Yale, and in his free time likes to read fiction, work out, and spend time with friends and family.

ABOUT THE AUTHORS